Essentials of Plastic Surgery

Essentials of Plastic Surgery

Edited by Archer Queen

hayle
medical

New York

Hayle Medical,
750 Third Avenue, 9th Floor,
New York, NY 10017, USA

Visit us on the World Wide Web at:
www.haylemedical.com

ISBN: 978-1-63241-767-1

Cataloging-in-Publication Data

Essentials of plastic surgery / edited by Archer Queen.
   p. cm.
Includes bibliographical references and index.
ISBN 978-1-63241-767-1
1. Surgery, Plastic. 2. Transplantation of organs, tissues, etc. I. Queen, Archer.
RD118 .E67 2019
617.95--dc23

Table of Contents

Permissions

List of Contributors

Index

Preface

The surgical specialty which is concerned with the restoration, alteration and reconstruction of the human body is known as plastic surgery. There are two categories of plastic surgery, i.e., reconstructive surgery and cosmetic surgery. Reconstructive surgery deals with the reconstruction of a specific body part to improve its functioning. Reconstructive surgery involves the treatment of burns, microsurgery, hand surgery and craniofacial surgery. Cosmetic surgery is a surgery concerned with both facial as well as body cosmetic surgery. It aims at improving the overall appearance of some specific body part or parts. This book unfolds the innovative aspects of plastic surgery which will be crucial for the progress of this field in the future. It provides significant information of this discipline to help develop a good understanding of plastic surgery and related fields. Doctors, experts and students actively engaged in this field, will find this book full of crucial and unexplored concepts.

This book has been the outcome of endless efforts put in by authors and researchers on various issues and topics within the field. The book is a comprehensive collection of significant researches that are addressed in a variety of chapters. It will surely enhance the knowledge of the field among readers across the globe.

It gives us an immense pleasure to thank our researchers and authors for their efforts to submit their piece of writing before the deadlines. Finally in the end, I would like to thank my family and colleagues who have been a great source of inspiration and support.

Editor

Breast Developmental Anomalies in Dormaa Municipality of Ghana: Prevalence and Impact on the Life of the Individual

P. Agbenorku,[1] E. Otupiri,[2] and S. Fugar[3]

[1] Reconstructive Plastic Surgery and Burns Unit, Komfo Anokye Teaching Hospital, School of Medical Sciences,
Kwame Nkrumah University of Science and Technology, Kumasi, Ghana
[2] Department of Community Health, School of Medical Sciences, Kwame Nkrumah University of Science and Technology,
Kumasi, Ghana
[3] Department of Surgery, Komfo Anokye Teaching Hospital, Kumasi, Ghana

Correspondence should be addressed to P. Agbenorku; pimagben@yahoo.com

Academic Editor: Nicolo Scuderi

Background. Breast developmental anomalies (BDAs) are abnormalities of breast tissue that arise during breast development. Some of the anomalies can have negative impact on the person's life. This study seeks to assess the prevalence of BDA in the Dormaa Municipality in Ghana and its impact on the life of the individual. *Materials and Methods.* A descriptive study involving 500 female respondents aged between 11 and 25 years from selected schools in the Dormaa Municipality using self-administered questionnaires and interviews. *Results.* From the study, it was found that the prevalence of BDA in the municipality was 12.8%. The commonest BDA was bilateral hypoplasia which accounted for 31.3% of the BDAs found in the study. Nine (14.1%) complained of the BDA affecting their lives with most being teased in school. Twenty-two (34.4%) girls out of the 64 with BDAs had a family member with a BDA. *Conclusion.* BDA is a worry; therefore, comprehensive educational programs for health workers and the general public are needed to increase awareness. Also, work should be done to include education on BDA when awareness is being raised about breast cancer and on the importance of breast self-Examination (BSE).

1. Introduction

Since the beginning of time, the female breast has been a symbol of feminism, and its presence is a major feature that delineates a man from a woman. A beautiful and attractive female breast is one which is symmetrically situated on the anterolateral chest wall and has soft but well-defined junctures with the chest, upper abdomen, and the axillae. The breast profile is a gentle downward vertical flow from the clavicle extending between the second and sixth ribs, vertically and horizontally between the lateral edge of the sternum and midaxillary line to the nipple-areola and forms a mildly convex curve from the nipple-areola to the inframammary crease [1, 2].

Budding of the breasts (thelarche), a sign of female secondary sexual characteristic, occurs at approximately 10-11 years, and the time it takes for the breast to reach maturity can be as short as 18 months or may take as long as nine years.

During this period of breast development, several processes or factors may go wrong leading to their abnormal growth. These include genetic, environmental, exposure to infectious agents, trauma, radiation, neoplastic, or endocrine conditions [3–7].

Some of these anomalies may arise purely in the breast tissue and these include amastia (absence of breast; occurs when mammary ridges fail to develop) [8], hypoplasia (underdeveloped breasts), macromastia (massive enlargement of one or both breasts; also defined as breast enlargement exceeding 600 grams) [9], and tuberous/tubular breast (breast with a tube-like shape; caused by an incomplete development of the mammary gland) [10]. Other breast anomalies are accessory nipples (polythelia) and accessory mammary glands (polymastia); these are believed to arise from an incomplete regression of the milk lines that arise embryologically [11].

Cases of BDAs have been recorded since the sixteen hundreds; one such case was described in 1670 where an autopsy performed on a patient who apparently died shortly after the onset of breast enlargement that weighed 64 pounds. Several other cases have been reported since then. One such case was described in 1993, in which a 12-year-old girl had abnormally large breast and developed marked kyphosis as a result. Apart from the physical impairment, the enlarged breast (hypertrophy) caused the girl intense psychological problems, incapacitating her in school activities and social relations [12]. Also, this form of large breasts has caused some people to stop engaging in normal daily activities because of the weight [13]. It has also been found that in the majority of these patients, they are young and healthy, but the psychological and social impacts of these conditions are crippling [14]. Other problems encountered by some women include physical disabilities such as constant back pain, scoliosis, as well as psychological problems as a result of insecurities about their beauty and feminism, and also teasing from peers [15].

Despite this long history of BDAs, there is a scarcity of research into these conditions. The importance of BDA has reached the point where centers are being set up in the US solely dedicated to management BDAs among adolescents [16]. Studies to investigate the awareness of breast anomalies such as performed by Agbenorku et al. in Jamasi revealed that the awareness of the breast anomaly was 83% among the people suffering from the BDA [17].

Diagnosis of BDAs is basically clinical and usually requires clinical examination of the breast. Careful breast examination is needed to prevent misdiagnosis because these anomalies may mimic breast malignances; so, it is important to rule them out [18]. Ultrasound is the ideal imaging modality in evaluating children's breasts [19]. Management of patients with BDAs requires a multidisciplinary approach which includes plastic surgeons, adolescent internists, endocrinologists, gynaecologists, psychiatrists, social workers and nutritionists. The whole team works primarily to fix any psychological problems that may exist first and secondly to correct the anomaly surgically if desired [20].

In patients with macromastia or gigantomastia, drugs are only marginally effective in reversing the condition; therefore, surgery (reduction mammaplasty) remains the mainstay of treatment [21]. When reduction mammaplasty is being considered in adolescent, surgery should be delayed until breast growth is completed, and this can be done by performing serial breast measurements [22]. Good skin care is also necessary in order to reduce breast crease inflammation and lessen the symptoms caused by moisture [23]. Tuberous breast can be treated by surgical procedures using tissue expansion methods [24]. Breast implants or reduction may be used to correct asymmetry.

Generally, the rate of patients who undergo surgery for BDA depends on the level of knowledge they have on the condition. Agbenorku et al. reported in their study that surgery and other forms of treatment such as counseling and regular followup assessment in patients with BDA were minimal, and in terms of treatment, 68% were ready to accept medication as the only treatment for their BDA [25].

1.1. Surgical Techniques for BDA Management. The most important aspects of the anatomy of the breast are the understanding of the blood supply and nerve supply to the nipple areola complex (NAC) [26]. It is also important to note that the inferior pedicle has been most associated with an inverted T- skin resection, a superior pedicle/supermedial pedicle with a vertical skin resection. The advent of pedicled techniques improved greatly NAC viability and improving cosmetics results [27]. Studies have shown that medial and superomedial pedicles have excellent postoperation nipple sensation [28]. Agbenorku et al. carried out bilateral reduction mammaplasty using the nipple-areola reposition technique which aims to preserve the nipples and some areolar tissue to retain sensibility and future breastfeeding. They reported in their study that reduction mammaplasty plays a significant role in the relief of pain and psychological distress of symptomatic macromastia patients, irrespective of available resources, technology, and country [25].

The technique employed is based on the individual patient's requirement. These include horizontal pedicle (which was the Strombeck pattern, with the blood supply coming from both sides) in which the dermal pedicle is sufficient to maintain nipple areolar viability but can cause nipple retraction and inclusion of glandular element in the pedicle which can make insetting difficult [29]. Inferior pedicle helps to maintain the NAC, and there is good circulation and sensation and breastfeeding possibility [30, 31]. Medial pedicle has good sensation and good blood supply and can be inserted relatively easy [32]. Lateral pedicle has good visibility and is based on the lateral thoracic artery perforators [33]. Superior pedicle has good circulation, but being a dermal pedicle, breastfeeding is impossible; it is not very easy to inset [34]. Central pedicle is a modification of the inferior pedicle with the removal of the dermal bridge [34]. Vertical bipedicle provided good blood supply and also easy inset [35].

1.2. Surgery and Psychology. The importance of psychological counseling of patients with BDA cannot be understated. It is important because in a study by Von Soest et al. amongst 130 Norwegian females who had cosmetic surgery, it was found that a high rate of preoperative psychological problems and low self-esteem were related to more negative psychosocial changes after the surgery as compared to those with better psychological health [36]. Thus, it is important to tackle the psychological aspect ideally even before the surgical correction takes place. Psychological management is also important because some of the individuals with these breast anomalies have an underlying body dysmorphic disorder [37].

2. Materials and Methods

2.1. Study Setting. Dormaa Municipal is located at the western part of the Brong-Ahafo Region of Ghana. It lies within longitudes 3° west and 3° 30′ west and latitudes 7° north and 7° 30′ north. Jaman and Berekum Districts, bound the district on the north, on the east by the Sunyani Municipal, in the south and southeast by Asunafo and Asutifi Districts respectively, in the southwest by Western Region, and in the west and northwest by Cote d'Ivoire. The municipal capital is Dormaa Ahenkro, located about 80 kilometers west of the regional capital, Sunyani [38]. The 2002 population census put Dormaa Municipality population at 150,229. It is estimated that Christians constitute the largest percentage of the district's population, accounting for 72% of the sampled population; Islam was 19%, while other religious groups represented 3%.

2.2. Materials and Methods. This descriptive study was conducted between February and April 2011. Consent was sought from the various leaders of the community and schools before the questionnaires were administered. The purpose of the study was explained to them after which the questionnaires were administered to a total of 500 hundred female students; 307 from senior high school (SHS) and 193 from junior high school (JHS) aged 11 to 25 in the municipality. The questionnaire used in the collection of data, developed from previous studies performed by Agbenorku et al. on BDAs at Jamasi and Sogakope, consisted of both open- and closed-ended questions [17, 28, 39]. Each respondent was shown 8 pictures of various BDAs (Figures 1, 2, 3, 4, 5, 6, 7, and 8).

They were then asked to state if their breasts were like any of them. If their breasts were not like any of the ones described, they then moved to a section to assess their satisfaction with their breasts and knowledge of any disease of the breast. If the respondent said that her breast was like one of those pictures, then she had to answer questions as to the kind of impact the BDA had on her life.

2.3. Data Analysis. Data from completed questionnaires were analyzed using data processing software, Statistical Package for Social Sciences (SPSS) 16th Edition.

3. Results

Figure 9 shows the distribution of the different anomalies. Out of the 500 respondents, 64 (12.8%) had BDA with the commonest being bilateral hypoplasia, 20 (31.3%), followed by macromastia 18 (28.1%). Figure 10 illustrates the age distribution of female students with BDA. Most of the respondents (78.4%) were between the age of 15 and 20 years; 53 (82.8%) of those with BDA were between 15 and 19 years. The mean age of the girls with bilateral hypoplasia was 16.75 years with the youngest and the oldest being 14 and 20 years, respectively.

3.1. Problems Faced by Affected Individuals in School and at Home. Out of the 64 respondents with BDA, 9 (5 of them had macromastia, while 4 had bilateral hypoplasia) complained that BDA affected their lives. The girls with the bilateral hypoplasia complained of being teased in school; however, their lives at home and in town were not affected in anyway. Three (3) girls out of the 5 with macromastia complained of the BDA affecting their life at home; when they had to do household chores, they developed back pain, and 2 complained of being shy in school because of the size of their breasts.

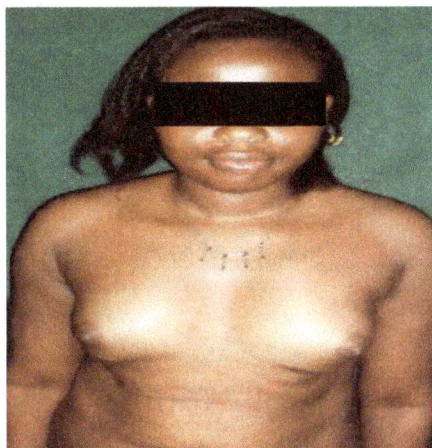

FIGURE 1: Bilateral hypoplasia in a 20-year-old.

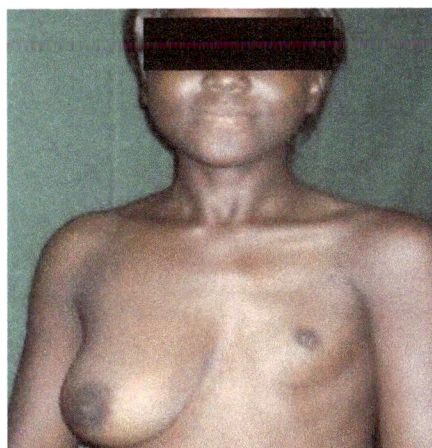

FIGURE 2: Left unilateral hypoplasia in a 22-year old.

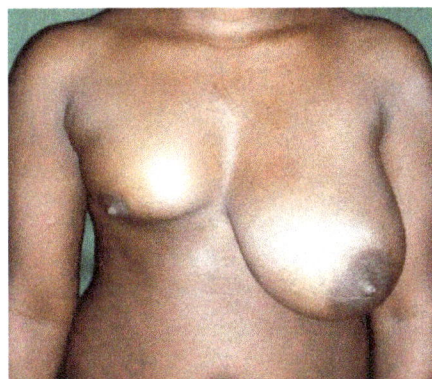

FIGURE 3: Left hyperplasia and right hypoplasia in a 16-year-old.

3.2. Reasons for Not Seeking Medical Treatment. None of the girls with a BDA had sought any treatment because 50 (78.1%) out of the 64 girls did not know that their conditions were considered abnormal. Three (3) girls with bilateral hypoplasia had researched into treatment options for people with small

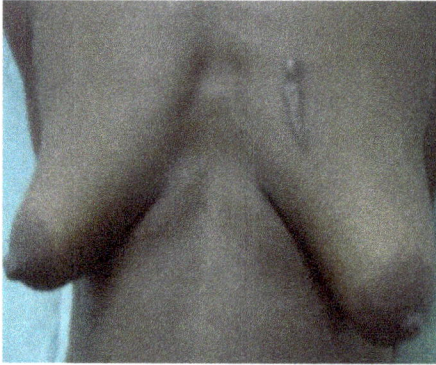

FIGURE 4: Bilateral tubular breasts in a 17-year-old.

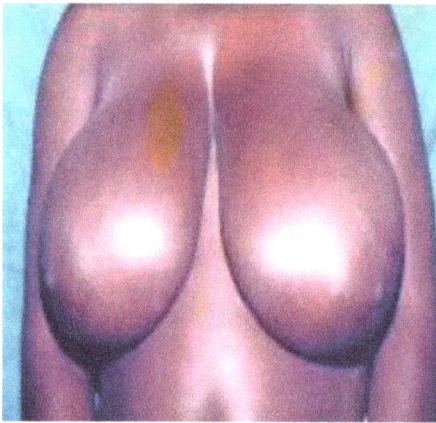

FIGURE 5: Bilateral juvenile macromastia in a 14-year-old.

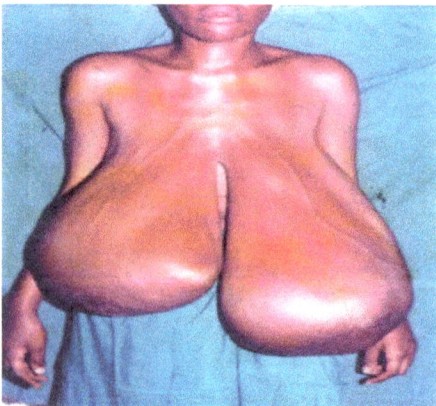

FIGURE 6: Bilateral breast hypertrophy in a 26-year-old.

breasts but were discouraged by the high cost of surgery. Also, 10 were not aware of any treatment available (Table 1).

3.3. Prevalence of BDA in the Family. Out of the 64 girls with BDA, 22 (34.4%) said they had a family member with a similar condition; 6 admitted to having seen the anomaly in their mothers, 22 in their sisters, 5 in their aunt, and 1 person admitted seeing it in her grandmother (Table 2).

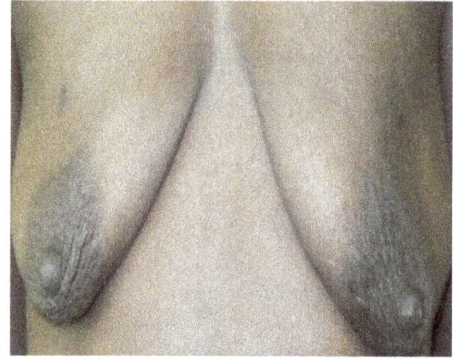

FIGURE 7: Bilateral accessory nipples in 45-year-old.

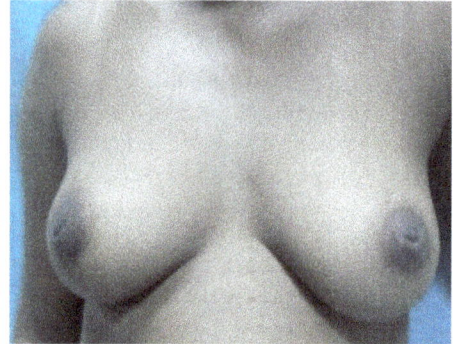

FIGURE 8: Bilateral nipple anomalies (Slit nipples) in a 23 year-old.

3.4. Attitude and Response of the Family and Community. Out of the 64 respondents, 14 of them were aware they had a BDA. Six (9.4%) openly complained to their families about the condition, and the family's response to all these respondents was that their condition was normal. Eight (12.5%) respondents failed to tell anyone about their condition because they felt too shy to tell anyone in their family.

3.5. Knowledge of Breast Diseases. Out of the 500 females interviewed, 134 (26.8%) girls were not satisfied with their breasts; 97 (72%) would be willing to have surgery performed to improve the look of their breasts. Thirty out of 97 wanted the size of their breasts to be increased, 65 wanted their breasts to be reduced, while the 2 wanted to fix the droopy nature of their breasts (augmentation). Thirty respondents out of the 64 (46.9%) with BDA were willing to have surgical correction of their anomaly. On knowledge of breast disease, 367 (73.4%) of the girls had heard of breast cancer; when asked whether they knew anyone apart of themselves or anyone in their family with BDA, 27 (5.4%) admitted knowing someone with a BDA.

4. Discussion

In this study, the prevalence of BDA was 12.8%. This is similar to findings done in other parts of the country where the prevalence recorded by Agbenorku et al. was 13% and 12.7% in Jamasi and Sogakope, respectively [17, 39]. More research

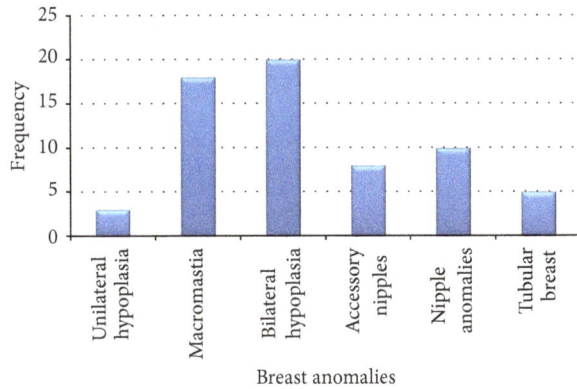

FIGURE 9: Forms of BDAs in respondents.

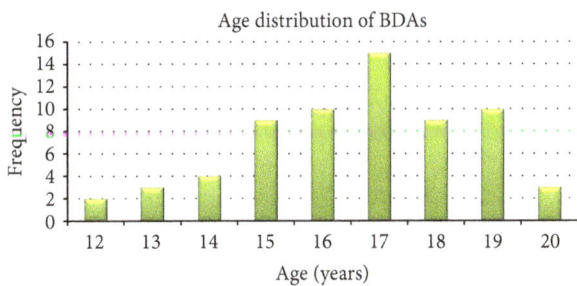

FIGURE 10: Age distribution of respondents with BDAs.

TABLE 1: Reasons for not seeking treatment.

Reason	Frequency	Percentage
Not aware of disease	50	78.1
Not aware of treatment	10	15.6
Too expensive	3	4.7
Has no time for treatment	1	1.6
Any other reason	0	0
Total	64	100%

TABLE 2: Prevalence of BDA in the family.

BDA	Total cases seen among respondents	People with the same condition in their family	% with occurrence in the family
Unilateral hypoplasia	3	0	0%
Macromastia	18	5	27.8%
Bilateral hypoplasia	20	8	40%
Accessory nipples	8	3	37.5%
Nipple anomalies	10	4	40.0%
Tubular breasts	5	2	20%
Totals	64	22	34.4%

on BDA has to be conducted, since prevalence in other areas could be high.

From this study, the commonest BDA found among the respondents was bilateral hypoplasia, followed by macromastia. Bilateral hypoplasia was reported much more frequently (30.7%) in this study than in other similar studies done in Ghana: 17.1% in Sogakope and 21.8% in Jamasi. In a study carried out by Simmons [16] among adolescents in the US, it revealed that polythelia and asymmetry were the most common BDAs. The prevalence of BDAs in this present study and other studies in Ghana was relatively higher than that found among Japanese where studies on young females revealed a prevalence of accessory nipples to be 5% [40, 41]. Some people may be of the view that breasts of the girls had not begun developing explaining the high prevalence of bilateral hypoplasia, but this cannot be the reason for the high rate of breast hypoplasia because the average age of the girls with bilateral hypoplasia was 16.75 years when in general most girls' breasts begin to develop between the ages of 10 and 11 years; therefore, the higher rate of breast hypoplasia may be attributed to other factors. One possible factor is that it could have arisen from the fact that this study design was a subjective design and unlike the other studies performed in the other areas where there was actual breast examination by the research team; so, the person's perception of their own breasts played a huge role in determining their choice.

Macromastia accounted for 28.1% of the BDAs. This value is not as high as those from other studies done in Ghana by Agbenorku et al. in Jamasi and Sogakope where macromastia accounted for 43.6% and 40.0%, respectively [17, 39].

A total of 34.4% of the respondents with a BDA had a family member with a similar condition (Table 2). This is similar to 31% reported by Agbenorku et al. in Jamasi [17]. This could mean that there is likely a genetic predisposition to the inheritance of BDA. Haagensen reported that there is a genetic element to BDAs when he noticed that the occurrence of polymastia or polythelia was inheritable condition [42].

In this study, 21.9% were aware that they had a BDA. This is quite low as compared to the awareness level of 63% recorded by Agbenorku et al. in Jamasi [17]. Awareness on BDA needs to be put in place in order to sensitize the general public. Regular breast self-examination (BSE) could result in early detection of these anomalies. A study conducted in Saudi Arabia revealed only 30.3% of the women had heard about BSE and 18.7% reported they practiced BSE within the previous year [43]. Also, a similar study undertaken in Nigeria by Okobia et al. showed that women lacked enough knowledge about breast cancer; 34.9% claimed to have ever-practiced BSE [44].

From the study, 67% wanted a reduction of their breasts. However, this is in contrast to a survey undertaken by Frederick on 26,703 American female adults where it was found that 70% of females were dissatisfied with their breasts and wanted more ample breasts [45]. This in response between the Ghanaians and Americans could be as a result of the fact that society plays a major role dictating the "ideal breast size," and this perception would strongly influence their decision to either reduce or increase their breasts. In the United States, there is constant social and media pressure for women to have big breasts.

Surgery is the best treatment option for BDA. As much as 46.9% respondents wanted to have surgical correction of their breasts. This rate is much higher than that seen in the study in Jamasi, where 20.5% of the girls with the BDA were willing to have surgical correction of their breasts [17]. The higher rates of acceptance of surgery in this study may arise from the fact that in this study the girls were not given any other treatment option such as drugs as a method of treatment which was an option in the Jamasi study. The treatment options were limited to surgical management because drug therapy is not effective.

BDA could have such negative impacts on the lives of people. From this present study, 14.1% ($n = 9$) said that the anomaly was affecting their life in school or at home negatively. However, the situation in this present study differs from a similar study conducted by Agbenorku et al. at Jamasi which revealed that among those with BDA, it had no effect on their school and family life [17]. Benditte-Klepetko et al. carried out a study on 50 women with various breast sizes and concluded that that high breast weight has a negative influence on the physical and psychological morbidity of women [46]. Gözü et al. also stated in his study on a 12-year-old girl suffering from breast hypertrophy that although the deformity is benign, it affects patients physically and psychologically [47]. Somma et al. reported a case of a 12-year old girl with juvenile hypertrophy of breast which caused her intense psychological problems, incapacitating her in school activities and social relations [18]. More education is therefore needed to help persons with BDA to develop a positive self image.

5. Conclusion

The study revealed that the prevalence of breast developmental anomalies in the Dormaa Municipality is high. The study also showed that some girls are negatively affected by this condition; hence, education on BDA should be promoted to increase awareness of the condition. This form of education should also enlighten the public on treatment measures available. People should also be educated and encouraged to practice breast self-examination.

Ethical Approval

The appropriate ethical approval was obtained from the Committee on Human Research, Publications and Ethics of the Kwame Nkrumah University of Science and Technology, School of Medical Sciences and Komfo Anokye Teaching Hospital, Kumasi.

References

[1] J. Bostwick, "Breast augmentation, reduction, and mastopexy," in *Plastic Surgery Principles and Practice*, M. J. Jurkiewicz, T. J. Krizek, S. J. Mathes, and Ariyan, Eds., pp. 458–467, Mosby, St. Louis, Mo, USA, 1990.

[2] M. A. Shermak, "Congenital and developmental abnormalities of the breast," in *Management of Breast Diseases*, I. Jatoi and M. Kaufmann, Eds., pp. 37–49, Springer, New York, NY, USA, 1st edition, 2010.

[3] L. S. Neinstein, "Breast disease in adolescents and young women," *Pediatric Clinics of North America*, vol. 46, no. 3, pp. 607–629, 1999.

[4] R. N. Matthews and F. T. Khan, "A seat belt injury to the female breast," *British Journal of Plastic Surgery*, vol. 51, no. 8, p. 653, 1998.

[5] N. S. Rosenfield, J. O. Haller, and W. E. Berdon, "Failure of the development of the growing breast after radiation therapy," *Pediatric Radiology*, vol. 19, no. 2, pp. 124–127, 1989.

[6] S. A. Bloom and M. Y. Nahabedian, "Gestational macromastia: a medical and surgical challenge," *Breast Journal*, vol. 14, no. 5, pp. 492–495, 2008.

[7] D. Ravichandran and S. Naz, "A study of children and adolescents referred to a rapid diagnosis breast clinic," *European Journal of Pediatric Surgery*, vol. 16, no. 5, pp. 303–306, 2006.

[8] M. J. Arca and D. A. Caniano, "Breast disorders in the adolescent patient," *Adolescent Medicine Clinics*, vol. 15, no. 3, pp. 473–485, 2004.

[9] K. Sharma, S. Nigam, N. Khurana, and K. U. Chaturvedi, "Unilateral gestational macromastia-a rare disorder," *The Malaysian journal of pathology.*, vol. 26, no. 2, pp. 125–128, 2004.

[10] C. J. Gabka, H. Bohmert, and P. N. Blondeel, *Plastic and Reconstructive Surgery of the Breast*, Thieme Publishing Group, New York, NY, USA, 2009.

[11] T. Sadler and L. J. Langman, *Medical Dictionary*, Lippincott Williams & Wilkins, Philadelphia, Pa, USA, 2006.

[12] M. Tadaoki, K. Komaki, T. Mori et al., "Juvenile Gigantomastia: report of a case," *Surgery Today of Japan*, pp. 260–264, 1993.

[13] L. Blomqvist, A. Eriksson, and Y. Brandberg, "Reduction mammaplasty provides long-term improvement in health status and quality of life," *Plastic and Reconstructive Surgery*, vol. 106, no. 5, pp. 991–997, 2000.

[14] D. Kulkarni and M. Dixon, "Congenital Abnormalities of the breast," *Women's Health*, pp. 75–88, 2012.

[15] W. Chromiński, B. Madej, R. Maciejewski, K. Torres, R. Ciechanek, and F. Burdan, "A development anomaly of the mammary glands-gigantomastia. A case report," *Folia Morphologica*, vol. 62, no. 4, pp. 517–518, 2003.

[16] P. S. Simmons, "Anomalies of the adolescent breast," *Paediatrics and Child Health*, vol. 18, no. 1, pp. S5–S7, 2008.

[17] P. Agbenorku, M. Agbenorku, A. Iddi et al., "Awareness of breast developmental anomalies: a study in Jamasi, Ghana," *Aesthetic Plastic Surgery*, vol. 35, no. 5, pp. 745–749, 2011.

[18] F. Somma, C. Calzoni, S. Arleo et al., "Polythelia and supernumerary breast. Personal experience and review of the literature," *Annali Italiani di Chirurgia*, vol. 83, no. 2, pp. 109–112, 2012.

[19] C. J. García, A. Espinoza, V. Dinamarca et al., "Breast US in children and adolescents," *Radiographics*, vol. 20, no. 6, pp. 1605–1612, 2000.

[20] Pediatric Views, "Retrieved January 30, 2012, from Children's Hospital, Boston," 2007, http://www.childrenshospital.org/views/august07/finding_solutions_to_adolescent_breast_problems.html.

[21] G. A. Rahman, I. A. Adigun, and I. F. Yusuf, "Macromastia: a review of presentation and management," *The Nigerian Postgraduate Medical Journal*, vol. 17, no. 1, pp. 45–49, 2010.

[22] J. O. Schorge, J. I. Schaffer, L. M. Halvorson et al., *Williams Gynecology*, McGraw-Hill, New York, NY, USA, 2008.

[23] Breast Reduction, "Retrieved January 30, 2012, from Wikipedia," 2012, http://en.wikipedia.org/wiki/Breast_reduction.

[24] A. D. Versaci and A. A. Rozzelle, "Treatment of tuberous breasts utilizing tissue expansion," *Aesthetic Plastic Surgery*, vol. 15, no. 4, pp. 307–312, 1991.

[25] P. Agbenorku, G. Agamah, M. Agbenorku, and M. Obeng, "Reduction mammaplasty in a developing country: a guideline for plastic surgeons for patient selection," *Aesthetic Plastic Surgery*, vol. 36, no. 1, pp. 91–96, 2011.

[26] J. Bostwick, *3rd Plastic and Reconstructive Breast Surgery*, vol. 1, 2000.

[27] M. S. Ahmed, "A simplified superior pedicle technique for reduction mammaplasty," *Journal of Plastic, Reconstructive & Aesthetic Surgery*, vol. 30, no. 1, pp. 57–61, 2006.

[28] M. Y. Nahabedian and M. M. Mofid, "Viability and sensation of the nipple-areolar complex after reduction mammaplasty," *Annals of Plastic Surgery*, vol. 49, no. 1, pp. 24–32, 2002.

[29] J. O. Strömbeck, "Mammaplasty: report of a new technique based on the two-pedicle procedure," *British Journal of Plastic Surgery C*, vol. 13, pp. 79–90, 1960.

[30] P. Regnault, "Reduction mammaplasty by the "B" technique," *Plastic and Reconstructive Surgery*, vol. 53, p. 19, 1974.

[31] T. H. Robbins, "A reduction mammaplasty with the areola nipple based on an inferior dermal pedicle," *Plastic and Reconstructive Surgery*, vol. 59, no. 1, pp. 64–67, 1977.

[32] H. Moustapha, H. C. Dennis, and N. Foad, *Vertical Scar Mammaplasty*, Spring, Berlin, Germany, 2005.

[33] T. Skoog, "A technique for breast reduction: transposition of the nipple on a cutaneous vascular pedicle," *Acta chirurgica Scandinavica*, vol. 126, pp. 453–465, 1963.

[34] E. Courtiiss and R. Goldwyn, "Reduction mammaplasty by the inferior pedicle technique," *Plastic & Reconstructive Surgery*, vol. 59, no. 1, pp. 64–67, 1977.

[35] P. K. McKissock, "Reduction mammaplasty with a vertical dermal flap," *Plastic and Reconstructive Surgery*, vol. 49, no. 3, pp. 245–252, 1972.

[36] T. Von Soest, I. Kvalem, K. Skolleborg et al., "Psychosocial changes after cosmetic surgery: a 5-year follow-up study," *Plastic and Reconstructive Surgery*, vol. 128, no. 3, pp. 765–772, 2011.

[37] D. J. Castle, R. J. Honigman, and K. A. Phillips, "Does cosmetic surgery improve psychosocial wellbeing?" *Medical Journal of Australia*, vol. 176, no. 12, pp. 601–604, 2002.

[38] Dormaa Municipal Assembly, "municipality info. Retrieved January 5, 2012, from Dormaa Municipal," 2006, http://www.dormaa.ghanadistricts.gov.gh/.

[39] P. Agbenorku, M. Agbenorku, A. Iddi et al., "Incidence of breast developmental anomalies: a study at Sogakope, Ghana," *Nigerian Journal of Plastic Surgery*, vol. 6, no. 1, pp. 1–5, 2010.

[40] M. Clement-Jones, S. Schiller, E. Rao et al., "The short stature homeobox gene SHOX is involved in skeletal abnormalities in Turner syndrome," *Human Molecular Genetics*, vol. 9, no. 5, pp. 695–702, 2000.

[41] M. Lee, "Growth Hormone deficiency as the only identidable cause for primary amennorrhea," *Journal of Pediatric and Adolescent Gynecology*, vol. 13, no. 2, pp. 93–95, 2000.

[42] C. D. Haagensen, "Breasts," in *Handbook of Congenital Malformation*, A. Rubin, Ed., pp. 398–401, WB Saunders Co, Philadelphia, Pa, USA, 1967.

[43] S. Jahan, A. M. Al-Saigul, and M. H. Abdelgadir, "Breast cancer. Knowledge, attitudes and practices of breast self examination among women in Qassim region of Saudi Arabia," *Saudi Medical Journal*, vol. 27, no. 11, pp. 1737–1741, 2006.

[44] M. N. Okobia, C. H. Bunker, F. E. Okonofua, and U. Osime, "Knowledge, attitude and practice of Nigerian women towards breast cancer: a cross-sectional study," *World Journal of Surgical Oncology*, vol. 4, p. 11, 2006.

[45] D. A. Frederick, A. Peplau, and J. Lever, "The barbie mystique: satisfaction with breast size and shape across the lifespan," *International Journal of Sexual Health*, vol. 20, no. 3, pp. 200–211, 2008.

[46] H. Benditte-Klepetko, V. Leisser, T. Paternostro-Sluga et al., "Hypertrophy of the breast: a problem of beauty or health?" *Journal of Women's Health*, vol. 16, no. 7, pp. 1062–1069, 2007.

[47] A. Gözü, F. N. Yoğun, Z. Özsoy, A. Özdemir, G. Özgürhan, and S. Tuzlali, "Juvenile breast hypertrophy," *Journal of Breast Health*, vol. 6, no. 3, pp. 122–124, 2010.

Skin-Sparing Mastectomy with Immediate Breast and Nipple Reconstruction: A New Technique of Nipple Reconstruction

Raffaele Serra,[1] Anna Maria Miglietta,[2] Sergio Abonante,[2] Vincent Giordano,[3] Gianluca Buffone,[1] and Stefano de Franciscis[1]

[1] *Department of Medical and Surgical Science, University Magna Graecia of Catanzaro, Viale Europa, 88100 Catanzaro, Italy*
[2] *Breast Unit, Annunziata Hospital, 87100 Cosenza, Italy*
[3] *Plastic Surgery Unit, Annunziata Hospital, 87100 Cosenza, Italy*

Correspondence should be addressed to Raffaele Serra; rserra@unicz.it

Academic Editor: Lee L. Q. Pu

Background. Most women with breast cancer today can be managed with breast conservation; however, some women still require mastectomy for treatment of their disease. Skin-sparing mastectomy (SSM) with immediate reconstruction has emerged as a favorable option for many of these patients. The authors combined the SSM technique with the preservation of a small part of the areola with immediate nipple together with with breast reconstruction. *Methods*. In an 8-year-period 155 female patients (age: 20–52 years old; mean age: 37.5 years) with extensive ductal intraepithelial neoplasia (DIN) or invasive breast cancer were treated with areola skin sparing mastectomy with immediate nipple and breast reconstruction. Patients were followed up prospectively by the breast surgeon, the plastic surgeon, and the oncologist for complications and recurrence. *Results*. After treatment, only 2 cases (1.29%) had a local recurrence. 8 out of 155 (5.5%) patients developed early complications (infections, seroma, haematoma), and 5 out of 155 patients (3.22%) developed delayed complications (implant rotation, aesthetic deterioration) in the post operative time period. The final aesthetic outcome was judged as positive in 150 out of 155 patients (96.78%). *Conclusion*. In our experience, immediate nipple reconstruction after skin-sparing mastectomy is a technically feasible procedure which can give excellent cosmetic results.

1. Introduction

Mastectomy represents the treatment of choice for approximately one-third of women with breast cancer due to aggressive, extensive, or multicentric tumour growth, contraindications for radiotherapy, or following the patient's wish.

To most of these cases, immediate breast reconstruction (IBR) can be offered to overcome the psychological burden caused by the disfigurement resulting from the loss of the breast [1].

Skin-sparing mastectomy (SSM) can be followed by immediate breast reconstruction (IBR) using autologous tissue and/or prosthetic implants, and this approach has been advocated as an effective treatment option for patients with early-stage breast cancer which is not amenable to breast-conserving therapy [2–4].

The presence of the nipples seems fundamental to marking the identity of the breast. Based on the psychological impact of nipple-areola complex (NAC) removal in classical mastectomy techniques, several authors have evaluated the risk of nipple areola involvement and investigated the possibility of nipple areola preservation, but the risk of cancer recurrence in the breast tissue preserved beneath the NAC for the blood supply is considered a major reason to avoid NAC conservation during the mastectomy [5].

The authors combined the SSM technique with the preservation of a small part of the areola with immediate nipple and breast reconstruction.

The most interesting part of the method used at the author's institution is precisely the particular new technique of nipple reconstruction that has not been previously described.

The authors reports their experience carried out in the last eight years in order to evaluate the oncological safety, postoperative morbidity and patients' satisfaction with this technique.

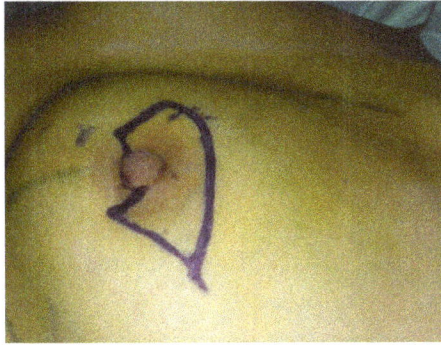

FIGURE 1: Incision line preserving part of the areola.

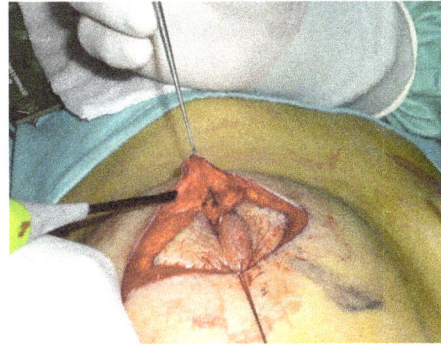

FIGURE 2: Surgical incision.

TABLE 1: Characteristics of patients.

Number of patients	155
Age of patients	20–52 (range), 37.5 (mean)
Followup (months)	12–96 (range), 47 (mean)
Tumor size	
Extensive DIN	23
T1	36
T2	96
Histology	
Ductal	137
Lobular	18
Nodal status	
N0	151
N1	4

2. Material and Methods

In an 8-year-period (2003–2010), 155 female patients (age: 20–52 years old; mean age: 37.5 years) with extensive ductal intraepithelial neoplasia (DIN) or invasive breast cancer (T1 and T2 tumors and an unfavorable breast to tumor ratio) were treated with areola skin-sparing mastectomy with immediate nipple and breast reconstruction.

Demographics and patient characteristics are shown in Table 1.

All patients were evaluated preoperatively by a multidisciplinary team, including the breast surgeon and the plastic surgeon, to define appropriate surgical procedure and to explain to the patient the advantages and possible disadvantages of the selected option.

Informed written consent was obtained and in this study the principles outlined in the Declaration of Helsinki have been followed.

The standard Stewart elliptical skin incision was performed around nipple/areola complex while preserving, as an originality of the tecnique, a small part of areola which will be used later for the reconstruction of the nipple (Figures 1 and 2). For oncological safety, the part of the areola to preserve is selected in order to be sufficiently distant from the tumor, and preferably on the opposite pole to it, but also to allow a symmetrical positioning with respect to the contralateral nipple.

Subsequent surgical procedures consisted of removal of mammary tissue and nipple-areola complex (NAC) with the preservation of the remaining breast skin envelope and the inframammary fold.

Once SSM has been completed, breast reconstruction commences with an incision along the lateral border of the pectoralis major muscle, and a submuscular pocket is created deep to both the pectoral and serratus muscles. To prevent cranial displacement of the implants and to allow for a more natural projection of the lower part of the reconstructed breast, the origin of the major pectoral muscle was detached from the lower costal arch and the caudal part of the sternum.

In this pocket, an appropriate size of the textured prosthesis (textured profile (anatomical) saline implants; mentor; california-USA) is placed.

The Closure of the pocket was achieved by using the pectoralis major muscle as coverage in its upper two-thirds and using the mastectomy skin flap as coverage in its lower third in order to avoid upper-pole hyperexpansion by virtue of decreased resistance to the forces of expansion in this area and a concomitant lower-pole elevation, leaving in this way the newly mammary fold by the curvature of the breast prosthesis.

Before suturing the skin reconstruction of the nipple begins, an absorbable suture is positioned at the base of the truncated cone formed by the residual areola, then a mattress stitch iss put between the new nipple edges. An intradermal continuous suture on the joining edges of the new nipple is performed, and at the end of the procedure, skin suturing is performed (Figure 3).

In our case series only unilateral reconstruction was performed.

All patients were followed during the postoperative period by the breast surgeon, the plastic surgeon and the oncologist. Followup was programmed every week for the first month, and monthly for the following 6 months, then every 6 months. The average followup was 4.5 years.

Patient satisfaction was estimated using a questionnaire (Table 3) administered at 1 year from the procedure.

The score was then totaled for a maximum of 10 points per patient as follows: "Excellent" (9-10 points), "Good" (7–8.5 points), "Acceptable" (5–6.5 points), and "Poor" (≤4.5 points).

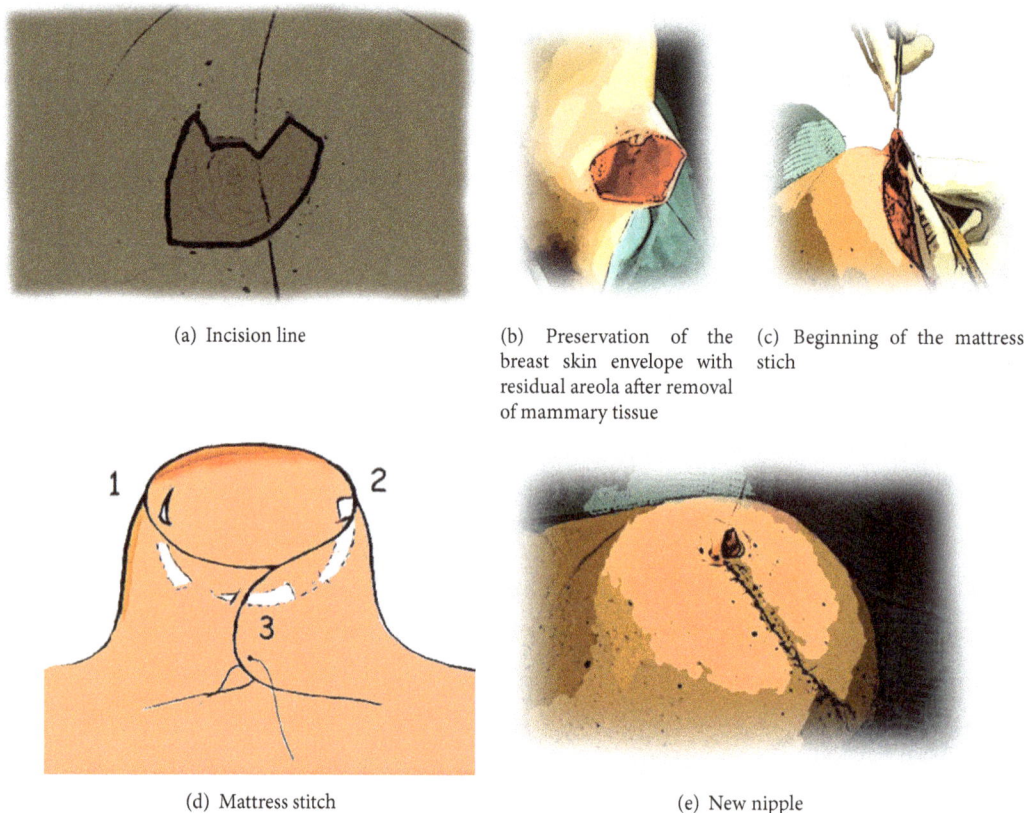

(a) Incision line

(b) Preservation of the breast skin envelope with residual areola after removal of mammary tissue

(c) Beginning of the mattress stich

(d) Mattress stitch

(e) New nipple

FIGURE 3: Scheme of the technique.

TABLE 2: Complications.

Early	
Infections	1 (0.64%)
Seroma	3 (1.93%)
Haematoma	4 (2.58%)
Delayed	
Implant rotation	2 (1.29%)
Aesthetic deterioration	3 (1.93%)

Objective data on the size, projection, and the symmetry with respect to the contralateral nipple were also collected.

The height and diameter of the reconstructed nipple were measured directly after the procedure and during follow-up controls.

After surgical procedure, 87 patients (56.12%) underwent adjuvant chemotherapy with FAC chemotherapy (5-fluorouracil, doxorubicin, cyclophosphamide) given 3 times weekly for 6 cycles, while 68 patients (49.15%) underwent long-term tamoxifen therapy for 5 years.

3. Results

After treatment, only 2 cases (1.29%) had a local recurrence.

Among the 155 patients who underwent SSM with immediate breast and nipple reconstruction, 8 (5.5%) patients developed early and 5 patients (3.22%) delayed complications in the postoperative time period; the complications have been collected and are reported in Table 2.

Given the thin nature of the residual areola tissue used for nipple reconstruction, there were, however, no instances of nipple necrosis as might be expected.

There were also no evidence of capsular contractures in the followup period.

The average diameter of the reconstructed nipple in the immediate postoperative period was 11.8 ± 1.1 mm compared with 12.1 ± 0.9 mm for the opposite nipple. After 1 year, the average diameter was 13.2 ± 1.3 mm.

The average projection of the nipple in the immediate postoperative period was 6.15 ± 0.6 mm, compared with 5.12 ± 1.35 mm for the opposite side. After one year the average projection of the new nipple was 4.16 ± 0.7 mm (−15.86%).

Symmetrization was achieved satisfactorily during first procedure for almost all patients. Only in two cases (1.29%), the symmetrization of the nipple compared with the contralateral nipple has not been satisfactory (due to the location of the tumor), and it was necessary to proceed with further intervention of repositioning of the nipple under local anesthesia after six months from the first procedure.

All patients completed aesthetic questionnaire.

The final aesthetic outcome was judged, according to questionnaire filled by all patients, as excellent in 98 patients (63.22%), good in 43 patients (27.74%), acceptable in 9

TABLE 3: Satisfaction Questionnaire.

Items	Very dissatisfied	Somewhat dissatisfied	Somewhat satisfied	Very satisfied
(A) How satisfied or dissatisfied have you been in the last 6 months with				
(1) the Shape of the breast	0.5	1	1.5	2
(2) the Scars of the breast	0.5	1	1.5	2
(3) the Sensibility of the breast	0.5	1	1.5	2
(4) the Appearence of the new nipple	0.5	1	1.5	2
(B) the overall surgical procedure fulfilled your expectations?				
	0.5	1	1.5	2

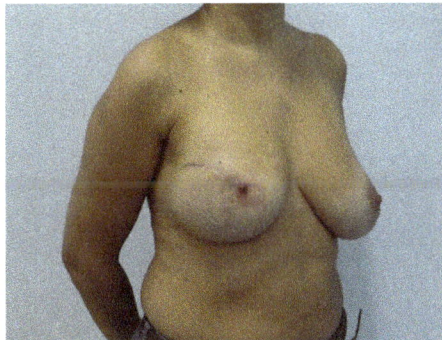

FIGURE 4: Outcome Example after 1 year.

patients (5.80%), and poor in 5 patients (3.22%). An example of positive result after 1 year is shown in Figure 4.

4. Discussion

Indications for mastectomy (with/without reconstruction) included tumor size >5 cm, central sector tumor unsuitable for breast conserving surgery (BCS), multiple tumor foci, relatively large tumor with respect to breast size, extensive high-grade in situ carcinoma, inflammatory cancer, history of prior cancer in the breast, where radiotherapy is contraindicated, and patient preference. In the absence of all these factors, BCS followed by adjuvant radiotherapy was the treatment of choice.

Historically, malignant involvement of the nipple-areola complex (NAC) in mastectomy specimens has been cited to be 5.6%–58%, thus leading many to suggest that NAC preservation is not a reasonable option [6, 7].

Concerned about local-regional recurrence from occult neoplastic involvement of the NAC, Petit and collegues performed the same nipple-sparing mastectomy and added intraoperative or postoperative brachytherapy to the preserved NAC. This resulted in equivalent oncologic results but higher rates of nipple necrosis and resection [8].

An alternative to NAC-sparing mastectomy is to remove the nipple, but preserve the areola (areola-sparing mastectomy), followed, in a second step, by nipple reconstruction using one of the conventional local flap techniques. Results are controversial [9].

In our personal experience, we preferred saline implants for breast reconstruction as they have a lower rate of revision surgery than silicone gel, and the overall rate of capsular contracture is lower for saline than silicone [10]. Further, the scar is shorter, as saline implants can be filled after they are placed, allowing a smaller incision, and there is no need for MRI, as silent rupture is not a concern.

The objectives of nipple reconstruction aim to create a nipple which is symmetrical to the contralateral nipple precisely in terms of shape, size, position, and projection in order to achieve patient satisfaction.

Numerous tecniques have been described for nipple reconstruction following mastectomy (e.g., local adipocutaneous flap, distant tissue flaps, cartilage grafts, local flaps as bell, skate flaps, star flaps, bilobed flaps, trilobed flpas, and C-V flap technique) but no one is entirely satisfactory. In fact, the most common problem following nipple reconstruction is that projection of the new nipple tends to shrink with time, and reported figures for percentage projection loss vary significantly [11, 12].

In our casuistry, we reported an increase of 12.1% in the diameter of the reconstructed nipple and a projection loss of 15.86% after 1 year.

In our experience the low rate of recurrences (1.29%) and complications (5.5% immediate and 3.22% late) with the positive aesthetic outcome of the procedures (96.76%) allows us to state that immediate nipple reconstruction after SSM is a technically feasible procedure which can give excellent cosmetic results.

Moreover, a recent paper showed that breast-conserving therapy nowadays can be offered as standard care with long-term results, in terms of survival, comparable to that of standard procedures [13].

In our experience, our unique stage surgery saves time in the surgical theatre and reduces the number of hospitalizations by giving to the patients the chance to complete the reconstruction in one stage without delaying the breast reconstruction and achieves, at the same time, excellent cosmetic results.

Ethical Approval

The authors have read and complied with the instructions to authors and in particular the policy of the journal on ethical consent.

Acknowledgments

A special thanks goes to Luisa Ruberto, Technical Designer at Lamezia Terme, Italy, for excellent technical assistance and for the scheme of Figure 3.

References

[1] R. Wirth and A. Banic, "Aesthetic outcome and oncological safety of nipple-areola complex replantation after mastectomy and immediate breast reconstruction," *Journal of Plastic, Reconstructive & Aesthetic Surgery*, vol. 63, no. 9, pp. 1490–1494, 2010.

[2] G. H. Cunnick and K. Mokbel, "Skin-sparing mastectomy," *American Journal of Surgery*, vol. 188, no. 1, pp. 78–84, 2004.

[3] S. E. Singletary and G. L. Robb, "Oncologic safety of skin-sparing mastectomy," *Annals of Surgical Oncology*, vol. 10, no. 2, pp. 95–97, 2003.

[4] R. M. Simmons and T. L. Adamovich, "Skin-sparing mastectomy," *Surgical Clinics of North America*, vol. 83, no. 4, pp. 885–899, 2003.

[5] A. K. Schecter, M. B. Freeman, D. Giri, E. Sabo, and J. Weinzweig, "Applicability of the nipple-areola complex-sparing mastectomy: a prediction model using mammography to estimate risk of nipple-areola complex involvement in breast cancer patients," *Annals of Plastic Surgery*, vol. 56, no. 5, pp. 498–504, 2006.

[6] H. A. Cense, E. J. T. Rutgers, M. Lopes Cardozo, and J. J. B. Van Lanschot, "Nipple-sparing mastectomy in breast cancer: a viable option?" *European Journal of Surgical Oncology*, vol. 27, no. 6, pp. 521–526, 2001.

[7] R. M. Simmons, M. Brennan, P. Christos, V. King, and M. Osborne, "Analysis of nipple/areolar involvement with mastectomy: can the areola be preserved?" *Annals of Surgical Oncology*, vol. 9, no. 2, pp. 165–168, 2002.

[8] J. Y. Petit, U. Veronesi, P. Rey et al., "Nipple-sparing mastectomy: risk of nipple-areolar recurrences in a series of 579 cases," *Breast Cancer Research and Treatment*, vol. 114, no. 1, pp. 97–101, 2009.

[9] N. Patani, H. Devalia, A. Anderson, and K. Mokbel, "Oncological safety and patient satisfaction with skin-sparing mastectomy and immediate breast reconstruction," *Surgical Oncology*, vol. 17, no. 2, pp. 97–105, 2008.

[10] K. Benediktsson and L. Perbeck, "Capsular contracture around saline-filled and textured subcutaneously-placed implants in irradiated and non-irradiated breast cancer patients: five years of monitoring of a prospective trial," *Journal of Plastic, Reconstructive & Aesthetic Surgery*, vol. 59, no. 1, pp. 27–34, 2006.

[11] B. Jamnadas-Khoda, R. Thomas, and S. Heppell, "The "cigar roll" flap for nipple areola complex reconstruction: a novel technique," *Journal of Plastic, Reconstructive & Aesthetic Surgery*, vol. 64, no. 8, pp. E218–E220, 2011.

[12] A. P. Jones and M. Erdmann, "Projection and patient satisfaction using the "Hamburger" nipple reconstruction technique," *Journal of Plastic, Reconstructive & Aesthetic Surgery*, vol. 65, no. 2, pp. 207–212, 2012.

[13] S. Litière, G. Werutsky, I. S. Fentiman et al., "Breast conserving therapy versus mastectomy for stage I-II breast cancer: 20 year follow-up of the EORTC 10801 phase 3 randomised trial," *The Lancet Oncology*, vol. 13, no. 4, pp. 412–419, 2012.

3

Nummular Eczema of Breast: A Potential Dermatologic Complication after Mastectomy and Subsequent Breast Reconstruction

Yoshiko Iwahira,[1] Tomohisa Nagasao,[2] Yusuke Shimizu,[3] Kumiko Kuwata,[4] and Yoshio Tanaka[1]

[1]Tokyo Breast Surgery Clinic, Japan
[2]Department of Plastic and Reconstructive Surgery, Faculty of Medicine/Graduate School of Medicine, Kagawa University, Kida County, Miki-Cho, Ikenobe 1750-1, Takamatsu, Kagawa 761-0793, Japan
[3]Department of Plastic and Reconstructive Surgery, Ryukyu University Hospital, Japan
[4]Department of Plastic Surgery, Aichi Children's Health and Medical Center, Japan

Correspondence should be addressed to Tomohisa Nagasao; nagasao@med.kagawa-u.ac.jp

Academic Editor: Nicolo Scuderi

Purposes. The present paper reports clinical cases where nummular eczema developed during the course of breast reconstruction by means of implantation and evaluates the occurrence patterns and ratios of this complication. *Methods.* 1662 patients undergoing breast reconstruction were reviewed. Patients who developed nummular eczema during the treatment were selected, and a survey was conducted on these patients regarding three items: (1) the stage of the treatment at which nummular eczema developed; (2) time required for the lesion to heal; (3) location of the lesion on the reconstructed breast(s). Furthermore, histopathological examination was conducted to elucidate the etiology of the lesion. *Results.* 48 patients (2.89%) developed nummular eczema. The timing of onset varied among these patients, with lesions developing after the placement of tissue expanders for 22 patients (45.8%); after the tissue expanders were replaced with silicone implants for 12 patients (25%); and after nipple-areola complex reconstruction for 14 patients (29.2%). Nummular eczema developed both in periwound regions (20 cases: 41.7%) and in nonperiwound regions (32 cases: 66.7%). Histopathological examination showed epidermal acanthosis, psoriasiform patterns, and reduction of sebaceous glands. *Conclusions.* Surgeons should recognize that nummular eczema is a potential complication of breast reconstruction with tissue expanders and silicone implants.

1. Introduction

Breast cancer is one of the most common cancers. For instance, in the United States, one out of eight females develops breast cancer in her life [1]. Total mastectomy is conducted for patients in whom the tumor extends to a large portion of the mammary gland. Since the breast symbolizes femininity, its loss can inflict serious psychological damage on patients. For this reason, reconstruction of the lost breast is generally performed. Methods of breast reconstruction are classified into two genres: reconstruction by the transfer of autologous tissues [2, 3] and reconstruction with artificial materials [4–6]. The latter genre is less invasive than the former. However, breast reconstruction with artificial materials is sometimes accompanied by postoperative complications. Well-known complications include exposure of expanders or silicone implants. Besides these complications, we have recognized that nummular eczema may develop on the skin of the reconstructed breast, although this is not widely noted. Nummular eczema is a skin lesion first reported by Marie Guillaume Alphonse Devergie in the 19th century [7–9]. The present paper aims to introduce clinical cases of nummular eczema that developed during the breast reconstruction process, and it discusses how we can prevent this complication.

2. Methods

A total of 1,662 patients operated on for breast reconstruction at Tokyo Breast Surgery Clinic between February 2008 and

October 2013 were surveyed. All these patients were Japanese females. Among these 1,662 patients, 48 patients developed lesions diagnosed by dermatologists as nummular eczema on the skin of the reconstructed breasts. These 48 patients were reviewed in the present study. This study was approved by the ethical committee of the institutional review board of Tokyo Breast Surgery Clinic, and written informed consent was obtained from all patients. Evaluation was performed regarding the following issues.

2.1. Onset. Breast reconstruction is performed in three steps. In the first step, tissue expanders are placed in the layer beneath the major pectoral muscle to expand the skin; in the second step, the expanders are replaced with silicone implants; in the third step, the nipple-areola complex is reconstructed using skin graft and local flaps. Based on at which of these three steps nummular eczema developed, the 48 patients were classified into the following three groups.

Group 1. This group included patients who developed nummular eczema after the placement of tissue expanders and before replacement with silicone implants.

Group 2. This group included patients who developed nummular eczema after implant placement and before reconstruction of the nipple-areola complex.

Group 3. This group included patients who developed nummular eczema after reconstruction of the nipple-areola complex.

The intervals between the operation preceding development and development of nummular eczema were evaluated for each of these groups.

2.2. Comorbidities and Medications. Comorbidities, medications, and absence/presence of atopic dermatitis were evaluated for each of the three groups.

2.3. Location of Lesion. Placement of the tissue expander and its subsequent replacement with an implant are conducted through the wound made in the initial mastectomy. The skin regions of the breast were divided into two regions: the region adjacent to the wound and the region away from the wound. The former region was termed the periwound region; the latter region was termed the nonperiwound region. For patients belonging to each of the three groups, the locations of lesions were evaluated based on this classification. For patients belonging to Group 3, the nonperiwound region was further subdivided into the nipple-areola complex and the other part, and the location of nummular eczema was evaluated.

2.4. Healing Time. All patients were treated with a vaseline-based ointment containing 0.12% betamethasone valerate. For the patients belonging to each of the three groups, the time needed to heal was evaluated.

2.5. Histopathological Evaluation. Harvesting skin pieces from the lesion to examine histological changes occurring in

TABLE 1: Ages, onset timing, and healing times. The figures in each column indicate averages and standard deviations. Onset timing means the interval between the development of nummular eczema and the last operation before onset.

	Age	Onset timing (weeks)	Healing time (weeks)
Group 1 ($n = 22$)	45.2 ± 9.0 SD	32.1 ± 21.5 SD	3.5 ± 1.4 SD
Group 2 ($n = 12$)	41.1 ± 7.7 SD	84.2 ± 107.4 SD	4.4 ± 2.6 SD
Group 3 ($n = 14$)	46.7 ± 11.5 SD	64.4 ± 61.9 SD	3.2 ± 2.8 SD

TABLE 2: Medication.

	Tamoxifen citrate	Anastrozole
Group 1 ($n = 22$)	13	2
Group 2 ($n = 12$)	3	0
Group 3 ($n = 14$)	2	0

the lesion of the skin was suggested to the 48 patients who developed nummular eczema. Two patients elected to receive the histopathological examination, and samples of the lesions were harvested from them. These samples were examined by means of haematoxylin-eosin staining and azan staining.

3. Results

3.1. Onset. The onset timing presented variation, with 28 cases (45.8%) developing nummular eczema after placement of tissue expanders (Group 1), 12 cases (25.0%) developing lesions after replacement of expanders with silicone implants (Group 2), and 14 cases (29.2%) developing lesions after reconstruction of the nipple-areola complex (Group 3). Pictures of representative cases for each of the three groups are provided in Figures 1–3, respectively.

Intervals between the development of nummular eczema and the nearest preceding operation are listed in Table 1.

3.2. Medication of the Patients

3.2.1. Comorbidities. Among the 48 patients who had nummular eczema, 47 patients had no comorbidities. One patient in Group 2 had rheumatoid arthritis. No patient had underlying dermatological disease, such as atopic dermatitis.

3.2.2. Medications. 18 patients were taking tamoxifen citrate; two patients were taking anastrozole. The distribution of these patients is shown in Table 2. The patient who had rheumatoid arthritis was taking prednisolone as treatment for the disease.

3.3. Location. Nummular eczema developed for both periwound regions (20 cases: 41.7%) and nonperiwound regions (32 cases: 66.7%). In four cases, the lesion extended to both regions. Distribution of the locations for each group is demonstrated in Table 3.

3.4. Healing Time. The average and standard deviation of the time the affected skin took to heal are presented in Table 1.

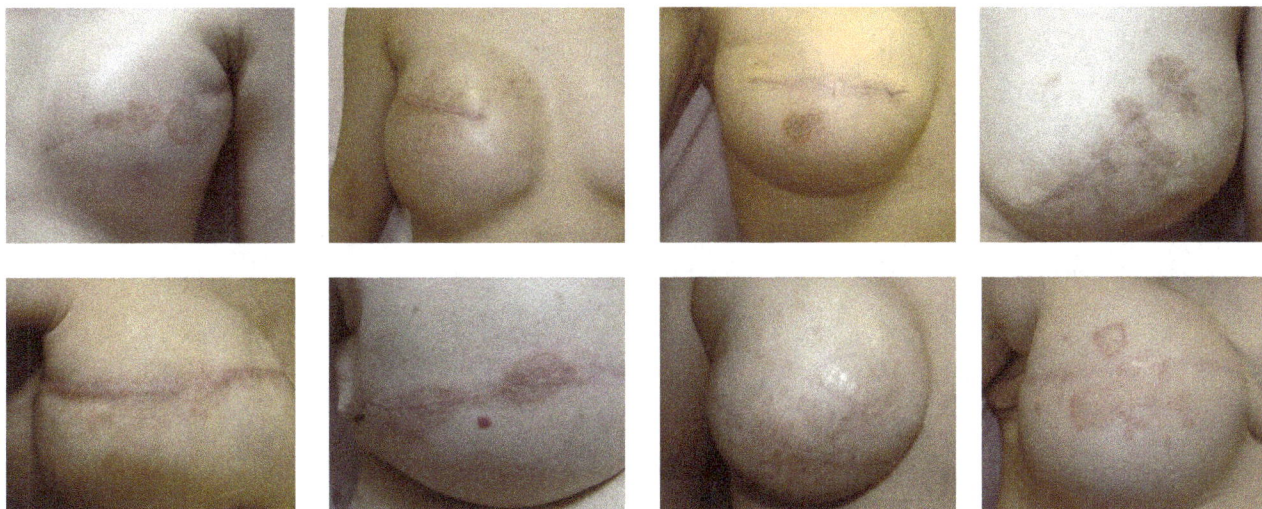

FIGURE 1: Representative cases of patients who developed nummular eczema after placement of tissue expanders and before replacement with silicone implants.

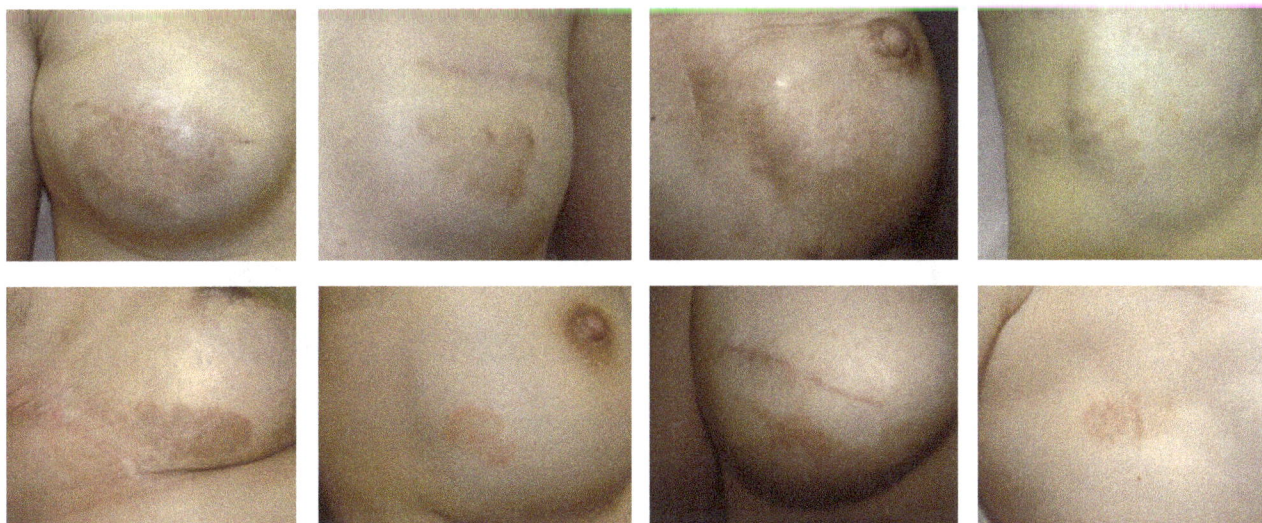

FIGURE 2: Representative cases of patients who developed nummular eczema after placement of silicone implants and before reconstruction of the nipple-areola complex.

In a majority of cases, nummular eczema healed within three to four weeks with the administration of steroid ointments (betamethasone valerate). In no cases did nummular eczema further deteriorate to cause ulceration or chronic infection after application of steroid ointment.

3.5. *Histopathological Findings.* Hematoxylin and eosin staining (Figure 4, left column) reveals significant epidermal acanthosis. Furthermore, psoriasiform patterns with hyperkeratosis, hypergranulosis, and minimal parakeratosis were also observed (Figure 4, left and right columns). Azan staining showed unidirectionally aligned collagen fibers, which formed the fibrosis.

4. Discussion

Nummular eczema is a discoid lesion of the skin that most frequently develops in the upper and lower extremities, as

TABLE 3: Location of lesions (since some patients had nummular eczema in more than one region, the sums of the columns do not necessarily match the patient's numbers for each group).

	Periwound region	Nonperiwound region	
Group 1 ($n = 22$)	9	15	
Group 2 ($n = 12$)	4	10	
Group 3 ($n = 14$)	7	Reconstructed nipple-areolar complex	7
		Non-NAC region	7

well as on the trunk, dorsum of the hand, face, and neck [10]. The etiological cause of nummular eczema remains unclear, and it is recognized as a multifactorial clinicomorphological entity, not an independent disease *per se* [8, 9]. Nummular

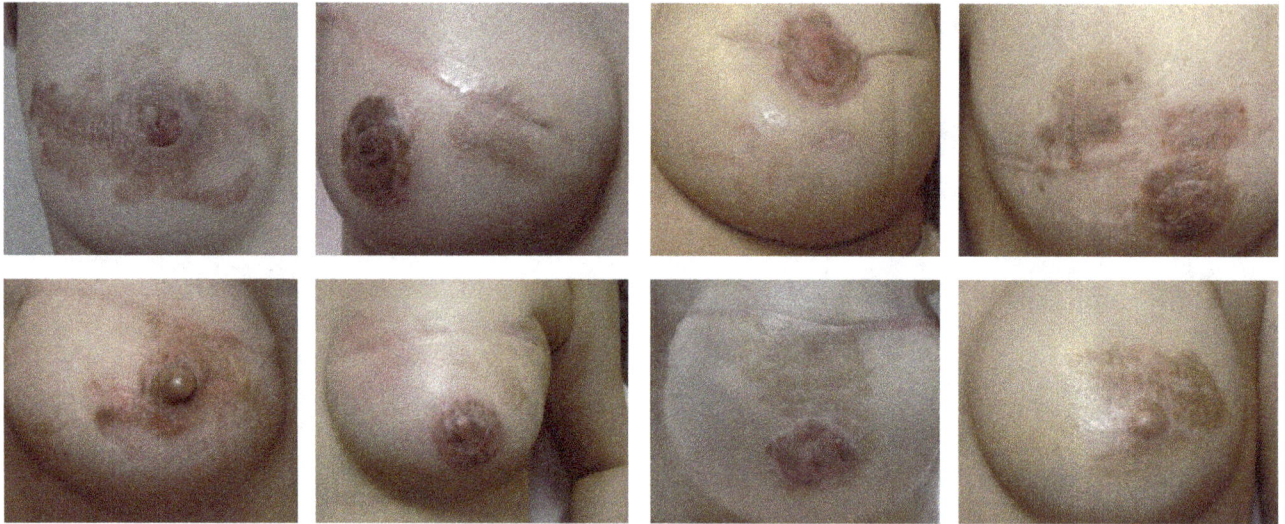

FIGURE 3: Representative cases of patients who developed nummular eczema after reconstruction of nipple-areola complex.

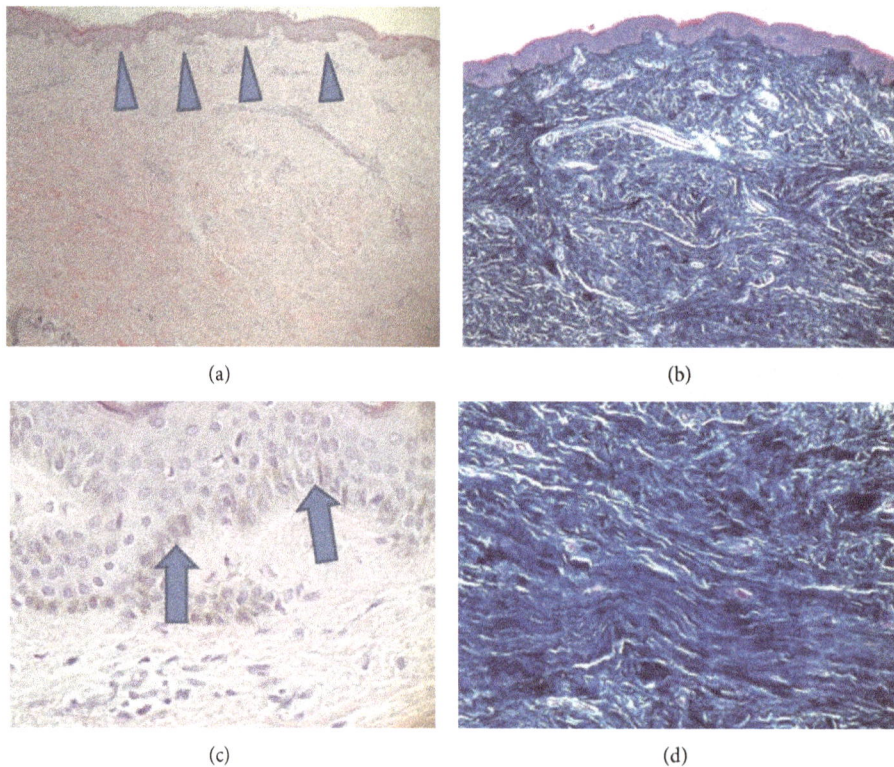

FIGURE 4: Histological findings of nummular eczema on the breast skin. (a) H-E staining magnified by 40 times. Epidermal acanthosis is shown (triangular arrows). (c) H-E staining magnified by 400 times. A psoriasiform pattern with hyperkeratosis (arrows), hypergranulosis, and minimal parakeratosis is observed. (b) Azan staining magnified by 40 times. Reduction of sebaceous glands is noted. (d) Azan staining magnified by 100 times. Randomly aligned hypertrophy of collagen fibers is observed.

eczema often takes a chronic and recursive course. Various causes such as atopic dermatitis, dry skin, mental stress, the weather, infection, and alcohol can induce nummular eczema [11–14].

Herein, the etiological causes of the nummular eczema in our series are discussed. Nummular eczema rarely occurs in the breast region, and it only develops there in limited situations, according to our review of the existing literature. Specifically, side effects caused by combined usage of interferon alfa-2b and ribavirin [15, 16], extramammary Paget's disease [17], and hematological diseases [18] are reported to have caused nummular eczema in the breast region. No patient in our series had any of these background factors. Among the 48 nummular eczema patients, 18 patients took

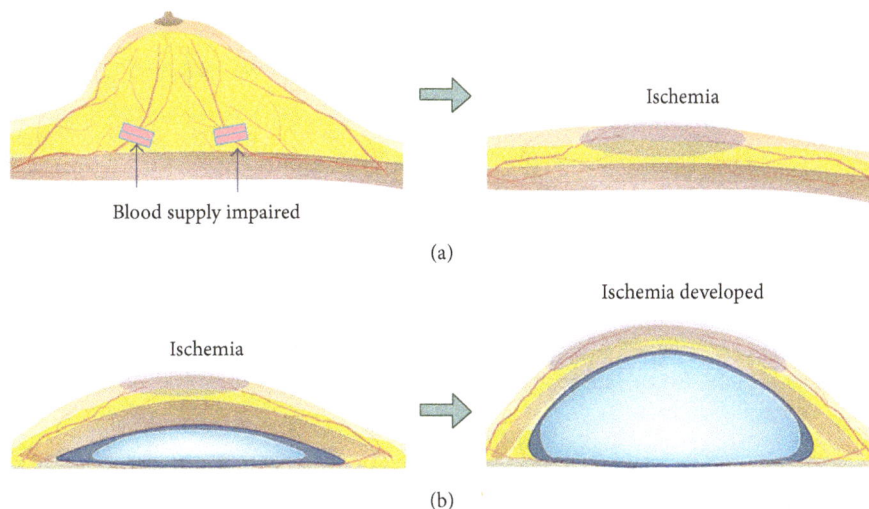

FIGURE 5: (a) Mastectomy impairs blood supply from the thoracic wall to the breast skin. (b) Embedment of an expander and expansion induces transient ischemia of the breast skin.

tamoxifen citrate, and two patients took anastrozole as supplemental medication for breast cancer. Review of the literature revealed no evidence of relationship between the intake of these drugs and the development of nummular eczema.

When foreign materials are placed in the human body, this induces an immunological response and provokes disorders, including skin lesions. This condition is called human adjuvant disease [19]. Since silicone implants are foreign to the human body, it is possible that the nummular eczema in our cases was a symptom of human adjuvant disease, which causes abnormal granulation to develop at sites where foreign material contacts the body. However, none of our patients developed such granulation. With human adjuvant disease, skin lesions do not heal as long as the foreign material remains in the human body. However, all our patients healed with application of steroid ointments, without removing the silicone implants. Hence, it seems unlikely that nummular eczema in our cases was caused by immunological response.

We speculate that nummular eczema was induced not by the intrinsic factors discussed above, but by structural change of the skin due to previous surgeries. When mastectomy is conducted, the skin of the breast region is impaired by two mechanisms. First, operative maneuvers damage the skin. Mastectomy is performed through a short incision for cosmetic reasons. When surgical approach is conducted through a short incision, the incision margin is strongly compressed with retractors to expose the operative field, damaging the skin at the margin of the incision. Second, the blood supply to the breast skin is reduced as a result of mastectomy. Usually, blood supply to the breast skin is provided through two routes. With the first route, the blood supply comes from regions surrounding the breast through vessels of the subdermal fat layer; with the second route, the blood supply comes from the thoracic wall through the mammary gland (Figure 5, top left). The second pathway is impaired by the removal of the mammary gland. Accordingly, ischemia occurs on the breast skin (Figure 5, top right).

Previously, we have conducted histopathological research regarding the effects on the breast skin of radiation for the treatment of breast cancer [20]. This study revealed that radiation induces hyperplasia of the epidermis, flattening of the papillary layer, atrophy of the dermal appendages, high density of dermal collagen fibers, and unidirectional alignment of dermal collagen fibers. On the other hand, the study also demonstrated that atrophy of dermal appendages, high density of dermal collagen fibers, and unidirectional alignment of dermal collagen fibers can also develop with the breast skin even when radiation is not used. Namely, whether radiated or not, skin of the breast region is damaged after mastectomy. It is speculated that the damage is caused by the reduction of blood supply induced by the two mechanisms described above.

Besides damage by the mastectomy, temporary ischemia due to subsequent expansion of the skin may be a causative factor for nummular eczema. Ischemia deteriorates the function of the sebaceous glands, making it difficult for the skin to retain its moisture. Hence, the skin becomes susceptible to mechanical stimulation caused by friction with underwear or clothes, increasing the risk of developing nummular eczema. Viewed this way, it is hypothesized that the thickness of the subdermal fat can also be an influential factor for the development of nummular eczema. In patients whose subdermal fat layers are thin, the blood supply to the breast skin may be significantly reduced as expansion proceeds. On the other hand, in patients who have thick fat layers, the blood supply to the skin is less likely to be reduced by skin expansion, because the thick subdermal layer functions as a shock absorber. The patients included in the present study were all Japanese females. Since fat layers are thinner in Asian patients than in Caucasian patients, it is possible that the occurrence ratio of nummular eczema is higher in the present study than it would be for other ethnicities. It is desirable that the influence of the patients' ethnicity be elucidated in future studies.

With all patients in our series, nummular eczema was successfully cured with the application of steroid ointments.

Infection of the embedded materials and skin necrosis are well known as major complications of breast reconstruction with tissue expanders and silicone implants. Nummular eczema might appear minor compared to these complications. However, patients with breast cancer are often nervous because of their uneasiness about the disease [21, 22]. Furthermore, an extended period—as long as six months—may be required for nummular eczema to heal in some patients (Table 2). Hence, even though nummular eczema does not directly lead to failure of the treatment, occurrence of this complication can negatively affect the relationship between the patient and physician. Breast surgeons and plastic surgeons should recognize nummular eczema as a potential complication of breast reconstruction—which we name Iwahira's eczema—and take measures to prevent its occurrence. For the prevention of nummular eczema, constant skin care with regular cleansing and moisturizers is recommended [23].

5. Conclusion

Nummular eczema can develop during breast reconstruction using tissue expanders and silicone implants. It is speculated that this dermatologic complication is induced by the deterioration of the sebaceous glands' functioning due to the change of the skin structure caused by surgical intervention. Breast surgeons and plastic surgeons should recognize nummular eczema as a potential complication of breast reconstruction using artificial materials.

References

[1] C. DeSantis, J. Ma, L. Bryan, and A. Jemal, "Breast cancer statistics, 2013," *CA—Cancer Journal for Clinicians*, vol. 64, no. 1, pp. 52–62, 2014.

[2] B. Kotti, "Optimizing the pedicled rectus abdominis flap: revised designs and vascular classification for safer procedures," *Aesthetic Plastic Surgery*, vol. 38, no. 2, pp. 387–394, 2014.

[3] A. Lindegren, M. Halle, A.-C. Docherty Skogh, and A. Edsander-Nord, "Postmastectomy breast reconstruction in the irradiated breast: a comparative study of DIEP and latissimus dorsi flap outcome," *Plastic and Reconstructive Surgery*, vol. 130, no. 1, pp. 10–18, 2012.

[4] G. T. Farias-Eisner, K. Small, A. Swistel, U. Ozerdem, and M. Talmor, "Immediate implant breast reconstruction with acellular dermal matrix for treatment of a large recurrent malignant phyllodes tumor," *Aesthetic Plastic Surgery*, vol. 38, no. 2, pp. 373–378, 2014.

[5] I. C. C. King, J. R. Harvey, and P. Bhaskar, "One-stage breast reconstruction using the inferior dermal flap, implant, and free nipple graft," *Aesthetic Plastic Surgery*, vol. 38, no. 2, pp. 358–364, 2014.

[6] B. Atiyeh, E. Zgheib, and P. Sadigh, "One-staged silicone implant breast reconstruction following bilateral nipple-sparing

[7] prophylactic mastectomy in patients at high risk for breast cancer," *Aesthetic Plastic Surgery*, vol. 37, no. 5, pp. 1063–1065, 2013.

[7] M. A. Cowan, "Nummular eczema. A review, follow-up and analysis of a series of 325 cases," *Acta Dermato-Venereologica*, vol. 41, pp. 453–460, 1961.

[8] L. Hellgren and H. Mobacken, "Nummular eczema—clinical and statistical data," *Acta Dermato Venereologica*, vol. 49, no. 2, pp. 189–196, 1969.

[9] M. G. Devergie, *Traité pratique des maladies de la peau*, V. Masson, Paris, France, 2nd edition, 1857.

[10] D. Bonamonte, C. Foti, M. Vestita, L. D. Ranieri, and G. Angelini, "Nummular eczema and contact allergy: a retrospective study," *Dermatitis*, vol. 23, no. 4, pp. 153–157, 2012.

[11] T. G. Rollins, "From xerosis to nummular dermatitis: the dehydration dermatosis," *The Journal of the American Medical Association*, vol. 206, no. 3, p. 637, 1968.

[12] P. D. Shenefelt, "Hypnosis in dermatology," *Archives of Dermatology*, vol. 136, no. 3, pp. 393–399, 2000.

[13] B. J. Bendl, "Nummular eczema of statis origin. The backbone of a morphologic pattern of diverse etiology," *International Journal of Dermatology*, vol. 18, no. 2, pp. 129–135, 1979.

[14] R. D. Carr, M. Berke, and S. W. Becker, "Incidence of atopy in the general population," *Archives of Dermatology*, vol. 89, pp. 27–32, 1964.

[15] M. M. Moore, D. J. Elpern, and D. J. Carter, "Severe, generalized nummular eczema secondary to interferon alfa-2b plus ribavirin combination therapy in a patient with chronic hepatitis C virus infection," *Archives of Dermatology*, vol. 140, no. 2, pp. 215–217, 2004.

[16] Y. Shen, J. Pielop, and S. Hsu, "Generalized nummular eczema secondary to peginterferon alfa-2b and ribavirin combination therapy for hepatitis C infection," *Archives of Dermatology*, vol. 141, no. 1, pp. 102–103, 2005.

[17] K. Dalberg, H. Hellborg, and F. Wärnberg, "Paget's disease of the nipple in a population based cohort," *Breast Cancer Research and Treatment*, vol. 111, no. 2, pp. 313–319, 2008.

[18] K. Eyerich, L. Cifaldi, L. D. Notarangelo et al., "Chronic eczema in a patient with Leukocyte Adhesion Deficiency (LAD) type I," *European Journal of Dermatology*, vol. 19, no. 1, pp. 78–79, 2009.

[19] K. Suzuki, M. Aoki, S. Takezaki et al., "A case of human adjuvant's disease with various symptoms simulating collagen diseases," *Journal of Nippon Medical School*, vol. 70, no. 3, pp. 283–287, 2003.

[20] Y. Iwahira, T. Nagase, G. Nakagami, L. Huang, Y. Ohta, and H. Sanada, "Histopathological comparisons of irradiated and non-irradiated breast skin from the same individuals," *Journal of Plastic, Reconstructive and Aesthetic Surgery*, vol. 65, no. 11, pp. 1496–1505, 2012.

[21] J. P. Fox, E. J. Philip, C. P. Gross, R. A. Desai, B. Killelea, and M. M. Desai, "Associations between mental health and surgical outcomes among women undergoing mastectomy for cancer," *Breast Journal*, vol. 19, no. 3, pp. 276–284, 2013.

[22] Y. Eltahir, L. L. C. H. Werners, M. M. Dreise et al., "Quality-of-life outcomes between mastectomy alone and breast reconstruction: comparison of patient-reported BREAST-Q and other health-related quality-of-life measures," *Plastic and Reconstructive Surgery*, vol. 132, no. 2, pp. 201e–209e, 2013.

[23] A. B. Gutman, A. M. Kligman, J. Sciacca, and W. D. James, "Soak and smear: a standard technique revisited," *Archives of Dermatology*, vol. 141, no. 12, pp. 1556–1559, 2005.

4

Aesthetic Surgery Training during Residency in the United States: A Comparison of the Integrated, Combined, and Independent Training Models

Arash Momeni,[1] Rebecca Y. Kim,[2] Derrick C. Wan,[1] Ali Izadpanah,[3] and Gordon K. Lee[1]

[1] Division of Plastic and Reconstructive Surgery, Stanford University Medical Center, 770 Welch Road, Suite 700, Palo Alto, CA 94305-5715, USA
[2] Division of General Surgery, Stanford University Medical Center, Stanford, CA 94305, USA
[3] Division of Plastic and Reconstructive Surgery, McGill University Health Centre, Montreal, Canada

Correspondence should be addressed to Arash Momeni; amomeni@stanford.edu

Academic Editor: Nicolo Scuderi

Background. Three educational models for plastic surgery training exist in the United States, the integrated, combined, and independent model. The present study is a comparative analysis of aesthetic surgery training, to assess whether one model is particularly suitable to provide for high-quality training in aesthetic surgery. *Methods.* An 18-item online survey was developed to assess residents' perceptions regarding the quality of training in aesthetic surgery in the US. The survey had three distinct sections: demographic information, current state of aesthetic surgery training, and residents' perception regarding the quality of aesthetic surgery training. *Results.* A total of 86 senior plastic surgery residents completed the survey. Twenty-three, 24, and 39 residents were in integrated, combined, and independent residency programs, respectively. No statistically significant differences were seen with respect to number of aesthetic surgery procedures performed, additional training received in minimal-invasive cosmetic procedures, median level of confidence with index cosmetic surgery procedures, or perceived quality of aesthetic surgery training. Facial aesthetic procedures were felt to be the most challenging procedures. Exposure to minimally invasive aesthetic procedures was limited. *Conclusion.* While the educational experience in aesthetic surgery appears to be similar, weaknesses still exist with respect to training in minimally invasive/nonsurgical aesthetic procedures.

1. Introduction

The American Board of Plastic Surgery currently approves two educational models for plastic surgery, the integrated and independent model [1]. As defined by the Board, residents in the former complete all training within the same training program, whereas residents in the independent model complete the prerequisite training outside of the plastic surgery residency process. A third model, the combined or coordinated model, represents a program in which residents complete the prerequisite general surgery training in the same institution as, but not within, the plastic surgery program [1]. While the integrated model was initially regarded as an experimental model of surgical training, the challenges of an ever increasing complexity of plastic surgery have resulted in

acknowledgment that more time should be spent in plastic surgery, thus resulting in an increasing popularity of the integrated model [2–4].

Advances in plastic surgery are seen not only in reconstructive but also in aesthetic surgery. In particular, minimally invasive/nonsurgical aesthetic procedures are in high demand, with a 231 percent increase from 1997 to 2009 [5]. Over 10 million minimally invasive aesthetic surgery procedures were performed in 2011 alone [6]. The challenges of mastering the expanding scope of aesthetic surgery upon graduation have resulted in an appreciation amongst leaders in the field that more emphasis should be placed on aesthetic surgery during residency training [7]. Despite the intuitive superiority of the integrated model, debate exists as to the ideal model for training of future plastic surgeons.

Previous studies by Morrison et al. and Oni et al shed light on the status of aesthetic surgery training among plastic surgery residents in the United States [5, 8]. However, no prior study has performed a head-to-head comparison of the training experience within the three existing plastic surgery training models. The present study represents a comparative analysis of aesthetic surgery training within these three training models to assess whether one model is superior in providing high-quality training in aesthetic surgery.

2. Methods

An online survey (SurveyMonkey, Menlo Park, CA) was developed to assess the quality of training in aesthetic surgery among plastic surgery residents in the United States. Content validity of the survey was determined by group consensus of the authors. Every question was critically assessed to minimize misinterpretation and ambiguity [9].

The 18-item survey had three distinct sections:

(1) demographic information (postgraduate year- (PGY-) level, type of training program (integrated, combined, and independent), and gender);

(2) current status of aesthetic surgery training, such as presence of a dedicated aesthetic surgery rotation, length of aesthetic surgery rotation (when offered), availability of resident aesthetic surgery clinics, number of aesthetic surgery procedures performed as primary surgeon, and predicted number of cosmetic surgery cases performed by the end of residency training;

(3) respondents' perception regarding the quality of aesthetic surgery training, such as areas in which further time should be spent to improve skills, level of confidence with different procedures, minimum number of cases that need to be performed to feel confident/competent, and need for additional training in aesthetic surgery (fellowship).

The survey focused on the following procedures: breast augmentation, rhinoplasty, blepharoplasty, liposuction, abdominoplasty, facelift, mastopexy, brachioplasty, and breast reduction [9, 10]. An additional focus was assessing the status of clinical training in the most commonly performed minimally invasive/nonsurgical cosmetic procedures. These included skin care, botulinum toxin A, soft-tissue fillers, chemical peel, and laser treatment. Data were collected via multiple-choice questions, Likert scale selections, "yes-no" answers, fill-in-the-blank questions, and areas for open-ended written comments [9].

Residency program coordinators were contacted in March 2011 and were asked to assist in distributing the survey via email. Data collection was completed in June 2011. Only completed surveys were included in the final analysis. Only plastic surgery residents were contacted, whereas program directors were intentionally not included in the study as it has been demonstrated that significant differences exist among these two groups with respect to the perceived quality of training, with a trend to overestimate the quality of training by program directors [8]. As such, we were mostly interested in the perceptions and opinions of plastic surgery residents.

Only the responses of senior residents (PGY-4 and above) were used for final analysis. A comparative analysis of residents in integrated, combined, and independent programs was performed.

3. Statistical Analysis

Final data analysis was performed in STATA 9.0 (STATA Corporation, College Station, TX, 2006). Exploratory analyses of continuous data included histograms, means, and standard deviations for normally distributed data and medians and interquartile ranges for nonnormally distributed data. Normality of the continuous variables was confirmed with the Shapiro-Wilk test using a critical P value of 0.05. For categorical data, tables were generated showing frequencies and percentages.

Bivariate analyses were conducted to assess the association between two variables. For the comparison of categorical versus continuous variables, Kruskal-Wallis test measured for differences in medians. n-by-n tables were generated to test for associations between categorical variables with the chi-squared test or Fisher's exact test.

4. Results

A total of 86 senior plastic surgery residents completed the survey. Of the respondents, 76.7 percent were male ($N = 66$) and 23.2 percent were female ($N = 20$). Twenty-three, 24, and 39 residents were in integrated, combined, and independent residency programs, respectively. The proportion of female residents was 26.1 percent ($N = 6$), 33.3 percent ($N = 8$), and 15.4 percent ($N = 6$) in integrated, combined, and independent programs, respectively ($P = 0.24$).

The majority of residents in integrated ($N = 15$; 65.2 percent) and independent ($N = 29$; 59 percent) programs reported having a dedicated aesthetic surgery rotation in contrast to 45.8 percent ($N = 11$) of residents in combined programs ($P = 0.38$). The median length of this rotation (when offered) was 4 months, 3 months, and 3 months in integrated, combined, and independent programs, respectively ($P = 0.07$). The majority of residents in integrated ($N = 16$; 69.6 percent), combined ($N = 20$; 83.3 percent), and independent ($N = 32$; 82.1 percent) programs reported that formal training in aesthetic surgery was incorporated in other rotations as well ($P = 0.44$). A statistically significant difference was seen with respect to the presence of resident cosmetic surgery clinics. Almost half of all residents in integrated ($N = 11$; 47.8 percent) and independent ($N = 19$; 48.7 percent) programs reported to have such a training opportunity in contrast to the majority of residents in combined programs ($N = 20$; 83.3 percent) ($P = 0.01$).

Although the majority of plastic surgery residents in combined programs ($N = 15$; 62.5 percent) reported to have performed more than 20 aesthetic surgery cases as the primary surgeon at the time of the survey compared to 34.8

percent and 41 percent for the integrated and independent programs, respectively ($P = 0.21$), the predicted number of aesthetic surgery cases performed upon completion of training was fairly similar among the three training models ($P = 0.98$) (Table 1).

Given the rise of minimally invasive/nonsurgical cosmetic procedures [5, 8], one focus of the present study was to assess how well senior residents were trained in these areas and whether differences existed among the various training models. No statistically significant differences were observed within the categories analyzed. The majority of residents in integrated, combined, and independent programs indicated to have additional training in administration of botulinum toxin A and use of fillers (Table 2).

As an indirect marker of quality of training, senior residents were asked to rate their level of confidence with each procedure using a Likert scale (1: not confident, 5: very confident). The highest median values were achieved for breast reduction and abdominoplasty with lowest values for rhinoplasty (Table 3). These findings were furthermore confirmed after subgroup analysis of residents who reported to be "confident" and "very confident" with the respective procedures (Table 4). Of note, the only statistically significant difference among the study groups was seen for "breast augmentation" with a significantly higher number of residents in combined programs reporting to be "confident" or "very confident" with this procedure ($P = 0.05$).

When offered the opportunity to spend more time to improve skills in any given area, "rhinoplasty" was the procedure chosen by the majority of senior residents (more than 87 percent). Interestingly, of the areas where additional training was desired 3 of the top 5 areas were nonsurgical, that is, skin care, chemical peels, and laser resurfacing. Senior residents in combined programs were significantly less likely to spend additional time in "breast augmentation" when compared to residents in integrated and independent programs ($P = 0.03$) (Table 5). This finding supports the previous finding; namely, residents in combined programs were significantly more likely to feel "confident" or "very confident" with this procedure.

Table 6 displays residents' opinion regarding the minimum number of aesthetic surgery cases required to achieve competency. No significant differences were seen among study groups. In almost all categories, residents felt that more than 8 cases as primary surgeon were necessary to provide sufficient training to allow competent execution of the procedure upon graduation.

When asked to rate the quality of aesthetic surgery training on a scale of 1 to 5 (1: poor, 5: excellent), a value of >4 was reported by 11 (47.8 percent), 15 (62.5 percent), and 20 (51.3 percent) residents in integrated, combined, and independent programs, respectively ($P = 0.58$). About a third of residents in each training model reported to have an interest in a predominantly aesthetic surgery practice (integrated: $N = 7$ (30.4 percent); combined: $N = 7$ (29.2 percent); independent: $N = 12$ (30.8 percent)) ($P = 0.99$). Similarly, a third of residents felt that additional training in aesthetic surgery (i.e., fellowship) was necessary (integrated: $N = 8$

(34.8 percent); combined: $N = 8$ (33.3 percent); independent: $N = 12$ (30.8 percent)) ($P = 0.94$).

5. Discussion

Advances in plastic surgery and the increasing complexity of the specialty have triggered discussions regarding the ideal training model in order to meet the challenges of providing adequate training in plastic and, in particular, aesthetic surgery [11, 12]. Consensus seems to exist that improving the quality of aesthetic surgery training during residency is critical [13]. Leaders in the field have commented that only through improvement in the quality of training will plastic surgery as a specialty continue to prosper [7]. Undoubtedly, without high-quality training, plastic surgeons will face difficulties distinguishing themselves from competing specialties. Specialties such as otolaryngology already have demonstrated great interest in incorporating aesthetic surgery into their specialty [14]. Studies from Brazil, Italy, Germany, England, and Canada emphasize the importance of comprehensive training in aesthetic surgery to prepare plastic surgeons for the demands and challenges ahead [9, 15–17].

The present study can be regarded as a follow-up study to the work by Morrison et al. and Oni et al. with the addition of a comparative analysis to assess whether differences exist among the three existing training models in the United States: integrated, combined, and independent models [5, 8]. This is in contrast to the previous studies which did not differentiate between the various existing training models [8].

Similar to previous studies, the majority of residents in this study were male, without any notable difference among the three training models. Further similarities include the length of dedicated aesthetic surgery rotations (when offered), with a typical duration of 3 to 4 months [5, 8, 9].

It is encouraging to notice that the majority of residents confirmed that formal training in aesthetic surgery was incorporated in other rotations as well. This certainly reflects the awareness that aesthetic surgery assumes a significantly greater role in plastic surgery training than in years past [18].

The educational value of resident clinics and the importance of hands-on experience have been discussed and demonstrated [19–21]. In fact, such clinics have been considered a "compulsory component of any training program" [22]. Similar to previous studies, our results indicate that 58.1 percent of all respondents had access to resident clinics [5, 8]; however, subgroup analysis revealed that this was significantly more likely to be the case for residents in combined programs. The observation that a similar experience was reported with respect to case numbers and confidence levels with aesthetic surgery procedures may be explained by the fact that residents in integrated and independent programs, in return, were more likely to have a dedicated aesthetic surgery rotation. Although some authors have argued that the combined training model combines weaknesses of the other two, this notion could not be supported by the findings of this study [4, 23].

Based on the results of the present study, exposure to techniques of minimally invasive/nonsurgical aesthetic procedures is still rather limited amongst all residents surveyed.

TABLE 1: Number of aesthetic surgery cases as primary surgeon at the time of the survey versus upon completion of training.

	Number of aesthetic surgery cases as primary surgeon at the time of the survey						Number of aesthetic surgery cases as primary surgeon upon completion of training					
	None	1-10	11-15	16-20	>20	P value	None	1-10	11-15	16-20	>20	P value
Integrated (N = 23) (%)	1 (4.4)	9 (39.1)	3 (13.0)	2 (8.7)	8 (34.8)		0 (0.0)	1 (4.4)	2 (8.7)	1 (4.4)	19 (82.6)	
Combined (N = 24) (%)	1 (4.2)	5 (20.8)	3 (12.5)	0 (0.0)	15 (62.5)	0.21	0 (0.0)	2 (8.3)	3 (12.5)	0 (0.0)	19 (79.2)	0.98
Independent (N = 39) (%)	5 (12.8)	9 (23.1)	9 (23.1)	0 (0.0)	16 (41.0)		1 (2.6)	4 (10.3)	3 (7.7)	2 (5.1)	29 (74.4)	

TABLE 2: Number of senior plastic surgery residents with additional training in minimally invasive/nonsurgical cosmetic procedures.

	Integrated ($n = 23$)	Combined ($n = 24$)	Independent ($n = 39$)	P value
Skin care (%)	9 (39.1)	4 (16.7)	8 (20.5)	0.16
Chemical peels (%)	7 (30.4)	5 (20.8)	7 (18.0)	0.57
Laser resurfacing (%)	10 (43.5)	7 (29.2)	16 (41.0)	0.54
Botox (%)	15 (65.2)	20 (83.3)	29 (74.4)	0.39
Fillers (%)	13 (56.5)	20 (83.3)	23 (59.0)	0.08

TABLE 3: Median level of confidence with various aesthetic surgery procedures (1: not confident, 5: very confident).

	Integrated ($n = 23$)	Combined ($n = 24$)	Independent ($n = 39$)	P value
Face lift (range)	3 (1–4)	3 (1–4)	2 (1–3)	0.39
Blepharoplasty (range)	3 (3-4)	4 (2.5–4.5)	3 (2–4)	0.76
Rhinoplasty (range)	2 (1-2)	2 (1–3)	2 (1–3)	0.19
Breast augmentation (range)	4 (3–5)	4.5 (4–5)	4 (2–5)	0.16
Breast reduction (range)	5 (4-5)	5 (4-5)	5 (4-5)	0.73
Mastopexy (range)	4 (3–5)	4 (3–5)	4 (3-4)	0.16
Abdominoplasty (range)	5 (4-5)	5 (4-5)	5 (4-5)	0.32
Brachioplasty (range)	4 (3-4)	3 (3-4)	3 (2–4)	0.44
Liposuction (range)	4 (4-5)	4 (4-5)	4 (3–5)	0.45

TABLE 4: Proportion of residents feeling "confident" or "very confident" with the procedures of interest.

	Integrated ($n = 23$)	Combined ($n = 24$)	Independent ($n = 39$)	P value
Face lift (%)	6 (26.1)	10 (41.7)	7 (18.0)	0.12
Blepharoplasty (%)	10 (43.5)	13 (54.2)	19 (48.7)	0.76
Rhinoplasty (%)	0 (0.0)	4 (16.7)	4 (10.3)	0.15
Breast augmentation (%)	14 (60.9)	20 (83.3)	21 (53.9)	0.05
Breast reduction (%)	20 (87.0)	21 (87.5)	30 (76.9)	0.54
Mastopexy (%)	14 (60.9)	17 (70.8)	21 (53.9)	0.41
Abdominoplasty (%)	19 (82.6)	22 (91.7)	33 (84.6)	0.73
Brachioplasty (%)	12 (52.2)	11 (45.8)	15 (38.5)	0.57
Liposuction (%)	18 (78.3)	19 (79.2)	26 (66.7)	0.52

TABLE 5: Areas in which senior plastic surgery residents would spend more time to improve their skills.

	Integrated ($n = 23$)	Combined ($n = 24$)	Independent ($n = 39$)	P value
Face lift (%)	**16 (69.6)**	**17 (70.8)**	**31 (79.5)**	0.62
Blepharoplasty (%)	9 (39.1)	9 (37.5)	13 (33.3)	0.89
Rhinoplasty (%)	**20 (87.0)**	**21 (87.5)**	**34 (87.2)**	1.00
Breast augmentation (%)	6 (26.1)	1 (4.2)	12 (30.8)	0.03
Breast reduction (%)	3 (13.0)	1 (4.2)	4 (10.3)	0.58
Mastopexy (%)	7 (30.4)	2 (8.3)	11 (28.2)	0.11
Abdominoplasty (%)	4 (17.4)	2 (8.3)	4 (10.3)	0.63
Brachioplasty (%)	7 (30.4)	6 (25.0)	13 (33.3)	0.79
Liposuction (%)	5 (21.7)	3 (12.5)	8 (20.5)	0.73
Skin care (%)	**11 (47.8)**	**13 (54.2)**	**23 (59.0)**	0.70
Chemical peels (%)	**12 (52.2)**	**15 (62.5)**	**27 (69.2)**	0.41
Laser resurfacing (%)	**10 (43.5)**	**13 (54.2)**	**23 (59.0)**	0.51
Botulinum toxin A (%)	6 (26.1)	8 (33.3)	15 (38.5)	0.65
Fillers (%)	9 (39.1)	12 (50.0)	18 (46.2)	0.75

TABLE 6: Residents' opinion regarding the minimum number of cosmetic surgery procedures required as primary surgeon during residency training to achieve competency.

		1–3	4–7	8–10	>10	P value
Face lift	Integrated ($N = 23$) (%)	0 (0.0%)	5 (21.7%)	8 (34.8%)	10 (43.5%)	
	Combined ($N = 24$) (%)	0 (0.0%)	6 (25.0%)	6 (25.0%)	12 (50.0%)	0.48
	Independent ($N = 39$) (%)	2 (5.1%)	7 (17.9%)	18 (46.2%)	12 (30.8%)	
Blepharoplasty	Integrated ($N = 23$) (%)	0 (0.0%)	7 (30.4%)	9 (39.1%)	7 (30.4%)	
	Combined ($N = 24$) (%)	1 (4.2%)	7 (29.2%)	5 (20.8%)	11 (45.8%)	0.25
	Independent ($N = 39$) (%)	2 (5.1%)	3 (7.7%)	17 (43.6%)	7 (17.9%)	
Rhinoplasty	Integrated ($N = 23$) (%)	0 (0.0%)	4 (17.4%)	3 (13.0%)	16 (69.6%)	
	Combined ($N = 24$) (%)	0 (0.0%)	2 (8.3%)	6 (25.0%)	16 (66.7%)	0.58
	Independent ($N = 39$) (%)	2 (5.1%)	3 (7.7%)	11 (28.2%)	23 (59.0%)	
Breast augmentation	Integrated ($N = 23$) (%)	0 (0.0%)	5 (21.7%)	8 (34.8%)	10 (43.5%)	
	Combined ($N = 24$) (%)	2 (8.3%)	4 (16.7%)	9 (37.5%)	9 (37.5%)	0.28
	Independent ($N = 39$) (%)	2 (5.1%)	12 (30.8%)	18 (46.2%)	7 (17.9%)	
Breast reduction	Integrated ($N = 23$) (%)	1 (4.3%)	6 (26.1%)	6 (26.1%)	10 (43.5%)	
	Combined ($N = 24$) (%)	1 (4.2%)	3 (12.5%)	10 (41.7%)	10 (41.7%)	0.51
	Independent ($N = 39$) (%)	0 (0.0%)	9 (23.1%)	17 (43.6%)	13 (33.3%)	
Mastopexy	Integrated ($N = 23$) (%)	1 (4.3%)	5 (21.7%)	8 (34.8%)	9 (39.1%)	
	Combined ($N = 24$) (%)	1 (4.2%)	6 (25.0%)	5 (20.8%)	12 (50.0%)	0.46
	Independent ($N = 39$) (%)	1 (2.6%)	12 (30.8%)	16 (41.0%)	10 (25.6%)	
Abdominoplasty	Integrated ($N = 23$) (%)	1 (4.3%)	11 (47.8%)	6 (26.1%)	5 (21.7%)	
	Combined ($N = 24$) (%)	2 (8.3%)	8 (33.3%)	8 (33.3%)	6 (25.0%)	0.78
	Independent ($N = 39$) (%)	3 (7.7%)	15 (38.5%)	16 (41.0%)	5 (12.8%)	
Brachioplasty	Integrated ($N = 23$) (%)	1 (4.3%)	10 (43.5%)	7 (30.4%)	5 (21.7%)	
	Combined ($N = 24$) (%)	2 (8.3%)	7 (29.2%)	10 (41.7%)	5 (20.8%)	0.78
	Independent ($N = 39$) (%)	5 (12.8%)	17 (43.6%)	12 (30.8%)	5 (12.8%)	
Liposuction	Integrated ($N = 23$) (%)	1 (4.3%)	12 (52.2%)	4 (17.4%)	6 (26.1%)	
	Combined ($N = 24$) (%)	4 (16.7%)	6 (25.0%)	8 (33.3%)	6 (25.0%)	0.13
	Independent ($N = 39$) (%)	3 (7.7%)	16 (41.0%)	16 (41.0%)	4 (10.3%)	

This is, furthermore, evidenced by the fact that of the areas where additional training was desired 3 of the top 5 areas were nonsurgical (i.e., skin care, chemical peels, and laser resurfacing). Notable exceptions are techniques in administration of botulinum toxin A and use of fillers. As such, although Oni et al. report on "increasing levels of resident confidence...in nonsurgical procedures," it appears that further improvement is warranted [5]. Interestingly, although minimally invasive/nonsurgical aesthetic procedures demonstrate the sector with the most rapid increase in demand, studies with focus on aesthetic surgery training frequently do not comment on this sector [15, 17, 20]. An increasing awareness and understanding that these techniques must be mastered by graduating plastic surgery residents is critical, as lack of familiarity with these techniques results in a substantial disadvantage after graduation.

More than half of all responders reported that they perceived their training in aesthetic surgery as either "very good" or "excellent." No significant differences were seen between residents in the different training models analyzed. The present study does, however, represent the first comparative analysis of the various training models leading to board certification in the United States. No objective (presence of dedicated aesthetic surgery rotations, number of aesthetic surgery cases performed, etc.) or subjective (level of confidence with aesthetic surgery procedures, perceived need for additional training, etc.) differences were seen among residents in integrated, combined, or independent programs. One may conclude that, at least with respect to aesthetic surgery training, an equivalent training experience seems to be provided. Any interpretation beyond this, however, is unsubstantiated. The results of this study should by no means be interpreted as proof that the quality of plastic surgery residency training is similar for the various training models.

6. Conclusion

The importance of aesthetic surgery training during residency has been recognized. The educational experience in aesthetic surgery among residents in integrated, combined, and independent residency programs is similar. Weaknesses still exist mainly with respect to training in minimally invasive/nonsurgical aesthetic procedures.

References

[1] The American Board of Plastic Surgery, https://www.abplsurg.org.

[2] L. Guo, J. Friend, E. Kim, S. Lipsitz, D. P. Orgill, and J. Pribaz, "Comparison of quantitative educational metrics between integrated and independent plastic surgery residents," *Plastic and Reconstructive Surgery*, vol. 122, no. 3, pp. 972–978, 2008.

[3] R. A. Chase, "The Stanford integrated plastic surgery program—history and philosophy," *Annals of Plastic Surgery*, vol. 7, no. 2, pp. 97–98, 1981.

[4] E. A. Luce, "Integrated training in plastic surgery: concept, implementation, benefits, and liabilities," *Plastic and Reconstructive Surgery*, vol. 95, no. 1, pp. 119–123, 1995.

[5] G. Oni, J. Ahmad, J. E. Zins, and J. M. Kenkel, "Cosmetic surgery training in plastic surgery residency programs in the United States: How have we progressed in the last three years?" *Aesthetic Surgery Journal*, vol. 31, no. 4, pp. 445–455, 2011.

[6] ASPS, "Plastic Surgery Procedural Statistics," 2011, http://www.plasticsurgery.org/news/plastic-surgery-statistics/2011-plastic-surgery-statistics.html.

[7] R. J. Rohrich, "The importance of cosmetic plastic surgery education: an evolution," *Plastic and Reconstructive Surgery*, vol. 105, no. 2, pp. 741–742, 2000.

[8] C. M. Morrison, S. C. Rotemberg, A. Moreira-Gonzalez, and J. E. Zins, "A survey of cosmetic surgery training in plastic surgery programs in the United States," *Plastic and Reconstructive Surgery*, vol. 122, no. 5, pp. 1570–1578, 2008.

[9] A. Momeni, S. M. Goerke, H. Bannasch, A. Arkudas, and G. B. Stark, "The quality of aesthetic surgery training in plastic surgery residency—a survey among residents in Germany," *Annals of Plastic Surgery*, vol. 70, no. 6, pp. 704–708, 2013.

[10] ASPS, "Plastic Surgery Statistics," 2010, http://www.plastic-surgery.org/news/plastic-surgery-statistics.html.

[11] A. Freiberg, "Challenges in developing resident training in aesthetic surgery," *Annals of Plastic Surgery*, vol. 22, no. 3, pp. 184–187, 1989.

[12] J. W. May Jr., "Aesthetic surgery 101: resident education in aesthetic surgery, the MGH experience," *Annals of Plastic Surgery*, vol. 50, no. 6, pp. 561–566, 2003.

[13] L. M. Krieger and W. W. Shaw, "The financial environment of aesthetic surgery: results of a survey of plastic surgeons," *Plastic and Reconstructive Surgery*, vol. 104, no. 7, pp. 2305–2311, 1999.

[14] S. A. T. Van Pinxteren, P. J. F. M. Lohuis, K. J. A. O. Ingels, and G. J. Nolst Trenité, "Interest in facial plastic and reconstructive surgery among otorhinolaryngologists: a survey in the Netherlands," *Archives of Facial Plastic Surgery*, vol. 7, no. 2, pp. 138–142, 2005.

[15] A. Sterodimas, F. Boriani, P. Bogetti, H. N. Radwanski, S. Bruschi, and I. Pitanguy, "Junior plastic surgeon's confidence in aesthetic surgery practice: a comparison of two didactic systems," *Journal of Plastic, Reconstructive & Aesthetic Surgery*, vol. 63, no. 8, pp. 1335–1337, 2010.

[16] A. Sterodimas, H. N. Radwanski, and I. Pitanguy, "Aesthetic plastic surgery: junior plastic surgeons' confidence in a training program," *Aesthetic Plastic Surgery*, vol. 33, no. 1, pp. 131–132, 2009.

[17] I. S. Whitaker, L. Mason, D. E. Boyce, and M. A. C. S. Cooper, "An analysis of 1361 aesthetic procedures from 2000 to 2005 in a large regional plastic surgery unit: implications for cosmetic surgery training," *Journal of Plastic, Reconstructive and Aesthetic Surgery*, vol. 60, no. 4, pp. 437–439, 2007.

[18] J. A. Persing, "Residency training in plastic surgery: a survey of educational goals. Discussion," *Plastic and Reconstructive Surgery*, vol. 112, no. 3, p. 730, 2003.

[19] K. C. Neaman, B. C. Hill, B. Ebner, and R. D. Ford, "Plastic surgery chief resident clinics: the current state of affairs," *Plastic and Reconstructive Surgery*, vol. 126, no. 2, pp. 626–633, 2010.

[20] M. Cueva-Galárraga, L. Cárdenas-Camarena, M. Boquín, J. A. Robles-Cervantes, and J. Guerrerosantos, "Aesthetic plastic surgery training at the jalisco plastic and reconstructive surgery institute: a 20-year review," *Plastic and Reconstructive Surgery*, vol. 127, no. 3, pp. 1346–1351, 2011.

[21] J. W. Pyle, J. O. Angobaldo, A. K. Bryant, M. W. Marks, and L. R. David, "Outcomes analysis of a resident cosmetic clinic: safety and feasibility after 7 years," *Annals of Plastic Surgery*, vol. 64, no. 3, pp. 270–274, 2010.

[22] A. T. Nguyen and J. E. Janis, "Discussion: Plastic surgery chief resident clinics: the current state of affairs," *Plastic and Reconstructive Surgery*, vol. 126, no. 2, pp. 634–635, 2010.

[23] E. A. Luce, "Comparison of quantitative educational metrics between integrated and independent plastic surgery residents," *Plastic and Reconstructive Surgery*, vol. 122, no. 3, pp. 979–981, 2008.

5

Philtral Columns and Nostril Shapes in Nigerian Children: A Morphometric and Aesthetic Analysis

Ibrahim Abdulrasheed and Asuku Malachy Eneye

Division of Plastic Surgery, Department of Surgery, Ahmadu Bello University Teaching Hospital, P.O. Box 06, Shika, Kaduna State, Zaria 810001, Nigeria

Correspondence should be addressed to Ibrahim Abdulrasheed; shidoibrahim@yahoo.com

Academic Editor: Francesco Carinci

Background. The upper lip-nose complex contributes significantly to the concept of symmetry and proportion of the face. A study of the morphology and aesthetic preferences of the lip-nose complex will provide a database that will serve as a guide for reconstruction. *Subjects and Methods.* Hundred Nigerian children participated in this study. Demographic data and standard photographs of the philtral column and nostrils were obtained. Sixty volunteers were recruited to evaluate the photographs. Each volunteer was asked to rank the photographs based on their aesthetic preference. *Results.* The morphology of the philtral columns was classified into four groups: (1) triangular, (2) concave, (3) flat, and (4) parallel. The nostril shape was also classified into four groups: (1) triangular, (2) round, (3) teardrop, and (4) rectangular. In both genders, the triangular shape of philtral column was the most common. There are significant age differences in the aesthetic rankings of philtral columns and nostril shapes. *Conclusion.* Our study establishes the basal values for the morphometric and aesthetic parameters of the lip-nose complex of 5- and 6-year-old children in Nigeria. We hope our results and reconstructive surgery will intersect at a point to treat disfigurements of the philtrum and nostrils successfully.

1. Introduction

The human face is one of the most attractive parts of the body [1]. It is central to many aspects of social interaction and the visual perception of the face is influenced by a complex combination of various factors such as appearance, expression, and symmetry. Earlier reports [2, 3] have shown that there is a proportional relationship between symmetry and attractiveness, and symmetrical faces are generally perceived as more attractive.

The upper lip-nose complex is an important aesthetic facial unit. It contributes significantly to the concept of symmetry, harmony, and proportion of the face [1, 4]. The philtrum is the central unit of the upper lip and plays a key role in the appearance of the lip and nostril [5, 6]. It consists of the dimple, two philtral ridges, the tubercle, and the white roll between the two high points of Cupid's bow. The philtrum is especially prominent during conversation and facial expression [7]. During labial movement, a dimple

is formed, with accentuation of the philtral ridges [5]. The nose is located in the middle of the face and is the most defining feature. Thus, it naturally attracts the gaze of the onlooker [4, 8]. The shape of the nostril is a signature indicating the ethnicity, race, age, and sex [9]. Given its importance and ability to change the appearance of the face, asymmetry of the nostrils will affect overall facial appearance [2, 10]. It is, however, also well recognized that disfigurements of the philtral columns and nostrils from congenital and acquired deformities causes significant emotional distress. This is because any deformity of the face has always been considered as one of the least desirable handicaps [3, 11].

Research provides evidence that the study of the morphology of the Lip-nose complex at various ages serves as a guideline for reconstruction [12–15]. Corresponding studies in Nigeria are very scarce. Furthermore, popular views of aesthetics of the face continue to evolve as our communities become more diverse and as the media and popular culture increasingly influence our tastes. A thorough understanding of current societal preferences will help guide surgical planning for aesthetic surgery of the face [16]. The purpose of this study is thus twofold: (1) to establish the morphology of philtral columns and nostril shape in Nigerian children, and (2) to identify the aesthetic preferences of philtral column and nostril shape in Nigerian children.

2. Subjects and Method

2.1. Morphology of Philtral Column and Nostrils. Subjects included in this study were required to be 5 or 6 years of age and both parents to be of Nigerian heritage. There were 100 Nigerian children (54 males, 46 females). The boys were aged 6 years (24 children) and 5 years (30 children) and the girls were aged 6 years (22 children) and 5 years (24 children). Other inclusion criteria included no history of craniofacial syndromes, major trauma, or previous plastic and reconstructive surgery of the face. We analyzed the shape of the philtral columns and nostrils and classified it into four groups. These groups are similar to those described by Mori et al. [13] Figure 1. Figure 1(a) triangular type: the origins of the philtral column are located near both sides of the medial crural footplates. The philtral dimple is approximately triangular. Figure 1(b) parallel type: the philtral columns originate from the nostril sills and exhibit an almost parallel shape with a prominent dimple along the upper lip. Figure 1(c) concave type: the philtral columns begin in the lower half of the upper lip and the dimple is emphasized. There is no philtrum dimple in the upper half of the upper lip. Figure 1(d) flat type: the philtral columns have almost no prominence with a vaguely delineated dimple. The nostril shapes were classified into four groups: Figure 2(a) round type, Figure 2(b) rectangular type, Figure 2(c) teardrop type, and Figure 2(d) triangular type (Figure 2).

Statistical evaluation of data was performed on SPSS 17.0 (SPSS Inc., Chicago, IL) statistical package program for Windows. Age and sex differences were evaluated using t-test and $P < 0.05$ was considered to be statistically significant.

2.2. Aesthetic Preferences of Philtral Column and Nostril Shape. Photographs of the philtral columns and nostril shape were obtained by the primary author (A.I.). Photographs were taken with a Canon IXUS 130 digital camera, 14.1 megapixels. (Canon United Kingdom). We took pictures of the philtrum and the upper lip in frontal view. The children had their head bent back, vertically exposing the nostrils. From this position, photographs of the nostril shape were obtained. We selected four photographs each, of the shape of the philtral columns and nostrils (Figures 3 and 4). The photographs were then placed onto two PowerPoint slides for viewing. We subsequently recruited 60 volunteers (30 professionals and 30 laypersons) to evaluate the photographs. The professionals consisted of consultant plastic surgeons, surgery residents, and nurses. The laypersons included members of the office staff of the department of surgery, friends, and relatives of patients at the surgical outpatient department. Each volunteer was asked to rank the photographs of the shape of the philtral column and nostril shape based on their aesthetic preference.

They were directed to rate each on a scale from 1 to 5, with 1 representing "very unattractive" and 5 as "very attractive."

On the basis of age, volunteers were divided into 2 groups: 35 years or older and younger than 35 years. Using Mann-Whitney tests, statistical comparisons based on volunteer age, sex, and profession were completed. $P < 0.05$ was considered as statistically significant.

3. Results

3.1. Morphology of Philtral Column and Nostrils. In both genders, the triangular type was the most common, and the parallel type was the second most common. The distribution of participants into groups regarding sex was not significantly different in the triangular group compared with the parallel, concave, and flat groups ($P = 0.207$). The result of the classification of the shape of the philtral column is shown in Table 1.

The teardrop-shaped nostrils were more common than the other types (Table 2). Triangular shaped nostril was the commonest in male while the teardrop shaped nostril was the commonest in females. This distribution was, however, not statistically significant, $P = 0.690$.

3.2. Aesthetic Preferences of Philtral Column and Nostril Shape. The professionals ranked the flat and parallel philtral columns higher while the laypersons scored the triangular and concave philtral columns more favorably. However, these differences are not statistically significant (Table 3). The distinction in the rankings between female and male volunteers was also less clear. Compared with females, males prefer the parallel and triangular shaped philtral column, whereas females ranked the flat and concave philtral shaped columns higher. This trend was also not statistically significant. The only statistically significant ranking was based on volunteer age, with volunteers less than 35 years preferring the concave shaped philtral column.

For nostril shape, the mean scores the professionals were slightly higher than the laypersons (Table 4). The mean scores for the professionals ranged 28.25–35.35 while the mean scores for the laypersons ranged 25.65–32.75. The aesthetic ranking of the triangular shaped nostril was statistically significant. $P = 0.025$ between the two groups. Comparisons of rating scores between male and female volunteers revealed higher mean scores by females (Females 30.56–31.08 versus Males 29.88–30.43). This distribution did not show a statistically significant difference. When comparing the aesthetic ratings of volunteers less than 35 years and those older than 35 years, the mean scores in the triangular and round shaped nostrils were statistically significant ($P = 0.015$ and $P = 0.025$).

4. Discussion

Objective evaluation of the face is based on measurements, proportions, and shapes. A great body of work in facial anthropometry is that of Farkas, who established a database of norms that are well accepted as linear, angular, and surface

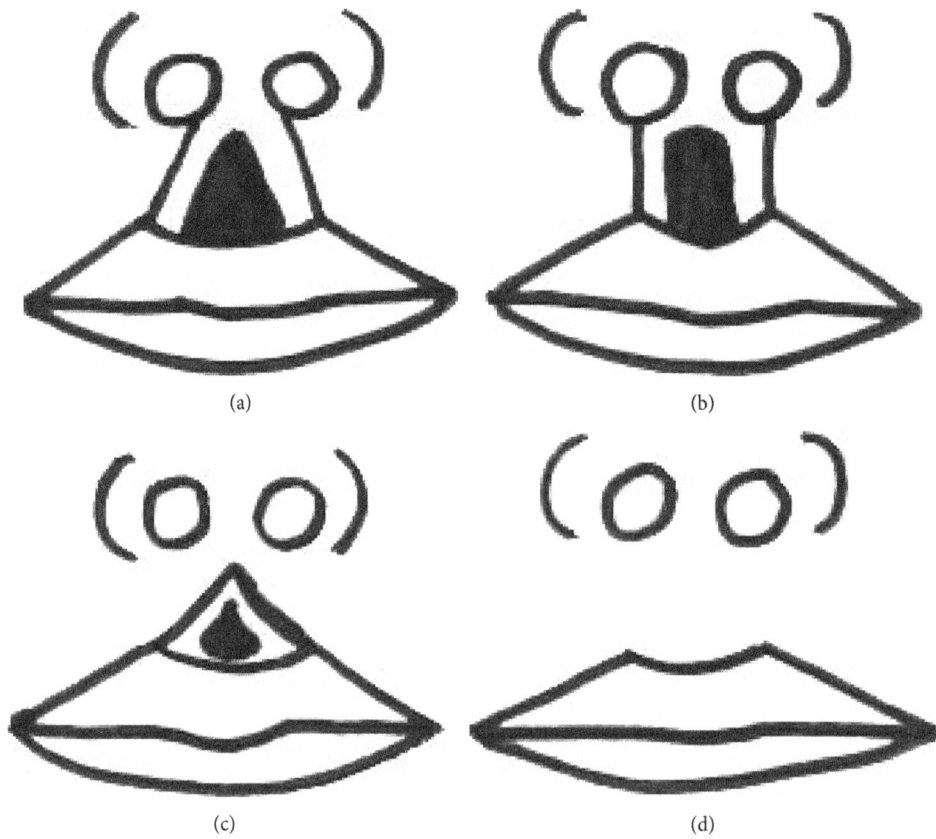

FIGURE 1: Diagram of philtral shape classification, Mori et al. [13]. (a) Triangular type, (b) parallel type, (c) concave type, and (d) flat type.

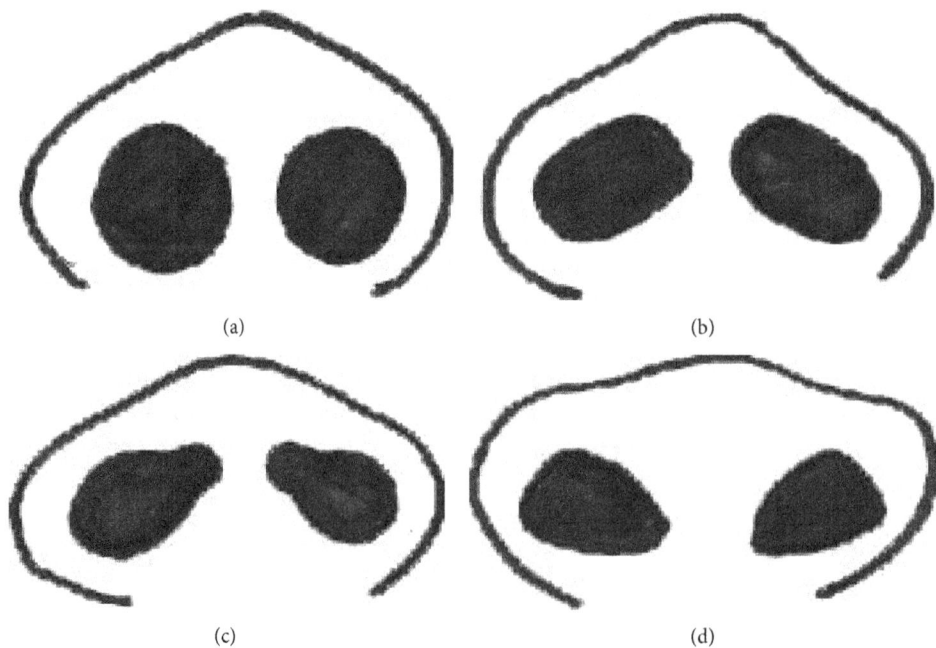

FIGURE 2: Diagram of nostril shape classification. (a) Round type, (b) rectangular type, (c) teardrop type, and (d) Triangular type.

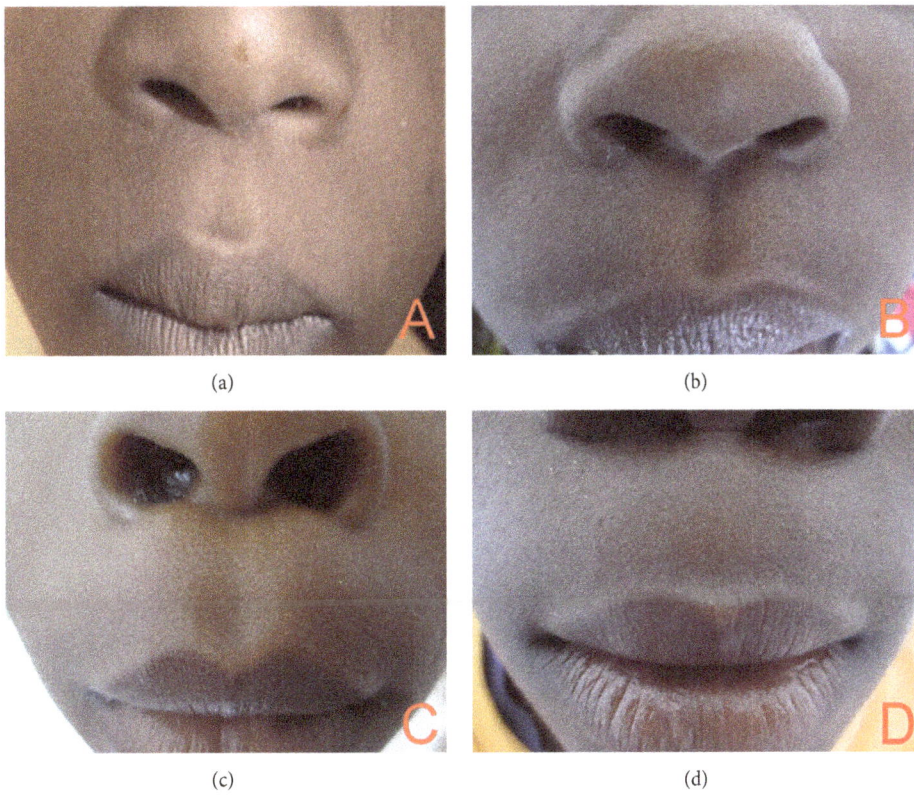

(a)

(b)

(c)

(d)

FIGURE 3: Pictures of philtral shape classification [13]. (a) Triangular type, (b) parallel type, (c) concave type, and (d) flat type.

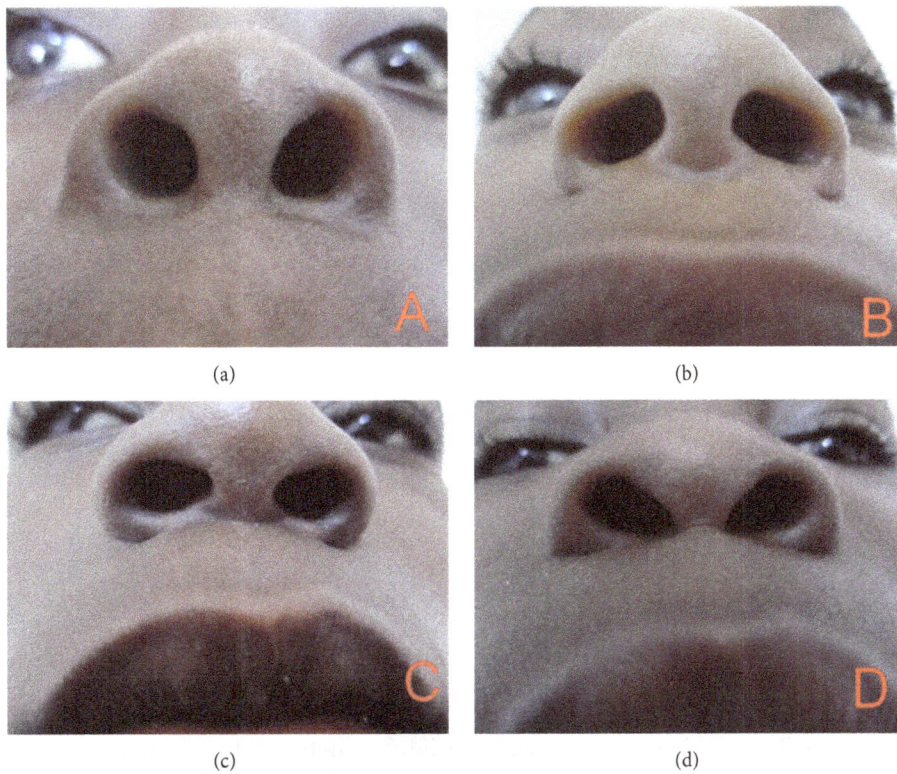

(a)

(b)

(c)

(d)

FIGURE 4: Pictures of nostril shape classification. (a) Round type, (b) rectangular type, (c) teardrop type, and (d) triangular type.

TABLE 1: The distribution of participants related to their sex and shape of philtral column.

Shape of philtrum	Total	Male		Female	
	N	N	%	N	%
Parallel	19	8	42.1	11	57.9
Triangular	55	34	61.8	21	38.2
Concave	12	4	33.3	8	66.7
Flat	14	8	57.1	6	42.9
Total	100	54		46	100

TABLE 2: The distribution of participants related to their sex and shape of the nostrils.

Shape of nostril	Total	Male		Female	
	N	N	%	N	%
Triangular	39	23	59	16	41
Round	13	7	53.8	6	46.2
Teardrop	42	22	52.4	20	47.6
Rectangular	6	2	33.3	4	66.7
Total	100	54		46	

contour reference values [9, 17]. Other reference values are from 2D cephalometric and photographic assessments [13, 18–21]. More recently, the laser scanning technique, the contact-type 3-dimensional measurement technique using facial plaster models, and the measurement technique using 3-dimensional computed tomography are considered to be able to 3-dimensionally measure the complicated shape of the face and to produce images on a computer screen [13, 20, 22].

The analysis obtained in this study was based on two-dimensional basal views and photographs of the philtral columns and the nostrils because they were economical, convenient, and noninvasive. Photographs were chosen to assess aesthetic preferences because they were proven to be reliable in previous studies [23, 24]. The strengths and limitations of photographic assessments must be appreciated. It is sensitive to the angle from which the photograph is taken and the position of the head. Because photographs are taken from varying distances with lenses of different focal lengths, the magnification of the final image is unknown. Therefore, it is unsuitable for absolute measurements, unless standardized procedures are followed to ensure a consistent, known magnification. However, it is ideally suited to the evaluation of proportions and shapes, as the magnification factor is eliminated [15].

The morphology of the philtral columns was classified into four types for Japanese children by Mori et al. in 2005 [13]. Amongst Nigerian children, in both genders, the triangular type was the most common, and the parallel type was the second most common. This contrasts the findings in Japanese children where the parallel type was the most common in both genders, and the triangular type was the second most common [13]. This corroborates the distinct differences in facial morphology further emphasizing the need for separate standards for facial analysis.

The characteristics and differences of the shapes of the nostrils have been studied in several racial groups [13–15, 18, 21, 25, 26]. Among the classifications of nostrils, Farkas' classification divides the shape of nostrils by the angle between the right and left long nostril axes [25]. We used 4 main nostril forms based on Farkas' classification in an earlier report [15] and replaced the heart shaped nostril with the rectangular shaped nostril in our classification. Our data was compared with Ofodile's data in African Americans [26], and the teardrop nostril was the commonest in both studies. However, the African American group also had a type III in females which accounted for 4%. The type III nostril shape was not present in this study.

Although the trend in this study demonstrates that female volunteers prefer the concave philtrum and triangular shaped nostril compared with male volunteers, these differences were not statistically significant. Furthermore, no differences were seen between professionals and laypersons volunteers for philtral column shape. Although some volunteers in this study were friends and relatives of patients in the hospital, most were graduate school students, a factor which introduces bias based on advanced educational level and urban residence [16]. In this study, it was found that the nostril shapes had higher aesthetic scores compared to the philtral columns shape. Two explanations for this finding are possible. First, the subjects were asked to not smile for an accurate assessment of philtral column shape. Rating pleasant, smiling lips may have resulted in higher aesthetic scores; however, this would have come with a price of decreased accuracy in philtral column assessment with the introduction of teeth and altered labial proportions. Another reason is that perhaps the ratings on photographs that are cropped are generally not a skill familiar to the volunteers and it may influence the results [27]. The difference in rating demonstrates the variance in what is perceived as attractive. Aesthetic judgments are subjective and may vary over time. It is therefore difficult to measure. Clinicians should thus develop patient-centered treatment goals through awareness of the aesthetic preference of their society [28, 29]. The acknowledgment of this is increasingly important in the modern era because our society continues to become more heterogeneous [16].

4.1. Clinical Correlates. Cleft lip and palate is one of the most common deformities of the upper lip-nose subunit in Nigeria [30]. One of the major goals of surgery is to improve the aesthetic appearance of the face and thereby improve the patient's social acceptability [4, 19, 31, 32]. Unfortunately, the nature of the unilateral and bilateral cleft lip and nasal deformity makes the asymmetry difficult to correct completely [5, 6, 27, 33–36]. A considerable number of children following cleft lip/nose repair in our institution had triangular shaped nostrils while others had heart shaped nostrils. Heart shaped nostrils are conventionally considered to be a typical nostril shape following cleft lip surgeries [13]. We also observed that the reconstruction of the cleft lip deformity (unilateral and bilateral) using modification of Millard's rotation advancement technique resulted in a parallel shape philtral column. A key feature of humans

TABLE 3: Mean scores of philtral column shape preferences based on volunteer professional status, sex, and age.

Philtral column shape	Professional status		P value	Sex		P value	Age		P value
	P*	L*		M	F		<35	>35	
Flat	32.40	28.60	0.362	29.57	31.37	0.666	28.73	33.79	0.247
Parallel	32.67	28.33	0.320	31.76	29.32	0.577	27.73	35.64	0.083
Triangular	30.38	30.62	0.957	31.40	29.66	0.691	30.29	30.88	0.898
Concave	27.40	33.60	0.153	28.17	32.68	0.299	33.95	24.10	0.030

P*: professional; L*: layperson.

TABLE 4: Mean scores of nostril shape preferences based on volunteer professional status, sex, and age.

Nostril shape	Professional status		P value	Sex		P value	Age		P value
	P*	L*		M	F		<35	>35	
Triangular	35.35	25.65	0.025	29.88	31.08	0.782	26.64	37.67	0.015
Rectangular	30.38	30.62	0.956	30.43	30.56	0.975	30.13	31.19	0.809
Tear drop	30.48	30.52	0.994	30.22	30.76	0.902	31.08	29.43	0.718
Round	28.25	32.75	0.308	29.97	31.00	0.815	34.13	23.76	0.025

P*: professional; L*: layperson.

is bilateral symmetry and the human eye is sensitive to differences in the two sides of paired structures [36]. Strict observation of hard and fast rules should, however, not blind us to the subtle uncertainty expressed by Picasso "art is not the appreciation of a canon of beauty but what instinct and the brain can conceive of outside the canon" [37]. Cleft lip surgeons must thus continue to be perfectionists and be willing to work in fractions of millimeters for the best possible results [9, 38].

5. Conclusion

Reconstruction of the upper lip and nostrils requires a thoughtful combination of art and science. We have contributed towards the science by describing the morphology of the philtral columns and nostrils and the aesthetic preferences in Nigerian children. We found that the triangular shaped philtral column is the commonest in boys and girls. There are significant age differences in the aesthetic rankings of philtral columns and nostril shapes. However, the aesthetic preferences are similar for professional status and gender. We hope that the results of our study and reconstructive surgery will intersect at a point to treat disfigurements of the upper lip-nose subunit in Nigerian children successfully.

References

[1] M. G. Bozkir, P. Karakas, and Ö. Oguz, "Vertical and horizontal neoclassical facial canons in Turkish young adults," *Surgical and Radiologic Anatomy*, vol. 26, no. 3, pp. 212–219, 2004.

[2] R. S. Gosla, V. Devarakonda, and R. R. Reddy, "Assessment of nostril symmetry after primary cleft rhinoplasty in patients with complete unilateral cleft lip and palate," *Journal of Cranio-Maxillofacial Surgery*, vol. 41, pp. 147–152, 2013.

[3] V. P. Sharma, H. Bella, M. M. Cadier, R. W. Pigott, T. E. E. Goodacre, and B. M. Richard, "Outcomes in facial aesthetics in cleft lip and palate surgery: a systematic review," *Journal of Plastic, Reconstructive & Aesthetic Surgery*, vol. 65, pp. 1233–1245, 2012.

[4] X. He, B. Shi, M. Kamdar, Q. Zheng, S. Li, and Y. Wang, "Development of a method for rating nasal appearance after cleft lip repair," *Journal of Plastic, Reconstructive and Aesthetic Surgery*, vol. 62, no. 11, pp. 1437–1441, 2009.

[5] B. C. Cho and B. S. Baik, "Formation of philtral column using vertical interdigitation of orbicularis oris muscle flaps in secondary cleft lip," *Plastic and Reconstructive Surgery*, vol. 106, no. 5, pp. 980–986, 2000.

[6] S. W. Kim, M. Oh, J. L. Park, A. K. Oh, and C. G. Park, "Functional reconstruction of the philtral ridge and dimple in the repaired cleft lip," *Journal of Craniofacial Surgery*, vol. 18, no. 6, pp. 1343–1348, 2007.

[7] N. Kishi, S. Tanaka, S. Iida, and M. Kogo, "The morphological features and developmental changes of the philtral dimple: a guide to surgical intervention in cases of cleft lip," *Journal of Cranio-Maxillofacial Surgery*, vol. 40, no. 3, pp. 215–222, 2012.

[8] S. O. P. Hofer and M. A. M. Mureau, "Improving outcomes in aesthetic facial reconstruction," *Perioperative Nursing Clinics*, vol. 6, no. 2, pp. 147–158, 2011.

[9] I. Ercan, A. Etoz, I. Guney et al., "Statistical shape analysis of nose in Turkish young adults," *Journal of Craniofacial Surgery*, vol. 18, no. 1, pp. 219–224, 2007.

[10] P. N. Broer, S. Buonocore, A. Morillas et al., "Nasal aesthetics: a cross-cultural analysis," *Plastic and Reconstructive Surgery*, vol. 130, pp. 843e–850e, 2012.

[11] F. Vegter and J. J. Hage, "Clinical anthropometry and canons of the face in historical perspective," *Plastic and Reconstructive Surgery*, vol. 106, no. 5, pp. 1090–1096, 2000.

[12] J. P. Porter, "The average African American male face: an anthropometric analysis," *Archives of Facial Plastic Surgery*, vol. 6, no. 2, pp. 78–81, 2004.

[13] A. Mori, T. Nakajima, T. Kaneko, H. Sakuma, and Y. Aoki, "Analysis of 109 Japanese children's lip and nose shapes using 3-dimensional digitizer," *British Journal of Plastic Surgery*, vol. 58, no. 3, pp. 318–329, 2005.

[14] B. Khandekar, S. Srinivasan, N. Mokal, and M. R. Thatte, "Anthropometric analysis of lip-nose complex in Indian population," *Indian Journal of Plastic Surgery*, vol. 38, no. 2, pp. 128–131, 2005.

[15] B. Q. Etöz, A. Etöz, and I. Ercan, "Nasal shapes and related differences in nostril forms: a morphometric analysis in young adults," *Journal of Craniofacial Surgery*, vol. 19, no. 5, pp. 1402–1408, 2008.

[16] J. A. Biller and D. W. Kim, "A contemporary assessment of facial aesthetic preferences," *Archives of Facial Plastic Surgery*, vol. 11, no. 2, pp. 91–97, 2009.

[17] L. G. Farkas, T. A. Hreczko, and C. K. Deutsch, "Objective assessment of standard nostril types—a morphometric study," *Annals of Plastic Surgery*, vol. 11, no. 5, pp. 381–389, 1983.

[18] T. Yamada, Y. Mori, K. Minami, K. Mishima, and Y. Tsukamoto, "Three-dimensional analysis of facial morphology in normal Japanese children as control data for cleft surgery," *The Cleft Palate-Craniofacial Journal*, vol. 39, pp. 517–526, 2002.

[19] C.-S. Chang, Y. C. Por, E. J.-W. Liou, C.-J. Chang, P. K.-T. Chen, and M. S. Noordhoff, "Long-term comparison of four techniques for obtaining nasal symmetry in unilateral complete cleft lip patients: a single surgeon's experience," *Plastic and Reconstructive Surgery*, vol. 126, no. 4, pp. 1276–1284, 2010.

[20] K. A. Russell, S. D. Waldman, B. Tompson, and J. M. Lee, "Nasal morphology and shape parameters as predictors of nasal esthetics in individuals with complete unilateral cleft lip and palate," *The Cleft Palate-Craniofacial Journal*, vol. 38, pp. 476–485, 2001.

[21] N. Kishi, S. Tanaka, S. Iida, and M. Kogo, "Comprehensive evaluation of three-dimensional philtral morphology," *Journal of Craniofacial Surgery*, vol. 22, no. 5, pp. 1606–1611, 2011.

[22] T. Yamada, Y. Mori, K. Minami, K. Mishima, T. Sugahara, and M. Sakuda, "Computer aided three-dimensional analysis of nostril forms: application in normal and operated cleft lip patients," *Journal of Cranio-Maxillofacial Surgery*, vol. 27, no. 6, pp. 345–353, 1999.

[23] P. Nechala, J. Mahoney, and L. G. Farkas, "Digital two-dimensional photogrammetry: a comparison of three techniques of obtaining digital photographs," *Plastic and Reconstructive Surgery*, vol. 103, no. 7, pp. 1819–1825, 1999.

[24] V. F. Ferrario, C. Sforza, G. Serrao, V. Ciusa, and C. Dellavia, "Growth and aging of facial soft tissues: a computerized three-dimensional mesh diagram analysis," *Clinical Anatomy*, vol. 16, no. 5, pp. 420–433, 2003.

[25] T.-S. Hwang and H.-S. Kang, "Morphometry of nasal bases and nostrils in Koreans," *Annals of Anatomy*, vol. 185, no. 2, pp. 189–193, 2003.

[26] F. A. Ofodile, F. J. Bokhari, C. Ellis, and W. E. Matory Jr., "The black American nose," *Annals of Plastic Surgery*, vol. 31, no. 3, pp. 209–219, 1993.

[27] L.-J. Lo, F.-H. Wong, S. Mardini, Y.-R. Chen, and M. S. Noordhoff, "Assessment of bilateral cleft lip nose deformity: a comparison of results as judged by cleft surgeons and laypersons," *Plastic and Reconstructive Surgery*, vol. 110, no. 3, pp. 733–738, 2002.

[28] J. Kunjur, T. Sabesan, and V. Ilankovan, "Anthropometric analysis of eyebrows and eyelids: an inter-racial study," *British Journal of Oral and Maxillofacial Surgery*, vol. 44, no. 2, pp. 89–93, 2006.

[29] N. S. Park, J. H. Park, M. Bayome, S. S. Mo, Y. Kim, and Y. A. Kook, "An evaluation of preferred lip positions according to different age groups," *International Journal of Oral and Maxillofacial Surgery*, vol. 42, 5, pp. 637–642, 2012.

[30] O. Adetayo, R. Ford, and M. Martin, "Africa has unique and urgent barriers to cleft care: lessons from practitioners at the Pan-African Congress on Cleft Lip and Palate," *The Pan African Medical Journal*, vol. 12, article 15, 2012.

[31] S. Stal, R. H. Brown, S. Higuera et al., "Fifty years of the millard rotation-advancement: looking back and moving forward," *Plastic and Reconstructive Surgery*, vol. 123, no. 4, pp. 1364–1377, 2009.

[32] N. Chaithanyaa, K. K. Rai, H. R. Shivakumar, and A. Upasi, "Evaluation of the outcome of secondary rhinoplasty in cleft lip and palate patients," *Journal of Plastic, Reconstructive and Aesthetic Surgery*, vol. 64, no. 1, pp. 27–33, 2011.

[33] J. S. Garfinkle, T. W. King, B. H. Grayson, L. E. Brecht, and C. B. Cutting, "A 12-year anthropometric evaluation of the nose in bilateral cleft lip-cleft palate patients following nasoalveolar molding and cutting bilateral cleft lip and nose reconstruction," *Plastic and Reconstructive Surgery*, vol. 127, no. 4, pp. 1659–1667, 2011.

[34] D. M. Fisher, R. Tse, and J. R. Marcus, "Objective measurements for grading the primary unilateral cleft lip nasal deformity," *Plastic and Reconstructive Surgery*, vol. 122, no. 3, pp. 874–880, 2008.

[35] E. Christofides, A. Potgieter, and L. Chait, "A long term subjective and objective assessment of the scar in unilateral cleft lip repairs using the Millard technique without revisional surgery," *Journal of Plastic, Reconstructive and Aesthetic Surgery*, vol. 59, no. 4, pp. 380–386, 2006.

[36] M. F. Grasseschi, "Minimal scar repair of unilateral cleft lip," *Plastic and Reconstructive Surgery*, vol. 125, no. 2, pp. 620–628, 2010.

[37] L. Ousehal, L. Lazrak, I. Serrhini, and F. Elquars, "Evaluation of facial esthetics by a panel of professionals and a lay panel," *International Orthodontics*, vol. 9, no. 2, pp. 224–234, 2011.

[38] C. J. Boorer, D. C. Cho, V. S. Vijayasekaran, and D. M. Fisher, "Presurgical unilateral cleft lip anthropometrics: implications for the choice of repair technique," *Plastic and Reconstructive Surgery*, vol. 127, no. 2, pp. 774–780, 2011.

6

Strategy of Surgical Management of Peripheral Neuropathy Form of Diabetic Foot Syndrome in Ghana

W. M. Rdeini,[1] P. Agbenorku,[2] and V. A. Mitish[3]

[1] *Seventh Day Adventist Hospital, Kumasi, Ghana*
[2] *Kwame Nkrumah University of Science & Technology, Kumasi, Ghana*
[3] *Russian Peoples' Friendship University of Russia, Moscow, Russia*

Correspondence should be addressed to P. Agbenorku; pimagben@yahoo.com

Academic Editor: Nicolo Scuderi

Introduction. Foot disorders such as ulceration, infection, and gangrene which are often due to diabetes mellitus are some major causes of morbidity and high amputation. *Aim.* This study aims to use a group of methods for the management of diabetic foot ulcers (DFU) in order to salvage the lower limb so as to reduce the rate of high amputations of the lower extremity. *Materials and Methods.* A group of different advanced methods for the management of DFU such as sharp debridement of ulcers, application of vacuum therapy, and other forms of reconstructive plastic surgical procedures were used. Data collection was done at 3 different hospitals where the treatments were given. *Results.* Fifty-four patients with type 2 diabetes mellitus were enrolled in the current study: females $n = 37$ (68.51%) and males $n = 17$ (31.49%) with different stages of PEDIS classification. They underwent different methods of surgical management: debridement, vacuum therapy (some constructed from locally used materials), and skin grafting giving good and fast results. Only 4 had below knee amputations. *Conclusion.* Using advanced surgical wound management including reconstructive plastic surgical procedures, it was possible to reduce the rate of high amputations of the lower limb.

1. Introduction

Diabetes mellitus is a condition characterized by a high blood glucose level occurring from inability of the pancreas to produce enough insulin or cells stop responding to the insulin that is produced [1]. It is a chronic disease that causes serious health complications including renal (kidney) failure, heart disease, stroke, and blindness. Symptoms include frequent urination, lethargy, excessive thirst, and hunger. There are several types of DM but under this study, the patients were under the type 2 DM. Type 2 DM occurs most often in people who are overweight and who do not exercise. The consequences of uncontrolled and untreated type 2 DM, however, are just as serious as those for Type 1 [1]. People with diabetes are usually older at presentation, usually above 30 years of age [2] and they may present with acute or chronic complications. The risk of a diabetic patient developing a foot ulcer may be as high as 25% [3] and can lead to considerable morbidity, amputation, and mortality [4]. Common

etiologies are neuropathy, trauma, deformity, high plantar pressures, and peripheral arterial disease [5].

1.1. Epidemiology. For the past years globally, there has been an increase growth of the number of patients suffering from diabetes mellitus (DM) of which Ghana is no exception. From the data of the International Diabetic Federation in 2012, Ghana registered 354.02 per 1000 persons of 20–79 years amounting to about 3.16% of the population [6], but persons suffering from DM and not diagnosed range from ages 20 to 79 years which are 292.42 per 1000 persons, which form 2.61% population [6], out of which 12–15% of the patients have diabetic foot syndrome with ulcer defects [7, 8]. That figure is expected to double over the next decade. Over time many diabetic patients will develop the chronic complications such as retinopathy, nephropathy, peripheral neuropathy, and atherosclerotic vascular disease. Loss of a leg as a consequence of peripheral neuropathy or ischemia is from a patient's perspective one of the most feared of these complications is [9].

Diabetes is the most common medical condition leading to lower limb amputation and 85% of amputations are preceded by foot ulcers that fail to heal [3]. The main risks from diabetes are peripheral ischemia and neuropathy (both sensory and motor).

1.2. Aetiology of Diabetic Foot Problems. The main underlying risk factors for foot ulcers in diabetic patients are peripheral neuropathy and ischemia. For the purpose and scope of this research the emphasis would be highlighted on the neuropathy.

1.2.1. Neuropathy. Prevalence of distal lower limb neuropathy affecting both type 1 and type 2 DM patients ranging from 30% to 50% has been reported in epidemiologic studies, a reason why more than 60% of diabetic patient foot ulcers are primarily due to underlying neuropathy [5, 10, 11]. The distal neuropathy of diabetes affects all components of the nervous system: sensory, motor, and autonomic, each of which contributes to foot ulcer development. Loss of nerve function correlates with chronic hyperglycaemia, as reflected in the mean level of glycosylated haemoglobin over time [7]. Ischemia of the endoneurial microvascular circulation induced by metabolic abnormalities from hyperglycaemia is believed to be the underlying mechanism for nerve deterioration [8].

1.2.2. Motor Nerve Involvement. Imbalance of the long flexor and extensor tendons is caused by loss of neural supply to the intrinsic muscles of the foot. The classic high-arched foot and claw-toe deformity usually seen in about 50% of diabetics is induced by contraction of the more powerful flexors of the lower limb [12]. Hyperextension of the toes with resultant overriding of the metatarsal-phalangeal joints forces the metatarsal heads downward, thereby increasing their prominence further displacing the metatarsal fat pads distally, reducing the natural cushioning of the metatarsal heads. These mechanical changes increase plantar pressures inducing callus formation and underlying skin breakdown. Foot becomes wider and thicker; hence, patient's shoes no longer fit; this is caused by broadening of the foot from loss of the intrinsic muscles in combination with disruption of the normal bony relationships [13].

1.2.3. Autonomic Neuropathy. Autonomic dysfunction of the foot from diabetic neuropathy results in loss of sweat and oil gland function. Anhidrosis leads to dry, fissured skin susceptible to bacterial invasion. Furthermore, loss of peripheral sympathetic vascular tone in the lower limb increases distal arterial flow and pressure, which, by damaging the capillary basement membrane, might contribute to peripheral oedema [6, 13]. Oedema increases the risk of foot ulceration by adding another element of minor trauma caused by wearing shoes that fit even more poorly as the oedema increases.

1.2.4. Sensory Neuropathy. The concurrent loss of protective sensation in the foot is the cause of extensive motor and autonomic neural abnormalities [14]. Normally, if the foot developed a fissure or blister, or if bony structures change, patients would feel the discomfort and take appropriate corrective measures. Unfortunately, with onset of the peripheral neuropathy of diabetes, this protective response diminishes and can eventually disappear with progressive reduction in nerve function. This sequence of events allows patients to walk with apparent comfort on ever-deepening ulcers. The lack of pain lulls patients, and often physicians, into a false sense of security, a misguided "but it does not hurt; therefore it cannot be a serious problem" mentality [14].

1.3. Management. This involves testing ankle reflexes and vibration threshold, determining the degree of protective sensation, evaluating circulation, X-ray examinations, and bone scans for osteomyelitis [15]. Management includes good blood sugar control, avoiding pressure or trauma with good shoes or a special total contact cast, treating infection, improving circulation, and using topical therapy. Management of patients with ulcer defects in diabetic foot syndrome has been a serious problem in Ghana [6]. Different methods had been used including conventional methods. The late seeking for medical attention is as a result of early use of herbal preparations due to poverty and lack of education on the disease [16]. Sometimes bad judgment from the medical officer and the patients has also contributed to that effect. This nonsystemic management has led to high amputation of the lower limb for many of patients. For the past few years a lot of advanced methods were developed in the treatment of diabetic wounds [17–20]. Starting with the control of hyperglycemia, aggressive wound debridement, using vacuum therapy, using Versa jet system, and auto-skin grafting have contributed immensely to increase the effectiveness of management of diabetic wounds thereby avoiding the gross complications such as amputation in most cases. Some of the effective methods are expensive and not easily available for patients in Ghana including the wound vacuum system. In Ghana, a vacuum system locally manufactured which provides similar negative pressure wound therapy which is affordable has been developed [21].

1.4. Grading of DFU and Their Management. PEDIS is a method of classification of lesions in patients with diabetic foot syndrome. PEDIS stands for perfusion, extent (size), depth, infection, and sensation [22]. This is the classification used in this study.

2. Patients and Methods

2.1. Study Setting. The *Komfo Anokye Teaching Hospital (KATH)* located in Kumasi, the second largest in the country, is a tertiary health facility and a referral center serving persons in the Northern, Upper East and West, Brong Ahafo and Ashanti Regions. Currently the hospital has 1000 bed capacity. The hospital attends to about 679,050 annually consisting of in and out patients with a bed capacity of 1,000.

(a) Necrotic tissue

(b) After debridement

(c) Complete healing after vacuum wound pressure system and skin grafting

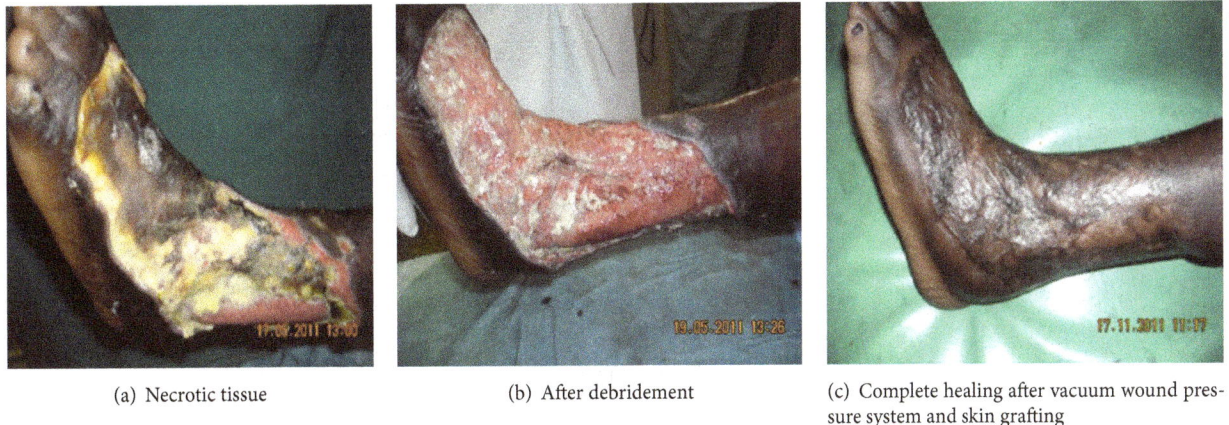

FIGURE 1: Example of PEDIS 2 DFU patients in the series.

Being a tertiary health facility, it is affiliated to the School of Medical Sciences (SMS) of Kwame Nkrumah University of Science and Technology (KNUST) [23].

The Seventh Day Adventist (SDA) Hospital is a district mission facility located in Kwadaso, a suburb of Kumasi. It was established in 1990 and has 84 patients' bed capacity [24].

Effiduase District Hospital is a district health facility in the Sekyere East District of the Ashanti Region; it was established in the 1950s to provide medical services to surrounding communities [25].

2.2. Data Collection. Data was collected based on patients' medical records at the three hospitals and the mode of treatment given to them by physicians and medical assistants. The work was based on the result of examinations and treatment of 54 patients with peripheral neuropathic form of diabetic foot syndrome (DFS) for the period January 1, 2011 till December 31, 2013.

2.3. Data Analysis. Data input was by MS excel and explained using qualitative analysis.

2.4. Ethical Clearance. Ethical clearance for this study was obtained from the KNUST School of Medical Sciences/KATH Committee on Human Research, Publication and Ethics, Kumasi.

2.5. Inclusion Criteria. Only patients who were diagnosed with type 2 diabetes were enrolled in the study.

2.6. Exclusion Criteria. Patients who had other types of diabetes mellitus were excluded from the study.

3. Results

3.1. Basic Data. In this series there were 54 DM patients: female $n = 37$ (68.5%), male $n = 17$ (31.5%); ages ranged 21–96 years; mean age = 54.9 years. The duration of DM from the day of diagnosis varied from few days to 26 years and the mean duration was 7.4 years. They were affected mostly on their feet and toes and other parts including the planter, dorsum, metatarsals, distal phalanges, and other parts below and above the ankle.

3.2. Categories of the DFU Patients and Their Management

3.2.1. PEDIS 1. This involves wound without inflammation or purulence. Patients are usually treated with topical antibiotics. There were no patients within this group during the study period.

3.2.2. PEDIS 2. There is purulence/erythema, pain, tenderness, and warmth/induration. There is cellulitis less than 2 cm around the ulcer and infection is limited to skin or subcutaneous tissue and usually not limb-threatening. This stage of diabetic ulcer included necrotizing inflammation, unhealed ulcers after amputation, gangrene, deep multiple chronic ulcers, leg cellulitis, wide deep necrotic ulcers, and septic wounds. Almost every patient had a multiple of these ulcerations. They were made up of 16 patients comprising 4 males and 12 females; their ages ranged 21–72 years living with their ulcers for at least 1 year and at most 15 years with a mean duration of 6.5 years. The ulcers were on their left or right foot, toes, and lateral and dorsal parts of their lower limbs. The ulcers were treated with debridement and excision of necrotic tissues and hyperkeratosis, wide excisions, and amputations of digits. All the patients were treated with povidone iodine daily dressings in combination with vaseline gauze and acetic acid dressings. Others also had daily foot baths. The wounds healed completely with 6 patients still under treatment (Table 1, Figure 1).

3.2.3. PEDIS 3. Infection, cellulitis greater than 2 cm, streaking, deep tissue abscess, gangrene (may be life-threatening in some), muscle, tendon, joint, and bone may be involved. Eleven (11) patients had this stage of ulcer comprising of 3 males and 8 females. They were characterized by gangrene, necrotic ulcers, cellulitis, and osteomyelitis. They were treated with debridement, amputation of some parts of the

TABLE 1: PEDIS 2 DFU patients in the series.

Age (years)	Duration of DM (years)	Operation
21	4	Debridement, fixing of vacuum wound pressure system, and skin grafting
42	15	Debridement of necrotic tissues several times, excision of hyperkeratosis
63	4	Debridement
49	6	Wide excision of phlegmon from dorsal and planter aspects of the right foot and excision of necrotic tissues
62	5	Amputation of 1st toe of the right foot
64	12	Debridement, fixing of vacuum wound pressure system
52	5	Debridement
72	2	Debridement, fixing of vacuum wound pressure system
64	15	Debridement
72	10	Debridement, incision and drainage of abscess
42	0 (newly diagnosed)	Wound debridement
28	1	Debridement
36	8	Debridement
53	3	Debridement, fixing of vacuum wound pressure system
Unknown	8	Debridement

TABLE 2: PEDIS 3 DFU patients in the series.

Age (years)	Duration of DM (years)	Operation
52	26	Debridement, amputation of 2nd toe
40	12	Debridement, amputation of 1st toe of right foot; debridement repeated 3 times, and skin grafting
62	20	Debridement, amputation of phalanges 2nd and 4th toes of left foot
43	10	Debridement amputation of 3rd and 4th toes, incision of phlegmon of the right foot, and dearticulation of 2nd toe of the right foot
45	13	Debridement, incision of phlegmon
56	10	Debridement
31	12	Debridement, sequestrectomy
57	21	Debridement, amputation of left 3rd toe
96	11	Dearticulation
54	15	Debridement, digital dearticulation of 1st big toe of the right foot
56	10	Debridement

foot, sequestrectomy, and dearticulation. Vacuum therapy and skin grafting were also done. Ulcers were managed with povidone iodine and normal saline daily dressings and metronidazole. One ulcer healed with contracture; four patients were still under treatment and the remaining 6 patients had their ulcers healing completely. The duration of patients' diagnosis of DM ranged from 10 to 26 years with a mean duration of 14.5 years; their ages ranged from 31 to 96 years. There was amputation involving the toes and metatarsal bones (Table 2, Figure 2).

3.2.4. PEDIS 4. Infection with systemic toxicity, chills, fever, tachycardia, vomiting, acidosis, hypotension, hyperglycemia, and confusion are usually life-threatening as infection is severe. This grade of DM ulcer was characterized with DFS gangrene, necrosis, and cellulitis and it affected the foot above the ankle and the toes; there were 3 males and 2 females; their

ages ranged 52–86 years. The duration of their DM ranged from 5 to 10 years with a mean duration of 4 years. Five patients were in this group and were treated by below knee amputations involving the tibia and fibula. Their ulcers were managed by daily dressing with povidone iodine and had no skin grafting. Four out of the 5 patients were discharged home with their amputated stumps well healed; one with ulcerated foot refused amputation and died a few days on admission (Table 3, Figure 3).

4. Discussion

The primary goal in the treatment of diabetic foot ulcers is to obtain wound closure. Presence of infection, severity, and vascularity determine the management of the foot ulcer [26, 27]. The first and most important procedure of ulcer therapy is debridement of all necrotic, callus and fibrous

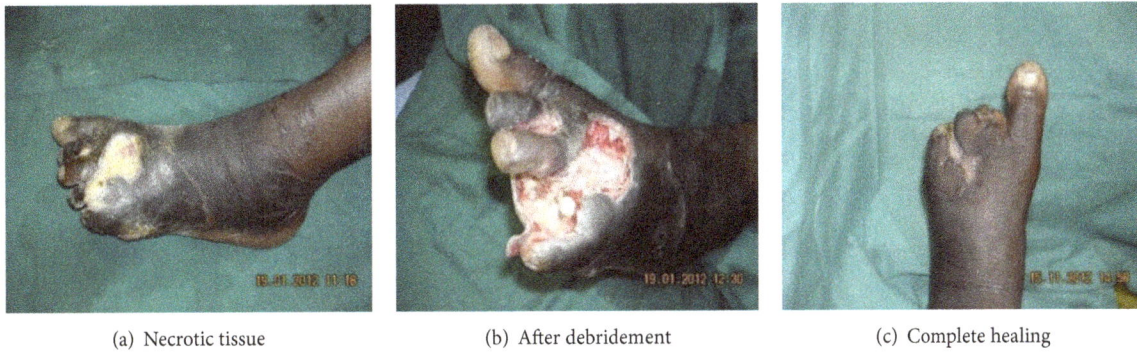

(a) Necrotic tissue   (b) After debridement   (c) Complete healing

FIGURE 2: Example of PEDIS 3 DFU patients in the series.

TABLE 3: PEDIS 4 DFU patients in the series.

Age (years)	Duration of DM (years)	Operation
75	0 (first diagnosed)	Debridement of dorsal and planter aspects of the right foot; patient refused amputation of necrotic toes; died a few days on admission
86	10	Below knee amputation
66	3	Below knee amputation
52	5	Below knee amputation
66	2	Below knee amputation

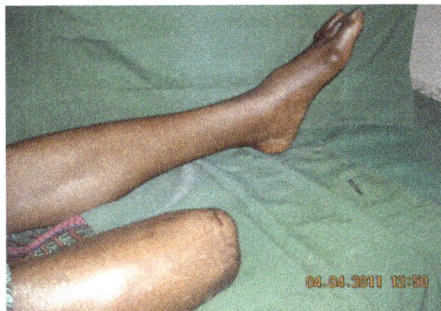

FIGURE 3: Example of PEDIS 4 DFU patients in the series: below knee amputation.

tissue [28–32] and this was applied to all degree of ulcers presented at the three hospitals. Unhealthy tissues of patients' ulcers were surgically debrided back to bleeding tissue to allow full visualization of the extent of the ulcer and detect underlying abscesses or sinuses. There was also excision of necrotic tissues and hyperkeratosis. It helped to reduce the rate of infection and provided an ideal healing environment by converting chronic wounds into acute; it also helped to reduce chronic inflammatory by-products as demonstrated by other authors in their studies [33–35].

Some researchers have reported toxification to healing of wounds by topical antiseptics such as povidone iodine [27, 29]; however in the current study povidone iodine was useful in wound dressing and facilitated healthy growth of ulcers in all patients.

Surgical drainage, deep debridement, or local partial foot amputations as done in some of the patients in the series are necessary adjuncts to antibiotic therapy of infections that are deep or limb-threatening; this was likewise proposed in some earlier studies by various authors [26, 36]. Hospitalization and surgical drainage becomes necessary when there is deep infection with abscess, cellulitis, gangrene, or osteomyelitis; foot infection and amputation as the major cause of hospitalization in diabetics have also been reported [37]. Also, in final healing of the foot ulcer especially in areas subject to exceedingly high plantar or shoe pressures, foot-sparing reconstructive procedures might be necessary [26, 38]. Antibiotics were subsequently tailored according to the clinical response of the patient and culture and sensitivity testing results. As in our current study, some other researches indicated that osteomyelitis is frequently present in patients with moderate to severe infections and requires aggressive bony incision of infected bone and joints followed by some weeks of culture-directed antibiotic therapy [38–41]. People with type 2 DM can control their condition with diet and oral medications. Insulin injections are sometimes necessary if treatment with diet and oral medication is not working [1]. Body exercise is also helpful [42].

Quality of life in patients with diabetic foot ulcers is low as the condition is related to comorbidity and in some cases fatalities [43, 44]. However, with the current study only one death was recorded as a result of patient's refusal to undergo surgery (amputation). Diabetic patients with foot ulcer compared to nondiabetics with foot ulcer have poor quality of life as well as survival rate [45]. However in the current study there was no such attempt to do any comparison with nondiabetic foot ulcers. Better management of patients could also be attained when there is proper grading of the patient, since it would help to determine the kind of treatment to be given out, since the likelihood of a patient to undergo surgery for amputation is highly dependent on the ulcer grade; thus, diabetic foot ulcers are complications of diabetes mellitus hence the earlier the detection implies avoidance of quick progression to the stage that may require amputation [46].

5. Conclusion

From the study, the use of advanced surgical wound management including reconstructive plastic surgical procedures made it possible to reduce the rate of amputations of the lower limb in patients. Early management of diabetic foot ulcers prevents complications which may require amputation of the affected person's limb as well as the quality of life.

Acknowledgments

The authors sincerely thank Miss Richcane Amankwa and Miss Juliet Afriyie both of Charis Missions International for helping to collect the data that formed the basis of this study; the authors are equally grateful to the several colleague doctors and the clinical nurses who helped in various ways in the management of these patients.

References

[1] Diabetes mellitus—medical dictionary—the free dictionary, hhttp://medical-dictionary.thefreedictionary.com/Diabetes+Mellitus.

[2] "Diabetes Mellitus," http://www.patient.co.uk/doctor/diabetes-mellitus.

[3] W. Clayton Jr. and T. A. Elasy, "A review of the pathophysiology, classification, and treatment of foot ulcers in diabetic patients," *Clinical Diabetes*, vol. 27, no. 2, pp. 52–58, 2009.

[4] E. H. Boyko, J. H. Ahroni, D. G. Smith et al., "Increased mortality associated with diabetic foot ulceration," *Diabetic Medicine*, vol. 13, pp. 967–972, 1996.

[5] R. G. Frykberg, "Diabetic foot ulcers: pathogenesis and management," *American Family Physician*, vol. 66, no. 9, pp. 1655–1662, 2002.

[6] International Diabetic Federation (IDF), *Diabetes Atlas*, 5th edition, 2012.

[7] G. R. Tennvall and J. Apelqvist, "Health-economic consequences of diabetic foot lesions," *Clinical Infectious Diseases*, vol. 39, no. 2, pp. S132–S139, 2004.

[8] J. B. Andrew, "The diabetic foot: a global view," *Diabetes/Metabolism Research and Reviews*, vol. 16, no. 1, pp. 2–5, 2000.

[9] H. I. Lippmann, "Must loss of limb be a consequence of diabetes mellitus?" *Diabetes Care*, vol. 2, no. 5, pp. 432–436, 1979.

[10] R. G. Frykberg, "Diabetic foot ulcers: current concepts," *Journal of Foot and Ankle Surgery*, vol. 37, no. 5, pp. 440–446, 1998.

[11] D. J. Margolis, L. Allen-Taylor, O. Hoffstad, and J. A. Berlin, "Diabetic neuropathic foot ulcers and amputation," *Wound Repair and Regeneration*, vol. 13, no. 3, pp. 230–236, 2005.

[12] L. C. Argenta, M. J. Morykwas, M. W. Marks, A. J. DeFranzo, J. A. Molnar, and L. R. David, "Vacuum-assisted closure: state of clinic art," *Plastic and Reconstructive Surgery*, vol. 117, no. 7, pp. 127–142, 2006.

[13] A. J. M. Boulton, R. S. Kirsner, and L. Vileikyte, "Neuropathic diabetic foot ulcers," *New England Journal of Medicine*, vol. 351, pp. 48–55, 2004.

[14] C. K. Bowering, "Diabetic foot ulcers: pathophysiology, assessment, and therapy," *Canadian Family Physician*, vol. 47, pp. 1007–1016, 2001.

[15] F. W. Wagner Jr., "The dysvascular foot: a system for diagnosis and treatment," *Foot and Ankle*, vol. 2, no. 2, pp. 64–122, 1981.

[16] J. Muha, "Local wound care in diabetic foot complications. Aggressive risk management and ulcer treatment to avoid amputation," *Postgraduate Medicine*, vol. 106, no. 1, pp. 97–102, 1999.

[17] L. P. Daronina, V. A. Mitish, and G. R. Galastyan, "Diabetes mellitus," *The Use of Hydro Surgical System Versa Jet in the Management of Diabetic Foot Syndrome*, vol. 3, no. 48, pp. 121–126, 2010.

[18] V. Jones, "Selecting a dressing for the diabetic foot: factors to consider," *Diabetic Foot*, vol. 1, pp. 48–52, 1998.

[19] A. M. Svetuchen, U. A. Amerslanof, and V. A. Mitish, "Reconstructive & plastic operations in septic surgery," in *Selection of Course Lectures in Septic Surgery*, pp. 64–76, 2007.

[20] B. M. Kostuchunok, Y. A. Kolkar, and V. A. Karalof, "Effect of vacuum in surgical treatment of septic wounds," *Sur News*, vol. 137, pp. 18–21.

[21] J. Yorke, J. Akpaloo, and P. Agbenorku, "Management of diabetic foot ulcers using negative pressure with locally available materials," *Modern Plastic Surgery*, vol. 3, pp. 84–88, 2013.

[22] PEDIS Classification, http://www.patient.co.uk/doctor/diabetes-mellitus.

[23] Komfo Anokye Teaching Hospital, http://www.kathhsp.org/aboutus1.php.

[24] Kwadaso Seventh-Day Adventist Hospital, http://www.adventistyearbook.org/default.aspx?page=ViewEntity&EntityID=20760.

[25] Sekyere East District, http://sekyereeast.ghanadistricts.gov.gh/?arrow=atd&_=25&sa=1082.

[26] R. G. Frykberg, D. G. Armstrong, J. Giurini et al., "Diabetic foot disorders: a clinical practice guideline. American College of Foot and Ankle Surgeons," *The Journal of Foot and Ankle Surgery*, vol. 39, supplement 5, pp. S1–S60, 2000.

[27] R. G. Frykberg, "Diabetic foot ulcerations," in *The High Risk Foot in Diabetes Mellitus*, R. G. Frykberg, Ed., pp. 151–95, Churchill Livingstone, New York, NY, USA, 1991.

[28] R. Kahn, "Consensus development conference on diabetic foot wound care: 7-8 April 1999, Boston, Massachusetts," *Diabetes Care*, vol. 22, no. 8, pp. 1354–1360, 1999.

[29] D. G. Armstrong and L. A. Lavery, "Diabetic foot ulcers: prevention, diagnosis and classification," *American Family Physician*, vol. 57, no. 6, pp. 1325–1332, 1998.

[30] R. Lewis, P. Whiting, G. ter Riet, S. O'Meara, and J. Glanville, "A rapid and systematic review of the clinical effectiveness and cost-effectiveness of debriding agents in treating surgical wounds healing by secondary intention," *Health Technology Assessment*, vol. 5, no. 14, pp. 1–131, 2001.

[31] D. G. Armstrong, L. A. Lavery, B. P. Nixon, and A. J. M. Boulton, "It's not what you put on, but what you take off: techniques for debriding and off-loading the diabetic foot wound," *Clinical Infectious Diseases*, vol. 39, no. 2, pp. S92–S99, 2004.

[32] D. L. Steed, "Debridement," *American Journal of Surgery*, vol. 187, no. 5, pp. 71S–74S, 2004.

[33] V. Falanga, "The chronic wound:impaired healing and solutions in the context of wound bed preparation," *Blood Cells, Molecules, and Diseases*, vol. 32, no. 1, pp. 88–94, 2004.

[34] B. C. Nwomeh, H. Liang, I. K. Cohen, and D. R. Yager, "MMP-8 is the predominant collagenase in healing wounds and nonhealing ulcers," *Journal of Surgical Research*, vol. 81, no. 2, pp. 189–195, 1999.

[35] E. B. Jude and A. A. Rogers, "Matrix metalloproteinase and tissue inhibitor of metalloproteinase expression in diabetic and venous ulcers," *Diabetologia*, vol. 44, supplement 1, article A3, 2001.

[36] M. Eneroth, J. Apelqvist, and A. Stenström, "Clinical characteristics and outcome in 223 diabetic patients with deep foot infections," *Foot and Ankle International*, vol. 18, no. 11, pp. 716–722, 1997.

[37] A. Yönem, B. Çakir, S. Güler, Ö. Azal, and A. Çorakçi, "Effects of granulocyte-colony stimulating factor in the treatment of diabetic foot infection," *Diabetes, Obesity and Metabolism*, vol. 3, no. 5, pp. 332–337, 2001.

[38] G. M. Caputo, P. R. Cavanagh, J. S. Ulbrecht, G. W. Gibbons, and A. W. Karchmer, "Current concepts: assessment and management of foot disease in patients with diabetes," *The New England Journal of Medicine*, vol. 331, no. 13, pp. 854–860, 1994.

[39] B. A. Lipsky, R. E. Pecoraro, and L. J. Wheat, "The diabetic foot. Soft tissue and bone infection," *Infectious disease clinics of North America*, vol. 4, no. 3, pp. 409–432, 1990.

[40] E. Caballero and R. G. Frykberg, "Diabetic foot infections," *Journal of Foot and Ankle Surgery*, vol. 37, no. 3, pp. 248–255, 1998.

[41] B. A. Lipsky, "Osteomyelitis of the foot in diabetic patients," *Clinical Infectious Diseases*, vol. 25, no. 6, pp. 1318–1326, 1997.

[42] L. J. Orozco, A. M. Buchleitner, G. Gimenez-Perez, M. Roqué I Figuls, B. Richter, and D. Mauricio, "Exercise or exercise and diet for preventing type 2 diabetes mellitus," *Cochrane Database of Systematic Reviews*, vol. 16, no. 3, p. CD003054, 2008.

[43] E. J. Boyko, J. H. Ahroni, D. G. Smith, and D. Davignon, "Increased mortality associated with diabetic foot ulcer," *Diabetic Medicine*, vol. 13, pp. 967–972, 1996.

[44] S. D. Ramsey, K. Newton, D. Blough et al., "Incidence, outcomes, and cost of foot ulcers in patients with diabetes," *Diabetes Care*, vol. 22, no. 3, pp. 382–387, 1999.

[45] O. Nelzen, D. Bergqvist, and A. Lindhagen, "Long-term prognosis for patients with chronic leg ulcers: a prospective cohort study," *European Journal of Vascular and Endovascular Surgery*, vol. 13, no. 5, pp. 500–508, 1997.

[46] S. O. O'Meara, N. Cullum, M. Majid, and T. Sheldon, "Systematic reviews of wound care management: (4) diabetic foot ulceration," *Health Technology Assessment*, vol. 4, no. 21, pp. 1–237, 2000.

7

Effects of Intense Pulsed Light on Tissue Vascularity and Wound Healing: A Study with Mouse Island Skin Flap Model

Trinh Cao Minh,[1] Do Xuan Hai,[1] and Pham Thi Ngoc[2]

[1]*Practical and Experimental Surgery Department, Vietnam Military Medical University (HVQY), K58, Hadong, Hanoi, Vietnam*
[2]*Veterinary Hygiene Department, National Institute of Veterinary Research (NIVR), Truong Chinh, Dong Da, Hanoi, Vietnam*

Correspondence should be addressed to Trinh Cao Minh; trinhcaominh@vmmu.edu.vn

Academic Editor: Nicolo Scuderi

Intense pulsed light (IPL) has been used extensively in aesthetic and cosmetic dermatology. To test whether IPL could change the tissue vascularity and improve wound healing, mice were separated into 4 groups. Mice in Group I were not treated with IPL, whereas, dorsal skins of mice in Groups II, III, and IV were treated with $35 \, \text{J/cm}^2$, $25 \, \text{J/cm}^2$, and $15 \, \text{J/cm}^2$ IPL, respectively. After 2 weeks, dorsal island skin flaps were raised, based on the left deep circumflex iliac vessels as pedicles; then, survival rate was assessed. Flaps in Group IV (treated with lowest dose of IPL) have a survival rate significantly higher than other groups. Counting blood vessels did not demonstrate any significant differences; however, vessel dilation was found in this group. The results show that IPL at the therapeutic doses which are usually applied to humans is harmful to mouse dorsal skin and did not enhance wound healing, whereas, IPL at much lower dose could improve wound healing. The possible mechanism is the dilation of tissue vasculature thanks to the electromagnetic character of IPL. Another mechanism could be the heat-shock protein production.

1. Introduction

Wound healing impairment is often encountered in surgery. There are many studies on this phenomenon, but many problems remain unknown and are subject to fierce debates.

To study wound healing, many research models have been developed [1]. In this study, the dorsal island skin flap model in the mouse has been used. This model has been pioneered by the author in the previous studies [2, 3]. The advantages and disadvantages of this model for wound healing study will be discussed along with relevant background information to help guide decision-making.

A wound is associated with the interruption of the blood supply (ischemia). The healing of a wound, besides many other mechanisms, is involved with the process of the resupply of blood (reperfusion). It is the decisive factor for healing.

Recently, it was found that electromagnetic radiation at low dose could improve the tissue perfusion of the irradiated tissue [4]. It has been known for long time that light can greatly affect the health. Light also has the character of the electromagnetic radiation. Therefore, it is reasonable to suggest that light might be able to affect the wound healing process.

Intense pulsed light (IPL) systems are high intensity pulsed sources that emit polychromatic light in a broad wavelength spectrum. The emitted broadband light is covering the spectrum from ultraviolet (UV) to infrared (IR). However, the most common systems emit radiations between 400 and 1,200 nm. When using IPL for cutaneous treatment, the reaction mechanism of the IPL sources is based on the principle of selective photothermolysis [5].

IPL devices are being used for a diverse range of treatments like photorejuvenation, for acne or cellulite and inflamed, and hypertrophic scars or keloids. It is safe and common that the novel, low-fluence, home-use IPL devices for hair removal have entered the consumer market [6].

IPL can make skin "stronger and younger," IPL has character of electromagnetic radiation, and IPL can induce heat-shock protein production [7]. Can IPL improve the wound healing in the skin? This study was carried out to check whether IPL could change the tissue vascularity and improve wound healing.

2. Materials and Methods

2.1. Animals. Adult, male, and ICR mice (30–40 gr) were acclimatized to their holding facility for at least 5 days before experimental manipulation. The animals were treated according to the Animal Regulations of the Vietnam Military Medical University published in 1989.

2.2. Experiment Protocol

2.2.1. Allocation of Animals. 160 mice were used and separated into 4 groups. Group I served as control. Two weeks before operation, dorsal skin of mice in Group II was treated with 35 J/cm^2 IPL, Group III with 25 J/cm^2, and Group IV with 15 J/cm^2.

40 mice (10 mice per group) were sacrificed for histological study; other 120 mice (30 mice per group) were used to create skin flaps.

2.2.2. Intense Pulsed Light (IPL) Treatment Parameters. Effect of IPL was investigated in 120 mice. Animals were randomly assigned to one of the 3 groups (Group II, Group III, and Group IV), 40 mice per group. Before receiving IPL treatment, mice were anesthetized with pentobarbital sodium (1 mg/mL), diluted 5 times with saline, and injected intraperitoneally (0.001 mg/gr). Dorsal hair was removed with electric clippers and depilatory cream. Dorsal skins were treated with a light emission apparatus of the Lumenis One IPL system with a Universal IPL handpiece in a single session. A 515 nm cut-off filter, triple pulse mode with pulse length of 5 ms and delay of 30 ms, was used for all treatment. However, mice in Group II, Group III, and Group IV were treated with different fluences of 35 J/cm^2, 25 J/cm^2, and 15 J/cm^2, respectively. The skin area was treated 3 times with 5-minute interval. During the procedure, chilled, colorless gel was used to aid in delivering the light uniformly onto the skin surface and to reduce the thermal effect of IPL. After IPL treatment, mice were observed daily for 2 weeks until the time of the skin flaps elevation.

2.2.3. Surgical Procedure and Flap Survival Assessment. 120 mice were used to create skin flaps. Among them, in Group I (control group), skin flaps were raised without IPL treatment, whereas in Group II, Group III, and Group IV, skin flaps were raised at the time of two weeks after IPL treatment.

Design and surgical technique for the elevation of the dorsal island skin flap in the mouse have been described in the author's previous studies [2, 3]. In brief, mice were anesthetized with pentobarbital sodium (1 mg/mL), diluted 5 times with saline, injected intraperitoneally (0.001 mg/gm), and supplemented as necessary. Dorsal hair was removed with electric clippers and depilatory cream. The entire dorsal island skin flap was elevated based on the left deep circumflex iliac vessels as pedicles (Figure 1(a)). Both halves of this flap

consisted of 2 adjacent vascular territories: the deep circumflex iliac artery and the lateral thoracic artery territories. If the vascular pattern deviated from the abovementioned pattern, the mouse was excluded from the study.

The flap was elevated from the cranial side to the caudal side. An operating microscope (Zeiss, Germany) was used for dissecting out the vascular pedicles. Flaps were then resutured in position using interrupted 6/0 nylon sutures.

Flap survival and necrosis were determined at the 6th postoperative day by the method described previously [8]. In brief, both outer and inner sides of the flap were checked. Skin necrosis was defined grossly by typical signs of tissue injury on the outer side: black color, dehydration, and eschar formation, and on the inner side, no vasculature (Figure 1(b)).

The total area of the flaps and the survival area were traced on clear acetate sheets and scanned as digital images. The digital images were analyzed using Adobe Photoshop CS3 Extended software (Adobe Systems, Inc., San Jose, CA) to calculate the percentage of the survival area. Measurements were performed twice, and mean values were used for statistical analysis. The survival rate was expressed as the percentage of the surviving area to the total skin flap area.

2.3. Histological Study. 40 mice of 4 groups (10 mice per group) were sacrificed for histological study. The skin samples were taken as 7×7 mm biopsies from the center of dorsal skin of mice in Group I (control group). The same was done with mice in Group II, Group III, and Group IV, but at the time of 2 weeks after IPL treatment.

Skin biopsies were stained with hematoxylin and eosin. Blood vessels were counted in histological sections by the method described elsewhere [9]. Blood vessels were evaluated in light microscopy at 200x magnification. Number of vessel was counted in five fields of each section. Results are presented as mean number of vessel per field ± SD. At the same time, vessel diameter was measured with the use of an eyepiece micrometer (reticle) and a stage micrometer. Results are presented as mean diameter of vessels per field ± SD.

2.4. Statistical Analysis. All data are presented as mean ± SD in the text and figures. The Student t-test was used to compare two means. Statistical significance was set at a $P < 0.05$ level.

3. Results

Table 1 shows the allocation of mice in the different groups of the study, as well as the number of excluded and participating animals.

Several vascular patterns of mouse dorsal skin have been recorded in this study. In the most frequently observed pattern, 114/120 (95%), the mouse dorsal skin was supplied by the two principal cutaneous perforators, which arose bilaterally from the deep circumflex iliac artery and the lateral thoracic artery.

6/120 (5%) mice have abnormal vasculature. Figure 2 shows an example of abnormal vasculature. In this case, the middle portion of dorsal skin in the left was supplied by

TABLE 1: Number of used and excluded mice in the study.

| Groups and IPL treatment fluences | Number of mice in each group | Number of mice used for histological Study | Number of mice used to create skin flaps and flap survival assessment | | | |
| | | | Excluded and reasons | | | |
			Abnormal vasculature	Pedicle not patent	Died	Used for study
Group I (control)	40	10	1	1	1	27
Group II (35 J/cm^2)	40	10	1		1	28
Group III (25 J/cm^2)	40	10	1			29
Group IV (15 J/cm^2)	40	10	3		1	26
Total	160	40	6	1	3	110

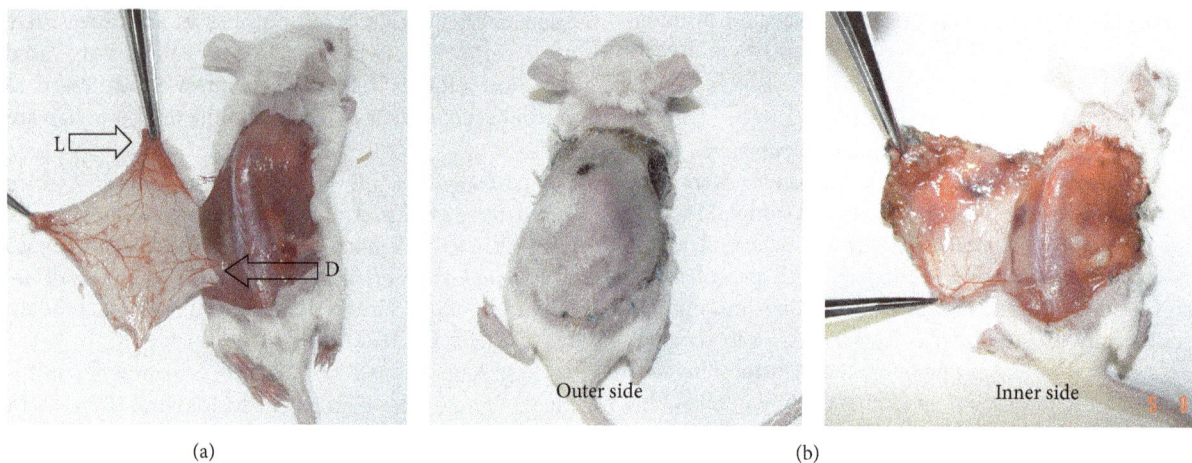

(a)   (b)

FIGURE 1: Dorsal island skin flap. (a) (D) the left deep circumflex iliac vessels as pedicle and (L) the left lateral thoracic vessels. (b) Flap survival and necrosis determination.

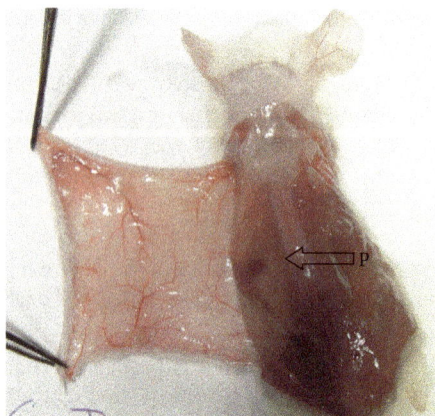

FIGURE 2: An example of abnormal vasculature. (P) a branch of the posterior intercostals arterial system.

a branch of the posterior intercostals arterial system. Such cases will be excluded from the study.

In 120 mice of IPL-treated groups, IPL with fluences of 35 J/cm^2 (Group II) has caused injury of the dorsal skin in 12/40 (30%) mice, whereas IPL with fluences of 25 J/cm^2 and 15 J/cm^2 has not caused any injury. The injury cannot be recognized immediately after IPL treatment. But it is able to be foreseen one day after IPL treatment and clearly seen four days after IPL treatment (Figure 3).

Table 2 shows the average survival rates of skin flaps from different groups of the study. Effect of IPL on wound healing was investigated based on the survival rates of skin flaps from different groups of the study.

In Group I (control group), skin flaps were raised without IPL treatment. At the 6th postoperative day, both outer and inner sides of the flap were checked. Change of vasculature was clearly seen at this day (Figure 4). Skin flaps average survival rate was 37.8 ± 10.6 (mean ± SD).

In Groups II and III, skin flaps survival rates are 35.2 ± 8.9 and 48.7 ± 12.5 respectively. There is no significant difference between these groups. Only in Group IV (mice treated with IPL fluences of 15 J/cm^2, lowest dose), skin flaps survival rate

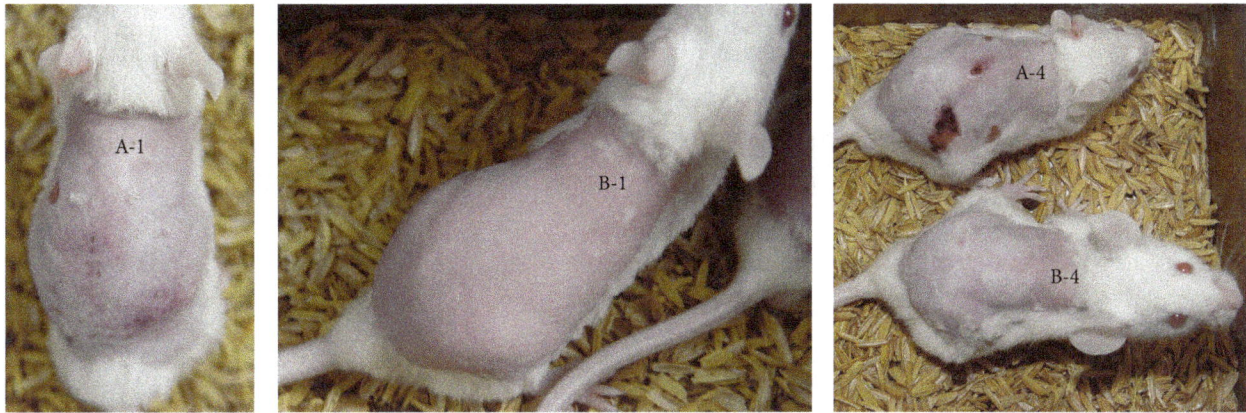

FIGURE 3: Injury caused by IPL. (A-1) mouse got 35 J/cm^2 IPL fluences, one day after treatment, (A-4) mouse got 35 J/cm^2 IPL fluences, 4 days after treatment, (B-1) mouse got 25 J/cm^2 IPL fluences, one day after treatment, and (B-4) mouse got 25 J/cm^2 IPL fluences, 4 days after treatment.

TABLE 2: Survival rates of skin flaps from different groups of the study.

Groups and IPL treatment fluences	Number of mice in each group	Number of mice used for flap survival assessment	Survival rate of skin flaps (%)
Group I (control)	40	27	37.8 ± 10.6 (mean ± SD)
Group II (35 J/cm^2)	40	28	35.2 ± 8.9 (mean ± SD)
Group III (25 J/cm^2)	40	29	48.7 ± 12.5 (mean ± SD)
Group IV (15 J/cm^2)	40	26	69.7 ± 15.9 (mean ± SD) **P < 0.05**
Total	160	110	

TABLE 3: Number of vessels and vessels diameter from different groups of the histological study.

Groups and IPL treatment fluences	Number of mice used for histological Study	Number of vessels per field	Diameter of vessels per field (μm)
Group I (control)	10	25.4 ± 6.2 (mean ± SD)	8.8 ± 3.6 (mean ± SD)
Group II (35 J/cm^2)	10	26.7 ± 7.1 (mean ± SD)	7.9 ± 4.2 (mean ± SD)
Group III (25 J/cm^2)	10	23.2 ± 8.3 (mean ± SD)	8.7 ± 2.5 (mean ± SD)
Group IV (15 J/cm^2)	10	25.7 ± 5.4 (mean ± SD)	14.7 ± 2.1 (mean ± SD) **P < 0.05**
Total	40		

is significantly higher than other groups: 69.7 ± 15.9 ($P < 0.05$).

Table 3 shows the number of vessels and vessels diameter from different groups of the histological study.

Histological study did not find any significant differences in vessels number of any groups, with or without IPL treatment. However, vessels dilation was found in Group IV; the group was treated with lowest dose of IPL (15 J/cm^2).

Hair regrowth is not primary consideration of this study. However, in 120 mice treated with IPL, it was recognized that hair regrowth did not follow any defined rule. Mice get the same treatment, but hair regrowth of each mouse is quite different (Figure 5).

4. Discussion

4.1. Mouse Island Skin Flap Model. Wound healing is a very complicated process. To study the basic mechanism of healing, to develop strategies for clinical treatment, and to evaluate the product safety and efficacy, a suitable animal wound model is indispensable [10]. Many different models have been devised [11]. An ideal wound model should reflect the wound pathogenesis and illustrate the clinical situation [1]. However, no ideal wound model could reflect all aspects of wound healing process [1, 11].

Blood supply to a wounded tissue is the prerequisite for normal tissue regeneration. Up to date, vascular change in the healing process of skin wounds is not fully understood. To study vascular change, installing a vital chamber to mouse dorsal skin is a good option, but it requires much expensive equipment [12].

In this study, our model can reflect one important factor of wound healing. It is the vascular change in the healing process of the ischemic skin flap. By counting the number of vessels in biopsies samples and looking to the vasculature from inner side of mouse skin (Figure 4), researchers can assess the neovascularization process. In this model, the neovascularization process was permitted to develop in the parallel way (from the proximal part to the distal part of the skin flap) instead of perpendicular way from wound bed as in other models.

(a)   (b)

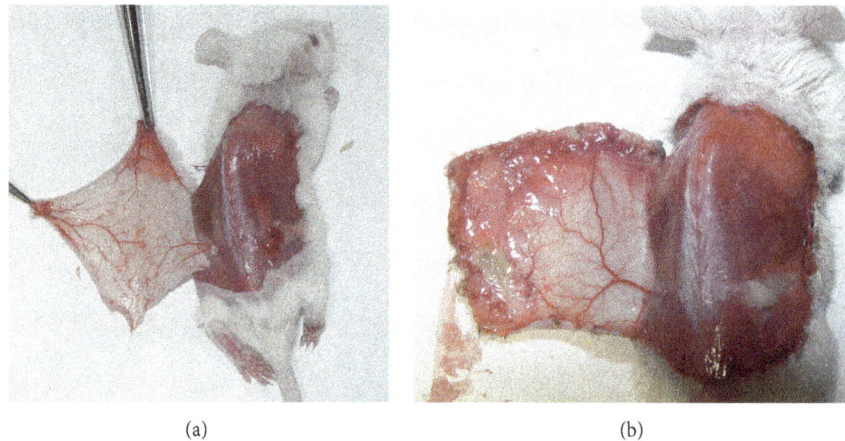

FIGURE 4: Changing of vasculature and neovascularization. (a) Vasculature at the time of flap elevation and (b) vasculature at the 6th postoperative day: changing and neovascularization could be clearly seen.

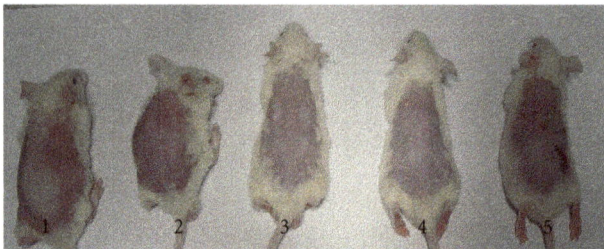

FIGURE 5: Hair reduction effect of IPL on mice.

Mice were used in this study. Skin flap models on dogs [13] and on rats [14] have been described. Flaps on mice offer clear advantage. Mice are inexpensive and easy to keep and gene modified mice are also available.

In comparison with the vital chamber model [12], this model is simple, cheap, and, therefore, suitable for less-equipped labs in developing countries. Obviously, continuous observation of vasculature is impossible. It is the disadvantage of this model.

4.2. Effect of IPL on Vascularity and Wound Healing. The novelty of this study is the effect of IPL on wound healing. We have not found any other reports about this particular approach to IPL use.

The results showed that the flap survival was significantly improved in the mice that had been treated with IPL fluences of 15 J/cm^2—the lowest dose. Interestingly, 15 J/cm^2 is a very low fluence in comparison with normal therapeutic fluences used on humans. We are not aware of any clinical studies using such low fluences. A higher dose (fluences of 35 J/cm^2 and 25 J/cm^2) did not produce any improvement on wound healing. Actually, fluences of 35 J/cm^2 have caused injury of the dorsal skin in 12/40 (30%) mice of Group II. By these results, one could say that the IPL effect is dose dependent. IPL can significantly improve the wound healing but only at low energy. The effect will be lost at high energy.

What is the mechanism of this phenomenon? Histological study has not found any tissue destruction after treatment with IPL fluences of 15 J/cm^2 (the effective dose). So, the possible mechanism must be different from tissue selective destruction mechanism which is generally used in human clinical situations [5].

Angiogenesis cannot be assumed to be the cause of wound healing improvement in this case. Vessel counting did not find any significant differences in vessel number of any groups, with or without IPL treatment (Table 3).

However, vessel dilation was found in Group IV; the group was treated with lowest dose of IPL and wound healing improved (Table 3). IPL produces heat in tissue. It is well known that, in the increased temperature, the cutaneous vessel becomes dilated as a way to expel the heat but this phenomenon will not last for long. Therefore, vessel dilation found 2 weeks after IPL treatment cannot be assumed to be caused by the heating effect of IPL. Possibly, it is due to the electromagnetic character of IPL. It was reported that the electromagnetic radiation at low dose could improve the tissue perfusion of the irradiated tissue [4].

Another possible explanation for wound healing enhancement of IPL treatment is the production of heat-shock protein after IPL treatment [7]. Then, heat-shock protein could protect tissue from ischemia injury and improve the healing [3].

It is not the main purpose of this study, but interestingly, it was found that hair reduction effect of IPL is not uniform from mouse to mouse (Figure 5). It resembles the clinical situation in humans. With the same IPL treatment, response of patients is quite different.

Results of this study cannot be supposed to be equally effective in human because of species differences. Mouse skin is much thinner than human skin. Even though IPL fluences of 15 J/cm^2 (which effectively improves wound healing) are just equal to the energy of home-use IPL devices that are freely available in the consumer market, such devices do not present any hazards according to currently available international standards [6].

5. Conclusion

In this study, we have shown that the dorsal island skin flap in the mouse is a suitable model for wound healing research purpose. This model is reliable and can offer some advantages for the study of wound healing where ischemia injury plays crucial role.

For the first time, the study has demonstrated that low-energy IPL augments wound healing. However, the exact mechanism is not clear at this stage of the study. Obviously, time and further research are needed to elucidate the true mechanism.

Therefore, we suggest using low-energy IPL as an adjuvant therapy to improve wound healing in humans because low-energy IPL devices are freely available for home use and do not present any hazard.

Disclosure

Do Xuân Hai and Pham Thi Ngoc are co-authors.

Acknowledgments

The authors would like to express their profound gratitude to Ms. Miranda Jane Tindill—Aukland University, New Zealand—Teacher of English, Language Link in Vietnam, for her English language editing. They sincerely thank all members of the Physiology Department, Vietnam Military Medical University, for their support and encouragement.

References

[1] F. Gottrup, M. S. Ågren, and T. Karlsmark, "Models for use in wound healing research: a survey focusing on in vitro and in vivo adult soft tissue," *Wound Repair and Regeneration*, vol. 8, no. 2, pp. 83–96, 2000.

[2] T. C. Minh, S. Ichioka, K. Harii, M. Shibata, J. Ando, and T. Nakatsuka, "Dorsal bipedicled island skin flap: a new flap model in mice," *Scandinavian Journal of Plastic and Reconstructive Surgery and Hand Surgery*, vol. 36, no. 5, pp. 262–267, 2002.

[3] T. C. Minh, S. Ichioka, T. Nakatsuka et al., "Effect of hyperthermic preconditioning on the survival of ischemia-reperfused skin flaps: a new skin-flap model in the mouse," *Journal of Reconstructive Microsurgery*, vol. 18, no. 2, pp. 115–119, 2002.

[4] B. Heissig, S. Rafii, H. Akiyama et al., "Low-dose irradiation promotes tissue revascularization through VEGF release from mast cells and MMP-9-mediated progenitor cell mobilization," *Journal of Experimental Medicine*, vol. 202, no. 6, pp. 739–750, 2005.

[5] R. R. Anderson and J. A. Parrish, "Selective photothermolysis: precise microsurgery by selective absorption of pulsed radiation," *Science*, vol. 220, no. 4596, pp. 524–527, 1983.

[6] E. Eadie, P. Miller, T. Goodman, and H. Moseley, "Assessment of the optical radiation hazard from a home-use intense pulsed light (IPL) source," *Lasers in Surgery and Medicine*, vol. 41, no. 7, pp. 534–539, 2009.

[7] V. G. Prieto, A. H. Diwan, C. R. Shea, P. Zhang, and N. S. Sadick, "Effects of intense pulsed light and the 1,064 nm Nd:YAG laser on sun-damaged human skin: histologic and immunohistochemical analysis," *Dermatologic Surgery*, vol. 31, no. 5, pp. 522–525, 2005.

[8] H. Ohara, K. Kishi, and T. Nakajima, "Rat dorsal paired island skin flaps: a precise model for flap survival evaluation," *Keio Journal of Medicine*, vol. 57, no. 4, pp. 211–216, 2008.

[9] H. Gustavsson, T. Tešan, K. Jennbacken, K. Kuno, J.-E. Damber, and K. Welén, "ADAMTS1 alters blood vessel morphology and TSP1 levels in LNCaP and LNCaP-19 prostate tumors," *BMC Cancer*, vol. 10, article 288, 2010.

[10] R. Perez and S. C. Davis, "Relevance of animal models for wound healing," *Wounds*, vol. 20, no. 1, pp. 3–8, 2008.

[11] J. M. Davidson, "Animal models for wound repair," *Archives of Dermatological Research*, vol. 290, pp. 1–11, 1998.

[12] S. Ichioka, T. C. Minh, M. Shibata et al., "In vivo model for visualizing flap microcirculation of ischemia-reperfusion," *Microsurgery*, vol. 22, no. 7, pp. 304–310, 2002.

[13] C. M. Trinh, V. L. Hoàng, T. N. Pham, and M. A. Hoàng, "Canine lateral thoracic fasciocutaneous flap: an experimental study," *International Journal of Surgery*, vol. 7, no. 5, pp. 472–475, 2009.

[14] F. Zhang, W. D. Sones, and W. C. Lineaweaver, "Microsurgical flap models in the rat," *Journal of Reconstructive Microsurgery*, vol. 17, no. 3, pp. 211–221, 2001.

8

Outcome of Split Thickness Skin Grafting and Multiple Z-Plasties in Postburn Contractures of Groin and Perineum: A 15-Year Experience

Wani Sajad[1] and Raashid Hamid[1,2]

[1] Department of Plastic Surgery, SKIMS, Srinagar, Jammu and Kashmir 190011, India
[2] Married Doctors Hostel, Block A, Room No. S2, SKIMS, Soura, Jammu and Kashmir 190011, India

Correspondence should be addressed to Raashid Hamid; drraashidhamid@gmail.com

Academic Editor: Nicolo Scuderi

Background. Groin and perineal burn contracture is a rare postburn sequel. Such postburn contractures causes distressing symptoms to the patients and in the management of these contractures, both functional and cosmetic appearance should be the primary concern. *Aims*. To study the outcome of surgical treatment (STSG and multiple Z-plasties) in postburn contractures of groin and perineum. *Material and Methods*. We conducted a study of 49 patients, with postburn groin and perineal contractures. Release of contracture with split thickness skin grafting (STSG) was done in 44 (89.79%) patients and release of contracture and closure by multiple Z-plasties was done in 5 (10.21%) patients. *Results*. Satisfactory functional and cosmetic outcome was seen in 44 (89.79%) patients. Minor secondary contractures of the graft were seen in 3 (6.81%) patients who were managed by physiotherapy and partial recurrence of the contracture in 4 (8.16%) patients required secondary surgery. *Conclusion*. We conclude that postburn contractures of the groin and perineum can be successfully treated with release of contracture followed by STSG with satisfactory functional and cosmetic results. Long term measures like regular physiotherapy, use of pressure garments, and messaging with emollient creams should not be neglected and should be instituted postoperatively to prevent secondary contractures of the graft and recurrence of the contracture.

1. Introduction

Perineum and groin constitute only 4–6% of total body surface area and are very important sites in the body anatomically and functionally. Isolated burns to the genitalia and perineum are not common [1–3]. These burns are of major concern to the patient as well as clinician [4]. Flame burns and scalds are common causes of perineal and genital burns [4–6]. Alcoholism is considered to be one of the leading predisposing factors in perineal and genital burns [7]. Child abuse is also a risk factor in perineal and genital burns [8]. "Chullah," an earthen made stove in which wood is used as fuel in the rural areas of India, is important cause for the perineal burns [2]. Use of loose clothes during cooking, spilling of kerosene on the clothes from a burning stove, or explosion of such stoves are also associated with perineal and genital burns [9, 10].

Patient usually presents with difficulty in squatting, walking, sitting, urination, defecation, and sexual intercourse in married persons [2]. Since the contracture is not in a stabilized position, recurrent ulceration may occur and in exceptional cases squamous cell carcinoma (Marjolin's ulcer) may develop [11]. Various complications of perineal burn contracture like intestinal obstruction, anal stenosis with megarectum, and gluteal pouching with total effacement of the gluteal folds and hooding of the rectum have also been reported [12–14].

In the management of these contractures, both functional and cosmetic appearances should be the primary concern. Various surgical procedures have been used for the release of these contractures which range from simple release and grafting to a number of different flap procedures.

2. Material and Methods

A total of 49 patients were evaluated, analysed, and treated from May 1996 to May 2011. All patients were studied in detail. A detailed history was recorded from each patient, laying special emphasis on the time since initial burn, causative agent, percentage of body surface area involved, presenting symptoms, and any associated illness. A detailed general physical, systemic, and local examination was carried out on all patients.

All patients were subjected to surgery under general anaesthesia and the following operative procedures were performed:

(1) release of contracture with split thickness skin grafting in 44 (89.79%) patients;

(2) release of contracture and closure by multiple Z-plasties in 5 (10.21%) patients. Z-plasties used included 5-flap Z-plasties for 2 patients and simple Z for 3 patients.

First dressing was seen on third or fourth postoperative day and percentage of graft take/loss was noted. Complications, if any, were recorded. Indwelling urinary catheter drainage was instituted for 3 to 4 days postoperatively. Once the graft stabilized, patients were discharged and advised to wear compression garments. Regular physiotherapy and messaging with emollient creams were advised in all cases to avoid any recurrence of the contracture. Operated patients were followed and the results were analyzed according to the functional and cosmetic outcome; patient's satisfaction regarding the operative procedure and need for any secondary surgeries were recorded.

3. Results

Majority of the patients, 23 (46.94%), were in the age group of 16–30 years. The patient's ages ranged from 3 to 70 years with mean age of 18 years. 35 (71.43%) were females and 14 (28.57%) were males. 40 (81.63%) patients belonged to the rural areas, where most of the people use Kangri during the winter months to keep themselves warm. In 77.56% of the patients, postburn contractures of the groin and perineum were because of Kangri burn. Other less common causes were hot water (8.16%), open chulla (8.16%), and flame burn (6.12%). In our series the meantime of sustaining the burn injury was 7.1 years with maximum 16 years and minimum 2 years. In our series, 25 (51.02%) patients had isolated burns of groin and perineum and, in 24 (48.98%) patients, burns to groin and perineum were associated with burns to surrounding areas including external genitalia, lower abdomen, and upper thighs. Majority of the patients were brought with complaints of difficulty in squatting (97.95%) followed by limitation of movements of hip joints (93.87%) and impairment of gait. External genitalia were hidden under the web in 21 (42.85%) patients having bilateral groin contractures associated with contractures of the surrounding areas. Ulcerations of the contracture scar were seen in 3 (6.12%) patients, out of which 1 (2.04%) patient had developed squamous cell carcinoma (Marjolin's ulcer). Unilateral groin contractures were seen in 25 (51.02%) of the patients and bilateral groin contractures were seen in 21 (42.86%) patients. In 3 (6.12%) of the patients contracture was confined to perineum only.

In our series of 49 patients two types of operative procedures were performed (Table 1):

(1) release of contracture with split thickness skin grafting;

(2) release of contracture and closure by multiple Z-plasties.

In our series of 49 patients, 44 (89.79%) patients underwent release of contracture and the resulting raw area was covered with split thickness skin graft and tie-over dressing was applied to immobilize the graft. Minor secondary contractures of the graft were managed by physiotherapy and pressure garments.

21 (42.85%) patients having bilateral groin contractures underwent release of contracture with split thickness skin grafting. Most of these patients had webbing over symphysis pubis which had hidden the external genitalia. Such webs were also released. 20 (40.82%) patients underwent release of unilateral groin contracture with split thickness skin grafting and 5 (10.21%) patients underwent release of unilateral groin contracture and closure by multiple Z-plasties. 3 (6.12%) patients with perineal contracture only underwent release of contracture with split thickness skin grafting.

Postoperative hematoma formation under the graft was seen in 2 (4.54%) patients. Minimal patchy graft loss was seen in 4 (9.09%) patients, which was managed conservatively. Minor secondary contractures of the graft were seen in 3 (6.81%) patient. Partial recurrence of the contracture was seen in 4 (8.16%) patients who required secondary surgeries.

Postoperative outcome was measured by comparing with contralateral groin where involvement was unilateral and with subjective assessment from patient satisfaction regarding function, mobility, exposed genitalia, improvements in movements at hip joint including gait, improvement in squatting, and cosmetic improvement. Objective assessment was made by the surgeon regarding the measurements of landmarks of groin.

Functional outcome was satisfactory in 44 (89.79%) patients; their squatting, walking, gait, and movements of the hip joints were improved and patients were able to perform all day to day activities of life and essential chores that require sitting or squatting position. In 4 (8.16%) patients functional outcome was not satisfactory. In these 4 patients partial recurrence of the contracture had occurred and required secondary surgeries. One patient died in follow-up due to road traffic accident. Cosmetic outcome was satisfactory in almost all except 4 (8.16%) patients, in which partial recurrence of the contracture had occurred (Figures 1, 2, 3, 4, 5, 6, 7, 8, 9, 10, and 11).

TABLE 1

Operative procedure	Number of patients	Percentage
Release of bilateral groin contracture with split thickness skin grafting	21	42.85
Release of unilateral groin contracture with split thickness skin grafting	20	40.82
Release of unilateral groin contracture and closure by multiple Z-plasties	5	10.21
Release of perineal contracture with split thickness skin grafting	3	6.12
Total	49	100.00

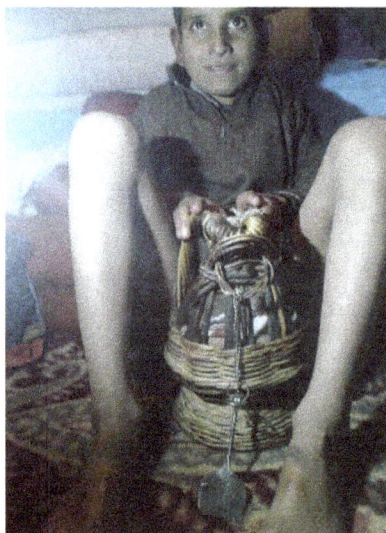

FIGURE 1: "Kangri" containing glowing charcoal, under a loose garment known as "Pheran" kept between medial aspect of thighs and lower abdomen in close proximity to groin.

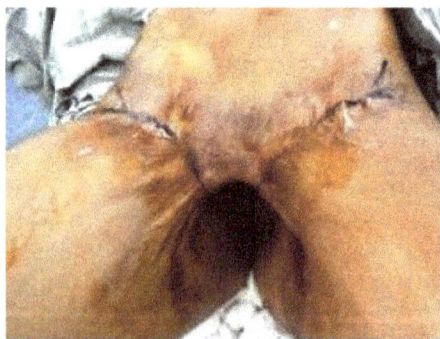

FIGURE 3: Raw area after release of contracture.

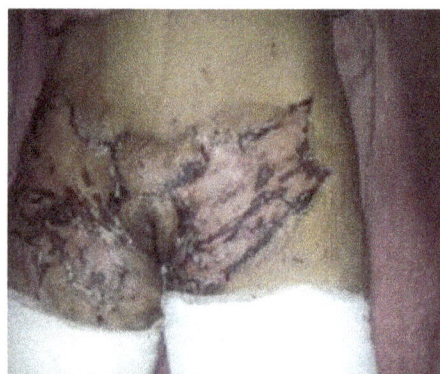

FIGURE 4: Split thickness skin graft in place in immediate postoperative view of patient shown in Figure 1.

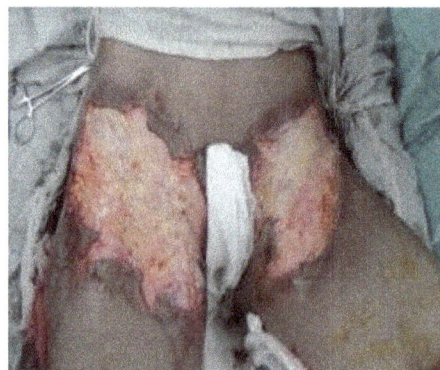

FIGURE 2: Bilateral postburn groin contracture with hidden genitalia under the web.

4. Discussion

Postburn contractures of groin and perineum are a rare burn sequel and such contractures are usually diagnosed late owing to the patient's negligence, ignorance, and shyness and delay can be extended until puberty and sometimes even later in females. The contracture band in the groin and across the symphysis pubis binds the thighs together, leading to functional problems like difficulty in squatting, walking, sitting, urination, defecation, and sexual function.

Squatting, a common posture adopted in India for urination and defecation, was the main complaint in all our patients.

The mode of burn injury in our series was different from that reported by other authors. Sawhney [9] reported perineal burns sustained by spilling of kerosene on the clothes from a burning stove or due to explosion of such stoves. Bangma et al. [5] reported burns to the perineum and genitals due to scalds, explosion, open fire, or electricity. Balakrishnan et al. [7] reported perineal burns due to hot water, chemicals, and grease in males secondary to spouse abuse. Kumar et al. [6] reported scalds, flames, and electric burns as the most common contributors to burn injury. Michielsen et al. [4] reported burn injury to the genitalia and perineum

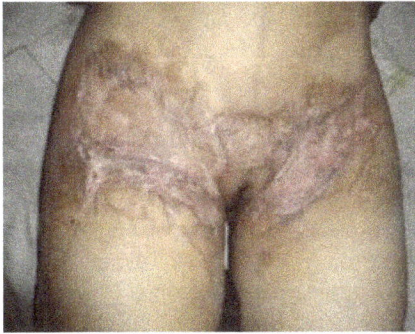

FIGURE 5: The same patient shown in Figure 1 in follow-up period. Genitalia exposed.

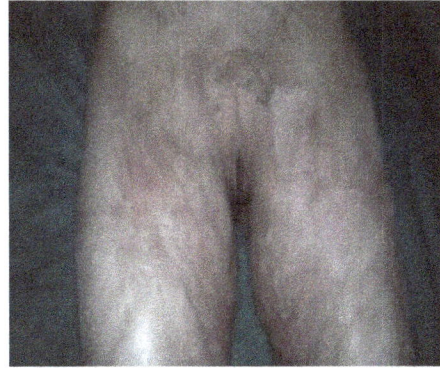

FIGURE 8: The same patient in Figure 5 on follow-up.

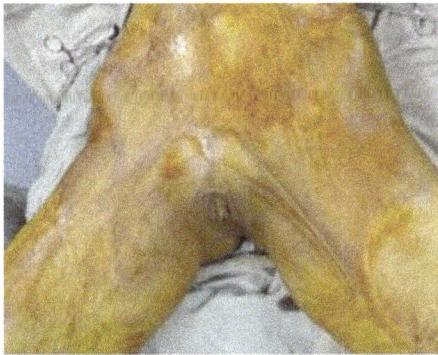

FIGURE 6: Bilateral postburn groin contracture.

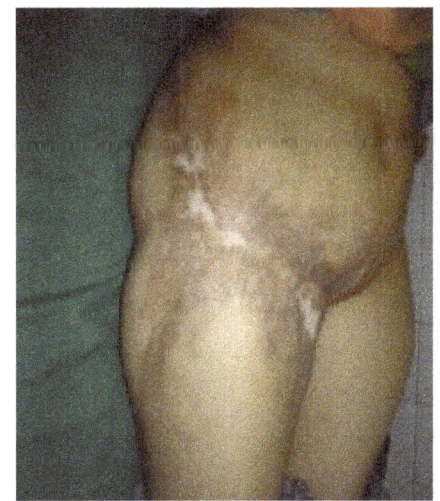

FIGURE 9: Right groin contracture with scarring.

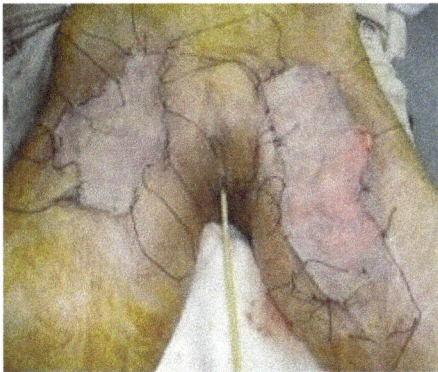

FIGURE 7: Split thickness skin grafting of raw area in Figure 5.

mostly due to scalds, flames, and chemicals. Abdel-Razek [1] reported accidental chemical (sulphuric acid) burns to the genitalia. Thakur et al. [2] reported perineal burns caused by fire wood used in open "chullah." In our series burns to the groin and perineum were mostly due to "Kangri" use (77.56%), open "chullah" (8.16%), hot water (8.16%), and flames (6.12%).

Because of the cold climate and poor economic conditions, majority of the people in Kashmir use "Kangri" to keep themselves warm during the winter months. "Kangri"

is an earthen bowl containing glowing charcoal. It is used under a loose garment known as "Pheran" and is kept between medial aspect of thighs and lower abdomen in close proximity to groin and perineum. In majority of our patients (77.56%), accidental "Kangri" burn injury to groin and perineum was the mode of injury. Because these burns were not managed properly in acute phase, they had healed with the development of contractures of groin and perineum.

Perineal and genital burns are mostly part of large body surface injuries and isolated burns to perineum and genitalia are uncommon as reported by Abdel-Razek [1], Peck et al. [15], Bangma et al. [5], and Thakur et al. [2]. In patients with isolated burns to groin and perineum, "Kangri" was the sole causative agent responsible. This contradictory observation was due to the habitual use of "Kangri" in our state during the winter months.

Limitation of the movements of hip joints was seen in 46 (93.87%) patients. This limitation of movements of the hip joints had led to impairment of gait in 42 (85.71%) patients. Most of these patients had long standing contractures of groin. The findings are in agreement with the observations made by other investigators [2, 11, 16, 17].

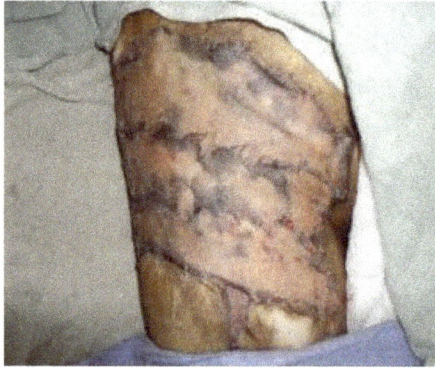

FIGURE 10: Immediate postoperative view after STSG of patient shown in Figure 8.

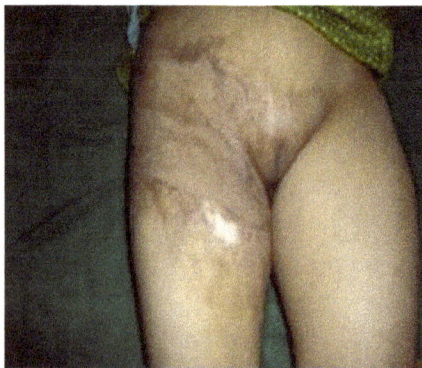

FIGURE 11: Follow-up view of the same patient shown in Figure 8.

As perineal burn contractures are not in a stabilized position, recurrent ulcerations may occur and, in exceptional cases, Marjolin's ulcer (squamous cell carcinoma) may develop [11]. Darzi and Chowdri [18] reported recurrent ulceration in 30 (41.66%) patients with postburn scar carcinoma. In our series we have seen recurrent ulcerations in 3 (6.12%) patients. Among these three patients, one patient, a 70-year-old male, had developed squamous cell carcinoma.

As reported by Sawhney [9], Rutan [19], and Thakur et al. [2], long term measures have to be instituted postoperatively to prevent skin graft contraction such as wearing tightly fitting undergarments. In our study also patients were advised to wear compression garments postoperatively. Regular physiotherapy and messaging with emollient creams were also advised in all cases to prevent any recurrence of the contracture. Postoperative follow-up ran smoothly with adequate healing. Squatting ability improved in 44 (89.79%) patients and they were able to perform essential chores that require squatting position. There were no donor site complications. Thus split thickness skin grafting was safe, less time consuming, and technically easy with good functional and cosmetic results. It can be done safely in patients having unilateral or bilateral postburn groin contractures and postburn perineal contractures of any severity.

Release of contracture and closure by multiple Z-plasties was done in 5 (10.21%) patients having minor unilateral postburn groin contractures in the form of linear bands. The functional and cosmetic results were satisfactory. Ye [20] found satisfactory results with local Z-plasty in 32 (82.05%) patients with postburn perianal scar contracture. Thus patients having minor postburn groin contractures, release of contracture and closure of wound by multiple Z-plasties can be done safely with shorter operative and recovery time and satisfactory functional results.

Besides graft and various types of Z-plasty used for release of groin contracture, the other clinical scenarios like extensive wounds after release of contracture, proximity to the anus and urethra, and wounds involving groin with exposure of femoral vessels after release of contracture may necessitate the use of flap cover. The sartorius muscle is transposed medially into groin for coverage of exposed femoral vessels. The gracilis muscle can be used to cover groin. The tenser fascia lata is useful for groin reconstruction. The rectus musculocutaneous flap based on its inferior pedicle provides a reliable flap cover. Free tissue transfer with anastomosis around femoral vessels remains a choice in difficult cases.

In our study satisfactory functional and cosmetic results were seen with split thickness skin grafts in patients having postburn contractures of groin and perineum. Our observations were consistent with the observations of other authors [1, 2, 4, 9, 11, 21].

References

[1] S. M. Abdel-Razek, "Isolated chemical burns to the genitalia. Analysis of 12 patients," *Annals of Burns and Fire Disasters*, vol. 19, no. 3, pp. 148–154, 2006.

[2] J. S. Thakur, C. G. S. Chauhan, V. K. Diwana, D. C. Chuahan, and A. Thakur, "Perineal burn contractures: an experience in tertiary hospital of a Himalayan state," *Indian Journal of Plastic Surgery*, vol. 41, no. 2, pp. 190–194, 2008.

[3] E. M. Weiler-Mithoff, M. E. Hassall, and D. A. Burd, "Burns of the female genitalia and perineum," *Burns*, vol. 22, no. 5, pp. 390–395, 1996.

[4] D. Michielsen, R. van Hee, C. Neetens, C. Lafaire, and R. Peeters, "Burns to the genitalia and the perineum," *Journal of Urology*, vol. 159, no. 2, pp. 418–419, 1998.

[5] C. H. Bangma, A. B. M. van der Molen, and H. Boxma, "Burns to the perineum and genitals—management, results and function of the thermally injured perineum in a 5-year-review," *European Journal of Plastic Surgery*, vol. 18, no. 2-3, pp. 111–114, 1995.

[6] P. Kumar, P. T. Chirayil, and R. Chittoria, "Ten years epidemiological study of paediatric burns in Manipal, India," *Burns*, vol. 26, no. 3, pp. 261–264, 2000.

[7] C. Balakrishnan, L. L. Imel, A. T. Bandy, and J. K. Prasad, "Perineal burns in males secondary to spouse abuse," *Burns*, vol. 21, no. 1, pp. 34–35, 1995.

[8] C. Angel, T. Shu, D. French, E. Orihuela, J. Lukefahr, and D. N. Herndon, "Genital and perineal burns in children: 10 years of experience at a major burn center," *Journal of Pediatric Surgery*, vol. 37, no. 1, pp. 99–103, 2002.

[9] C. P. Sawhney, "Management of burn contractures of the perineum," *Plastic and Reconstructive Surgery*, vol. 72, no. 6, pp. 837–842, 1983.

[10] R. B. Ahuja and S. Bhattacharya, "ABC of burns: burns in the developing world and burn disasters," *British Medical Journal*, vol. 329, no. 7463, pp. 447–449, 2004.

[11] S. Erguns, D. I. Cek, and M. Ulay, "Reconstruction of vulva in a female patient having long-standing genital burn contracture with severe web and Marjolin's ulcer: a case report," *Annals of Burns and Fire Disasters*, vol. 12, pp. 36–39, 1999.

[12] J. S. Thakur, C. G. S. Chauhan, V. K. Divana, and A. Thakur, "Extrinsic post burn peri-anal contracture leading to subacute intestinal obstruction: a case report," *Cases Journal*, vol. 1, pp. 117–119, 2008.

[13] A. Sagi, E. Freud, A. J. Mares, P. Ben-Meir, Y. Ben-Yakar, and D. Mahler, "Anal stenosis with megarectum: an unusual complication of a perineal burn," *Journal of Burn Care and Rehabilitation*, vol. 14, no. 3, pp. 350–352, 1993.

[14] A. A. Alghanem, R. L. McCauley, and M. C. Robson, "Gluteal pouching: a complication of perineal burn scar contracture: a case report," *Journal of Burn Care and Rehabilitation*, vol. 11, no. 2, pp. 137–139, 1990.

[15] M. D. Peck, M. A. Boileau, B. J. Grube, and D. M. Heimbach, "The management of burns to the perineum and genitals," *Journal of Burn Care and Rehabilitation*, vol. 11, no. 1, pp. 54–56, 1990.

[16] V. M. Grishkevich, "Postburn perineal obliteration: elimination of perineal, inguinal, and perianal contractures with the groin flap," *Journal of Burn Care and Research*, vol. 31, no. 5, pp. 786–790, 2010.

[17] S. Eo, D. Kim, and N. F. Jones, "Microdissection thinning of a pedicled deep inferior epigastric perforator flap for burn scar contracture of the groin: case report," *Journal of Reconstructive Microsurgery*, vol. 21, no. 7, pp. 447–450, 2005.

[18] M. A. Darzi and N. A. Chowdri, "Post burn scar carcinoma in Kashmiris," *Burns*, vol. 22, no. 6, pp. 477–482, 1996.

[19] R. L. Rutan, "Management of perineal and genital burns," *Journal of ET Nursing*, vol. 20, no. 4, pp. 169–176, 1993.

[20] E.-M. Ye, "Clinical experience in treatment of peri-anal scar contracture in children," *Burns*, vol. 25, no. 8, pp. 760–761, 1999.

[21] G. P. Pisarski, D. G. Greenhalgh, and G. D. Warden, "The management of perineal contractures in children with burns," *Journal of Burn Care and Rehabilitation*, vol. 15, no. 3, pp. 256–259, 1994.

9

Hypospadias Repair: A Single Centre Experience

Mansoor Khan, Abdul Majeed, Waqas Hayat, Hidayat Ullah, Shazia Naz, Syed Asif Shah, Tahmeedullah Tahmeed, Kanwal Yousaf, and Muhammad Tahir

Plastic & Reconstructive Surgery, Hayatabad Medical Complex, IV Hayatabad, P.O. Box 25100, Peshawar, Pakistan

Correspondence should be addressed to Mansoor Khan; drkhanps@yahoo.com

Academic Editor: Nicolo Scuderi

Objectives. To determine the demographics and analyze the management and factors influencing the postoperative complications of hypospadias repair. *Settings.* Hayatabad Medical Complex Peshawar, Pakistan, from January 2007 to December 2011. *Material and Methods.* All male patients presenting with hypospadias irrespective of their ages were included in the study. The data were acquired from the hospital's database and analyzed with Statistical Package for Social Sciences (SPSS). *Results.* A total of 428 patients with mean age of 8.12 ± 5.04 SD presented for hypospadias repair. Midpenile hypospadias were the most common. Chordee, meatal abnormalities, cryptorchidism, and inguinal hernias were observed in 74.3%, 9.6%, 2.8%, and 2.1% cases, respectively. Two-stage (Bracka) and TIP (tubularized incised urethral plate) repairs were performed in 76.2% and 20.8% of cases, respectively. The most common complications were edema and urethrocutaneous fistula (UCF). The complications were significantly lower in the hands of specialists than residents (P-value = 0.0086). The two-stage hypospadias repair resulted in higher complications frequency than single-stage repair (P value = 0.0001). *Conclusion.* Hypospadias surgery has a long learning curve because it requires a great deal of temperament, surgical skill and acquaintance with magnifications. Single-stage repair should be encouraged wherever applicable due to its lower postoperative complications.

1. Introduction

Hypospadias is the most common congenital abnormality of the urethra affecting 1 : 300 live male births worldwide. The incidence is on the rise with the increasing environmental pollution as the suspected cause [1]. In 1993, the Birth Defects Monitoring Program (BDMP) has reported a doubling of the rates of hypospadias since 1970s in the United States [2]. Hypospadias is the abnormal location of the urethra on the ventral surface of the penis with variable association with the aborted development of the urethral spongiosum, ventral prepuce, and penile chordee [3]. By meatal location hypospadias is classified as anterior (glanular and subcoronal), midpenile (distal penile, midshaft, and proximal penile), and posterior (penoscrotal, scrotal, and perineal) accounting for 50%, 30%, and 20%, respectively [4]. Those cases in which multiple procedures are performed with suboptimal results are termed "crippled cases" [5]. One fourth of the hypospadias are associated with chordee [6]. Devine and Horton classified chordee into type I (skin tethering), type II (fibrotic dartos and buck's fascia), type III (corporal disproportion), and type IV (congenital short urethra) [7, 8].

In the management of hypospadias preoperative assessment is of prime importance which should include measurement of the size of the phallus, glans cleft (flat, incomplete, or complete), location and size of the meatus (type of hypospadias and meatal stenosis or mega-meatus), urethral plate width (<1 cm or ≥1 cm), type of chordee, prepuce (complete, incomplete, circumcised), penile torsion (clockwise, anticlockwise), shape of the scrotum (normal, penoscrotal transposition), and associated anomalies (cryptorchidism, inguinal hernia, persistent Mullerian structures) [4, 9]. Hypospadias can be associated with other urogenital tract anomalies such as pelviureteric junction (PUJ) obstruction, vesicoureteric reflux and renal agenesis which should be excluded by ultrasonographic scan in every hypospadias patient [4, 10, 11]. Proximal hypospadias with cryptorchidism, enlarged utricle, or penile size <2.5 cm should be investigated for intersex disorders by ultrasonography, hormonal profile, and karyotyping [12].

Timing of surgery is decided on the basis of anaesthesia's risk, penile size, and psychosocial development of the infant. The tolerance to anaesthesia is good at the age of 6 months.

The difference in the penile length at one year and preschool age is 8 millimetre only. After 18 months the children enter a behavioural phase of development uncooperative for hospitalization. In the background of these facts, using microsurgical instruments and magnification, 6–18 months is the most suitable age for hypospadias repair. If the surgery is not performed during this age then the next window of surgery is preschool age (3-4 years) when the child starts cooperating with treatment [4, 13].

Minimal tissue trauma, minimal/pin-point use of cautery, and well-vascularised tension free repair of all layers with epithelial inversion are the general principles of hypospadias repair. The goal of hypospadias repair is to build confidence in the child by creating a straight penis with a slit-like meatus at the tip of the glans and a urethra of uniform calibre and adequate length, reconstructing a symmetrical glans and penile shaft and achieving projectile stream and normal erection [4].

In patients with chordee the curvature is quantified per-operatively by Horton test after degloving the penis into mild (10°–20°), moderate (30°–40°), and severe (>50°). Most of the hypospadiologists do not address the mild chordee although they agree on correcting the moderate and severe forms through dorsal (plication) and ventral approach (excising the fibrous tissue), respectively [14, 15]. The chordee correction starts by penile degloving, and urethral plate and proximal urethral mobilization. The persistent chordee after these maneuvers is either due to urethral plate tethering or corporal disproportion. The former is corrected by urethral plate transaction while the later anomaly requires dorsal plication/Nesbit procedure [13]. The dorsal nerve branches from 11 and 1 o'clock positions to the 5 and 7 o'clock positions, making the 12 o'clock position ideal for dorsal plication during correction of the chordee [16]. In cases of hypoplastic penis where dorsal plication can unacceptably shorten the length then tunica release and dermal or tunica grafts can be considered [13].

The choice of the procedure is based on the characteristics of the urethral plate irrespective of the meatal location. The hypospadias repairs can be classified into single-stage procedures and two-stage urethral plate substitution procedure (Bracka's repair). The single-stage procedures are (a) urethral plate tubularization (glanular approximation and Snodgrass repair) and (b) urethral plate augmentation (onlay flap and Snodgraft repair) [13].

When the urethral plate does not need transaction then it can be tubularized either by Zaonz's GAP (glanular approximation procedure) when the plate is wide and deep or by Snodgrass's TIP in cases of narrow, shallow urethral plates with occasional bands. In cases of inelastic urethral plate where the midline releasing incision is not expected to widen the plate then substantial augmentation can be performed either by Duckett's onlay preputial island flap or a more popular Snodgraft repair by quilting a full thickness preputial skin graft in the dorsal defect after the releasing midline incision. The Snodgraft repair is also indicated in conical glans where the Snodgrass (TIP) midline incision is extended beyond the distal limit of the glans groove to achieve an apical meatus, inciting meatal stenosis unless grafted [13].

The urethral substitution procedures come into play when the chordee is corrected by urethral plate transaction. Due to the long term complications of Transverse Preputial Island Flap (Duckett's procedure) for the substitution of the whole circumference of the transacted urethra has fallen out of favour for the Bracka's two-stage repair where full thickness preputial skin graft is used [13].

Despite the controversial status, most of the hypospadiologists favour the urinary diversion and postoperative dressing. The penile block along with the general anaesthesia should be used to achieve successful postoperative analgesia.

Follow-up protocol after hypospadias repair is designed to institute a balance between its pros (early detection of complications) and cones (psychological concerns by repeatedly reminding with the patient the abnormality). After removal of the stent at one week postoperatively the patient is followed for 1, 3 and 6 months intervals and then yearly for two years. For the assessment of long term results patient can be followed up to midteen age [4, 13].

Biotechnology development in hypospadias surgery is directed toward the application of LASER shouldering (to replace conventional suturing techniques), robotics (for removal of human errors, e.g., hand tremors), tissue engineering (for urethral regeneration), and the use of tubular acellular collagen seeded with urothelial cells [17, 18].

Hypospadias surgery has a long learning curve. A reliable operator has the temperament for the hypospadias surgery, with an annual case load of at least 40–50, and has mastered six common techniques [4, 13]. This paper is aimed to present and analyze the demographics, protocols, techniques, complication of hypospadias repair, and its effect modifiers at our centre.

2. Material and Methods

After approval of the study protocol from the ethical committee, all male patients, irrespective of their age, managed for hypospadias from January 2007 to December 2011 at the Plastic and Reconstructive Surgery Department of Hayatabad Medical Complex Peshawar, Pakistan, were included in the study. Patients with comorbidities (coagulation disorders, diabetes mellitus, and disorders of sex development) and those patients who were lost in the followup were excluded from the study population to omit bias from the study results. All the demographic, clinical presentation, laboratory studies, surgical treatment, complications, and their management data were collected from the department's record sheets. To stratify the results, surgeons were divided into two groups; residents (trainees) and specialists (fellow plastic surgeons). Residents performed surgeries under direct or indirect supervision of the specialist. The data were organized, analyzed, and presented with the help of Statistical Package for Social Sciences (SPSS). The qualitative variables were presented as frequencies and percentages while quantitative variables were analyzed as means ± SD. All the important variables were stratified against age, type and severity of hypospadias, duration of surgery, type of surgical procedure, and experience of the surgeon to see the effect modifiers. The results were projected as tables and figures.

3. Results

A total of 428 male patients consisting of 96.3% primary cases and 3.7% secondary cases fulfilled the inclusion criteria. Patients with age ranging from 1 to 40 years with mean age of 8.12 ± 5.04 SD presented for hypospadias repair. Thirty-seven (8.6%) patients had the positive family history for hypospadias. Increasing trend of hypospadias patients presenting for surgery was observed during the study period with the highest of 103 (24.1%) patients presented in 2011. Only 1.87% and 34.6% patients were operated in 1-2 years, 3–5-year age windows while the rest presented in ≥6 years of age.

Mid-penile hypospadias (distal penile, midshaft, and proximal penile) was the most common type in the study population accounting for 48.6% ($n = 208$) patients followed by anterior hypospadias (glanular and subcoronal) in 36.4% ($n = 156$) cases, which is consistent for all geographical locations of the study population (Figure 1). Of the total study population, 74.3% ($n = 318$) of the hypospadias was associated with some degree of chordee. The most common type of chordee was the mild degree (<20°) with a count of 51.4% ($n = 220$) cases. Severe chordee was found in 7.5% ($n = 32$) cases. The chordee was present in 100% cases of penoscrotal and perineal hypospadias and the least common for glanular hypospadias accounting for 54.8% cases (Figure 2). Meatal abnormalities associated with the hypospadias were observed in 9.6% ($n = 41$) patients. Meatal stenosis was the most common meatal abnormality affecting 9.1% ($n = 39$) patients while mega-meatus was observed in 0.5% ($n = 2$) cases. Perineal and glanular hypospadias were the most commonly associated with meatal stenosis in 16.7% and 16.1% cases, respectively. Cryptorchidism was observed in 2.8% ($n = 12$) cases. A total of 2.1% ($n = 9$) hypospadias were associated with inguinal hernias.

Of the total 428 cases, 76.2% ($n = 326$) patients' hypospadias were repaired in two stages (Bracka) while 20.8% ($n = 89$) were subjected to TIP repair. Two-stage hypospadias repair was the predominant surgical procedure for all types of the hypospadias. For 110 cases without chordee, 53.6% ($n = 59$) hypospadias were managed by different single-stage repairs with TIP the predominant procedure performed in 54 (49.1%) cases. Two-stage (Bracka) repair was performed in 46.4% ($n = 51$) in 110 hypospadias without chordee for narrow urethral plate and incomplete glans cleft.

Of the total 428 hypospadias, 66.1% ($n = 283$) were performed by specialist plastic surgeons while 33.9% ($n = 145$) were operated on by residents. Specialists performed two-stage (Bracka) and single-stage (i.e., TIP, MAGPI, and Mathieu's) repairs in 67.14% and 32.9% cases, respectively. While residents performed two-stage (Bracka) and TIP repair in 93.8% and 6.2% cases.

For 50.7% ($n = 217$) cases duration of surgical procedure was >60 minutes. Duration of surgical procedure for specialists was ≤60 minutes in 58.7% cases while for the residents it

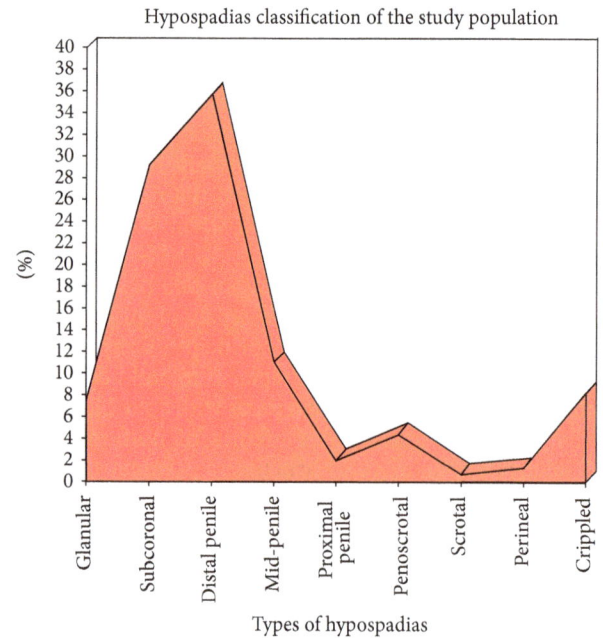

FIGURE 1: Hypospadias classification of the study population.

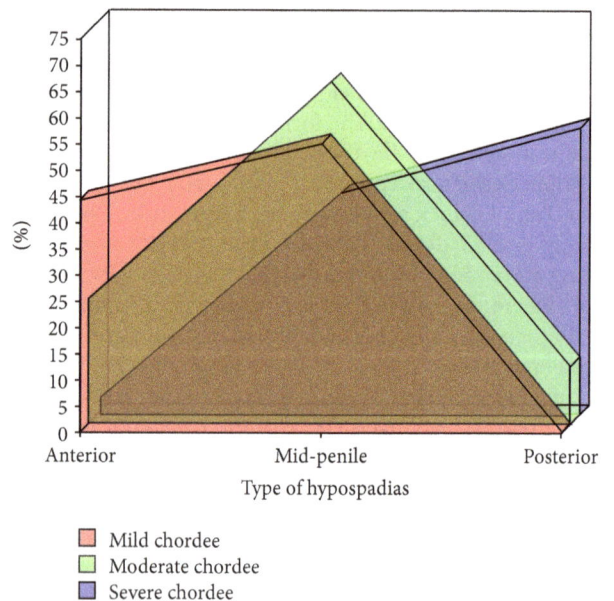

FIGURE 2: Type of hypospadias and degree of chordee.

was >60 minutes in 68.7% cases. In 90% ($n = 385$) cases the hospital stay was 3 days.

The frequency of postoperative acute complications was edema (28.3%), bleeding (4.4%), surgical site infection 4.2%, wound dehiscence (4.2%), and partial graft (1.4%) loss, which were successfully managed conservatively (Table 1).

The most common chronic complication was UCF which was initially observed in 38.8% ($n = 166$), of which 50.6% ($n = 84$) and 15.1% ($n = 25$) were managed by single surgical procedure and multiple surgical procedures, respectively. While 31.33% ($n = 52$) closed spontaneously during one to

TABLE 1: Complications for different procedures.

Procedure	Complications				Total
	Nil	Acute complications	Chronic complications	Acute and chronic	
Two-stage repair	108 (33.1%)	72 (22.1%)	82 (25.1%)	64 (19.6%)	**326**
TIPS	50 (56.2%)	12 (13.5%)	19 (21.3%)	8 (8.9%)	**89**
Mathieu's repair	1 (50%)	0 (0%)	1 (50%)	0 (0%)	**2**
MAGPAI	6 (54.54%)	0 (0%)	5 (45.45%)	0 (0%)	**11**
Total	**165**	**84**	**107**	**72**	**428**

three months postoperatively leaving the corrected frequency of UCF as 26.6%. The second most common chronic complication was meatal stenosis observed in 5.6% ($n = 24$) patients. The UCF frequency was the highest for proximal hypospadias (scrotal, penoscrotal and perineal) as projected in Table 2.

The overall complication frequencies for specialists and residents were 56.9% ($n = 161$) and 70.34% ($n = 102$) which is statistically very significant with a P value of 0.0086 with a confidence interval of 95%, calculated by Fisher's exact test (Table 3). The corrected fistula rates (excluding those which healed spontaneously) for specialists and residents were 23.32% ($n = 66$) and 33.10% ($n = 48$), respectively, which is statistically significant with a P-value of 0.0374, calculated by Fisher's exact test with a confidence interval of 95% (Table 4).

The frequencies of complications for two-stage hypospadias repair and single-stage repair were 66.9% ($n = 218$) and 44.1% ($n = 45$), respectively, which is statistically extremely significant with a P value of 0.0001, calculated by Fischer's exact test with a confidence interval of 95% (Table 5, Figure 3). The frequencies of UCF for two-stage repair and single-stage repair were 28.8% ($n = 94$) and 19.6% ($n = 20$), respectively, which is not statistically significant with P-value of 0.0728, calculated with Fischer's exact test with a confidence interval of 95% (Table 6).

4. Discussion

Hypospadias surgery is continuously evolving since its description by Celsius and Galen in the first and second centuries AD to improve suboptimal functional and cosmetic results. In spite of the achievements made in terms of establishing surgical protocols and improvements of short term results over the past 2 decades, the long term results are yet to be established. In the current study we evaluated the protocols, results, and effect modifiers of hypospadias repair at our centre.

In the current study only 1.87% and 34.6% patients were operated on in 1-2-year and 3–5-year age windows while the rest presented in ≥6 years of age. These are in contrary to the guidelines of the timing of hypospadias repair in the age of 6–18 months [4, 13]. The reason of low number of patients operated on in the 1st therapeutic window (6–18 months of age) is that we prefer hypospadias repair at preschool age (3-4 years) at our centre. The high ratio of patients presenting at age ≥6 years is due to lack of public awareness about the conditions and financial restraints.

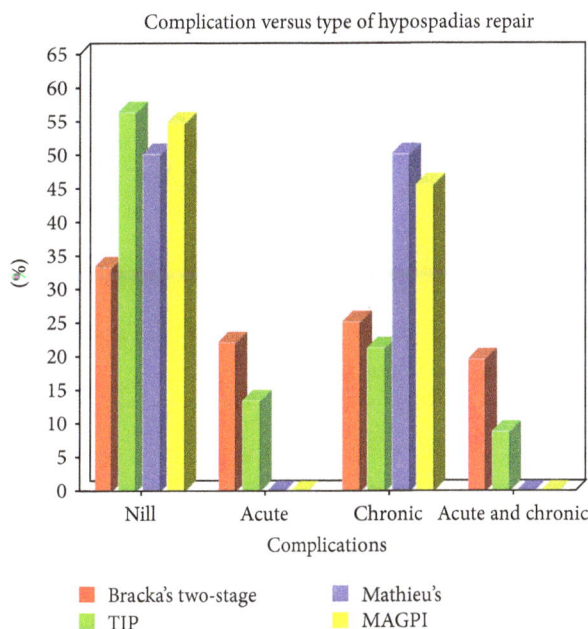

FIGURE 3: Complications versus type of hypospadias repair.

TABLE 2: Cross-tabulation of types of hypospadias and urethrocutaneous fistula.

Type of hypospadias	Urethrocutaneous fistula		Total
	Nil	Yes	
Glanular	25 (80.6%)	6 (19.4%)	**31**
Subcoronal	93 (74.4%)	32 (25.6%)	**125**
Distal penile	116 (75.8%)	37 (24.21%)	**153**
Midshaft	33 (70.2%)	14 (29.8%)	**47**
Proximal penile	6 (75%)	2 (25%)	**8**
Scrotal	1 (33.3%)	2 (66.7%)	**3**
Penoscrotal	10 (52.63%)	9 (47.34%)	**19**
Perineal	4 (66.7%)	2 (33.3%)	**6**
Crippled	26 (72.2%)	10 (27.8%)	**36**
Total	**314 (73.4%)**	**114 (26.6%)**	**428**

Of the total study population 8.6% had positive family history for hypospadias. Akin et al. [19] observed positive family history in patients with hypospadias in 26.5% cases in their study in Turkey. Abdelrahman et al. [20] also observed 12% hypospadias patients with positive family history for this condition. Biased family history due to social stigma of

TABLE 3: Cross-tabulation of complications versus level of expertise.

Level of expertise	Complications		Total
	Yes	No	
Specialists	161 (56.9%)	122 (43.11%)	**283**
Residents	102 (70.34%)	43 (29.65%)	**145**
Total	**263**	**165**	**428**

P value = 0.0086 with a confidence interval of 95%, calculated by Fisher's exact test.

TABLE 4: Level of expertise versus corrected urethrocutaneous fistula cross-tabulation.

Level of expertise	Fistula		Total
	Nil	Yes	
Specialists	217 (76.7%)	66 (23.32%)	**283**
Residents	97 (66.9%)	48 (33.10%)	**145**
Total	**314 (73.4%)**	**114 (26.6%)**	**428**

P value = 0.0374, calculated by Fisher's exact test with a confidence interval of 95%.

TABLE 5: Type of surgical procedure versus complications cross-tabulation.

Type of surgical procedure	Complications		Total
	Yes	No	
Two-stage repair	218 (66.9%)	108 (33.1%)	**326**
Single-stage repair	45 (44.1%)	57 (55.9%)	**102**
Total	**165 (38.6%)**	**263 (61.4%)**	**428**

P value = 0.0001, calculated by Fisher's exact test with a confidence interval of 95%.

TABLE 6: Type of surgical procedure versus urethrocutaneous fistula cross-tabulation.

Type of surgical procedure	Fistula		Total
	Yes	No	
Two-stage repair	94 (28.8%)	232 (71.2%)	**326**
Single-stage repair	20 (19.6%)	82 (80.4%)	**102**
Total	**114 (26.6%)**	**314 (73.4%)**	**428**

P value = 0.0728, calculated by Fisher's exact test with a confidence interval of 95%.

hypospadias may be the reason behind this low frequency familial association in our study population.

Mid-penile hypospadias was the most common type followed by anterior hypospadias. Abdelrahman et al. [20] and Prat et al. [21] reported anterior hypospadias to be the most common type in their studies. In contrary to this Wu et al. [22] observed proximal hypospadias in 65.7% of their study population in China.

Chordee was associated with 74.3% of the hypospadias of the present study population and mild chordee was the most common type. Abdelrahman et al. [20] reported similar results with positive chordee in 88% cases.

Meatal abnormalities were associated with 9.6% cases of the hypospadias in the current study.

In contrast to 2.8% patients with hypospadias associated with cryptorchidism, Akin et al. [19] reported 14.7% patients of hypospadias with cryptorchidism. Abdelrahman et al. [20] observed this positive relationship between hypospadias and

cryptorchidism in 20%. Wu et al. [22] also observed the same association in 7.3% cases.

In our study population 2.1% patients had inguinal hernia which is consistent with the results of Abdelrahman et al. [20] from Sudan who reported it in 2% of their study population. In contrast to our observations Wu WH et al. [22] observed inguinal hernia in 12.4% of hypospadias patients.

Two-stage (Bracka) repair was the most common procedure performed in 76.2% of cases. In 46.4% cases without chordee two-stage repair was performed for narrow urethral plate and incomplete glans cleft. Snodgrass' TIP was the second most common procedure performed in 20.8% cases. Abdelrahman et al. [20] performed MAGPI in most cases in their study population. Prat et al. [21] also performed single-stage procedure in most of their study population. The highest ratio of operators was the residents for two-stage repair (Bracka's). This overall high number of two-stage repairs is due to relative low expertise and awareness about single-stage procedures and relative short learning curve for two-stage repair.

The most common postoperative complication was edema observed in 28.3% cases. This high rate of postoperative edema may be due to prolonged tourniquet and inadvertent bipolar cautery use. UCF was noticed in 26.6% cases in the current study. Bhat and Mandal [23] observed UCF as the most common complication followed by edema in their PubMed literature review. Similar frequencies of UCF were reported by Chung et al. [24] in their study. Relatively lower frequency of 14.6% for UCF was observed by Huang et al. [25] in their study population. Bush et al. [26] reported UCF of 11.5% in their series of TIP repair. Snodgrass and Yucel [27] observed UCF of 33% and 10% for patients undergoing TIP with chromic catgut single layer closure and polyglactin subepithelial 2-layer closure, respectively. This relatively high frequency of UCF in our study population may be due to lack of routine use of magnification and microvascular instruments.

The overall frequency of complication and UCF was significantly higher for residents than specialist plastic surgeons which signify the long learning curve for hypospadias repair. Horowitz and Salzhauer [28] also reported results consistent with our observation about the learning curve of hypospadias repair.

The UCF frequency was higher for proximal hypospadias (penoscrotal, scrotal, and perineal) as compared to distal hypospadias which is consistent with the results of Chung et al. [24] study.

The overall frequency of complications was significantly high for two-stage repair than for single-stage repair. This may be because subjecting the patient to two surgeries 6 months apart prolongs psychological stress in the most vulnerable stage of life and cumulative donor site morbidity of the skin graft site. The two-stage repair of hypospadias also subjects patient to different operators at different level of expertise. There was no statistically significant difference noted in the frequency of UCF for single- and two-stage hypospadias repair.

To assess the long term outcome of hypospadias repair is a challenging job due to the difficulties in acquiring data.

MacNeily et al. [29] reported excellent long term functional (voiding, sexual function, psychosexual adjustment, and self-appraisal) results despite initial higher frequencies of complications with a satisfaction rate of 86%.

To improve the outcome of hypospadias management we advocated the revision of existing institutional guidelines as repair of hypospadias in the initial window of 6–18 months, mandatory use of perioperative magnification, and increasing the threshold for two-stage Bracka's repair by revising its indications as severe degree of chordee, crippled cases with residual chordee, and fibrosed narrow urethral plate not correctable with Snodgraft repair. The expertise development in problem solving with single-stage repairs of hypospadias should be encouraged to minimize the psychological trauma and postoperative complications. In view of dedication required for management of hypospadias, the culture of casual hypospadias surgery should be abandoned and hypospadiology should be developed as separate surgical subspecialty.

5. Conclusion

Hypospadias surgery has a long learning curve because it requires a great deal of temperament, surgical skill, and acquaintance with magnifications along with knowledge of surgical anatomy. The most common type of hypospadias in the current study was distal penile and most of it was associated with chordee in our set-up. The most common complications were edema and UCF with a slightly higher prevalence than the ideal frequencies. The prevalence of postoperative complications can be reduced by establishing strict guidelines as operating within the recommended therapeutic windows, use of intraoperative magnifications and microsurgical instruments, strict direct supervision while residents are operating, and switching the preference and developing skills of single-stage repairs for more proximal hypospadias, hypospadias associated with mild to moderate chordee, and crippled cases. Regular periodic audit should also be performed to improve the outcome of the hypospadias repair.

References

[1] N. Djakovic, J. Nyarangi-Dix, A. Ozturk, and M. Hohenfellner, "Hypospadias," *Advances in Urology*, vol. 2008, Article ID 650135, 7 pages, 2008.

[2] L. J. Paulozzi, J. D. Erickson, and R. J. Jackson, "Hypospadias trends in two US surveillance systems," *Pediatrics*, vol. 100, no. 5, pp. 831–834, 1997.

[3] T. Iqbal, U. Nasir, M. Khan et al., "Frequency of complication in the snodgrass repair and its risk factors," *Pakistan Journal of Surgery*, vol. 27, no. 3, pp. 188–193, 2011.

[4] A. Bhat, "General considerations in hypospadias surgery," *Indian Journal of Urology*, vol. 24, no. 2, pp. 188–194, 2008.

[5] S. L. Baskin, "Hypospadias, anatomy, embryology and reconstructive techniques," *Brazilian Journal of Urology*, vol. 26, pp. 621–629, 2000.

[6] S. Montag and L. S. Palmer, "Abnormalities of penile curvature: chordee and penile torsion," *TheScientificWorldJournal*, vol. 11, pp. 1470–1478, 2011.

[7] Y.-M. Tang, S.-J. Chen, L.-G. Huang, and M.-H. Wang, "Chordee without hypospadias: report of 79 Chinese prepubertal patients," *Journal of Andrology*, vol. 28, no. 4, pp. 630–633, 2007.

[8] G. Dipaola, M. Spalletta, T. Balducci et al., "Surgical treatment of chordee without hypospadias," *European Urology*, vol. 38, no. 6, pp. 758–761, 2000.

[9] A. T. Hadidi, *Hypospadias Surgery*, Springer, Heidelberg, Germany, 2004.

[10] Y. Hayashi and Y. Kojima, "Current concepts in hypospadias surgery," *International Journal of Urology*, vol. 15, no. 8, pp. 651–664, 2008.

[11] D. Manski, "Hypospadias: causes, diagnosis and treatment [Internet]," 2012, http://www.urology textbook.com/hypospadias.html.

[12] C. Kuschel and J. Hamill, "hypospadias [Internet]," 2005, http://www.adhb.govt.nz/newborn/Guidelines/Anomalies/Hypospadias.htm.

[13] G. Manzoni, A. Bracka, E. Palminteri, and G. Marrocco, "Hypospadias surgery: when, what and by whom?" *BJU International*, vol. 94, no. 8, pp. 1188–1195, 2004.

[14] R. A. Bologna, T. A. Noah, P. F. Nasrallah, and D. R. McMahon, "Chordee: varied opinions and treatments as documented in a survey of the American Academy of Pediatrics, Section of Urology," *Urology*, vol. 53, no. 3, pp. 608–612, 1999.

[15] A. Springer, W. Krois, and E. Horcher, "Trends in hypospadias surgery: results of a worldwide survey," *European Urology*, vol. 60, no. 6, pp. 1184–1189, 2011.

[16] G. Mingin and L. S. Baskin, "Management of chordee in children and young adults," *Urologic Clinics of North America*, vol. 29, no. 2, pp. 277–284, 2002.

[17] A. Atala, "Recent developments in tissue engineering and regenerative medicine," *Current Opinion in Pediatrics*, vol. 18, no. 2, pp. 167–171, 2006.

[18] T. G. Kwon, J. J. Yoo, and A. Atala, "Autologous penile corpora cavernosa replacement using tissue engineering techniques," *Journal of Urology*, vol. 168, no. 4, pp. 1754–1758, 2002.

[19] Y. Akin, O. Ercan, B. Telatar, F. Tarhan, and S. Comert, "Hypospadias in Istanbul: incidence and risk factors," *Pediatrics International*, vol. 53, no. 5, pp. 754–760, 2011.

[20] M. Y. H. Abdelrahman, I. A. Abdeljaleel, E. Mohamed, A.-T. O. Bagadi, and O. E. M. Khair, "Hypospadias in Sudan, clinical and surgical review," *African Journal of Paediatric Surgery*, vol. 8, no. 3, pp. 269–271, 2011.

[21] D. Prat, A. Natasha, A. Polak et al., "Surgical outcome of different types of primary hypospadias repair during three decades in a single center," *Urology*, vol. 79, no. 6, pp. 1350–1354, 2012.

[22] W.-H. Wu, J.-H. Chuang, Y.-C. Ting, S.-Y. Lee, and C.-S. Hsieh, "Developmental anomalies and disabilities associated with hypospadias," *Journal of Urology*, vol. 168, no. 1, pp. 229–232, 2002.

[23] A. Bhat and A. K. Mandal, "Acute postoperative complications of hypospadias repair," *Indian Journal of Urology*, vol. 24, no. 2, pp. 241–248, 2008.

[24] J. W. Chung, S. H. Choi, B. S. Kim, and S. K. Chung, "Risk factors for the development of urethrocutaneous fistula after hypospadias repair: a retrospective study," *Korean Journal of Urology*, vol. 53, no. 10, pp. 711–715, 2012.

[25] L. Huang, Y. Tang, M. Wang, and S. Chen, "Tubularized incised plate urethroplasty for hypospadias in children," *Zhongguo Xiu Fu Chong Jian Wai Ke Za Zhi*, vol. 20, no. 3, pp. 226–228, 2006.

[26] N. C. Bush, M. Holzer, S. Zhang, and W. Snodgrass, "Age does not impact risk for urethroplasty complications after tubularized incised plate repair of hypospadias in prepubertal boys," *Journal of Pediatric Urology*, vol. 9, no. 3, pp. 252–256, 2013.

[27] W. Snodgrass and S. Yucel, "Tubularized incised plate for mid shaft and proximal hypospadias repair," *Journal of Urology*, vol. 177, no. 2, pp. 698–702, 2007.

[28] M. Horowitz and E. Salzhauer, "The "learning curve" in hypospadias surgery," *BJU International*, vol. 97, no. 3, pp. 593–596, 2006.

[29] A. E. MacNeily, C. C. Hoag, G. T. Gotto, K. B. Morrison, and G. U. Coleman, "Long-term functional outcome and satisfaction of patients with hypospadias repaired in childhood," *Journal of the Canadian Urological Association*, vol. 2, no. 1, pp. 23–31, 2008.

10

Free Flap Transfer to Preserve Main Arterial Flow in Early Reconstruction of Open Fracture in the Lower Extremity

Mitsuru Nemoto, Shinsuke Ishikawa, Natsuko Kounoike,
Takayuki Sugimoto, and Akira Takeda

Department of Plastic and Reconstructive Surgery, Kitasato University Hospital, 1-15-1 Kitasato, Minami-ku, Sagamihara,
Kanagawa 252-0374, Japan

Correspondence should be addressed to Mitsuru Nemoto; mnemoto@med.kitasato-u.ac.jp

Academic Editor: Nicolo Scuderi

The selection of recipient vessels is crucial when reconstructing traumatized lower extremities using a free flap. When the dorsalis pedis artery and/or posterior tibial artery cannot be palpated, we utilize computed tomography angiography to verify the site of vascular injury prior to performing free flap transfer. For vascular anastomosis, we fundamentally perform end-to-side anastomosis or flow-through anastomosis to preserve the main arterial flow. In addition, in open fracture of the lower extremity, we utilize the anterolateral thigh flap for moderate soft tissue defects and the latissimus dorsi musculocutaneous flap for extensive soft tissue defects. The free flaps used in these two techniques are long and include a large-caliber pedicle, and reconstruction can be performed with either the anterior or posterior tibial artery. The preparation of recipient vessels is easier during the acute phase early after injury, when there is no influence of scarring. A free flap allows flow-through anastomosis and is thus optimal for open fracture of the lower extremity that requires simultaneous reconstruction of main vessel injury and soft tissue defect from the middle to distal thirds of the lower extremity.

1. Introduction

Reconstruction of a traumatized lower extremity using a free flap carries a greater risk of developing complications compared to reconstruction of other sites [1–4]. Many investigators have reported the importance of selecting an appropriate recipient vessel when reconstructing the lower extremity by free flap transfer [5–7]. To enhance the success rate of free flap transfer in open fractures of the lower extremity, anastomosis with healthy recipient vessels that have not been affected by the trauma must be performed. Chen et al. [8] recommended using the posterior tibial artery as the recipient vessel, since the anterior tibial artery is injured more frequently than the posterior tibial artery in open fracture of the lower extremity. Several investigators have performed vascular anastomosis distal to the zone of injury, since main vessels in the distal third of the lower extremity pass through a superficial layer [9, 10]. Kolker et al. [11] reported no differences in operative outcomes between use of vascular anastomosis proximal or distal to the zone of injury.

This retrospective study examined recipient vessels and vascular anastomosis techniques in 18 consecutive patients who underwent free flap transfer at an early stage after suffering open fracture of the lower extremity.

2. Patients and Methods

We performed free flap transfer within 1 week after injury in 18 consecutive patients (15 men and 3 women) who suffered Gustilo type IIIB open fracture of the lower extremity between January 2002 and December 2008. Mean age at the time of surgery was 31.9 years (range, 18–58 years). The causes of injury were a traffic accident in 15 cases and an occupational accident in 3 cases. Data on fracture site, transferred flaps, vessels selected for anastomosis, anastomosis techniques, and postoperative complications were obtained

TABLE 1: Patients summary.

Number	Age	Sex	Fracture site	Free flap	Recipient artery	Anastomotic type	Complications	Result	Comments
1	51	M	Distal	ALT	Anterior tibial a.	Flow-through		Successful	
2	53	M	Distal	ALT	Posterior tibial a.	Flow-through		Successful	
3	31	M	Middle	ALT	Anterior tibial a.	Flow-through		Successful	
4	21	M	Distal	ALT	Anterior tibial a.	Flow-through		Successful	
5	18	M	Proximal	ALT	Medial inferior genicular a.	End-to-end		Successful	
6	34	F	Middle	ALT	Posterior tibial a.	End-to-side	Congestion	Reexploration	Survival
7	25	M	Middle	ALT	Anterior tibial a.	End-to-side		Successful	
8	58	F	Middle	ALT	Anterior tibial a.	Flow-through		Successful	
9	50	M	Middle	LD	Posterior tibial a.	End-to-side		Successful	
10	22	M	Distal	ALT	Anterior tibial a.	Flow-through		Successful	
11	19	M	Distal	ALT	Posterior tibial a.	Flow-through		Successful	
12	33	M	Middle	LD	Anterior tibial a.	Flow-through		Successful	
13	24	M	Middle	LD	Anterior tibial a.	Flow-through		Successful	
14	32	M	Distal	ALT	Posterior tibial a.	End-to-side		Successful	
15	30	M	Proximal	LD	Popliteal a.	End-to-side	Deep infection	Debridement	Survival
16	22	M	Distal	ALT	Posterior tibial a.	Flow-through	Congestion	Reexploration	Survival
17	21	M	Middle	ALT	Anterior tibial a.	Flow-through		Successful	
18	30	F	Middle	LD	Anterior tibial a.	Flow-through		Successful	

ALT: anterolateral thigh flap, LD: latissimus dorsi musculocutaneous flap.

from medical records. Mean duration of follow-up was 41 months (range, 7–86 months).

3. Results

The fracture sites were the proximal third of the lower extremity in 2 cases, the middle third of the lower extremity in 7, and the distal third of the lower extremity in 9. The transferred free flaps were an anterolateral thigh flap in 13 cases and a latissimus dorsi musculocutaneous flap in 5. The anastomosed recipient arteries were the anterior tibial artery in 10 cases, the posterior tibial artery in 6, the popliteal artery in 1, and the superior medial genicular artery in 1.

The vascular anastomosis techniques used were flow-through anastomosis in 12 cases, end-to-side anastomosis in 5, and end-to-end anastomosis in 1. Postoperative complications were congestion due to thrombosis in 2 patients who subsequently underwent reexploration and deep infection that subsided with additional debridement in 1 patient. Free flaps survived in all patients, including the 3 patients who underwent reoperation (Table 1).

4. Case Reports

4.1. Case 1. A 58-year-old woman suffered open fracture injury to the lower right extremity in a traffic accident. On the day of injury, debridement and external fixation of the open fracture of the lower extremity were performed. On day 6 after injury, reconstruction was performed using intramedullary fixation and a free anterolateral thigh flap. On preoperative medical examination, the dorsalis pedis artery and posterior tibial artery were palpable. In surgery, the anterior tibial artery was carefully dissected to confirm

the absence of injury. End-to-side anastomoses of the lateral circumflex femoral artery and anterior tibial artery with the anterolateral thigh flap were performed to preserve arterial blood flow. The anterolateral thigh flap survived without postoperative complications (Figure 1).

4.2. Case 2. A 21-year-old man suffered open fracture injury to the lower right extremity in an occupational accident at a construction site. At the initial surgery, debridement and external fixation were performed. Two days later, open fracture of the lower right extremity was reconstructed with intramedullary fixation and free anterolateral thigh flap. Since the anterior tibial artery had been injured in the open fracture of the lower right extremity, the anterior tibial artery was reconstructed by interposing the lateral circumflex femoral artery of the anterolateral thigh flap. Lateral circumflex femoral veins were anastomosed with the concomitant and great saphenous veins using end-to-end anastomosis. The anterolateral thigh flap survived without postoperative complications. Four months after injury, autologous bone grafting was performed for the bone defect in the open fracture of the lower extremity. Bone union was achieved by 18 months after injury, and the patient has since returned to his original occupation (Figure 2).

5. Discussion

The selection of recipient vessels is crucial when reconstructing traumatized lower extremities with free flap. Since the anterior tibial artery is prone to injury in lower extremity trauma, the posterior tibial artery is often selected as the recipient vessel [8]. For recipient vessel selection, in

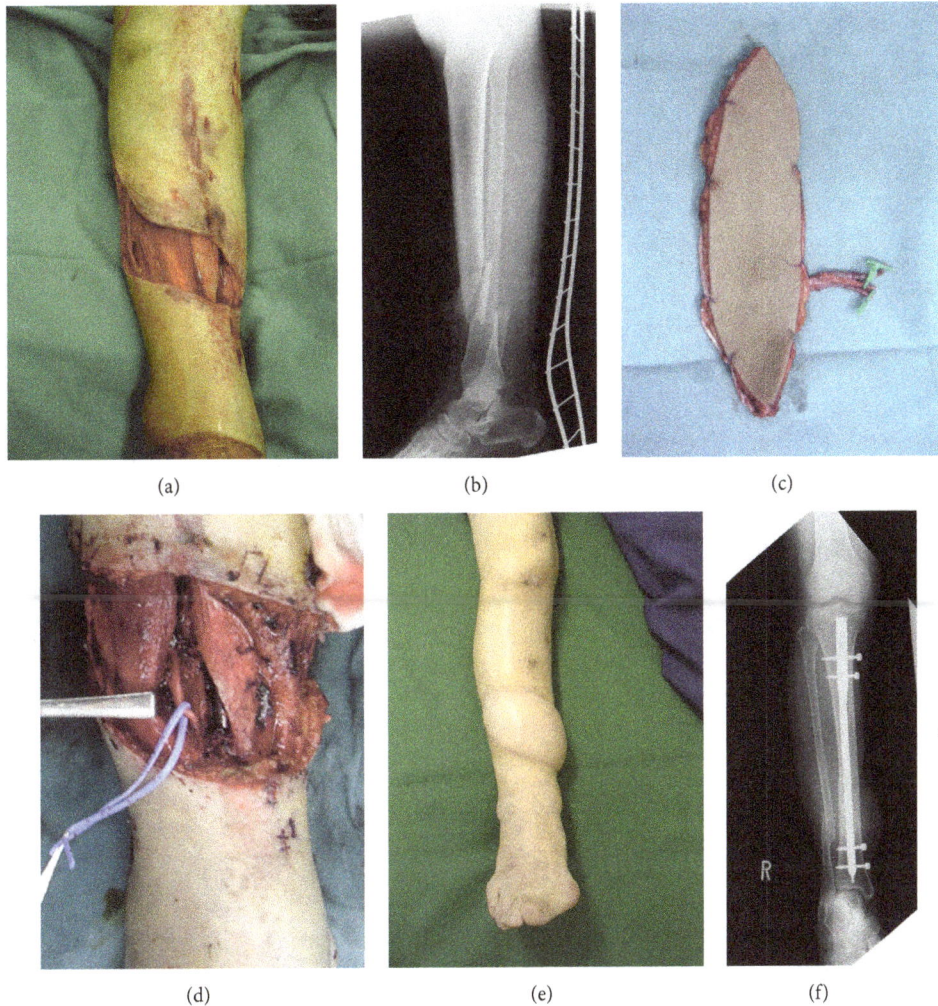

FIGURE 1: (a) Open fracture of the lower extremity is accompanied by an moderate soft tissue defect on the anterior lower extremity. (b) X-ray findings. (c) Anterolateral thigh flap harvested from the same side. (d) The anterior tibial artery was selected for end-to-side anastomosis. (e) Appearance at 7 months postoperatively. (f) X-ray findings at 7 months postoperatively, showing bone union.

addition to intraoperative examination, preoperative palpation, Doppler flowmetry, and angiography were conducted. Isenberg and Sherman [12] reported that if no problems are seen with the dorsalis pedis artery and posterior tibial artery based on palpation, Doppler flowmetry, and Allen's test, preoperative angiography is unnecessary. Lutz et al. [13] also indicated that preoperative angiography should be applied only when pedal pulses of both the dorsalis pedis and posterior tibial arteries are not palpable and that routine preoperative angiography is unnecessary. On the other hand, Duymaz et al. [14] recommended computed tomography angiography as the first-stage diagnostic procedure, as this method is superior for visualizing the hemodynamics of the traumatized lower extremity. When the dorsalis pedis artery and/or posterior tibial artery are not palpable, we conduct computed tomography angiography to confirm the vascular injury site prior to free flap transfer.

The anterior lower extremity is often injured in open fracture of the lower extremity, and recipient vessels pass through a deeper layer in parts more proximal to the zone of injury, making vascular anastomosis increasingly difficult. For this reason, Stompro and Stevenson [9] conducted free flap transfer with distally based anastomosis for surgery performed in the distal third of the lower extremity, where recipient vessels pass through the superficial layer. Minami et al. [10] also stated that distally based anastomosis is useful in reconstruction of the anterior lower extremity with free flap transfer. Kolker et al. [11] reported that the outcomes of free flap transfer do not differ between distal and proximal anastomosis, stating that distal anastomosis is appropriate when proper hemodynamics are maintained in the zone of injury.

Godina et al. [15] reported a posterior approach to the recipient vessels. Specifically, they described the usefulness of the posterior approach, which can ensure a sufficient surgical field of view and healthy recipient vessels. Park and Eom [16] recommended the superior medial genicular vessels and descending genicular vessels as recipient vessels around the knee. In the two patients who suffered fracture in the proximal third of the lower extremity, recipient arteries were

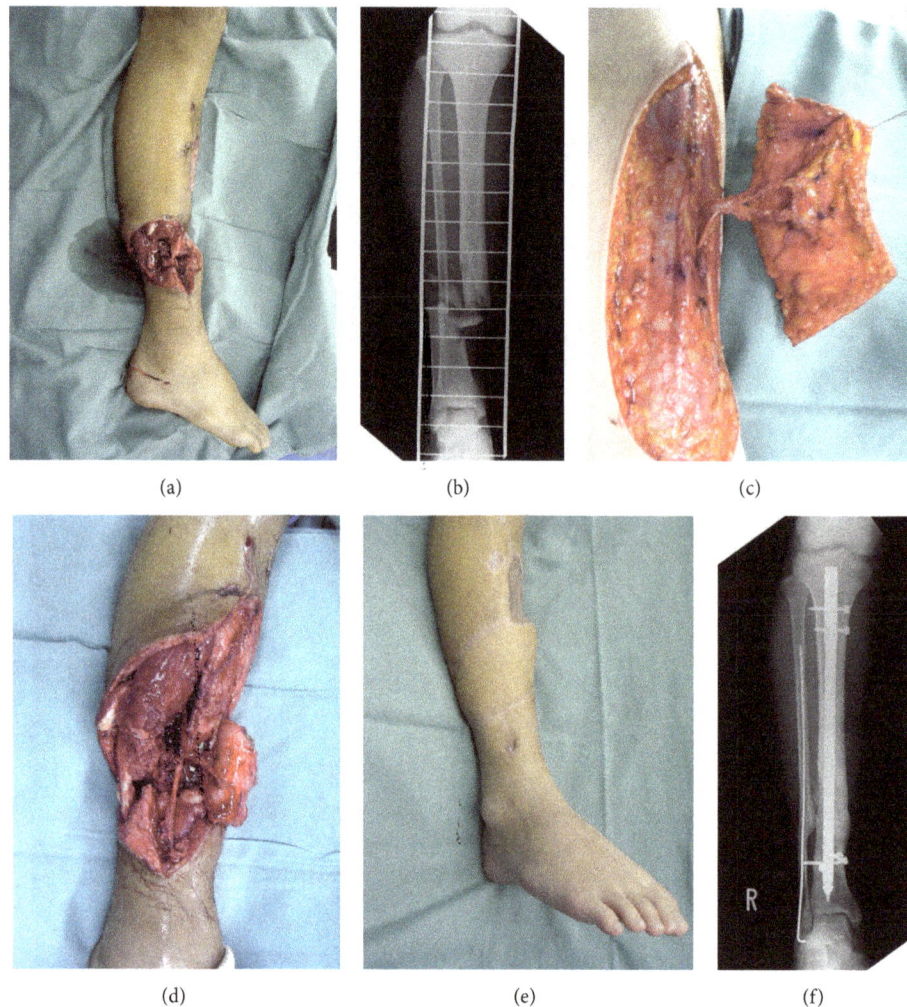

FIGURE 2: (a) Open fracture is located in the distal third of the lower extremity, accompanied by injury to the anterior tibial artery. (b) X-ray findings. The open fracture is accompanied by a bone defect. (c) The flow-through type anterolateral thigh flap harvested from the same side. (d) The anterior tibial artery is reconstructed by flow-through anastomosis with the lateral circumflex femoral artery. (e) Appearance at 18 months postoperatively. (f) X-ray findings at 18 months postoperatively, showing that union of the bone defect occurred after autologous bone grafting.

the superior medial genicular artery in 1 patient and the popliteal artery via a posterior approach in the other patient. Only a few recipient vessels around the knee are available for free flap transfers from the proximal third of the lower extremity, and both arteries have proven useful as recipient arteries.

For vascular anastomosis, to preserve the main arterial flow, we fundamentally perform end-to-side anastomosis or flow-through anastomosis. Various outcomes of end-to-side anastomosis have been reported [2, 9, 17, 18]. Godina [17] reported favorable outcomes from end-to-side anastomosis. However, Khouri and Shaw [2] reported that end-to-side anastomosis is prone to thrombosis. Samaha et al. [7] demonstrated a lack of differences in outcomes between end-to-end anastomosis and end-to-side anastomosis and reported that outcomes are influenced by recipient vessel selection and the condition of blood perfusion from distal areas.

To preserve main arterial flow in open fracture of the lower extremity, we perform end-to-side anastomosis if no obvious injuries to the main artery are present and flow-through anastomosis whenever possible if the fracture is accompanied by injuries to the main artery. Koshima et al. [19] reported several advantages of flow-through anastomosis, indicating that the damaged main vessels can be reconstructed simultaneously with large skin defects, while double artery inflow using both ends of the pedicle artery ensures safe blood circulation in the flap, and two concomitant pedicle veins interposed into the damaged recipient concomitant veins can be used as a drainage system in extremities with severe edema. We perform flow-through anastomosis using lateral circumflex femoral vessels of the anterolateral thigh flap and thoracodorsal vessels of the latissimus dorsi musculocutaneous flap. In the acute phase when the influences of scarring are absent, the dissection is relatively easy even in the anterior tibial artery, which is highly likely to be injured. We, therefore, performed anterior tibial artery reconstruction with flow-through anastomosis as much as possible. Free flap with flow-through anastomosis fundamentally entails a flap with stable blood flow. Although 1 patient who underwent flow-through type anterolateral thigh flap developed partial congestion, the flap ultimately survived reexploration. Free flap transfer with flow-through anastomosis does not cause vascular insufficiency as long as the surgery is performed meticulously and the proper recipient vessels are selected. When the dorsal pedis and the posterior tibial arteries are palpable, a flow-through anastomosis is not indicated.

With an open fracture of the lower extremity, we utilize an anterolateral thigh flap with the pedicle descending branch of the lateral femoral circumflex artery for the moderate soft tissue defect and the latissimus dorsi musculocutaneous flap with the pedicle thoracodorsal artery and the serratus branch for the extensive soft tissue defect. These two techniques are long and include a large-caliber pedicle, and reconstruction can be performed with either the anterior or posterior tibial artery. Preparation of recipient vessels is easier during the acute phase when the influences of scarring have not yet manifested. Free flap, which allows flow-through anastomosis, is thus optimal for simultaneous reconstruction of the main vessel injury and soft tissue defect from the middle to distal thirds of the lower extremity.

6. Conclusions

When injury to the anterior or posterior tibial artery is suspected in open fracture of the lower extremity, we perform computed tomography angiography to evaluate the arterial injury. In open fracture of the lower extremity without arterial injury, we perform free flap transfer with end-to-side anastomosis to preserve the main vessels. When the arterial injury is present from the middle to distal thirds of the lower extremity in open fracture of the lower extremity, we perform free flap transfer with flow-through anastomosis as much as possible. Free flap transfer with flow-through anastomosis is a useful method that can simultaneously reconstruct soft tissue defects and the main artery.

References

[1] T. Harashina, "Analysis of 200 free flaps," *British Journal of Plastic Surgery*, vol. 41, no. 1, pp. 33–36, 1988.

[2] R. Khouri and W. W. Shaw, "Reconstruction of the lower extremity with microvascular free flaps: a 10-year experience with 304 consecutive cases," *Journal of Trauma*, vol. 29, no. 8, pp. 1086–1094, 1989.

[3] E. G. Melissinos and D. H. Parks, "Post-trauma reconstruction with free tissue transfer: analysis of 442 consecutive cases," *Journal of Trauma*, vol. 29, no. 8, pp. 1095–1103, 1989.

[4] R. K. Khouri, "Avoiding free flap failure," *Clinics in Plastic Surgery*, vol. 19, no. 4, pp. 773–781, 1992.

[5] R. D. Acland, "Refinements in lower extremity free flap surgery," *Clinics in Plastic Surgery*, vol. 17, no. 4, pp. 733–744, 1990.

[6] J. A. Goldberg, B. S. Alpert, W. C. Lineaweaver, and H. J. Buncke, "Microvascular reconstruction of the lower extremity in the elderly," *Clinics in Plastic Surgery*, vol. 18, no. 3, pp. 459–465, 1991.

[7] F. J. Samaha, A. Oliva, G. M. Buncke, H. J. Buncke, and P. P. Siko, "A clinical study of end-to-end versus end-to-side techniques for microvascular anastomosis," *Plastic and Reconstructive Surgery*, vol. 99, no. 4, pp. 1109–1111, 1997.

[8] H.-C. Chen, C.-C. Chuang, S. Chen, W.-M. Hsu, and F.-C. Wei, "Selection of recipient vessels for free flaps to the distal leg and foot following trauma," *Microsurgery*, vol. 15, no. 5, pp. 358–363, 1994.

[9] B. E. Stompro and T. R. Stevenson, "Reconstruction of the traumatized leg: use of distally based free flaps," *Plastic and Reconstructive Surgery*, vol. 93, no. 5, pp. 1021–1027, 1994.

[10] A. Minami, H. Kato, N. Suenaga, and N. Iwasaki, "Distally-based free vascularized tissue grafts in the lower leg," *Journal of Reconstructive Microsurgery*, vol. 15, no. 7, pp. 495–499, 1999.

[11] A. R. Kolker, A. K. Kasabian, N. S. Karp, and J. J. Gottlieb, "Fate of free flap microanastomosis distal to the zone of injury in lower extremity trauma," *Plastic and Reconstructive Surgery*, vol. 99, no. 4, pp. 1068–1073, 1997.

[12] J. S. Isenberg and R. Sherman, "The limited value of preoperative angiography in microsurgical reconstruction of the lower limb," *Journal of Reconstructive Microsurgery*, vol. 12, no. 5, pp. 303–306, 1996.

[13] B. S. Lutz, F.-C. Wei, H.-G. Machens, U. Rhode, and A. Berger, "Indications and limitations of angiography before free-flap transplantation to the distal lower leg after trauma: prospective study in 36 patients," *Journal of Reconstructive Microsurgery*, vol. 16, no. 3, pp. 187–192, 2000.

[14] A. Duymaz, F. E. Karabekmez, T. J. Vrtiska, S. Mardini, and S. L. Moran, "Free tissue transfer for lower extremity reconstruction: a study of the role of computed angiography in the planning of free tissue transfer in the posttraumatic setting," *Plastic and Reconstructive Surgery*, vol. 124, no. 2, pp. 523–529, 2009.

[15] M. Godina, Z. M. Arnez, and G. D. Lister, "Preferential use of the posterior approach to blood vessels of the lower leg in microvascular surgery," *Plastic and Reconstructive Surgery*, vol. 88, no. 2, pp. 287–291, 1991.

[16] S. Park and J. S. Eom, "Selection of the recipient vessel in the free flap around the knee: the superior medial genicular vessels and the descending genicular vessels," *Plastic and Reconstructive Surgery*, vol. 107, no. 5, pp. 1177–1182, 2001.

[17] M. Godina, "Preferential use of end-to-side arterial anastomoses in free flap transfers," *Plastic and Reconstructive Surgery*, vol. 64, no. 5, pp. 673–682, 1979.

[18] J. L. Frodel, R. Trachy, and C. W. Cummings, "End-to-end and end-to-side microvascular anastomoses: a comparative study," *Microsurgery*, vol. 7, no. 3, pp. 117–123, 1986.

[19] I. Koshima, S. Kawada, H. Etoh, S. Kawamura, T. Moriguchi, and H. Sonoh, "Flow-through anterior thigh flaps for one-stage reconstruction of soft-tissue defects and revascularization of ischemic extremities," *Plastic and Reconstructive Surgery*, vol. 95, no. 2, pp. 252–260, 1995.

11

Funding for Postbariatric Body-Contouring (Bariplastic) Surgery in England: A Postcode Lottery

Samrat Mukherjee,[1] Sachin Kamat,[1] Samuel Adegbola,[1] and Sanjay Agrawal[1,2]

[1] *Bariatric Surgery Unit, Homerton University Hospital, Homerton Row, Homerton, London E9 6SR, UK*
[2] *Centre for Digestive Diseases, Blizard Institute, Queen Mary University of London, London E1 2AT, UK*

Correspondence should be addressed to Sanjay Agrawal; sanju_agrawal@hotmail.com

Academic Editor: Bishara S. Atiyeh

Background. With the increase in bariatric surgery in the UK, there has been a substantial increase in patients undergoing massive weight loss (MWL) seeking postbariatric body-contouring (bariplastic) surgery. However, there is a wide variation of availability on the National Health Service (NHS). *Aims.* To (1) review the funding policies of Primary Care Trusts (PCTs) in England for bariplastic surgery and (2) analyse the number of procedures funded in two consecutive financial years. *Methods.* We sent out questionnaires to all PCTs in England regarding their funding policies for bariplastic surgery and requested the number of procedures funded in 2008-09 and 2009-10. *Findings.* 121/147 (82%) PCTs replied to our questionnaires. 73 (60%) excluded all bariplastic procedures. 106/121 (87.6%) PCTs had referral guidelines for plastic surgery. 46/121 (38%) PCTs provided the total number of funded abdominoplasty-apronectomy (A-A) in the two financial years: total number of A-A applicants rose from 393 to 531, but approval for funding fell from 24.2% to 19.6%. Only 3 (2%) PCTs indicated increase in their future spending on bariplastic procedures in the next 5 years, with 67% planning to decrease or unsure about future funding. *Conclusion.* There exists a postcode lottery for bariplastic surgery in England and we feel the need for guidelines on provision of bariplastic procedures following MWL.

1. Introduction

Paralleling the increasing prevalence of obesity, there has been an exponential rise in bariatric surgery worldwide. A recent report showed a 70% rise in bariatric procedures in England in 2009-10 compared to 2008-09 [1]. Following bariatric surgery, most patients lose about 60–70% of their excess body weight in the initial 2 years. However, their skin does not contract with this massive weight loss (MWL) [2]. It often leads to disheartening ptotic skin envelopes which cause intertriginous infections, struggles with hygiene, impairment of mobility, interference with sexual intimacy, and personal distress because of appearance. These often lead to psychosocial problems which negatively affect the patients' quality of life [3] and may also hamper further weight loss or even lead to weight regain [4]. The term "bariplastic surgery" was proposed by Joseph O'Connell to encompass all body contouring procedures after bariatric surgery like apronectomy, abdominoplasty, mastopexy, brachioplasty, and buttock and thigh lift [5]. It resides at a perplexing intersection between cosmetic and functional surgery. Bariplastic surgery addresses the problems of redundant skin and has also shown to improve the quality of life and body image in these unique subgroup of patients [6–8].

In England, the National Health Service (NHS) is a publicly funded healthcare system and treatment on the NHS is free of cost at the point of delivery, but spending is presently controlled by the Primary Care Trusts (PCTs). Each PCT serves patients within a defined geographical area and decides independently how to allocate its budget. Bariplastic surgery is often regarded by the PCT as cosmetic and therefore of low priority, which means funding is either unavailable or subject to various criteria as determined by the PCT. In this age of economic constraints and rationing within the modern NHS, it is widely acknowledged that such treatments would be less available to patients on the NHS. As the PCTs make these difficult decisions independently of each other, treatments that are available in one trust may not be available in another.

The "Action on Plastic Surgery" (AoPS) document was produced by the NHS Modernisation Agency in 2005 (in association with the British Association of Plastic, Reconstructive and Aesthetic Surgeons, BAPRAS) [9]. This document provides guidance for commissioners of plastic surgery services regarding explicit criteria for referral and treatment thresholds for plastic surgical procedures that should be available on the NHS (Index 1).

Index 1. (AoPS guidance on who should be offered abdomino-plasty-apronectomy (A-A)).

AoPS recommends that A-A may be offered to the following groups of people:

(i) those who are undergoing treatment for morbid obesity and have excessive skin folds,

(ii) previously obese patients who have achieved significant weight loss and have maintained their weight loss for at least two years,

(iii) stable BMI between 18 and 27 Kg/m^2,

and

(iv) suffering from severe functional problems with the following:

(a) recurrent intertrigo between the skin folds,

(b) activities of daily living, for example, ambulatory problems,

(c) surgical scarring leading to poor appearance and resulting in disabling psychological distress,

(d) poorly fitting stoma bags.

The aims of this study were (1) to review the funding policies of PCTs in England for bariplastic surgery; (2) to evaluate the degree to which the AoPS guidelines are followed; and (3) to look at the total number of bariplastic procedures funded in England in the two consecutive financial years, 2008-09 and 2009-10. We also asked PCTs about their plans for expenditure on bariplastic surgery in the next 5 years. This study is the first comprehensive review of funding policies for bariplastic surgery in England.

2. Methods

We sent out a detailed questionnaire electronically to all 147 PCTs in England asking about their funding criteria for bariplastic surgery and whether they used the AoPS guidelines while drafting their policies. We also asked for the number of bariplastic procedures being funded in the two consecutive financial years, 2008-09 and 2009-10. We requested information on abdominoplasty, breast reduction and augmentation, facelift, and buttock, arm, and thigh lift postbariatric surgery (see the Supplementary Material available online at http://dx.doi.org/10.1155/2014/153194).

Many PCTs were part of regional groups that had been established to develop and manage policies such as funding criteria. Where a reply clearly represented a group policy, its data was applied to all PCTs in that group. In the cases where

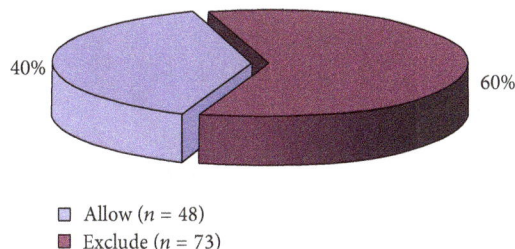

FIGURE 1: Pie chart showing the proportions of Primary Care Trusts ($n = 121$) that allow or exclude bariplastic surgery on the National Health Service.

a PCT replied with its own policy and also was part of a group, its own policy was recorded.

PCTs that did not respond by 8 weeks were followed up with reminder emails and also by telephone wherever possible. The freedom of information act (2000) (FOI) was used where the information was withheld. The data was collected over ten months, from February to November 2011. Data was collated and analysed on Microsoft Excel spreadsheet.

3. Results

Out of 147 PCTs, responses were received from 121 (82.3%) PCTs. 4 PCTs acknowledged our request but refused to use the FOI to provide us with the data.

Of the 121 PCTs, 48 (40%) PCTs fund bariplastic surgery on the NHS. The remaining 73 (60%) PCTs excluded all bariplastic surgery (Figure 1). Of these, 67 PCTs included a disclaimer for "exceptional circumstances" (EC); that is, individual patients could apply for "exceptional" funding and be considered for these procedures even if their guidelines excluded them from that particular treatment. The remaining 6 PCTs do not fund bariplastic procedures under any circumstances.

106 out of 121 (87.6%) PCTs had a guideline for plastic surgery procedures. Of these, 5 PCTs (4.7%) followed the AoPS guidelines exactly and 46 PCTs (43.4%) had guidelines similar to it. Of the rest, 25 PCTs (23.6%) had their own guidelines that did not match the AoPS and 30 PCTs (28.3%) were unsure or did not specify in the reply whether they followed the AoPS (Figure 2).

The AoPS guidelines mention 27 Kg/m^2 as the upper limit of BMI for abdominoplasty-apronectomy (A-A). Of the 106 PCTs which had guidelines for A-A, 79/106 (74.5%) had specific body mass index (BMI) targets, ranging from 25 Kg/m^2 to 30 Kg/m^2, which the patient needed to achieve to be eligible for the procedure (Figure 3). Only 8/106 (7.6%) PCTs acknowledged the fact that, in the postbariatric surgery patients, it is difficult to attain the target BMI, because of the weight of the apron itself, and have put in a criterion of 50% excess weight loss to be eligible for A-A. The AoPS guidelines mention that the patients should have maintained their weight loss for at least 2 years following MWL. 62/106 (58.5%) PCTs required the weight loss to be maintained for a duration ranging from 6 months to 2 years before undergoing

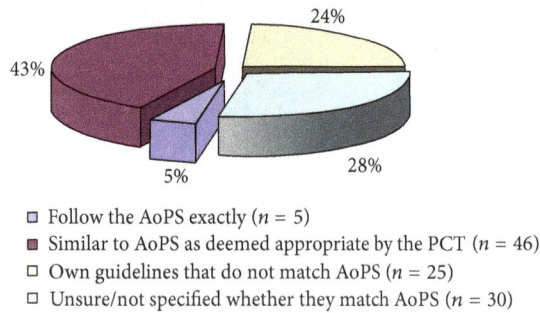

- ▫ Follow the AoPS exactly ($n = 5$)
- ▪ Similar to AoPS as deemed appropriate by the PCT ($n = 46$)
- ▫ Own guidelines that do not match AoPS ($n = 25$)
- ▫ Unsure/not specified whether they match AoPS ($n = 30$)

FIGURE 2: Pie chart showing the proportion of Primary Care Trusts ($n = 106$) having guidelines for plastic surgery procedures. AoPS is "Action on Plastic Surgery" document.

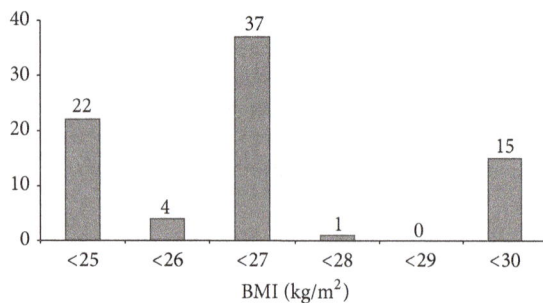

FIGURE 4: Chart showing length of time the Primary Care Trusts (PCTs) ($n = 62$) required patients to maintain their weight loss before being eligible for abdominoplasty-apronectomy. y-axis is the number of PCTs.

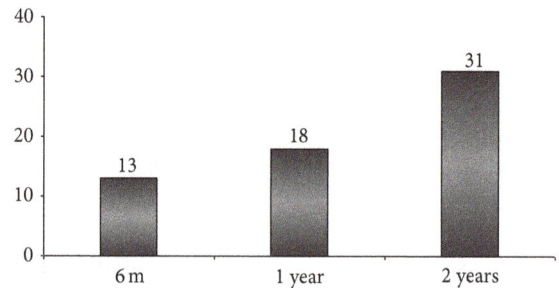

FIGURE 3: Chart showing specific body mass index (BMI) targets set by Primary Care Trusts (PCTs) ($n = 79$) that must be reached by patients seeking abdominoplasty-apronectomy. y-axis is the number of PCTs. The AoPS recommends a BMI < 27 Kg/m^2.

4. Discussion

There is very little in the literature on the prevalence of bariplastic surgery after bariatric surgery. According to a study by Mitchell et al. 33, out of 70 (47%) patients underwent bariplastic procedures after gastric bypass surgery [10]. Gusenoff et al. reported 11.3% of their 926 patients undergoing a body contouring procedure after gastric bypass [11]. A similar study from Austria suggested 21% of 252 patients had undergone body contouring surgery at least 1 year after gastric bypass surgery [12]. Assuming a conservative estimate of 20% needing bariplastic surgery, there would be a need for commissioning of more than 1600 body-contouring procedures in 2012-13 based on 8000 bariatric surgeries performed in the year 2010-11 in the UK [13]. This means large numbers of MWL patients will present for bariplastic surgery in the coming years.

Despite successful weight loss following bariatric surgery, the patients' body image and psychological state may actually deteriorate following the soft tissue deflation noted with MWL [3, 14]. Bariplastic surgery has been shown to improve the quality of life and body image of patients who have undergone MWL and optimize results achieved from bariatric surgery [6–8, 15]. As with burn surgery or cancer reconstruction, the body contouring procedures should be viewed as aesthetic as well as functional procedures. However, its role is still underestimated and often viewed as a cosmetic adjunct to bariatric surgery by the funding bodies [11].

The PCTs act independently of each other while drawing up their guidelines for the purposes of rationing. This leads to variability in funding for procedures in different regions within the NHS. Wraight et al., in 2007, showed a variation in guidelines across Trusts in the UK, amounting to a "postcode lottery" for patients seeking breast reduction [16]. More recent work by Henderson in 2009 [17] and Goodson et al. in 2011 [18] has shown that there does exist a disparity between PCTs for plastic surgery procedures, despite national guidelines. This has also been demonstrated for in vitro fertilisation (IVF) treatment in a report in 2009 [19]. In our study, 73/121 (60%) PCTs excluded all bariplastic procedures. It is also evident from our survey that majority (101/106, 95.3%) of PCTs have their own guidelines and individual cut-off points for referrals leading to a postcode lottery for

bariplastic surgery. This is summarised in Figure 4. The remaining 44 PCTs did not specify any timescale criteria.

75/106 (70.7%) PCTs specifically required the patients to have functional problems in the form of ambulatory difficulties, and 51/106 (48.1%) PCTs required the patients to have troublesome intertrigo, refractory to medical treatment from a period ranging from 6 weeks to 1 year. 8/106 (7.5%) PCTs required the abdominal apron to hang below the symphysis pubis and 9 (8.5%) required the patients to stop smoking to be allowed the A-A. Specific conditions imposed by the PCTs are shown in Figure 5.

The most common bariplastic procedure performed was A-A. The PCTs did not provide analyzable data on the other bariplastic procedures like mastopexy, brachioplasty, and buttock and thigh lift. 46/121 (38%) PCTs provided the total number of funded A-A in the two financial years (2008-09 and 2009-10). The total number of A-A applicants rose from 393 to 531, but the approval rate for funding fell from 24.2% to 19.6% consecutively in the two financial years (Figure 6).

On future service provision and expenditure, only 3/121 (2%) PCTs indicated that they would increase their spending on bariplastic procedures in the next 5 years, with 37/121 (31%) maintaining the current level of spending and the rest (67%) either planning to decrease or unsure about the future level of funding (Figure 7).

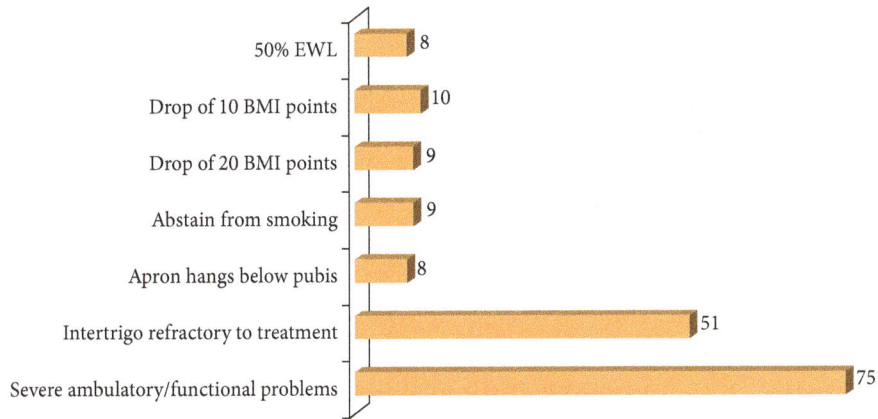

FIGURE 5: Chart showing the number of Primary Care Trusts that use a variety of additional assessment criteria to determine eligibility for patients requesting abdominoplasty-apronectomy. EWL = excess weight loss; BMI = body mass index.

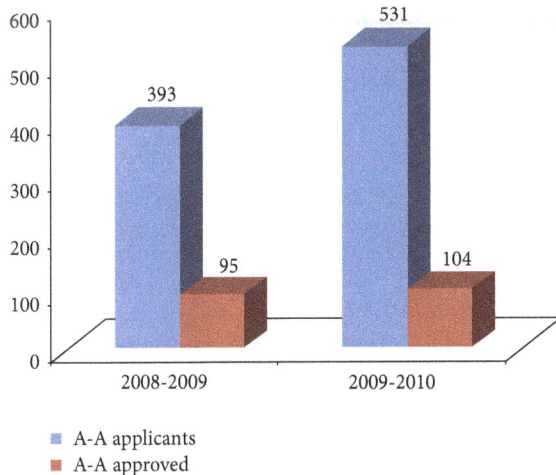

FIGURE 6: Chart showing current trend of abdominoplasty-apronectomy (A-A) being funded across England. y-axis is the number of patients.

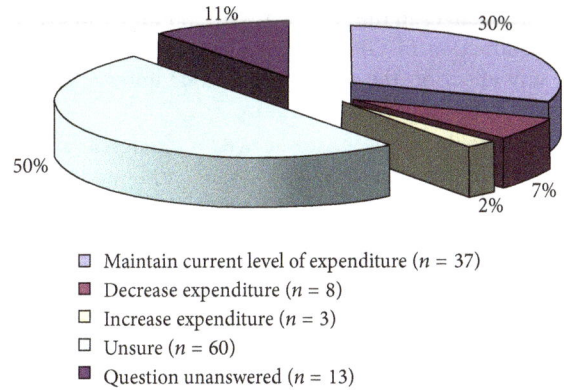

FIGURE 7: Pie chart showing the expenditure plans of the Primary Care Trusts for bariplastic surgery in the next five years.

bariplastic surgery. This is specially highlighted by the target BMIs and timescales following surgery set by the individual PCTs for patients seeking A-A.

At the present time there is no clear BMI cut-off above which bariplastic surgery should not be performed, but higher BMIs have been associated with increased complications [20]. A-A is generally avoided in those with a BMI > 35 Kg/m^2 for these reasons [2, 21, 22]. The AoPS sets the upper limit of BMI as 27 Kg/m^2 for A-A, but stricter criteria are being set by many PCTs as a means of rationing. Of the 79 PCTs who had specific BMI targets, 26 (32.9%) PCTs had criteria stricter than AoPS, but 15 (18.9%) PCTs have set a higher BMI cut-off at 30 Kg/m^2 and acknowledge the fact that it might be difficult for these patients to lose further weight because of the intrinsic weight of the abdominal apron itself. In fact, Dafydd et al. have shown that the weight of the abdominal pannus in patients undergoing MWL may affect their BMI and exclude them from bariplastic procedures.

They have therefore recommended that these patients should be considered for surgery even if their BMI is within 1-2 BMI points from the cut-off [23].

The ideal timing for the bariplastic procedure is when the weight loss has plateaued, the catabolism has ceased, and there has been an improvement in the comorbidities [24]. However, if a patients' weight loss has plateaued, waiting beyond 18 months before bariplastic procedures can sometimes be counterproductive [21]. The AoPS recommends that A-A could be offered to previously obese patients who have achieved significant weight loss and maintained their weight loss for at least two years. In our study we noted that, of the 62 PCTs who had specific criteria relating to timing of the A-A, 18 (29%) PCTs allow A-A in patients in whom the weight loss has been maintained for 1 year and 13 (21%) PCTs have reduced the timing to 6 months only leading to a wide variation in England.

Bariplastic surgery should be regarded as an integral component of the total care of the obese patient [2]. The National Institute for Health and Clinical Excellence (NICE) guidelines recommend that patients undergoing bariatric surgery should have information on, or access to, plastic surgery (such as A-A) where appropriate [25]. A recent survey of bariatric surgeons in the UK revealed that 41% reported that their patients did not have access to a plastic surgeon and a further 37% reported restricted access dependent on locally determined criteria. 96% felt that bariplastic surgery should be funded on the NHS in selected cases [14].

In our study 46 PCTs provided us with the actual number of A-A funded in consecutive years. The number of A-A funded was 95 and 104 in the two consecutive years which means at most on average each PCT was funding about 2 A-A in a year. This means a huge proportion of MWL patients are being denied A-A even at this present moment.

A recent survey from the UK, commissioned by the BAPRAS, shows that, of 1000 GPs questioned, 45% support NHS funding for bariplastic surgery [26]. We propose that postbariatric surgery patients should have easier access to the bariplastic procedures more in keeping with the pathway followed by breast cancer patients who are automatically funded for their oncoplastic procedures. It would be interesting to see if the changes in the NHS with the abolition of PCTs and the introduction of GP led clinical commissioning groups have any effect on the existing "postcode lottery" for these procedures in England in the future.

Our study had a response rate of 82% which is a very good response for this type of questionnaire study and provides a good estimation of the current postcode lottery for these procedures in England. Our questionnaire looked into the funding criteria for bariplastic procedures in England and further studies should be undertaken to compare the availability of these procedures in Wales, Scotland, and Northern Ireland where the healthcare is devolved.

5. Conclusion

This study shows that there exists a postcode lottery for bariplastic surgery in England. There is a strong need for national guidelines on the provision of body contouring procedures following MWL for the comprehensive treatment of these patients.

Ethical Approval

Ethical approval was not needed for this study. This study was registered with the Research and Development department of the Homerton University Hospital.

Disclosure

This study was presented at the 3rd Annual Scientific meeting of the British Obesity and Metabolic Surgery Society in Bristol, January 2012, and at the 5th Congress of the International Federation for the Surgery of Obesity and Metabolic Disorders European Chapter (IFSO-EC) in Barcelona, April 2012. It was published as an abstract in the British Journal of Surgery 2012; 99(S2):6, and in Obesity Surgery 2012, Volume 22 (8):1144-1205.

References

[1] The NHS Information Centre, "Statistics on obesity, physical activity and diet: England, 2011," Lifestyles Statistics, 2011.

[2] A. S. Colwell, "Current concepts in post-bariatric body contouring," *Obesity Surgery*, vol. 20, no. 8, pp. 1178–1182, 2010.

[3] R. Y. Chandawarkar, "Body contouring following massive weight loss resulting from bariatric surgery," *Advances in Psychosomatic Medicine*, vol. 27, pp. 61–72, 2006.

[4] H. B. Zuelzer and N. G. Baugh, "Bariatric and body-contouring surgery: a continuum of care for excess and lax skin," *Plastic Surgical Nursing*, vol. 27, no. 1, pp. 3–13, 2007.

[5] J. B. O'Connell, "Bariplastic surgery," *Plastic and Reconstructive Surgery*, vol. 113, no. 5, p. 1530, 2004.

[6] W. Cintra Jr., M. L. A. Modolin, R. Gemperli, C. I. C. Gobbi, J. Faintuch, and M. C. Ferreira, "Quality of life after abdominoplasty in women after bariatric surgery," *Obesity Surgery*, vol. 18, no. 6, pp. 728–732, 2008.

[7] E. S. J. van der Beek, W. te Riele, T. F. Specken, D. Boerma, and B. van Ramshorst, "The impact of reconstructive procedures following bariatric surgery on patient well-being and quality of life," *Obesity Surgery*, vol. 20, no. 1, pp. 36–41, 2010.

[8] A. Y. Song, J. P. Rubin, V. Thomas, J. R. Dudas, K. G. Marra, and M. H. Fernstrom, "Body image and quality of life in post massive weight loss body contouring patients," *Obesity*, vol. 14, no. 9, pp. 1626–1636, 2006.

[9] NHS Modernisation Agency, "Action on plastic surgery. Information for commissioners of plastic surgery services. Referrals and guidelines in plastic surgery," http://www.institute.nhs.uk/index.php?option=com_joomcart&Itemid=194&main_page=document_product_info&products_id=223.

[10] J. E. Mitchell, R. D. Crosby, T. W. Ertelt et al., "The desire for body contouring surgery after bariatric surgery," *Obesity Surgery*, vol. 18, no. 10, pp. 1308–1312, 2008.

[11] J. A. Gusenoff, S. Messing, W. O'Malley, and H. N. Langstein, "Temporal and demographic factors influencing the desire for plastic surgery after gastric bypass surgery," *Plastic and Reconstructive Surgery*, vol. 121, no. 6, pp. 2120–2126, 2008.

[12] H. B. Kitzinger, S. Abayev, A. Pittermann et al., "The prevalence of body contouring surgery after gastric bypass surgery," *Obesity Surgery*, vol. 22, no. 1, pp. 8–12, 2012.

[13] The NHS Information Centre, http://www.hscic.gov.uk/article/1728/Weight-loss-stomach-surgery-up-12-per-cent-in-a-year-says-new-report.

[14] L. Highton, C. Ekwobi, and V. Rose, "Post-bariatric surgery body contouring in the NHS: a survey of UK bariatric surgeons," *Journal of Plastic, Reconstructive & Aesthetic Surgery*, vol. 65, no. 4, pp. 426–432, 2012.

[15] C. C. Lazar, I. Clerc, S. Deneuve, I. Auquit-Auckbur, and P. Y. Milliez, "Abdominoplasty after major weight loss: improvement of quality of life and psychological status," *Obesity Surgery*, vol. 19, no. 8, pp. 1170–1175, 2009.

[16] W. M. Wraight, S. K. L. Tay, C. Nduka, and J. A. Pereira, "Bilateral breast reduction surgery in England: a postcode lottery," *Journal of Plastic, Reconstructive & Aesthetic Surgery*, vol. 60, no. 9, pp. 1039–1044, 2007.

[17] J. Henderson, "The plastic surgery postcode lottery in England," *International Journal of Surgery*, vol. 7, no. 6, pp. 550–558, 2009.

[18] A. Goodson, B. Khoda, and C. Nduka, "Funding criteria for common procedures: a postcode lottery in NHS plastic surgery," *Journal of Plastic, Reconstructive & Aesthetic Surgery*, vol. 64, no. 3, pp. 417–419, 2011.

[19] G. Shapps, "All your eggs in one basket. A comprehensive study into the continuing postcode lottery in IVF provision through the NHS," 2011, http://www.nursingtimes.net/Journals/1/Files/2009/8/6/All-your-eggs-in-one-basket.pdf.

[20] J. A. Gusenoff and J. P. Rubin, "Plastic surgery after weight loss: current concepts in massive weight loss surgery," *Aesthetic Surgery Journal*, vol. 28, no. 4, pp. 452–455, 2008.

[21] D. Hurwitz, "Plastic surgery following weight loss," in *Minimally Invasive Bariatric Surgery*, P. R. Schauer, B. D. Schirmer, and S. Brethauer, Eds., pp. 485–488, Springer, New York, NY, USA, 2007.

[22] K. C. Neaman and J. E. Hansen, "Analysis of complications from abdominoplasty: a review of 206 cases at an university hospital," *Annals of Plastic Surgery*, vol. 58, no. 3, pp. 292–298, 2007.

[23] H. Dafydd, A. Juma, P. Meyers, and K. Shokrollahi, "The contribution of breast and abdominal pannus weight to body mass index: implications for rationing of reduction mammaplasty and abdominoplasty," *Annals of Plastic Surgery*, vol. 62, no. 3, pp. 244–245, 2009.

[24] T. P. Sterry and J. Sacks, "Plastic surgery after excessive weight loss," in *Laparoscopic Bariatric Surgery*, W. B. Inabet, E. J. DeMaria, and S. Ikramuddin, Eds., pp. 314–324, Lippincott Williams & Wilkins, Baltimore, Md, USA, 2007.

[25] National Institute for Health and Clinical Excellence, "Obesity: guidance on the prevention, identification, assessment and management of overweight and obesity in adults and children," http://www.nice.org.uk/nicemedia/live/11000/30365/30365.pdf.

[26] Research conducted on behalf of BAPRAS by MedeConnect with 1,000 GPs in November 2011, http://www.bapras.org.uk/news.asp?id=909.

12

Second Generation Self-Inflating Tissue Expanders: A Two-Year Experience

Jamal Omran Al Madani

Plastic Surgery Unit, Plastic Surgery Resident, Security Forces Hospital, Riyadh, Saudi Arabia

Correspondence should be addressed to Jamal Omran Al Madani; dr_jmadani@hotmail.com

Academic Editor: Stephen M. Warren

Background. Tissue expansion is a well-established surgical technique that produces an additional amount of normal skin to cover a defect. This technique is appealing because the skin quality and color are from the patient's own. The widely used injectable expanders are of great reliability but carry the disadvantage of being painful during injection and most of the time require multiple clinic visits. So the idea of self-inflation became attractive and hydrogel expanders were developed and became widely known for being painless during clinic visit and decrease number of visits. The first generation expanders were modified by adding an enclosing plastic shell to decrease the unopposed expansion that occurred in the first generation expanders, which lead to pressure necrosis of the skin flaps. This made it an attractive option for tissue expansion in children and some adult patients. *Patients, Materials, and Methods*. Charts of 17 patients were retrospectively reviewed, all of them had second generation self-inflating expanders implanted over a 2-year period for one of two purposes, the treatment of giant nevi or burn scars. *Results*. Fifteen patients were females and 2 were males. The indication was large burn scar in 14 cases (14/17), in which 47/55 expanders were implanted, and giant nevus in 3/17 cases in which 8/55 expanders were implanted. Extrusion of the expander occurred in 8/55 expanders (14.5%), which occurred in 6/14 patients. The highest percentage of extrusion occurred in the neck in which two out of three expanders extruded; otherwise this complication does not seem to be related to the indication, gender, nor age of the patients. It seems to be that it is technical in nature. The patients did not have to get any injections to fill the tissue expanders, which made the expansion process less painful and more convenient. *Conclusion*. This seems to be currently the largest published review in which second generation expanders were used. Those expanders seem to offer a desirable advantage of being painless for children, also they do not require repeated visits to the surgeon's clinic, which is of great value for patients living in the periphery.

1. Introduction

Tissue expansion is an important tool in the plastic surgeon's toolbox. First report of this method was in 1957, when Neumann used a rubber balloon to expand skin in the temporooccipital area to reconstruct a traumatized ear [1]. At that time it seemed like a sporadic idea it did not get a lot of publicity. Twenty years later, the idea resurfaced by Radovan and Argenta who used a silicon inflatable expander in breast reconstruction. Afterwards this technique gained a lot of attention [2, 3].

Injectable (conventional) expanders were regularly used for this purpose. The expander needs to be filled manually through an external filling port. This lead to a couple of major disadvantages, the filling process is usually painful when the surgeon introduces the needle into the port underneath the skin and the patient must come to a medical facility regularly in most cases, unless they were trusted with their expanders to be filled by them at their homes.

In 1982 Austad and Rose developed the first self-inflating tissue expander composed of hypertonic, saturated saline, which was abandoned. The reason was the increased risk of skin necrosis when the fluid leaked from its shell [4]. In 1993, Weise tested a newer hydrogel self-inflating expander on rats, that gave a new horizon for tissue expansion [5]. In 1999 Osmed (Ilmenau, Germany) introduced the self-inflating tissue expanders giving a new option for tissue expansion. The expanders are made from a solid material called hydrogel, vinyl pyrrolidone, and methyl methacrylate material that absorbs the surrounding tissue fluid and increase in size over

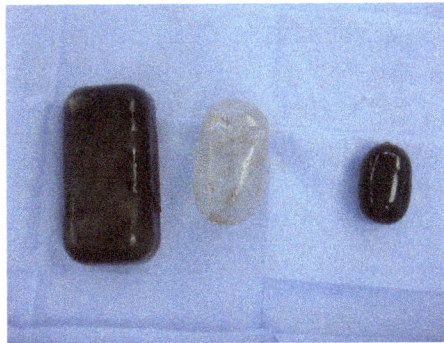

FIGURE 1: Left expander that has expanded in size beyond the expected size, middle ruptured envelop of the expander on the left, right, expander that expanded to the calculated volume and did not extrude.

a period of 6–8 weeks. The company marketing the expander claims that it increases to 10 times the original size, but the increase in size measured in a clinical report on human was 6.9 times the original size in the second generation expanders [6] (see Figure 1).

The first generation expanders rapidly increased in size and extruded outside the body. This caused pressure necrosis over the overlying skin flap. So they were modified by adding an envelope to decrease the unopposed expansion. The envelope is made of silicone and had pores to allow the fluid in. Hence those second generation tissue expanders had a better outcome [7].

This study is a single-center experience, in which 55 rectangular second generation self-inflating tissue expanders were used.

2. Materials and Methods

2.1. Patients. Seventeen patients had implantation of 55 expanders over a 2-year period, from April, 2010, to April, 2012. All the patients that had tissue expander implanted records were retrospectively reviewed. The data collected included age, gender, indication, site, number of surgeries including insertion and both elective and emergency removal, size of the expanders, and number of days the expander remained in the body. Out of the 17 patients included in the study 15 patients were females and 2 were males. The indication was large burn scar in 14 cases (14/17), in which 47/55 expanders were implanted, and giant nevus in 3/17 cases in which 8/55 expanders were implanted. Three patients were of pediatric age group (less than 14 years) and the remaining were adults. Age ranged from 9 to 40 years and mean age was 19.14 years. The use of those expanders was preferred in pediatrics and in patients living far from Riyadh, the capital of Saudi Arabia, referred from the peripheral hospital in their regions. The aim was to decrease the sessions of painful inflations and the number of visits for patients living away from the hospital. Selection of patients depended on the surgeons' and patients' preference.

2.2. Expanders. All expanders were second generation self-inflating tissue expanders produced by Osmed GmbH,

Ilmenau, Germany. All used expanders were rectangular in shape. Sizes were 60, 75, 130, 200, and 300 cc predicted final volume as per company box (for details see Table 1).

2.3. Course

2.3.1. Implantation. All elective surgeries were performed by a team of two plastic surgery consultants. All were under general anesthesia; preoperatively the normal skin next to the lesion to be removed is marked in a way to create a subcutaneous pocket in which the expander would be inserted. The dimensions of the pocket would be equal to the final dimensions that the expander is supposed to reach as indicated on the company box. This was done in an attempt to make the expander get a bigger room to expand under and to decrease the unopposed pressure on the overlying skin to prevent ischemia and extrusion.

In cases of large lesion that would require the insertion of more than one expander on one side, separate pockets were created to disallow any potential infection to spread from one expander to another in case any infection occurs 2-3 weeks postoperatively. The aim is to keep the uninfected expanders and utilize them later if they did not reach their final predicted volume yet which happens after around 6 weeks.

The surgery would begin by making a 3-4 cm cut inside the lesion territory perpendicular to the expander's pocket; infiltration of around 30–40 cc of tumescent fluid containing epinephrine would follow. Dissection of the pocket using metzenbaum scissors is done leaving a 1 cm thick skin. Atraumatic dissection of the pocket follows. The expander is inserted and the skin is closed using continuous sutures. A course of oral antibiotic for 5 days was given. The implantation process would take around 20 minutes.

2.3.2. Elective Removal. All surgeries were performed under GA. An incision is made in the line between the normal skin and the lesion, the pocket is opened and the expander is removed, and the capsule may be scored if the desired stretch was not achieved. The surface area of the lesion that can be removed is estimated and the skin flaps are advanced; a drain is inserted, which is usually removed after 1-2 days according to the output.

2.3.3. Removal of the Extruded Expanders. When extrusions occurred the patients were admitted through the emergency. Intravenous antibiotics were started at the time of admission, and were taken to the operating room as soon as possible. A similar technique to electively remove the expander is used, but the pocket is thoroughly irrigated and cleaned. In case the expander was inserted together with other expanders the pocket would be inspected to make sure that the infection did not spread to another expander; drains were left in place like other elective cases. In all the cases the infection did not spread and the decision of removing the other expanders electively was made depending on whether the uninfected expander reached a reasonable volume or not. Antibiotics (cefuroxime, dose according to weight) were used regularly to prevent the spread of the infection. Cultures showed

TABLE 1: Patients and expanders data.

Patient order	Age in years	Gender	Other illnesses	Indication	Order of implantation surgery	Final size of the expander (cc)	Duration (days)	Location	Extruded
1	38	Female	Sickle cell anemia	Burn scar	1st	130	47	Arm	No
						130	47	Arm	No
					2nd	130	100	Arm	No
						75	100	Arm	No
2	21	Female	None	Burn scar	1st	75	102	Chest	Yes
						60	171	Chest	No
						60	171	Chest	No
3	10	Male	None	Nevus	1st	60	52	Neck	Yes
4	9	Female	None	Nevus	1st	60	42	Chest	No
						60	42	Chest	No
						130	42	Neck	Yes
5	29	Female	None	Burn scar	1st	75	126	Forearm	No
						75	126	Forearm	No
6	25	Female	None	Burn scar	1st	75	69	Neck	No
7	11	Female	None	Burn scar	1st	130	63	Chest	No
						200	63	Chest	No
8	18	Female	None	Burn scar	1st	200	46	Shoulder	No
9	38	Female	None	Burn scar	1st	75	167	Arm	No
						130	167	Arm	No
10	40	Male	None	Burn scar	1st	200	99	Forearm	No
						200	99	Forearm	No
11	28	Female	None	Burn scar	1st	300	165	Shoulder	No
						200	165	Shoulder	No
						130	165	Shoulder	No
						130	165	Shoulder	No
12	11	Female	None	Nevus	1st	75	102	Chest	No
						130	102	Chest	No
						60	102	Arm	No
						60	102	Arm	No
13	11	Female	None	Burn scar	1st	60	112	Chest	No
						60	112	Chest	No
						60	112	Chest	Extruded
						75	112	Chest	No
						75	112	Chest	No
						130	112	Chest	No
						300	30	Arm	Yes
14	33	Female	None	Burn scar	1st	60	105	Shoulder	No
15	21	Female	None	Burn scar	1st	75	86	Forearm	No
						75	86	Forearm	No
16	15	Female	None	Burn scar	1st	75	85	Back	No
						300	85	Back	No
						130	85	Back	No
						130	55	Back	Yes
						200	85	Back	Yes

TABLE 1: Continued.

Patient order	Age in years	Gender	Other illnesses	Indication	Order of implantation surgery	Final size of the expander (cc)	Duration (days)	Location	Extruded
						130	120	Thigh	No
						130	120	Thigh	No
						200	120	Thigh	No
	12				1st	200	120	Thigh	No
17		Female	None	Burn scar		75	120	Thigh	No
						75	120	Thigh	No
						300	120	Thigh	No
						300	29	Thigh	Yes
	13				2nd	300	52	Thigh	No
						60	52	Thigh	Yes

TABLE 2: Patients and expanders of complicated cases.

Duration (days)	Size (cc)	Age	Gender	Indication	Location	Extruded	Other illnesses
102	75	21	Female	Burn scar	Chest	Yes	None
52	60	10	Male	Nevus	Neck	Yes	None
42	130	9	Female	Nevus	Neck	Yes	None
30	300	11	Female	Burn scar	Arm	Yes	None
55	130	15	Female	Burn scar	Back	Yes	None
85	200	15	Female	Burn scar	Back	Yes	None
29	300	12	Female	Burn scar	Thigh	Yes	None
52	65	12	Female	Burn scar	Thigh	Yes	None

staphylococci uniformly. Patients left the hospital after 3–5 days, after the cellulitis has subsided.

3. Results

3.1. Patients. All patients described were healthy. Only one patient had another illness, which was sickle cell anemia, and no complications occurred during the management of that patient. Two of the patients had the implantation twice due to the very large surface area of the lesion. A minimum of one expander and a maximum of 7 expanders in each patient were implanted. The size of the expanded skin in those self-inflating tissue expanders was similar to the conventional expanders (details of the patients and implanted expanders are in Table 1.)

3.2. Complication. All patients reported minimal discomfort and were discharged from the hospital a day after surgery. Extrusion of the expander occurred in 8/55 expanders (14.5%), which occurred in 6/17 patients. Six happened when the indication was burn scar management (75%) and 2 happened when the indication was giant nevus (25%). The extrusion occurred between 30 days and 102 days after implantation with mean of 55.87 days. Out of the eight expanders 2 were inserted in the thigh, 2 in the chest, 1 in the back, 1 in the arm, 2 in the neck, and none in the shoulder or the forearm. Average age in the whole study was 19.14 years; in the group in which the expanders extruded the average was 13.12 years while in the group in which complication did not occur it

TABLE 3: Rate of complications in relation to site.

Location	Count	%
Arm	1	12.5
Forearm	0	0
Chest	1	12.5
Neck	2	25
Shoulder	0	0
Back	2	25
Thigh	2	25

was 20.19 years. All patients did not have other complications during surgeries and postoperatively until seen in the clinic at least one month later. Neither superficial infection nor ulceration occurred (Details of the patients and the extruded expanders are in Table 2 and rate of complications in relation to site is in Table 3).

4. Discussion

After the introduction of the self-inflating tissue expanders many reports were published about the use and versatility of these expanders which included unpphalmia, breast reconstruction, free flap reconstruction, giant nevi and burn scars [6, 7].

The center in which this study was done is a government referral center, in Riyadh, the capital of Saudi Arabia, receiving many patients from smaller peripheral hospitals. Concerning conventional expander to be inserted and the process of expansion to be carried out the surgeon has 2 choices the first is to bring the patient and maybe the family of a child weekly to the clinic. This carries a large number of work and school absences because the clinic time is during the day working hours only. The other choice is to trust the family with the expander and teach them how to inflate it at home, which for many surgeons is not a very reliable option, as it would potentially carry a higher risk of extrusion and infection.

So, this second generation expander came in hand for many patients especially the ones living away from the center and for children. The implantation is usually uncomplicated. Postoperative pain is minimal as the incision is usually small. The number of days in which the expander electively stayed was primarily decided by the social factors for the patients and the availability of operation theater time for the surgeon as well, but it was not less than 42 days and an average (99.1) days.

Extrusion apparently occurs due to pressure necrosis from the unopposed expansion from expander, causing failure of the envelope surrounding the expander. This can be explained by the necrosis of the skin flap seen at the time of removal and debridement.

Extrusion rate for the first generation tissue expanders was as high as 35% in some reports [8, 9], until the second generation that is enclosed by a silicone fenestrated envelop was introduced, after which the complication rate has decreased to some extent. Ronert et al. [7] reported a success rate of 93.3% for tubular breast management, 83.3% for other reconstructions, and 91% for all 26 second generation expanders. While Obdeijn et al. in 2009 reported a lesser success rate which was 70%, they had 20 expanders implanted, but in their experience 2 of the 6 extrusions happened in radiated fields [6]. An impressive 96.2% success rate was reported in 2010 by Böttcher-Haberzeth et al. in a study that was carried on pediatric population in which 53 expanders were implanted; the surgery was short and the expansion process was painless, because the patient did not have to get injections of fluid to fill the expander. No radiation was given to any of the patients but this alone is not the cause of this greater success rate an oversized pocket potentially played an important factor in decreasing the extrusion rate [10].

The results in this study are similar to those reported as the extrusion rate is 14.5%. The extrusion from anatomical areas other than the neck is not remarkable, whereas from the neck 66.6% expanders extruded, which is a limitation in our study, but making this a definitive conclusion is difficult as only 3 expanders were inserted in which 2 extruded. Furthermore in the previous studies [7, 9, 10] no implantations were done in the neck.

Looking at the gender in this study, most of the implantations were carried out in females (52/55) as they would present for cosmetic concerns more than the males who are less concerned about the appearance especially in areas usually covered with clothes. Only 3 expanders were implanted in males. One of those three expanders extruded (33%), and seven out of fifty two (14.3%) in females. There are no previous

reports about increased extrusion in either gender with any type of expanders and the number of male patients is very small to make a definite conclusion.

Similarly the indication also does not seem to play a role. Two out of eight expanders extruded in 2 different giant nevi patients but those 2 were in the neck, unlike the other 6 that did not extrude which were implanted in the chest (4/8) and arm (2/8).

In the presented data the pediatrics (less than 14 years) were 6 (in Table 1 their numbers are 3, 4, 7, 12, 13, and 17) and had 27 expanders implanted, 4 of them extruded (14.8%) which is similar to the whole patient group and does not signify an increased risk contrary to the fact that the average age of patients in which the expander extruded was 13.1 years. This number is not as impressive as the one reported before in pediatrics [10].

Two patients had expansion by self-inflating expander twice (patients number 1 and 17 in Table 1). One had an uncomplicated course and the implantation surgeries were around a year apart. The other had 7 expanders implanted and removed without any problems in the first surgery; the patient remained without any expanders for 11 months; then 3 expanders were inserted again in the right thigh and the patient had a complication in the second time with two of the three expanders; the first was removed alone and the second extruded expander when removed was with the last and third expander that did not extrude at all. This is similar to what was reported by Obdeijn et al. [9] in one of their cases where 3 expanders were implanted in a previously expanded area and 1 of them extruded.

Extrusion occurred in a similar rate in the 5 different sizes used (60, 75, 120, 200, and 300 cc). In all the cases the flaps created by the extruded expander were advanced and utilized safely. Extrusion occurred between 29 to 102 days and average 55.8; days the average number of days in which the expander remained without any later complication was 94 days.

At this stage creation of an oversized pocket is advised, similar to the one described by Böttcher-Haberzeth et al. [10]. This was not done in the current study. In this study the pockets dimensions and designs did not account for the vertical height that the expander would reach; only 2 dimensions of the expander were measured and maybe this caused the extrusion.

The disadvantages of this type of expander are that the process is uncontrolled and that the expander cannot be deflated nor reused.

5. For Future Studies

The state in which the expanders were found during removal was not documented; in at least one of the cases that was not complicated the expander was outside the enclosing envelop, and in at least one of the cases that were complicated the expander was found in a similar state, which may have caused the extrusion in that patient. But the envelope was intact in some other complicated cases. Important data to be documented is the final size that the expander actually reached and the color the expander got stained with, as some of the expanders were red-color stained which may mean that the blood altered the osmotic inflation process, which are all were lacking in our study and psychological trauma. There is some inconsistency in the reports with regard to the final volume reached in vivo between 10 times and 6.5 times [8, 9, 11]. In a study about hydrogel expansion Weise et al. addressed different inflation behavior in different media in vitro only and responses to blood and serous fluid were not tested [12], which places the final volume proposed by the company on its boxes in doubt. Cost effectiveness cannot be determined in this center because it is a government facility and care including the expanders, nurse clinic, and operating theater time is for free. Nonfinancial benefit in terms of absence of pain are psychological trauma and missing school classes weekly for inflating the expander maybe evaluated in a comparative study.

6. Conclusion

(1) Second generation tissue expanders look very attractive for burn scar and giant nevi reconstruction. (2) The neck maybe an area for a high extrusion risk, but this needs to be looked at after more cases are done in the neck. Other anatomical areas like age, gender, size of the expander, and indication do not seem to play a role in extrusion. (3) An oversized pocket is advised. (4) The expander can stay for around 100 days without extrusion, but removal as soon as the expander reaches the required size is advised. (5) If extrusion occurs the expanded skin can still be utilized. (6) Reexpansion seems safe but should be further studied and evaluated.

Acknowledgments

The author would like to thank Dr. Osama Shareefi and Dr. Maimouna Alomawi as they were the consultants that operated on the patients and gave the chance to do this research.

References

[1] C. G. Neumann, "The expansion of an area of skin by progressive distension of a subcutaneous balloon," *Plastic and Reconstructive Surgery*, vol. 19, no. 2, pp. 124–130, 1957.

[2] C. Radovan, "Development of adjacent flaps using a temporary expander," *Plastic Surgery Forum*, vol. 2, article 62, 1979.

[3] L. C. Argenta, "Reconstruction of the breast by tissue-expansion," *Clinics in Plastic Surgery*, vol. 11, no. 2, pp. 257–264, 1984.

[4] E. D. Austad and G. L. Rose, "A self-inflating tissue expander," *Plastic and Reconstructive Surgery*, vol. 70, no. 5, pp. 588–594.

[5] K. G. Wiese, "Osmotically induced tissue expansion with hydrogels: a new dimension in tissue expansion? A preliminary report," *Journal of Cranio-Maxillo-Facial Surgery*, vol. 21, no. 7, pp. 309–313, 1993.

[6] M. C. Obdeijn, J. P. A. Nicolai, and P. M. N. Werker, "The osmotic tissue expander: a three-year clinical experience," *Journal of Plastic, Reconstructive and Aesthetic Surgery*, vol. 62, no. 9, pp. 1219–1222, 2009.

[7] M. A. Ronert, H. Hofheinz, E. Manassa, H. Asgarouladi, and R. R. Olbrisch, "The beginning of a new era in tissue expansion: self-filling osmotic tissue expander—four-year clinical experience," *Plastic and Reconstructive Surgery*, vol. 114, no. 5, pp. 1024–1031, 2004.

[8] S. Chummun, P. Addison, and K. J. Stewart, "The osmotic tissue expander: a 5-year experience," *Journal of Plastic, Reconstructive and Aesthetic Surgery*, vol. 63, no. 12, pp. 2128–2132, 2010.

[9] M. C. Obdeijn, J. P. A. Nicolai, and P. M. N. Werker, "The osmotic tissue expander: a three-year clinical experience," *Journal of Plastic, Reconstructive and Aesthetic Surgery*, vol. 62, no. 9, pp. 1219–1222, 2009.

[10] S. Böttcher-Haberzeth, S. Kapoor, M. Meuli et al., "Osmotic expanders in children: no filling—no control—no problem?" *European Journal of Pediatric Surgery*, vol. 21, no. 3, pp. 163–167, 2011.

[11] P. Lohana, N. S. Moiemen, and Y. T. Wilson, "The use of Osmed (TM) tissue expanders in paediatric burns reconstruction," *Annals of Burns and Fire Disasters*, vol. 25, no. 1, pp. 38–42, 2012.

[12] K. G. Weise, D. E. Heinemann, D. Ostermeier, and J. H. Peters, "Biomaterial properties and biocompatibility in cell culture of a novel self-inflating hydrogel tissue expander," *Journal of Biomedical Materials Research*, vol. 54, no. 2, pp. 179–188, 2001.

13

Vascular Waveform Analysis of Flap-Feeding Vessels Using Color Doppler Ultrasonography

Akihiro Ogino and Kiyoshi Onishi

Department of Plastic and Reconstructive Surgery, 6-11-1, Omori-nishi, Ota-ku, Tokyo 143-8541, Japan

Correspondence should be addressed to Akihiro Ogino; ogino0613@aol.com

Academic Editor: Yoshihiro Kimata

We performed vascular waveform analysis of flap-feeding vessels using color Doppler ultrasonography and evaluated the blood flow in the flaps prior to surgery. Vascular waveform analysis was performed in 19 patients. The analyzed parameters included the vascular diameter, flow volume, flow velocity, resistance index, pulsatility index, and acceleration time. The arterial waveform was classified into 5 types based on the partially modified blood flow waveform classification reported by Hirai et al.; in particular, D-1a, D-1b, and D-2 were considered as normal waveforms. They were 4 patients which observed abnormal vascular waveform among 19 patients (D-4 : 1, D-3 : 1, and Poor detect : 2). The case which presented D-4 waveform changed the surgical procedure, and a favorable outcome was achieved. Muscle flap of the case which presented D-3 waveform was partially necrosed. The case which detected blood flow poorly was judged to be the vascular obstruction of the internal thoracic artery. In the evaluation of blood flow in flaps using color Doppler ultrasonography, determination of not only basic blood flow information, such as the vascular distribution and diameter and flow velocity, but also the flow volume, vascular resistance, and arterial waveform is essential to elucidate the hemodynamics of the flap.

1. Introduction

For the evaluation of blood flow in flap-feeding vessels in the field of plastic and reconstructive surgery, various methods are used, such as angiography, MRA, and MDCT, and stable results are obtained; but these methods can be confirmed the presence and distribution of a flap-feeding vessels, and the details, such as the flow velocity and flow volume and vascular resistance, cannot be evaluated. Since color Doppler ultrasonography can be visualized noninvasively and easily, relative low cost of the microblood vessels has recently been used to identify flap-feeding vessels, particularly perforating arteries, and its usefulness has been reported [1–3]. We performed vascular waveform analysis of flap-feeding vessels using color Doppler ultrasonography and evaluated the blood flow in the flaps prior to surgery. In the present study, we introduce an overview of the tests and report on its usefulness.

2. Subjects and Methods

Vascular waveform analysis was performed in 19 patients who underwent reconstructive surgery with pedicle flap (9 patients males and 10 patients females; age was 33~79; mean age was 59 years). Primal disease was 7 patients of mediastinitis, 7 patients of malignant tumor, 2 patients of esophagus skin fistula, 1 patient of scar contracture after burn, 1 patient of abdominal wall incisional herniatis, and 1 patient of vagina defect. Transplanted flap was 8 patients of latissimus dorsi musculocutaneous flap, 6 patients of rectus abdominis musculocutaneous flap, 3 patients of pectoralis major musculocutaneous flap, and 2 patients of tensor fascia lata musculocutaneous flap (Table 1).

No underlying severe disease, such as diabetes mellitus, atherosclerosis obliterans, or chronic renal disease, was observed in any patient.

TABLE 1: Clinical characteristics of patients. Vascular waveform analysis of thoracodorsal artery was performed in 8 patients, deep inferior epigastric artery in 2 patients, superior epigastric artery in 6 patients, thoracoacrominal artery in 3 patients, and lateral circumflex femoral artery in 2 patients.

Patient	Age	Sex	Disease	Selected flap	Vascular waveform analysis
1	67	M	Mediastinitis	LDMC	SEA and TDA
2	36	F	Breast cancer	LDMC	TDA
3	33	F	Breast cancer	LDMC	TDA
4	59	M	Esophageal fistula	LDMC	TDA
5	44	F	Breast cancer	LDMC	TDA
6	41	F	Breast cancer	LDMC	TDA
7	55	F	Scar contracture after burn	LDMC	TDA
8	79	F	Mediastinitis	LDMC	TDA
9	55	M	Mediastinitis	RAMC	SEA
10	78	F	Mediastinitis	RAM	SEA
11	69	M	Rectal cancer anal invasion	RAMC	DIEA
12	67	M	Mediastinitis	RAMC	SEA
13	67	F	Vaginal defect	RAMC	DIEA
14	48	F	Breast cancer	RAMC	SEA
15	68	M	Esophageal fistula	PMMC	TAA
16	67	M	Mediastinitis	PMMC	TAA
17	57	M	Mediastinitis	PMM	SEA & TAA
18	71	M	Gallbladder cancer abdominal wall invasion	TFLMC	LCFA
19	71	F	Abdominal wall incisional herniatis	TFLMC	LCFA

LDMC: lattisimus dorsi musculocutaneous flap; RAMC: rectus abdominis musculocutaneous flap; RAM: rectus abdominis muscle flap; PMMC: pectoralis major musculocutaneous flap; PMM: pectoralis major muscle flap; TFLMC: tensor fascia lata musculocutaneous flap; TDA: thoracodorsal artery; SEA: superior epigastric artery; DIEA: deep inferior epigastric artery; TAA: thoracoacrominal artery; LCFA: lateral circumflex femoral artery.

TABLE 2: Reference values of epigastric artery and subscapular-thoracodorsal artery. The standard values for the superior epigastric artery were: vascular diameter, 0.8 mm or greater; FV, 7 mL/min or faster; V_{max}, 15 cm/sec or greater; RI, 0.7 or greater; PI, 2.2 ± 0.8; and AT, ≦100 msec. Those for the deep inferior epigastric artery were: vascular diameter, 1.3 mm or greater; FV, 10 mL/min or faster; V_{max}, 25 cm/sec or greater; RI, 0.7 or greater; PI, 2.7 ± 1; and AT, ≦100 msec. Those for the subscapular artery were: vascular diameter, 2 mm or greater; FV, 20 mL/min or faster; V_{max}, 30 cm/sec or greater; RI, 0.7 or greater; PI, 4 ± 2; and AT, ≦100 msec. Those for the thoracodorsal artery were: vascular diameter, 1 mm or greater; FV, 5 mL/min or faster; V_{max}, 20 cm/sec or greater; RI, 0.7 or greater; PI, 4 ± 2; and AT, ≦100 msec.

	Superior epigastric artery ($N = 9$)	Deep inferior epigastric artery ($N = 20$)	Subscapular artery ($N = 12$)	Thoracodorsal artery ($N = 12$)
Diameter (mm)	0.8 mm or more	1.3 mm or more	2 mm or more	1 mm or more
FV (mL/min)	7 mL/min or more	10 mL/min or more	20 mL/min or more	5 mL/min or more
V_{max} (cm/sec)	15 cm/sec or more	25 cm/sec or more	30 cm/sec or more	20 cm/sec or more
RI	0.7 or more	0.7 or more	0.7 or more	0.7 or more
PI	2.2 ± 0.8	2.7 ± 1	4 ± 2	4 ± 2
AT	≦100 msec	≦100 msec	≦100 msec	≦100 msec

The XARIO SSA-660A -770A (Toshiba) as an ultrasonic diagnosis system and a high frequency linear surface probe (7.5–10 MHz) was used.

Concerning items of vascular waveform analysis, the vascular diameter, flow volume (F-V), maximum flow velocity (V_{max}), minimum flow velocity (V_{min}), mean flow velocity (V_{mean}), and resistance index (RI), pulsatility index (PI), and acceleration time (AT: time reaching a peak during systole) based on arterial waveforms were measured. F-V was calculated by multiplying the time integral value of V_{mean} by the cross-sectional area of the vessel assumed to be a circle. RI was calculated as $(V_{max} - V_{min})/V_{max}$ and PI as $(V_{max} - V_{min})/V_{mean}$. The vascular waveform was measured at a site of the flap-feeding vessels after branching within 3 cm. The incidence angle of ultrasound during vascular waveform analysis was ≤60° in principle.

Blood flow evaluation of flap feeding vessels was performed referring to the standard value of superior epigastric artery, deep inferior epigastric artery, subscapular artery, and thoracodorsal artery which we set up before [4] (Table 2).

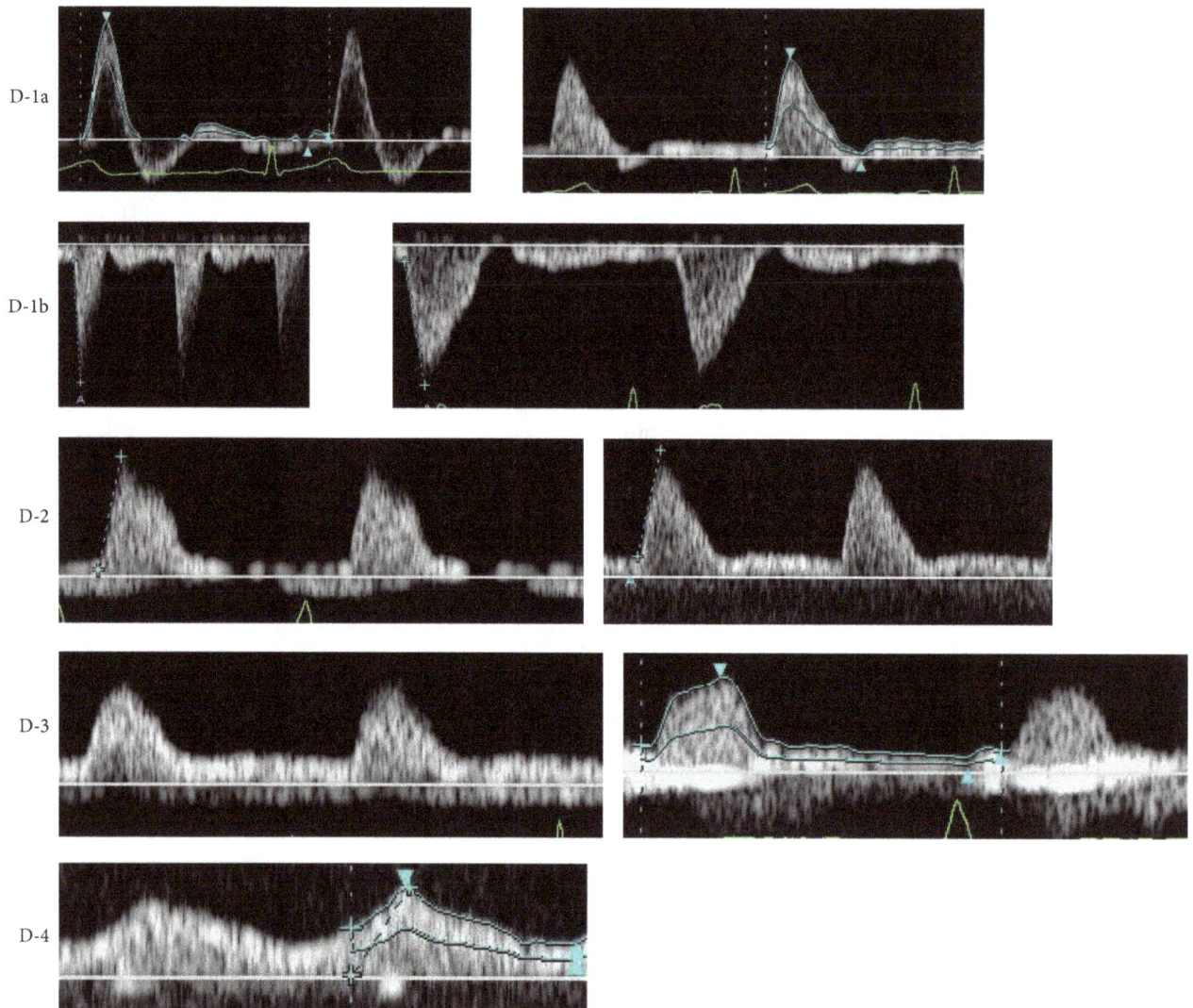

FIGURE 1: Novel classification of the vascular waveform of flap-feeding vessels in Doppler ultrasonography. D-1a type: normal waveforms in which systolic crests rise steeply, followed by reflux components; D-1b type: normal waveforms in which systolic crests rise steeply but reflux components are lost, and a notch is noted between systolic and diastolic waves; D-2 type: peaks are formed, but the width of systolic crests is wider than normal, reflux components are lost, and no notch is present between systolic and diastolic waves; D-3 type: systolic crests are moderate and form no peak; and D-4 type: moderate continuous waveforms.

Arterial waveforms were classified into the following 5 types using a partially modified blood flow waveform classification reported by Hirai et al. [5] (Figure 1).

D-1a, D-1b, and D-2 waveforms were regarded as normal; D-3 and D-4 were regarded as abnormal.

Moreover, venous blood flow was confirmed by visualize the running of the vessel and venous waveform.

This study was approved by the Ethics Committee of Toho University Omori Medical Center (number: 24026) and performed after obtaining comprehension from the patients with sufficient informed consent.

3. Results

It was 4 patients which observed abnormal vascular waveform among 19 patients which performed vascular waveform analysis of flap-feeding vessels using color Doppler ultrasonography prior to surgery (D-4: 1 patient, D-3: 1 patient, and Poor detect: 2 patients). An abnormal D-4 waveform was noted in a case in which superior epigastric arterial waveform analysis was performed before surgery for sternal osteomyelitis (Patient 1). The V_{max} was 15.6 cm/sec, being slower than the standard; RI was 0.34, and PI was 0.50, being lower than the standard. Since the waveform of internal thoracic artery was a normal waveform, a part of internal thoracic artery was damaged on the occasion of sternum debridement, and a possibility of angiostenosis was suspected (Figure 2). Therefore the surgical procedure was changed to one using latissimus dorsi musculocutaneous flap, and a favorable outcome was achieved. The case which presented D-3 waveform planned reconstruction by rectus abdominis muscle flap to mediastinitis and vascular waveform analysis

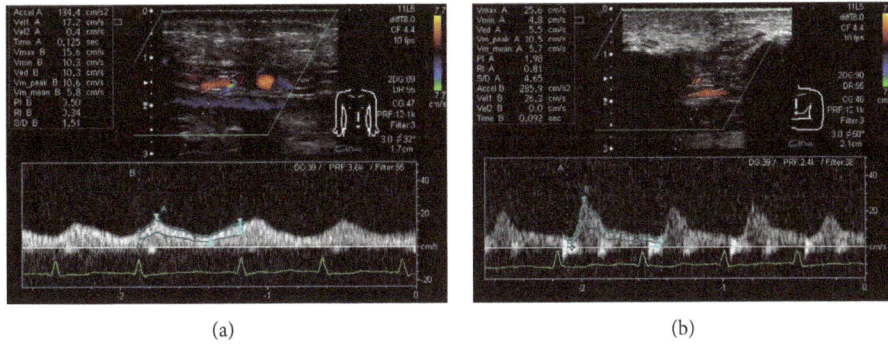

(a)   (b)

FIGURE 2: (a) Patient 1. Waveform of the superior epigastric artery (Type D-4). The $V_{\max}$ was 15.6 cm/sec, the lower limit of the standard value, and RI and PI were 0.34 and 0.50, respectively, apparently lower than the standard values. (b) Patient 1. Waveform of the internal thoracic artery (Type D-2). The waveform was a normal waveform.

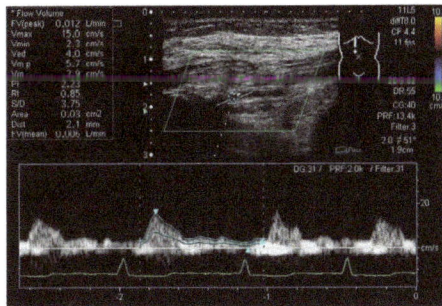

FIGURE 3: Patient 10. Waveform of the superior epigastric artery (Type D-3). The rectus abdominis musculocutaneous flap was partially necrosed.

of the superior epigastric artery was performed. However, the $V_{\max}$ was 15.0 cm/sec, being lower than the standard, and the muscle flap was partially necrosed (Figure 3). The case which detected blood flow poorly planned reconstruction by rectus abdominis musculocutaneous flap to mediastinitis and vascular waveform analysis of the superior epigastric artery was performed. However blood flow detection of the internal thoracic artery to the superior epigastric artery was poor. The blood vessel which flows into rectus abdominis muscle was confirmed in the direction of the outside; we performed blood flow evaluation by vascular waveform analysis. Although the vessel diameter was slightly as thin as about 1 mm, the vascular waveform was normal as D-2 waveform. Therefore we judged that the flap transplantation was possible and performed reconstruction using rectus abdominis musculocutaneous flap which was planned. The flap was partially necrosed after the operation. It was guessed to be because the tension of the flap distal part was strong in order to cover the defect of the chest upper part. Patient 17 was judged to be the vascular obstruction of the internal thoracic artery and was changed into reconstruction using omentum and pectoralis major muscle flap. Other 15 patients were valued with sufficient blood flow volume and flow velocity, and the vascular waveform was also normal waveform and the flap completely survived (Table 3).

Pedicled rectus abdominis musculocutaneous flaps supplied by the superior epigastric artery and vein were transplanted in 4 patients. The waveform type was D-1b in 1 patient and D-2 in 2 patients and D-3 in 1 patient. One of 2 flaps prepared with D-2 waveform vessels was completely survived, but the other flap was partially necrosed. One flap prepared with D-3 waveform vessels was partially necrosed.

Pedicled rectus abdominis musculocutaneous flaps supplied by the deep inferior epigastric artery and vein were transplanted in 2 patients. The waveform type was D-1b in 1 patient and D-2 in 1 patient, and all flaps were completely survived.

Pedicled latissimus dorsi musculocutaneous flaps supplied by the thoracodorsal artery and vein were transplanted in 8 patients. The waveform type was D-1a in 3 and D-1b in 3 and D-2 in 2 patients, and all flaps were completely survived.

Pedicled pectoralis major musculocutaneous flaps supplied by the thoracoacrominal artery and vein were transplanted in 3 patients. The waveform type was D-1b in 3 patients, and all flaps were completely survived.

Pedicled tensor fascia lata musculocutaneous flaps supplied by the lateral circumflex femoral artery and vein were transplanted in 2 patients. The waveform type was D-1b in 1 and D-2 in 1 patient, and all flaps were completely survived (Table 4).

All surgeries were performed by the same operator.

4. Discussion

To plan reconstruction with a vascularized flap, it is necessary to investigate the hemodynamics of feeding vessels before surgery in consideration of individual differences, vascular mutation, angiostenosis, and vascular obstruction. For the evaluation of blood flow in flap-feeding vessels in the field of plastic and reconstructive surgery, various methods are used, such as Doppler probe, angiography, MRA, and MDCT [6, 7].

Doppler probe has many advantages, such as simple operation, low cost, and short time of inspection. On the other hand, since the depth of the detected blood vessel cannot be judged, there is a risk of detecting a blood vessel deeper or shallower than the target blood vessel by mistake [6].

TABLE 3: Vascular waveform analysis of flap-feeding vessels. They were 4 patients which observed abnormal vascular waveform among 19 patients which performed vascular waveform analysis of flap-feeding vessels by using color Doppler ultrasonography prior to surgery (D-4: 1 patient, D-3: 1 patient, and Poor detect: 2 patients).

Patient	Vascularity	Side	Diameter	FV	V_{max}	V_{min}	V_{mean}	RI	PI	AT	Wave form
1	SEA	Lt	1.3 mm		15.6 cm/sec	10.3 cm/sec	10.6 cm/sec	0.34	0.50	125 msec	D-4
	TDA	Rt	1.6 mm		25.6 cm/sec	2.9 cm/sec	10.4 cm/sec	0.81	1.98	92 msec	D-2
2	TDA	Lt	1.3 mm	20 mL/min	35.3 cm/sec	6.8 cm/sec	14.2 cm/sec	0.81	2.01	66 msec	D-1b
3	TDA	Rt	2.0 mm	14 mL/min	26.0 cm/sec	2.6 cm/sec	7.6 cm/sec	0.90	3.08	25 msec	D-1a
4	TDA	Lt	1.3 mm	6 mL/min	23.5 cm/sec	2.8 cm/sec	7.1 cm/sec	0.81	2.68	58 msec	D-1b
5	TDA	Rt	0.7 mm	2 mL/min	22.6 cm/sec	0 cm/sec	6.6 cm/sec	1.00	3.42	50 msec	D-2
6	TDA	Rt	1.8 mm	14 mL/min	56.5 cm/sec	0 cm/sec	9.4 cm/sec	1.00	6.01	54 msec	D-1a
7	TDA	Rt	2.3 mm	37 mL/min	53.3 cm/sec	4.4 cm/sec	14.8 cm/sec	0.92	3.30	58 msec	D-1b
8	TDA	Rt	1.7 mm	20 mL/min	40.5 cm/sec	4.6 cm/sec	14.6 cm/sec	0.89	2.46	63 msec	D-1b
9	SEA	Lt	1.1 mm		24.3 cm/sec	4.7 cm/sec	10.1 cm/sec	0.81	1.94	62 msec	D-1b
10	SEA	Rt	2.1 mm	12 mL/min	15.0 cm/sec	2.3 cm/sec	5.7 cm/sec	0.85	2.23	75 msec	D-3
11	DIEA	Rt	1.8 mm	15 mL/min	42.3 cm/sec	1.2 cm/sec	12.9 cm/sec	0.87	2.86	71 msec	D-1b
12	SEA	Lt	1.0 mm	4 mL/min	19.1 cm/sec	4.4 cm/sec	7.6 cm/sec	0.81	2.04	71 msec	D-2
13	DIEA	Lt	1.3 mm	27 mL/min	81.1 cm/sec	16 cm/sec	34 cm/sec	0.8	1.91	45 msec	D-1b
14	SEA	Lt	1.3 mm	7 mL/min	25.8 cm/sec	3.6 cm/sec	9.7 cm/sec	0.86	2.29	46 msec	D-2 (ITA: poor detect)
15	TAA	Rt	1.8 mm	21 mL/min	45.5 cm/sec	4.7 cm/sec	13.9 cm/sec	0.94	3.07	62 msec	D-2
16	TAA	Lt	2.2 mm	19 mL/min	51.1 cm/sec	5.9 cm/sec	8.4 cm/sec	0.88	5.38	58 msec	D-1b
17	TAA	Lt	1.9 mm	28 mL/min	51.5 cm/sec	4.9 cm/sec	9.1 cm/sec	0.87	2.69	62 msec	D-1b (SEA: poor detect)
18	LCFA	Rt	1.7 mm	18 mL/min	37.9 cm/sec	6.3 cm/sec	13.4 cm/sec	0.74	2.10	70 msec	D-2
19	LCFA	Rt	1.7 mm	12 mL/min	32.4 cm/sec	2.4 cm/sec	8.8 cm/sec	0.93	3.41	54 msec	D-1b

TDA: thoracodorsal artery; SEA: superior epigastric artery; DIEA: deep inferior epigastric artery; TAA: thoracoacrominal artery; LCFA: lateral circumflex femoral artery.

TABLE 4: Vascular waveform classification and survival of the transplanted musculocutaneous flaps. For the survival of the transplanted musculocutaneous flaps, two cases of superior epigastric artery pedicled rectus abdominis musculocutaneous flaps were completely survived in four cases, two cases were partial necrosis. Two cases of deep inferior epigastric artery pedicled rectus abdominis musculocutaneous flaps were completely survived. Eight cases of thoracodorsal artery pedicled latissimus dorsi musculocutaneous flaps were completely survived. Three cases of thoracoacrominal artery pedicled pectoralis major musculocutaneous flaps were completely survived. Two cases of lateral circumflex femoral artery pedicled tensor fascia lata musculocutaneous flaps were completely survived.

	Superior epigastric artery		Deep inferior epigastric artery		Thoracodorsal artery		Thoracoacrominal artery		Lateral circumflex feroral artery	
	Number	Outcome	Number	Outcome	Number	Outcome	Number	Outcome	Number	Outcome
D-1a	0		0		3	S: 3	0		0	
D-1b	1	S	1	S	3	S: 3	3	S: 3	1	S
D-2	2	S: 1 PN: 1	1	S	2	S: 2	0		1	S
D-3	1	PN: 1	0		0		0		0	
D-4	0		0		0		0		0	

PN: partial necrosis; S: survive.

Although angiography is suitable for blood-flow evaluation of medium sized artery, it has problems, such as high invasion, radioactive exposure, and a high cost. Moreover, the special technique of image processing method is needed for imaging a thin artery like perforating vessels. Since MRA and MDCT have high contrast resolution, not only blood vessels and bones can be visualized, but also muscles and the surrounding soft tissue. Moreover, a perforating vessel less than 1 mm [7] also can be visualized. Thus, although highly precise image is obtained by low invasion, condition setting is necessary in order to enable the imaging of perforating vessels, such as to squeeze the particular vessel and to reduce the slice thickness of the image. In addition, the available facilities are limited because equipment is expensive.

On the other hand, color Doppler ultrasonography can be visualized noninvasively and easily, relative low cost the micro blood vessels compared to these tests, it has recently been used to identify flap-feeding vessels, particularly perforating arteries, and its usefulness has been reported [1–3]. Recently, the detectability of low-speed blood flow

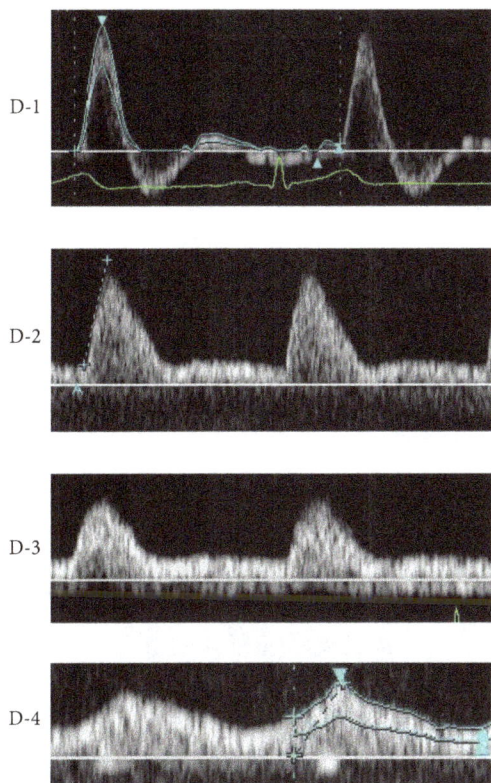

FIGURE 4: Hirai's classification of the vascular waveform. Hirai classified vascular waveforms into 4 types (D-1 to D-4).

employing the Doppler method has markedly improved with advancement in ultrasonographic diagnostic devices, and the accuracy has also markedly improved. In particular, the introduction of the power Doppler method, which is excellent for detecting low velocity blood flow, has allowed the visualization of peripheral vessels, which was conventionally difficult, and its application has expanded to many departments.

Regarding vascular waveform analysis of peripheral blood vessels, analysis is applied to diagnose lower limb occlusive arterial diseases. Hirai et al. [5] applied it for the screening of pelvic and lower limb occlusive arterial diseases, and classified the vascular waveforms into 4 types: D-1 to D-4 (Figure 4). Baba et al. [8] performed vascular waveform analysis of severely ischemic lower limbs and observed that whether the waveform type is D-1 or not could be determined following the waveform classification reported by Hirai et al.; but classification of the other types was difficult in many cases. They classified waveforms based on the presence or absence of diastolic components and direction (antegrade/retrograde) into the following 3 types: Type A to C (Figure 5). However, some arterial waveforms were difficult to classify employing the classifications reported by Hirai et al. and Baba et al. in our patients: systolic waves rose steeply but were not followed by reflux components in diastole, a notch was present between the systolic and diastolic waves, and anterograde diastolic waves were observed. No reflux component was noted in diastolic waves in many cases, even

though the vascular resistance was high and systolic waves showed a favorable steep rise in flap-feeding arteries, because these are peripheral arteries with a smaller diameter than those of the distal external iliac artery and proximal region of the popliteal artery involved in the waveform classification reported by Hirai et al. Thus, we considered it inappropriate to classify all these waveforms as D-2 and classified them as D-1b when a notch was noted between systolic and diastolic waves and designated the original D-1 as D-1a (Figure 1).

Hirai et al. regarded the D-1 type as a normal waveform with no significant stenosis on the proximal side and suggested the presence of a stenosis lesion on the proximal side in D-2, D-3, and D-4 waveforms. However, these are applied to arterial waveforms in the pelvis and thighs but difficult to apply to peripheral arteries unless some modification is made. In peripheral arteries, diastolic waveforms are lost because peripheral vascular resistance is high, and V_{min} is nearly 0 in many waveforms. Since these waveforms may also be normal in peripheral arteries, we regarded D-1a, D-1b, and D-2 as normal waveforms in the classification.

As parameters for the quantification of pulsative waveforms, based on V_{max}, V_{min}, and V_{mean}, the A/B ratio calculated as V_{max}/V_{min}, RI as $(V_{max} - V_{min})/V_{max}$, PI as $(V_{max} - V_{min})/V_{mean}$, and AT have been used. High and low values of A/B ratio, RI, and PI indicate high and low peripheral vascular resistances, respectively. The A/B ratio and RI are simply calculated from V_{max} and V_{min}, and the reproducibility is superior because values with relatively small errors are used, showing that these are practical parameters. However, the A/B ratio reaches infinity when V_{min} comes close to 0, and the RI can be calculated even when peripheral vascular resistance is markedly high and no diastolic blood flow component is observed in waveforms, but the value becomes RI = 1 regardless of the waveform shape. On the other hand, the PI value has no problem because of the use of V_{mean} even when no diastolic blood flow component is observed, but the calculation is not simple because the mean flow rate is calculated by tracing blood flow waveforms. Moreover, its calculation accuracy is inferior to that of RI due to technical errors. AT is an index reflecting changes in the time axis. Its calculation is simple, and an element in the time axis direction is added, for which improvement of the accuracy of blood flow evaluation is expected. In this study, we used RI, PI, and AT as indices for quantification of the pulsating waveforms of blood flow.

We performed vascular waveform analysis of the flap-feeding vessels of about 40 patients and reported the established reference values based on measurement values of vascular diameter, F-V, RI, PI, and AT [4] (Table 2). Now it is applied as an index of the blood flow in the flaps prior to surgery. Although there is some difference by the kind of flap-feeding vessels about the standard value for judged whether the transplantation of the skin flap is safe; vascular diameter $\geqq 1$ mm; FV $\geqq 5$ mL/min; $V_{max} \geqq 15$ cm/sec; RI $\geqq 0.7$; and AT $\leqq 100$ msec.

On a comparison of the results of vascular waveform analysis in actual cases of flap transplantation with the established standard values, the vascular waveform were normal (D-1a or D-1b or D-2) in cases which achieved complete survival,

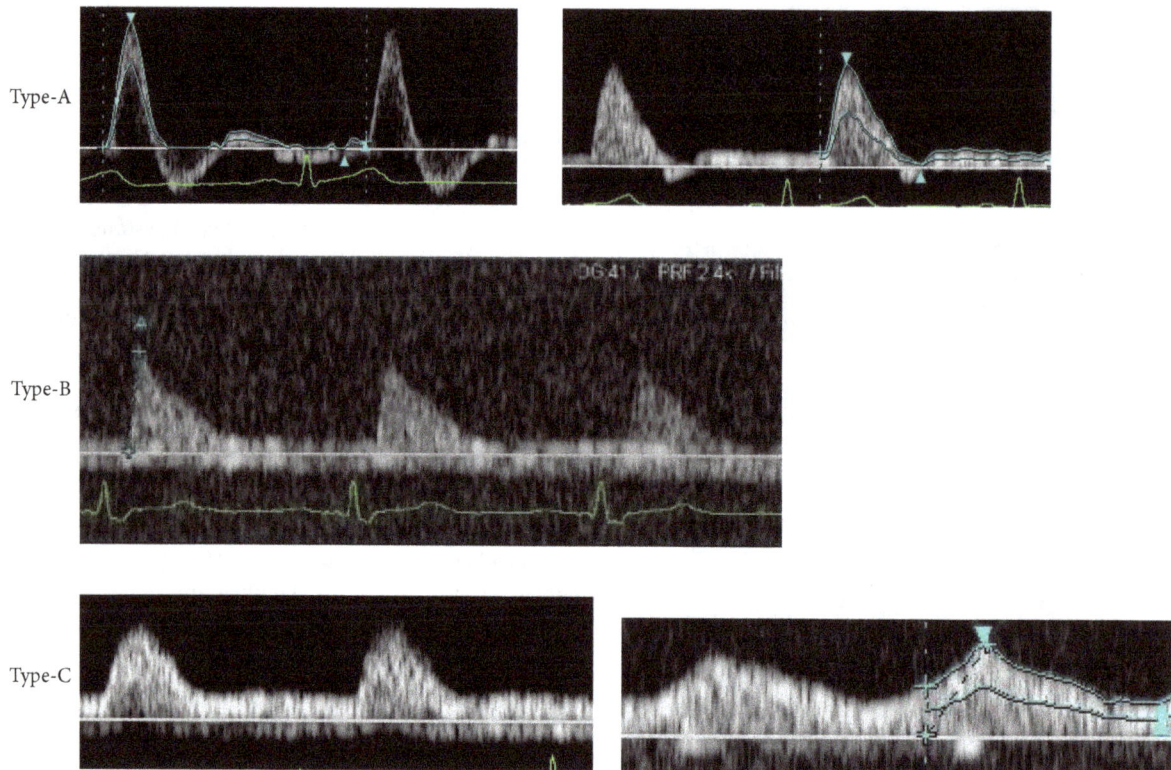

FIGURE 5: Baba's classification of the vascular waveform. Baba classified vascular waveforms into 3 types: type A: systolic waves rise steeply and are followed by reflux components in diastole, type B: the waveform is comprised of only systolic waves and diastolic waves are lost, and type C: systolic waves rise slowly and continue antegradely in diastole.

the diameter, FV, and V_{max}, were higher than the established values, indicating favorable blood flow, and the RI, PI, and AT were within the standard value ranges.

On the other hand, an abnormal D-4 waveform was noted in a case in which superior epigastric arterial waveform analysis was performed before surgery for sternal osteomyelitis. The V_{max} was 15.6 cm/sec, being slower than the standard; RI was 0.34, and PI was 0.50, being lower than the standard (Figure 2). The surgical procedure was changed to one using lattisimus dorsi musculocutaneous flap, and it was possible to perform a safe operation. In the case in which the pedicled flap containing the superior epigastric artery was partially necrosed, the waveform was abnormal D-3, and the V_{max} was 15.0 cm/sec, being lower than the standard (Figure 3).

The case which detected blood flow poorly, the vascular obstruction of the internal thoracic artery, was able to be judged prior to surgery, and it was possible to perform safe operation by changing into the reconstruction using omentum and pectoralis major muscle flap. The above clinical findings reflected the usefulness of the established standards.

The following advantages can be mentioned in the color Doppler ultrasonography. (1) It can be visualized the vessels at the same time as the fascia and muscle, adipose tissue, bone, it is possible to understand the detailed running of flap-feeding vessels. (2) We can select the skin flap with good blood flow more by measuring vessel diameter, flow volume, and flow velocity. (3) In the free flap transplant patients, postoperative patency confirmation of vascular anastomosis is easy; it can

be observed noninvasively and frequent times. (4) Therefore, it is useful for early detection of vascular occlusion such as postoperative thrombosis. (5) Quantitative observation of blood flow velocity of the anastomotic vessels after surgery is possible. However, technical skills, such as the skill of acquiring vascular images and experience in device operation are necessary. To perform vascular waveform analysis by visualizing the vascular distribution in detail and measuring the vascular diameter, F-V, RI, PI, and AT, collaboration with technologists is necessary, which will take time to conduct tests to some extent. To identify the distribution of a flap-feeding vessels and detailed hemodynamics, that is, for preoperative evaluation to perform safe surgery, it may be necessary for an operator familiar with vascular anatomy to attend to the tests and collaboration with technologists for the operation and setting of the ultrasonography system.

5. Conclusions

As preoperative blood flow assessment of the flap-feeding vessels, we performed vascular waveform analysis using color Doppler ultrasonography. Based on arterial waveform of the flap-feeding vessels, F-V, RI, PI, and AT were measured and classified vascular waveforms into 5 types partially modifying the blood flow waveform classification of Hirai et al. Although skills are necessary for the manipulation and setting of the ultrasonography system, and collaboration with clinical technologists is required, it is important to evaluate not only basic blood flow information of the vascular distribution, vascular diameter, and flow velocity, but also the flow volume, vascular resistance, and arterial waveform in analyzing the hemodynamics of the vascularised flaps and essential in performing Doppler ultrasonography.

Acknowledgment

The authors are grateful to Mr. Yakuwa, technologist at the Clinical Physiological Laboratory, Toho University Omori Medical Center, for his cooperation with this study.

References

[1] G. G. Hallock, "Evaluation of fasciocutaneous perforators using color duplex imaging," *Plastic and Reconstructive Surgery*, vol. 94, no. 5, pp. 644–651, 1994.

[2] P. N. Blondeel, G. Beyens, R. Verhaeghe et al., "Doppler flowmetry in the planning of pertorator flaps," *British Journal of Plastic Surgery*, vol. 51, no. 3, pp. 202–209, 1998.

[3] A. Ogino, Y. Maruyama, K. Onishi, K. Kanda, and T. Muro, "Preoperative colorDoppler assessment for identifying vascular of skin flaps," *the Japan Society for Simulation Surgery*, vol. 30, no. 2, pp. 45–51, 2010.

[4] A. Ogino, K. Onishi, and Y. Maruyama, "Vascular waveform analysis of vascularized flaps using color Doppler ultrasonography," *Journal of Japan Society of Plastic and Reconstructive Surgery*, vol. 19, no. 3, pp. 1–11, 2011.

[5] T. Hirai, H. Ohishi, K. Kichikawa, H. Yoshimura, and H. Uchida, "Ultrasonographic screening for arterial occlusive disease in the pelvis and lower extremities," *Radiation Medicine—Medical Imaging and Radiation Oncology*, vol. 16, no. 6, pp. 411–416, 1998.

[6] G. I. Taylor, M. Doyle, and G. McCarten, "The doppler probe for planning flaps: anatomical study and clinical applications," *British Journal of Plastic Surgery*, vol. 43, no. 1, pp. 1–16, 1990.

[7] J. Pauchot, S. Aubry, A. Kastler, O. Laurent, B. Kastler, and Y. Tropet, "Preoperative imaging for deep inferior epigastric perforator flaps: a comparative study of computed tomographic angiography and magnetic resonance angiography," *European Journal of Plastic Surgery*, vol. 35, pp. 795–801, 2012.

[8] R. Baba, K. Minowa, A. Kawamoto, M. Katayama, N. Handa, and Y. Kaneko, "Usefullness of the doppler wave form analysis in doppler ultrasonography: screening for critical limb ischemia," *Journal of Japanese College of Angiology*, vol. 48, no. 2, pp. 203–211, 2008.

14

Biologic Collagen Cylinder with Skate Flap Technique for Nipple Reconstruction

Brian P. Tierney,[1] Jason P. Hodde,[2] and Daniela I. Changkuon[2]

[1] *Tierney Plastic Surgery, 2011 Church Street, Suite 805, Nashville, TN 37203, USA*
[2] *Cook Biotech Incorporated, 1425 Innovation Place, West Lafayette, IN 47906, USA*

Correspondence should be addressed to Daniela I. Changkuon; dchangkuon@cookbiotech.com

Academic Editor: Nicolo Scuderi

A surgical technique using local tissue skate flaps combined with cylinders made from a naturally derived biomaterial has been used effectively for nipple reconstruction. A retrospective review of patients who underwent nipple reconstruction using this technique was performed. Comorbidities and type of breast reconstruction were collected. Outcome evaluation included complications, surgical revisions, and nipple projection. There were 115 skate flap reconstructions performed in 83 patients between July 2009 and January 2013. Patients ranged from 32 to 73 years old. Average body mass index was 28.0. The most common comorbidities were hypertension (39.8%) and smoking (16.9%). After breast reconstruction, 68.7% of the patients underwent chemotherapy and 20.5% underwent radiation. Seventy-one patients had immediate breast reconstruction with expanders and 12 had delayed reconstruction. The only reported complications were extrusions (3.5%). Six nipples (5.2%) in 5 patients required surgical revision due to loss of projection; two patients had minor loss of projection but did not require surgical revision. Nipple projection at time of surgery ranged from 6 to 7 mm and average projection at 6 months was 3–5 mm. A surgical technique for nipple reconstruction using a skate flap with a graft material is described. Complications are infrequent and short-term projection measurements are encouraging.

1. Introduction

In 2013, the American Cancer Society estimated that 232,340 new cases of invasive breast cancer would be diagnosed in women. Nipple-areola reconstruction is the last stage in a long and multifaceted journey to restore the presurgical appearance of a person's breast following mastectomy. The presence of a nipple on a reconstructed breast has been shown to be psychologically significant for women who have had mastectomies [1, 2]. Numerous techniques exist for nipple reconstruction, but no method has reliable and consistent aesthetic results [3–13]. Recently, a surgical technique using local tissue flaps combined with cylinders made from a naturally derived biomaterial has been used effectively.

The Biodesign Nipple Reconstruction Cylinder (NRC; COOK Inc., Bloomington, IN) is a rolled cylinder of extracellular matrix collagen derived from porcine small intestinal submucosa (SIS) and is intended for implantation to reinforce soft tissue in plastic and reconstructive surgery of the nipple (Figure 1). Like dermis or fascia, SIS is composed of fibrillar collagens and adhesive glycoproteins which serve as a scaffold into which cells can migrate and multiply. Once implanted, the NRC material allows for angiogenesis as well as connective and epithelial tissue growth and differentiation. Furthermore, the material allows cells to migrate into the device and form an organized extracellular matrix (ECM) through the deposition of collagen and other proteins. Over time, this remodeling results in the formation of tissue that is histologically similar to the tissue at the implant site. Eventually, the body metabolizes the device, leaving behind only naturally augmented patient tissue [14–16].

Although some patients decide not to proceed with nipple-areolar reconstruction, the nipple is considered to be a well-defined anatomic marker that contributes significantly to the shape and symmetry of the breast [17]. This retrospective case series describes a skate-flap reconstruction technique in combination with the Biodesign NRC that can be safely performed over breast implants.

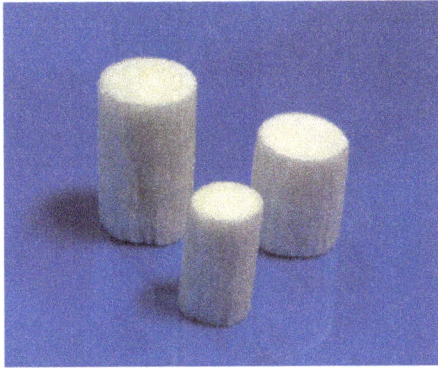

FIGURE 1: Image of the Biodesign Nipple Reconstruction Cylinder (COOK Inc., Bloomington, IN). Cylinders have a length of either 1.0 cm or 1.5 cm and a diameter of either 0.7 cm or 1.0 cm. All sizes can be trimmed prior to implantation.

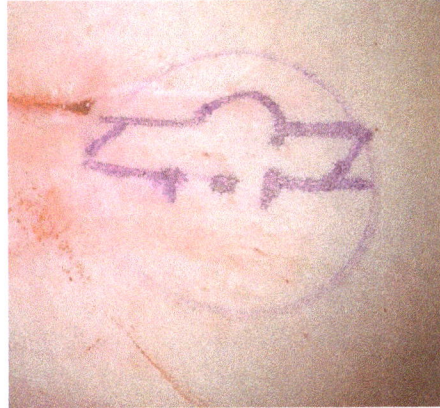

FIGURE 2: Skate-flap pattern drawn onto the patient's breast to guide the creation of the skin flap.

2. Methods

A retrospective, single-center, single-surgeon, chart review was performed on all postmastectomy breast reconstruction patients who underwent skate-flap nipple reconstruction in combination with a Biodesign NRC between July 2009 and January 2013. Patient demographic data including age, weight, indication for surgery, and cancer stage were collected. Other risk factors, including smoking, preoperative and postoperative chemotherapy, and radiation therapy, were also collected and analyzed. The surgery dates, types of mastectomy, and types of breast reconstruction were recorded for every patient. Outcome evaluations included complications, the need for surgical revision, and nipple projection measurements.

2.1. Surgical Technique. Nipple cylinder diameter (0.7 cm or 1.0 cm) and length (1 cm or 1.5 cm) were selected to closely match the contralateral nipple. If a contralateral nipple was not present, the overall size of the reconstructed breast, the presence or absence of a well-vascularized skin flap, and/or the patient's desired final appearance were considered when determining the cylinder size, allowing for some shrinkage following implant. The position of the nipple was determined with the patient seated in a relaxed position. Using a surgical marker, a skate-flap pattern (Figure 2) was drawn onto the patient's breast to guide the creation of the skin flaps. The NRC was allowed to rehydrate for no greater than 10 seconds before it was placed underneath the appropriate skin flaps, ensuring that an adequate blood supply reached the device. This placement allowed for maximum contact with healthy, well-vascularized tissue and encouraged cell in-growth and tissue remodeling (Figure 3). The cylinder was then secured into place with a combination of 3-0 Vicryl (Ethicon, Somerville, NJ) and 4-0 Monocryl (Ethicon, Somerville, NJ) sutures at the base of the nipple reconstruction to prevent migration of the cylinder into the subcutaneous region beneath the flaps. After reconstruction, incisions were closed with a combination of inverted dermal 3-0 Vicryl sutures and simple interrupted 4-0 Monocryl sutures. The reconstructed

nipple was protected using a hard plastic shield, which was left in place for up to 4 weeks. Topical antibiotic cream was not routinely used following surgery, but patients were instructed to use triple antibiotic and return to the clinic if signs of infection were observed when cleansing the area. The areola was later pigmented by tattoo according to standard practice.

3. Results

There were 83 women who underwent postmastectomy breast reconstruction and subsequent nipple reconstruction. The average age was 50.4 years (range: 32–73 years) and average body mass index was 28.0 (range: 15.8–48.4). Thirty-three patients (39.8%) had a diagnosis of hypertension, 14 (16.9%) used tobacco products, and 9 (10.8%) had type II diabetes at the time of reconstruction (see Table 1). Indications for mastectomy included infiltrating carcinoma in 40 patients (48.2%), ductal carcinoma in situ in 35 patients (42.2%), 1 case (1.2%) each of lobular carcinoma, Paget's disease of the nipple, BRCA+ and high risk benign mass, and 4 patients (4.8%) with unknown indications. Fifteen patients (18.1%) underwent both radiation and chemotherapy, 42 (50.6%) had adjuvant chemotherapy alone, 2 (2.4%) underwent radiation alone, 8 (9.6%) had no adjuvant therapy, and for 16 (19.3%) patients, adjuvant therapy was unknown. Out of the 83 patients, 71 (85.5%) chose to have immediate 2-stage breast reconstruction after mastectomy. The process involved the placement of tissue expanders immediately following mastectomy and a second surgery to replace the expanders with permanent implants. The remaining 12 patients (14.5%) had delayed breast reconstruction, also with tissue expanders.

Using a skate-flap and graft technique in combination with the Biodesign NRC, the total number of nipple reconstructions was 115 (61 unilateral reconstructions and 27 bilateral reconstructions). The only reported complications included 4 cases (3.5%) of NRC extrusion and 5 patients (4 unilateral and 1 bilateral reconstructions, 5.2%) who required surgical revision due to loss of nipple projection (see Table 2). Additionally, two patients reported minor loss of projection but did not require surgical revision. No postoperative cases

(a)

(b)

(c)

(d)

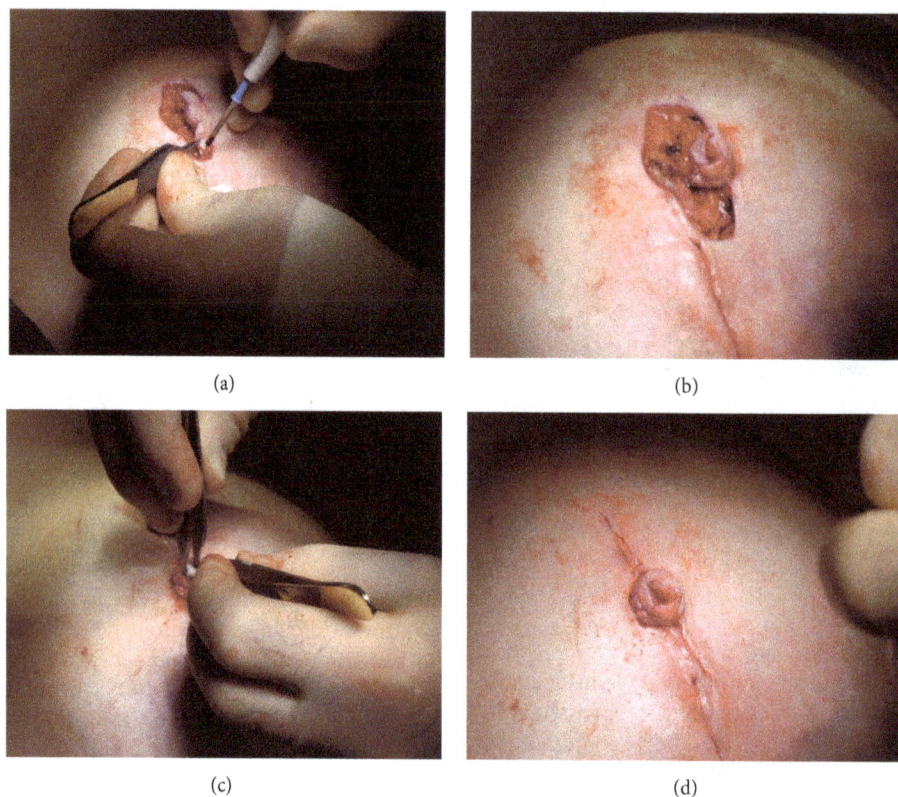

FIGURE 3: Intraoperative pictures. (a) Skate flap comprised of skin and fatty tissue is cut and lifted along the surgical markings; (b) the ends of the flap are brought together and sutured to allow for cylinder placement; (c) the cylinder is carefully placed inside the flap, (d) resulting in the cylinder being securely wrapped by vascularized skin tissue.

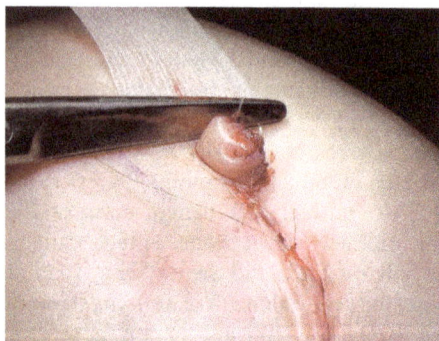

FIGURE 4: Nipple projection at time of surgery ranged from 6 to 7 mm.

of infection or allergic reaction to the cylinder were reported. Nipple projection at time of surgery ranged from 6 to 7 mm (see Figure 4) and average projection at 6 months was 3–5 mm. An example of long-term results can be seen in Figure 5.

4. Discussion

Published information for nipple-areola reconstruction reveals numerous surgical techniques and variable long-term results in terms of patient satisfaction and sustained nipple projection. Some of the different techniques and local flaps

that are used for nipple reconstruction, besides the skate-flap, are the Marshall technique [4], the button-hole technique [5], the C-V flap [6], silicone rods [7], the star-flap [8], the cigar roll flap [9], the hamburger technique [10], the arrow-flap [11], the top-hat-flap [12], the Swiss Roll flap [13], and others. One of the main limitations to this retrospective case review is that it only evaluates the skate-flap technique in combination with the Biodesign NRC; however, this is the senior author's surgical technique of choice and this series demonstrates that the procedure is safe and reliable, with very low complication rates.

Surgeon preference is usually what determines the surgical method of choice for nipple reconstruction. It is difficult to conclude if there is one method that yields superior results than others because very few evidence-based comparisons have been published. It is expected, however, that with every surgical technique for nipple reconstruction that exists today there will be variations in the results, complications, and some degree of projection loss with time. Modifications of current surgical techniques and new device technologies are continuously being developed and tested for lower complication rates and longer lasting nipple projection.

The only cases in this series that required surgical revision were due to loss of nipple projection or cylinder extrusion. The cause of the loss of nipple projection is unknown but may be related to individual patient characteristics or noncompliance in wearing the plastic shield following surgery.

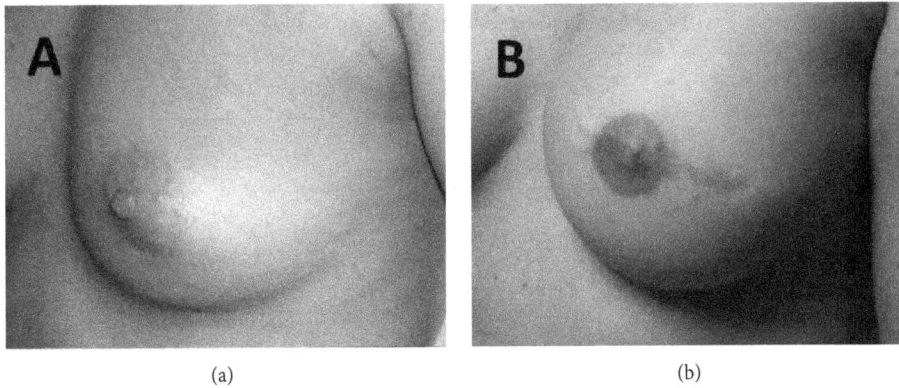

FIGURE 5: (a) Patient before breast and nipple reconstruction. (b) Same patient after breast and nipple reconstruction.

TABLE 1: Patient demographics.

Total number of patients = 83	
Age	Range: 32–73 years old
	Mean: 50.4 years old
BMI	Range: 15.8–48.4
	Mean: 28.0
Indication for surgery	IC = 40 patients (48.2%)
	DCIS = 35 patients (42.2%)
	LC = 1 patient (1.2%)
	Paget's = 1 patient (1.2%)
	BRCA+ = 1 patient (1.2%)
	Benign mass = 1 patient (1.2%)
	Unknown = 4 patients (4.8%)
Diabetes (Type II)	9 patients (10.8%)
Hypertension	33 patients (39.8%)
Smoking (or tobacco products)	14 patients (16.9%)
Preoperative chemotherapy	22 patients (26.5%)
Postoperative chemotherapy	48 patients (57.8%)
Chemotherapy alone (no radiation)	42 patients (50.6%)
Preoperative radiation	6 patients (7.2%)
Postoperative radiation	14 patients (16.9%)
Radiation alone (no chemotherapy)	2 patients (2.4%)
Combined chemotherapy and radiation	15 patients (18.1%)
No adjuvant cancer treatment	8 patients (9.6%)
Unknown cancer treatment	16 patients (19.3%)

IC: infiltrating carcinoma, DCIS: ductal carcinoma in situ, LC: lobular carcinoma, Paget's: Paget's disease of the nipple, and BRCA+: positive breast cancer gene.

Four patients suffered from extrusion of the Biodesign NRC between 2 and 4 weeks after surgery but only 1 patient required further surgical revision. The most likely reason for cylinder extrusion was tension on the sutures that lead to a small degree of tissue ischemia and necrosis of part of the flap.

Other risks of nipple reconstruction reported in the literature include localized tip/flap necrosis, partial flap loss, complete flap loss/infection, dehiscence, seroma formation, and an overall expected complication rate of approximately 12% in all patients [17–19]. While all of these risks are applicable when implanting the NRC, this case series did not present any of the aforementioned complications. The limited use of the NRC in patients to date does not allow for an accurate account of the extent of these risks beyond those associated with the surgical procedure alone.

The intended goal of this retrospective case series was to describe a successful skin flap technique and device combination that could be used to reconstruct the nipple-areola complex following the removal and reconstruction of breast tissue. The potential clinical benefits to the subjects are a surgery that can be performed quickly and with minimal morbidity, providing safe, predictable, and long-lasting aesthetic results. Seventy-eight out of 83 patients (94.0%) underwent skate-flap nipple reconstruction in combination with the Biodesign NRC and had no complications. At the time of surgery, average nipple projection ranged from 6 to 7 mm and average projection at 6 months was 3–5 mm, representing a 30%–50% percent loss of projection, which is similar to the projection loss noted following local skin flap nipple reconstruction without graft material augmentation [11]. This loss of projection over time is an important consideration when attempting to decide what size of implant to choose for surgery. It is acknowledged that the relatively short follow-up time of 6 months does not allow us to comment on long-lasting aesthetic outcome at this time.

Alternative treatments to the nipple cylinder for reconstruction include cosmetic tattooing of the areola only, local skin flap nipple reconstruction without graft material augmentation, autologous or composite grafts (i.e., contra lateral nipple, fat grafting, or cartilage) [17, 20, 21], or the use of other biologic materials like human dermis, hyaluronic acid [22], or poly-lactic acid [23].

Currently, more comparative clinical studies are needed to optimize the procedures used to reconstruct the nipple-areola complex following mastectomy. With the use of the Biodesign NRC, there is a potential for reducing patient complications, providing longer-lasting nipple projection

TABLE 2: Nipple reconstruction complications.

Patient	Date of nipple reconstruction	Surgery procedure used	NRC: L, R, or bilateral	Complications
1	7/10/2009	Skate + NRC	Left	Lost projection, surgical revision required
	10/16/2009	Revision with second NRC		
2	1/19/2011	Skate + NRC	Bilateral	Lost projection, surgical revision required
	4/5/2011	Revision with second NRC		
3	4/12/2011	Skate + NRC	Right	Cylinder extrusion 3 weeks post-op; projection still viable, no surgical revision required
4	3/28/2011	Skate + NRC	Right	Patient displeased with projection, surgical revision required
	7/26/2011	Revision with second NRC		
5	5/18/2011	Skate + NRC	Left	Cylinder extrusion 2 weeks post-op; projection still viable, no surgical revision required
6	2/7/2012	Revision with NRC	Right	Loss of projection due to radiation therapy; cylinder extrusion 3 weeks post-op; projection still viable, no surgical revision required
7	9/30/2011	Skate + NRC	Right	Lost projection, surgical revision required
	10/26/2012	Revision with second NRC		
8	10/5/2011	Skate + NRC	Left	Cylinder extrusion 4 weeks post-op; lost projection, surgical revision required
	3/9/2012	Revision with second NRC		
9	10/14/2012	Skate + NRC	Left	Lost projection, surgical revision required
	2/24/2012	Revision with second NRC		

Skate: skate-flap nipple reconstruction technique and NRC: Biodesign Nipple Reconstruction Cylinder.

and achieving higher patient satisfaction than either autologous graft procedures or flap procedures alone. A combined surgical technique for nipple reconstruction that used a skate flap and an off-the-shelf biologic graft material that resulted in comparable aesthetic results to alternative treatments and promising long-lasting projection was presented. Complications are infrequent and short-term projection measurements are encouraging. Longer-term followup is needed to determine if nipple projection is sustained for longer periods of time and if the added cost of the cylinder is justified by long-term aesthetic outcome.

Disclosure

This paper is not currently under consideration, in press, or published elsewhere. This paper is truthful original work without fabrication, fraud, or plagiarism.

Authors' Contribution

All authors have made an important scientific contribution to this study, are familiar with the primary data, and have read the entire paper and take responsibility for its content.

References

[1] S. C. J. Goh, N. A. Martin, A. N. Pandya, and R. I. Cutress, "Patient satisfaction following nipple-areolar complex reconstruction and tattooing," *Journal of Plastic, Reconstructive and Aesthetic Surgery*, vol. 64, no. 3, pp. 360–363, 2011.

[2] S. L. Spear, A. D. Schaffner, M. R. Jespersen, and J. A. Goldstein, "Donor-site morbidity and patient satisfaction using a composite nipple graft for unilateral nipple reconstruction in the radiated and nonradiated breast," *Plastic and Reconstructive Surgery*, vol. 127, no. 4, pp. 1437–1446, 2011.

[3] K. C. Shestak, A. Gabriel, A. Landecker, S. Peters, A. Shestak, and J. Kim, "Assessment of long-term nipple projection: a comparison of three techniques," *Plastic and Reconstructive Surgery*, vol. 110, no. 3, pp. 780–786, 2002.

[4] J. Skillman, O. Ahmed, A. R. Rowsell, and B. Dheansa, "The Marshall technique: an economic one-stage technique for nipple-areola reconstruction," *British Journal of Plastic Surgery*, vol. 55, no. 6, pp. 504–506, 2002.

[5] S. Hamilton and M. D. Brough, "The button-hole technique for nipple-areola complex reconstruction," *Journal of Plastic, Reconstructive and Aesthetic Surgery*, vol. 59, no. 1, pp. 35–39, 2006.

[6] L. Valdatta, P. Montemurro, F. Tamborini, C. Fidanza, A. Gottardi, and S. Scamoni, "Our experience of nipple reconstruction using the C-V flap technique: 1 year evaluation," *Journal of Plastic, Reconstructive and Aesthetic Surgery*, vol. 62, no. 10, pp. 1293–1298, 2009.

[7] J. Jankau, J. Jaśkiewicz, and A. Ankiewicz, "A new method for using a silicone rod for permanent nipple projection after breast reconstruction procedures," *The Breast*, vol. 20, no. 2, pp. 124–128, 2011.

[8] Y. Yamamoto, H. Furukawa, A. Oyama et al., "Two innovations of the star-flap technique for nipple reconstruction," *British Journal of Plastic Surgery*, vol. 54, no. 8, pp. 723–726, 2001.

[9] B. Jamnadas-Khoda, R. Thomas, and S. Heppell, "The "cigar roll" flap for nipple areola complex reconstruction: a novel technique," *Journal of Plastic, Reconstructive and Aesthetic Surgery*, vol. 64, no. 8, pp. E218–E220, 2011.

[10] A. P. Jones and M. Erdmann, "Projection and patient satisfaction using the "hamburger" nipple reconstruction technique," *Journal of Plastic, Reconstructive and Aesthetic Surgery*, vol. 65, no. 2, pp. 207–212, 2012.

[11] C. Rubino, L. A. Dessy, and A. Posadinu, "A modified technique for nipple reconstruction: The 'arrow flap'," *British Journal of Plastic Surgery*, vol. 56, no. 3, pp. 247–251, 2003.

[12] M. H. Cheng, M. Ho-Asjoe, F. C. Wei, and D. C. Chuang, "Nipple reconstruction in Asian females using banked cartilage graft and modified top hat flap," *British Journal of Plastic Surgery*, vol. 56, no. 7, pp. 692–694, 2003.

[13] C. R. Macdonald, A. Nakhdjevani, and A. Shah, "The "Swiss-Roll" flap: a modified C-V flap for nipple reconstruction," *Breast*, vol. 20, no. 5, pp. 475–477, 2011.

[14] R. F. Centeno, "Surgisis acellular collagen matrix in aesthetic and reconstructive plastic surgery soft tissue applications," *Clinics in Plastic Surgery*, vol. 36, no. 2, pp. 229–240, 2009.

[15] A. Wiedemann and M. Otto, "Small intestinal submucosa for pubourethral sling suspension for the treatment of stress incontinence: first histopathological results in humans," *Journal of Urology*, vol. 172, no. 1, pp. 215–218, 2004.

[16] S. F. Badylak, K. Park, N. Peppas, G. McCabe, and M. Yoder, "Marrow-derived cells populate scaffolds composed of xenogeneic extracellular matrix," *Experimental Hematology*, vol. 29, no. 11, pp. 1310–1318, 2001.

[17] M. Cheng, E. D. Rodriguez, J. M. Smartt, and A. Cardenas-Mejia, "Nipple reconstruction using the modified top hat flap with banked costal cartilage graft: Long-term follow-up in 58 patients," *Annals of Plastic Surgery*, vol. 59, no. 6, pp. 621–628, 2007.

[18] D. M. Otterburn, K. E. Sikora, and A. Losken, "An outcome evaluation following postmastectomy nipple reconstruction using the C-V flap technique," *Annals of Plastic Surgery*, vol. 64, no. 5, pp. 574–578, 2010.

[19] K. El-Ali, M. Dalal, and C. C. Kat, "Modified C-V flap for nipple reconstruction: our results in 50 patients," *Journal of Plastic, Reconstructive and Aesthetic Surgery*, vol. 62, no. 8, pp. 991–996, 2009.

[20] R. W. Bernard and S. J. Beran, "Autologous fat graft in nipple reconstruction," *Plastic and Reconstructive Surgery*, vol. 112, no. 4, pp. 964–968, 2003.

[21] A. B. Guerra, K. Khoobehi, S. E. Metzinger, and R. J. Allen, "New technique for nipple areola reconstruction: arrow flap and rib cartilage graft for long-lasting nipple projection," *Annals of Plastic Surgery*, vol. 50, no. 1, pp. 31–37, 2003.

[22] K. Lennox and K. R. Beer, "Nipple contouring with hyaluronics postmastectomy.," *Journal of Drugs in Dermatology*, vol. 6, no. 10, pp. 1030–1033, 2007.

[23] L. A. Dessy, A. Troccola, R. L. M. Ranno, M. Maruccia, C. Alfano, and M. G. Onesti, "The use of poly-lactic acid to improve projection of reconstructed nipple," *Breast*, vol. 20, no. 3, pp. 220–224, 2011.

15

Stem Cell-Based Therapeutics to Improve Wound Healing

Michael S. Hu,[1,2,3] Tripp Leavitt,[1] Samir Malhotra,[1]
Dominik Duscher,[1,4] Michael S. Pollhammer,[4] Graham G. Walmsley,[1,2]
Zeshaan N. Maan,[1] Alexander T. M. Cheung,[1] Manfred Schmidt,[4]
Georg M. Huemer,[4] Michael T. Longaker,[1,2] and H. Peter Lorenz[1]

[1]*Hagey Laboratory for Pediatric Regenerative Medicine, Department of Surgery, Division of Plastic and Reconstructive Surgery, Stanford University School of Medicine, Stanford, CA 94305, USA*
[2]*Institute for Stem Cell Biology and Regenerative Medicine, Stanford University School of Medicine, Stanford, CA 94305, USA*
[3]*Department of Surgery, John A. Burns School of Medicine, University of Hawaii, Honolulu, HI 96813, USA*
[4]*Section of Plastic, Aesthetic and Reconstructive Surgery, Johannes Kepler University, Linz, Austria*

Correspondence should be addressed to Michael S. Hu; mhu2@stanford.edu

Academic Editor: Nicolo Scuderi

Issues surrounding wound healing have garnered deep scientific interest as well as booming financial markets invested in novel wound therapies. Much progress has been made in the field, but it is unsurprising to find that recent successes reveal new challenges to be addressed. With regard to wound healing, large tissue deficits, recalcitrant wounds, and pathological scar formation remain but a few of our most pressing challenges. Stem cell-based therapies have been heralded as a promising means by which to surpass current limitations in wound management. The wide differentiation potential of stem cells allows for the possibility of restoring lost or damaged tissue, while their ability to immunomodulate the wound bed from afar suggests that their clinical applications need not be restricted to direct tissue formation. The clinical utility of stem cells has been demonstrated across dozens of clinical trials in chronic wound therapy, but there is hope that other aspects of wound care will inherit similar benefit. Scientific inquiry into stem cell-based wound therapy abounds in research labs around the world. While their clinical applications remain in their infancy, the heavy investment in their potential makes it a worthwhile subject to review for plastic surgeons, in terms of both their current and future applications.

1. Introduction

Wound healing is a complex process involving several physiological mechanisms coordinated in an effective response to tissue injury. This process consists of several distinct, yet overlapping phases—hemostasis and inflammation, proliferation, and maturation—that result in scar formation under normal circumstances [1, 2]. Normal wound repair exists along a spectrum of outcomes resulting from tissue injury. These range from pathologic underhealing (i.e., chronic, nonhealing wounds) to pathologic overhealing (i.e., hypertrophic scars and keloids), with physiologic healing, including scar formation, somewhere in between. Interest in wound healing research continues to grow, with much focus now directed towards stem cell therapies to overcome limitations in our current wound management practices. To date, 45 published clinical studies and an additional 33 trials with as yet unpublished results have explored the potential for stem cells in addressing pathological underhealing (unpublished data). Thus, current research suggests that we are nearing a tipping point in the proliferation of stem cell-based therapies and the use of these therapies to treat disease. As such, a basic understanding of wound healing and the recent advances in stem cell therapies are important topics for plastic surgeons. Herein, we discuss the unmet need that stem cell therapies are purported to address, as well as their current uses in wound healing.

2. Importance of Wound Healing

The majority of the body's tissues are capable of undergoing wound repair following a disruption of tissue integrity [2]. Wound care is a major component of surgical practice both acutely (e.g., trauma, burns, and surgery) and chronically (e.g., pressure ulcers, venous ulcers, and diabetic ulcers). Upon healing, these wounds result in scar formation. Tens of billions of dollars are devoted to wound care each year [3]. Chronic wounds are especially costly, as they often require prolonged follow-up with repeated interventions and are not uncommonly resistant to therapy; it is estimated that 1% of the population at any given time is suffering from some form of chronic wound [4].

Pathological scar formation, including hypertrophic scars and keloids, is another concern in wound management. These conditions can be particularly problematic given the possibility for permanent functional loss as well as social stigma [5]. Hypertrophic scars are usually the result of traumatic injuries or burns, but surgery is another potential cause. In a given year, the 1 million burns and 2 million patients injured in motor vehicle accidents necessitating treatment, in addition to the millions of others undergoing invasive surgery, demonstrate the pressing nature of this issue [5, 6].z

3. Normal Wound Healing Physiology

As stated previously, wound healing is comprised of three overlapping stages: (1) inflammatory phase, (2) proliferation phase, and (3) maturation phase. It is important to understand the physiological mechanisms of wound healing to fully appreciate the abnormalities underlying various wound healing disorders in order to provide adequate treatment. Here we will briefly summarize the basic physiological mechanisms of wound healing. For more in-depth discussions of these processes beyond the scope of this paper, particularly in terms of the inflammatory response, the reader is directed to reviews by Gurtner et al. [2] and Eming et al. [1].

Tissue injury initiates the wound healing response, beginning with wound hemostasis as part of the inflammatory phase. Though blood flow is restricted at the wound bed itself, the adjacent tissue is subject to increased perfusion. Inflammatory mediators are produced in concert with the coagulation cascade, generating a local concentration gradient. This promotes fibrin matrix formation and neutrophil chemotaxis. Once the matrix is established, neutrophils enter to remove the dead tissue and attempt to control any potential infections via the innate immune response. These migrating cells further amplify the inflammatory response, themselves releasing proinflammatory cytokines, contributing to the swelling and erythema often observed in the initial stages of wound healing. This phase typically lasts for 4 days [7, 8].

In the ensuing proliferation phase, inflammatory cells release various cytokines and other signaling molecules to recruit fibroblasts and vascular endothelial cells to the site of injury. Fibroblasts produce collagen, which begins to replace the provisional fibrin matrix, increasing the mechanical strength of the wound. A portion of these fibroblasts also differentiates into myofibroblasts, which contribute to mechanical wound contraction. Migrating endothelial cells contribute revascularization of the wound bed via angiogenesis, helping to support the developing granulation tissue. Keratinocytes also migrate to the wound edge, where they undergo proliferation [7, 9]. Of note, destruction of hair follicles in larger wounds correlates with slower reepithelialization secondary to the loss of the epidermal stem cell niche, potentially necessitating skin graft placement to achieve complete closure [10].

It is during the final maturation phase that the wound undergoes reepithelialization. Scar formation allows the healed tissue to regain some, but not all, of its original tensile strength. However, tissue elasticity is dramatically reduced secondary to extensive fibrosis. As the intensity of the healing response deescalates in its final stages, the majority of the endothelial cells, macrophages, and myofibroblasts localized to the wound bed undergo apoptosis. The remaining scar will continue to undergo further remodeling over the subsequent months to years [7, 11].

4. Targets for Novel Cell-Based Therapies

In the United States, costs of chronic wound management alone are estimated to exceed $25 billion per annum [3]. Furthermore, these therapies are often supportive with suboptimal clinical outcomes, marking chronic wounds as important targets for novel therapies. While normal wound healing results in benign scar formation, impaired wound healing processes can result in aesthetically displeasing scar formation or even a chronic, nonhealing wound. Factors understood to perturb physiological healing include aging, sedentary lifestyle (characterized by little or no physical activity), psychological status, and smoking [12]. Chronic disease states share many of the modifiable risk factors associated with poor wound healing and are themselves impediments to the physiological healing process. For example, diabetes is tightly linked to chronic wound formation in the form of nonhealing diabetic ulcers [13]. Uncontrolled diabetes impairs neutrophil and macrophage migration to the wound bed. The resultant delay of wound healing predisposes patients to develop diabetic foot ulcers, which in turn may become infected and necessitate surgical debridement or amputation. A better understanding of chronic wound pathophysiology can help identify potential roles for stem cell-based therapies in nonhealing wounds [13]. Ultimately, the goal is to create cost-effective therapies that can significantly improve the quality of life for patients suffering from these conditions. Stem cells offer a promising means to this end with the potential to heal recalcitrant wounds and prevent costly sequelae of prolonged tissue defects [14].

At the opposite end of the wound healing spectrum exists pathological overhealing, subdivided into hypertrophic scarring and keloid formation. Hypertrophic scarring is attributed to the dysregulated proliferation of inflammatory cells and fibroblasts during the wound healing process, further contributing to a highly disorganized matrix structure that is characteristic of scars [15]. Hypertrophic scarring currently has no known cure; available treatments are inadequate at curbing scar formation or diminishing the resulting aesthetic defect. Excessive inflammation is a characteristic of both hypertrophic scar formation and chronic wound beds, the latter of which have been successfully managed through stem cell immunomodulation [16]. Stem cells may thus offer a means to address pathological scarring [17].

Keloid formation is a more extreme example of pathological scar formation. Often considered as separate from hypertrophic scars in terms of their pathophysiology, histological analysis has suggested that keloids may in fact simply be further along the pathological spectrum [18]. Keloids occur solely in humans following tissue injury, not uncommonly resulting from surgical incisions [19]. Both hypertrophic scarring and keloid formation involve abnormally high levels of scar formation. However, hypertrophic scars remain confined to within the wound margins, whereas keloids invade beyond them into the surrounding normal tissue. While hypertrophic scars characteristically regress over time, keloids can grow for years and almost never spontaneously regress, leading to more devastating cosmetic outcomes [20]. In fact, the amount of scar tissue formed does not correlate with the severity of the initial wounding, so even small wounds can have substantial aesthetic consequences. Although multiple types of treatments have been attempted to manage keloid scarring, none has yielded significant results [21, 22]. However, experimental studies have demonstrated the ability of stem cells to inhibit keloid growth, opening up new avenues for their treatment [23]. Unfortunately, these findings are not universal and more study is needed in terms of stem cell applications for keloid management [24].

5. Traditional Approaches to Wound Healing

In cases where tissue defects necessitate placement of a skin graft, surgeons can ideally utilize autologous tissue, foregoing any need for immunosuppression. However, autograft harvest is not possible in all cases, for example, due to insufficient tissue for harvest. In scenarios that preclude autologous tissue grafting, surgeons can utilize cadaveric tissue, termed allografts, or porcine xenografts. These are merely temporizing measures to provide growth factors for wound healing, as the host immune response causes transplant rejection in the weeks following implantation [25].

Tissue availability and graft immunogenicity are common issues in all areas of transplant medicine. Skin grafting is no exception, spurring the development of tissue engineered skin substitutes. The first of these substitutes were known as matrix-based products, which continue to be used today. These matrices are implanted at the wound bed, where they function as templates for revascularization and dermal regeneration. However, complete wound healing still often necessitates epidermal covering of the neodermis by skin graft or flap, though some small defects can be left to heal by secondary intention [26]. More recent developments in tissue engineering have led to the application of cell-based therapies. As opposed to harvesting areas of dermal tissue, keratinocytes can now be harvested from patients. Subsequent *ex vivo* expansion thereby allows for the production of an autologous epidermal graft. However, the product is very thin, fragile, and relatively expensive to produce [26].

It is clear that there have been multiple attempts to increase the effectiveness of wound healing techniques, as well as creating more efficient and reliable grafts. Unfortunately, even the most advanced engineered skin substitutes demonstrate limitations; they are very expensive, are not always effective, and cannot completely reconstitute skin appendages. A different approach to wound healing is therefore necessary to overcome current barriers in wound therapy and create more pragmatic and effective solutions to wound-related issues [27]. The pluripotent nature of stem cells suggests that they may provide a means to overcome at least some of the aforementioned barriers to optimal wound management.

6. Stem Cells and Wound Healing

In order for cells to be classified as stem cells, they must fulfill two criteria: they must have a prolonged capacity for self-renewal and they must be able to employ asymmetric division to differentiate into more specialized cell types [28]. These characteristics endow a set of unique abilities in these types of cells, which could be harnessed to aid the regeneration and repair process in damaged skin. Studies using models of tissue injury have shown severe injury has resulted in a dramatic increase in the number of stem cells circulating in blood [29]. Furthermore, circulating bone marrow-derived cells were found to localize to the wound site where they also differentiated into nonhematopoietic skin structures [30]. Other such findings also suggest that stem cells play a very important role in the process of wound healing, and further studies are needed to better understand the underlying mechanisms. This section will elaborate on notable findings in wound healing applications of various stem cell populations (Figure 1), such as mesenchymal stem cells (MSCs) (including adipose-derived stem cells (ASCs)), induced pluripotent stem cells (iPSCs), and embryonic stem cells (ESCs).

The majority of studies looking at potential stem cell-related wound healing therapies have centered on adult stem cells, specifically mesenchymal stem cells (MSCs). MSCs are able to self-renew and have shown great promise for treating tissue damage involving immune responses [31, 32]. MSCs can be harvested from a patient's bone marrow, adipose tissue, umbilical cord blood, and dermis [33]. Not only do autologous MSCs forgo the risks of transplant rejection, they are also understood to inhibit the inflammatory response at the wound bed, which can otherwise impair effective tissue regeneration [32, 34]. Moreover, bone marrow-derived MSCs (BM-MSCs) have been shown to synthesize higher amounts of collagen, growth factors, and angiogenic factors than the native dermal fibroblasts, which suggests that they could be implanted in wounds to increase the rate of healing without eliciting any immune response. One case study also demonstrated closure of a recalcitrant diabetic foot ulcer treated with a combination of direct BM-MSCs to the wound bed covered with a biograft composed of autologous skin fibroblasts in a collagen membrane [35]. Infection also often complicates management of chronic wounds, presenting a further issue to address in treatment. Another mechanism by

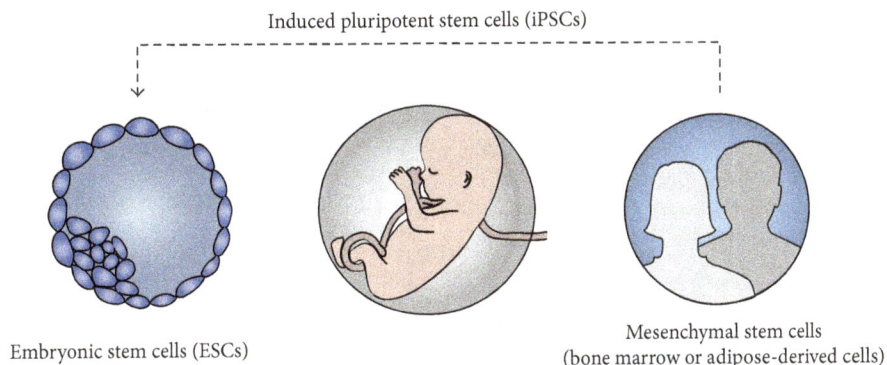

Induced pluripotent stem cells (iPSCs)

Embryonic stem cells (ESCs)

Mesenchymal stem cells
(bone marrow or adipose-derived cells)

FIGURE 1: Stem cell populations.

which MSCs can augment the wound healing response is via antimicrobial peptide secretion [36]. In targeting numerous aspects of wound healing, stem cells thus offer a versatile treatment for wounds that have not responded to standard care.

Though MSCs have demonstrated a consistent ability to increase the rate of wound healing in a variety of scenarios, there are still some drawbacks to these therapies. For example, MSCs are a practical approach to small wounds, but it is unfeasible to culture enough MSCs to apply to a large wound. In addition, the population of MSCs within humans decreases over time, possibly eliminating the option of using autologous MSCs for treatment in the older generations [37]. While MSCs have been observed to directly contribute to wound healing via transdifferentiation into keratinocytes [38], paracrine mechanisms are generally believed to play a much more important role [39]. Therefore, fewer cells may be required for clinical efficacy, circumventing potential limitations for stem cell-based wound therapies and maintaining them as exciting modalities to improve wound healing.

While surgical manipulation and harvest of adipose tissue are generally simple procedures, the tissue itself is complex. Adipose tissue is comprised of a plethora of cells including adipocytes, smooth muscle cells, fibroblasts, macrophages, endothelial cells, and lymphocytes, as well as adipose-derived stem cells (ASCs). ASCs are a class of MSCs, pluripotent cells able to differentiate into bone, cartilage, tendon, and fat, provided they are cultured under the necessary conditions. They share an almost equal potential with MSCs to differentiate into cells of mesodermal origin but are preferred due to their wide availability and relative ease of harvesting sufficient cell numbers [40]. ASCs have been shown to promote human dermal fibroblast proliferation at the wound site by secretion of paracrine factors, which ultimately increase the rate of wound healing [41]. Another study showed that ASCs, under hypoxic conditions due to inflammation, significantly increase levels of collagen synthesis and help reduce wound area. Further study showed that this was achieved by upregulation of imperative growth factors, vascular endothelial growth factor (VEGF) and basic fibroblast growth factor (bFGF) [42]. Such evidence demonstrates the immense promise of ASCs in future wound management.

Several issues have arisen in terms of MSC and ASC use. The small population of available MSCs and necessitation of painful invasive harvest procedures have in part been circumvented by shifting to ASC applications [43]. However, a number of other issues remain. The efficacy of any cell-based therapy requires that sufficient numbers of cells be administered, which has often led to ex vivo expansion of MSCs for clinical use. This may be problematic as long-term culture can result in epigenetic and phenotypic changes in cell populations, potentially affecting efficacy or worse, resulting in harmful mutations [44]. Closed-system bioreactors offer a means to increase cell numbers and reduce variability of culture methods, increasing the potential for large-scale clinical use [45]. Given the challenges of ex vivo stem cell culture, in addition to findings that once transplanted, MSC survival is often short-lived and their effects transient, technologies to improve their efficiency are also heavily sought after [16]. Various developments have occurred to improve means of administering cells, such as within fibrin sprays [46]. Enhancing the local microenvironment of transplanted stem cells, for example, by seeding them in human collagen matrices [47, 48], provides a means for optimization of cell delivery and survival. Stem cell enhancement is not limited to collagen scaffolds, as hydrogels and silk fibroin scaffolds have also improved wound healing characteristics of coadministered stem cells [49, 50]. New methods for targeting stem cells to desired tissues with peptide or antibody marking could potentially eliminate the need for direct administration [51]. Harnessing the potential of stem cells in wound therapy has created vast opportunities for innovation, in terms of both basic science research and commercialization of new technologies. As cell therapies continue to be optimized, more applications of adult stem cells such as ASCs and MSCs will be developed for use by plastic surgeons.

The astounding proliferative capacity of the embryo suggested that the study of embryonic stem cells (ESCs) might further our understanding of regenerative processes and provide more optimal wound treatments. While embryos had originally been regarded as a key source of pluripotent stem cells, ESCs have been a topic of extreme controversy in the United States, and access to these cells in the past has been very limited. ESCs are derived from the inner cell mass of the blastocyst, an early-stage preimplantation embryo.

Thus, ESCs cannot be harvested from the patient and their direct use would involve all the drawbacks of allografting, in addition to ethical concerns associated with embryonic tissue [52]. While ESCs themselves are less suitable for tissue grafting, they do provide the potential to augment physiological healing processes via paracrine mechanisms. For example, ESC-derived endothelial cells secrete a variety of cytokine factors leading to enhanced wound healing [53].

Finally, the landmark study conducted by Takahashi and Yamanaka in 2006 described a method of reprogramming adult cells back to an embryonic state, termed induced pluripotent stem cells (iPSCs) [54]. These cells opened up many new avenues in stem cell research by circumventing ethical controversy and issues associated with exogenous tissue rejection. One study managed to reprogram dermal fibroblasts into iPSCs, without use of a viral vector, which meant that iPSCs could be derived for the sick and/or elderly patients who most likely need them more [55]. Another study has shown that iPSC-derived fibroblasts show an increased production of extracellular matrix proteins that could also increase the rate of wound healing [56]. The role of iPSCs continues to expand across numerous fields of research, from the basic to translational sciences. In 2014, a Japanese team became the first to administer iPSCs clinically, in this case for the treatment of age-related macular degeneration. However, reliable iPSC-based therapies for wound management remain elusive, in part as we continue to await the results of their first clinical application. The administration of dedifferentiated pluripotent cells carries risks of subsequent tumor formation and thus long-term preliminary studies must be conducted prior to any proliferation in terms of their clinical use. We must continue to expand our understanding of how they can modulate the wound environment, while also improving our ability to manipulate them *in vitro* and *in vivo*. In this manner we can more effectively translate our discoveries from bench to bedside.

Issues pertaining to wound healing demonstrate a significant burden to the healthcare system as a whole, but their negative psychosocial impact on patients is immeasurable. Traditional wound healing technologies, including skin grafting and tissue engineered skin substitutes, remain invaluable in clinical practice. However, the growing prevalence of recalcitrant wounds goes hand-in-hand with the rise of chronic disease. It is thus imperative that older wound management techniques are augmented with novel cell-based therapies to address the limitations of current treatments.

Authors' Contribution

Michael S. Hu, Tripp Leavitt, and Samir Malhotra contributed equally to this work.

References

[1] S. A. Eming, T. Krieg, and J. M. Davidson, "Inflammation in wound repair: molecular and cellular mechanisms," *Journal of Investigative Dermatology*, vol. 127, no. 3, pp. 514–525, 2007.

[2] G. C. Gurtner, S. Werner, Y. Barrandon, and M. T. Longaker, "Wound repair and regeneration," *Nature*, vol. 453, no. 7193, pp. 314–321, 2008.

[3] C. K. Sen, G. M. Gordillo, S. Roy et al., "Human skin wounds: a major and snowballing threat to public health and the economy," *Wound Repair and Regeneration*, vol. 17, no. 6, pp. 763–771, 2009.

[4] G. Crovetti, G. Martinelli, M. Issi et al., "Platelet gel for healing cutaneous chronic wounds," *Transfusion and Apheresis Science*, vol. 30, no. 2, pp. 145–151, 2004.

[5] S. Aarabi, M. T. Longaker, and G. C. Gurtner, "Hypertrophic scar formation following burns and trauma: new approaches to treatment," *PLoS Medicine*, vol. 4, no. 9, article e234, 2007.

[6] P. A. Brigham and E. McLoughlin, "Burn incidence and medical care use in the United States: estimates, trends, and data sources," *Journal of Burn Care and Rehabilitation*, vol. 17, no. 2, pp. 95–107, 1996.

[7] C. Harvey, "Wound healing," *Orthopaedic Nursing*, vol. 24, no. 2, pp. 143–157, 2005.

[8] R. Grose and S. Werner, "Wound-healing studies in transgenic and knockout mice," *Molecular Biotechnology*, vol. 28, no. 2, pp. 147–166, 2004.

[9] J. M. Rhett, G. S. Ghatnekar, J. A. Palatinus, M. O'Quinn, M. J. Yost, and R. G. Gourdie, "Novel therapies for scar reduction and regenerative healing of skin wounds," *Trends in Biotechnology*, vol. 26, no. 4, pp. 173–180, 2008.

[10] I. Pastar, O. Stojadinovic, N. C. Yin et al., "Epithelialization in wound healing: a comprehensive review," *Advances in Wound Care*, vol. 3, no. 7, pp. 445–464, 2014.

[11] A. Szabowski, N. Maas-Szabowski, S. Andrecht et al., "c-Jun and JunB antagonistically control cytokine-regulated mesenchymal-epidermal interaction in skin," *Cell*, vol. 103, no. 5, pp. 745–755, 2000.

[12] A. Cole-King and K. G. Harding, "Psychological factors and delayed healing in chronic wounds," *Psychosomatic Medicine*, vol. 63, no. 2, pp. 216–220, 2001.

[13] D. Duscher, R. C. Rennert, M. Januszyk et al., "Aging disrupts cell subpopulation dynamics and diminishes the function of mesenchymal stem cells," *Scientific Reports*, vol. 4, article 7144, 2014.

[14] R. Blakytny and E. Jude, "The molecular biology of chronic wounds and delayed healing in diabetes," *Diabetic Medicine*, vol. 23, no. 6, pp. 594–608, 2006.

[15] A. J. Singer and R. A. F. Clark, "Cutaneous wound healing," *The New England Journal of Medicine*, vol. 341, no. 10, pp. 738–746, 1999.

[16] A. Nuschke, "Activity of mesenchymal stem cells in therapies for chronic skin wound healing," *Organogenesis*, vol. 10, no. 1, pp. 29–37, 2014.

[17] Y.-L. Liu, W.-H. Liu, J. Sun et al., "Mesenchymal stem cell-mediated suppression of hypertrophic scarring is p53 dependent in a rabbit ear model," *Stem Cell Research & Therapy*, vol. 5, no. 6, article 136, 2014.

[18] C. Huang, S. Akaishi, H. Hyakusoku, and R. Ogawa, "Are keloid and hypertrophic scar different forms of the same disorder?

A fibroproliferative skin disorder hypothesis based on keloid findings," *International Wound Journal*, vol. 11, no. 5, pp. 517–522, 2014.

[19] G. P. Yang, I. J. Lim, T.-T. Phan, H. P. Lorenz, and M. T. Longaker, "From scarless fetal wounds to keloids: molecular studies in wound healing," *Wound Repair and Regeneration*, vol. 11, no. 6, pp. 411–418, 2003.

[20] H. P. Ehrlich, A. Desmoulière, R. F. Diegelmann et al., "Morphological and immunochemical differences between keloid and hypertrophic scar," *The American Journal of Pathology*, vol. 145, no. 1, pp. 105–113, 1994.

[21] F. B. Niessen, P. H. M. Spauwen, J. Schalkwijk, and M. Kon, "On the nature of hypertrophic scars and keloids: a review," *Plastic and Reconstructive Surgery*, vol. 104, no. 5, pp. 1435–1458, 1999.

[22] S. T. O'Sullivan, M. O'Shaughnessy, and T. O'Connor, "Aetiology and management of hypertrophic scars and keloids," *Annals of the Royal College of Surgeons of England*, vol. 78, part 1, no. 3, pp. 168–175, 1996.

[23] C.-Y. Fong, A. Biswas, A. Subramanian, A. Srinivasan, M. Choolani, and A. Bongso, "Human keloid cell characterization and inhibition of growth with human wharton's jelly stem cell extracts," *Journal of Cellular Biochemistry*, vol. 115, no. 5, pp. 826–838, 2014.

[24] A. I. Arno, S. Amini-Nik, P. H. Blit et al., "Effect of human Wharton's jelly mesenchymal stem cell paracrine signaling on keloid fibroblasts," *Stem Cells Translational Medicine*, vol. 3, no. 3, pp. 299–307, 2014.

[25] C. Pham, J. Greenwood, H. Cleland, P. Woodruff, and G. Maddern, "Bioengineered skin substitutes for the management of burns: a systematic review," *Burns*, vol. 33, no. 8, pp. 946–957, 2007.

[26] Y. M. Bello, A. F. Falabella, and W. H. Eaglstein, "Tissue-engineered skin: current status in wound healing," *American Journal of Clinical Dermatology*, vol. 2, no. 5, pp. 305–313, 2001.

[27] A. Burd, K. Ahmed, S. Lam, T. Ayyappan, and L. Huang, "Stem cell strategies in burns care," *Burns*, vol. 33, no. 3, pp. 282–291, 2007.

[28] I. L. Weissman, "Stem cells: Units of development, units of regeneration, and units in evolution," *Cell*, vol. 100, no. 1, pp. 157–168, 2000.

[29] M. Kucia, J. Ratajczak, R. Reca, A. Janowska-Wieczorek, and M. Z. Ratajczak, "Tissue-specific muscle, neural and liver stem/progenitor cells reside in the bone marrow, respond to an SDF-1 gradient and are mobilized into peripheral blood during stress and tissue injury," *Blood Cells, Molecules, and Diseases*, vol. 32, no. 1, pp. 52–57, 2004.

[30] E. V. Badiavas, M. Abedi, J. Butmarc, V. Falanga, and P. Quesenberry, "Participation of bone marrow derived cells in cutaneous wound healing," *Journal of Cellular Physiology*, vol. 196, no. 2, pp. 245–250, 2003.

[31] H. Nakagawa, S. Akita, M. Fukui, T. Fujii, and K. Akino, "Human mesenchymal stem cells successfully improve skin-substitute wound healing," *British Journal of Dermatology*, vol. 153, no. 1, pp. 29–36, 2005.

[32] Y. Shi, G. Hu, J. Su et al., "Mesenchymal stem cells: a new strategy for immunosuppression and tissue repair," *Cell Research*, vol. 20, no. 5, pp. 510–518, 2010.

[33] Y. Dai, J. Li, J. Li et al., "Skin epithelial cells in mice from umbilical cord blood mesenchymal stem cells," *Burns*, vol. 33, no. 4, pp. 418–428, 2007.

[34] S. Bajada, I. Mazakova, J. B. Richardson, and N. Ashammakhi, "Updates on stem cells and their applications in regenerative medicine," *Journal of Tissue Engineering and Regenerative Medicine*, vol. 2, no. 4, pp. 169–183, 2008.

[35] J. Vojtassák, L. Danisovic, M. Kubes et al., "Autologous biograft and mesenchymal stem cells in treatment of the diabetic foot," *Neuro Endocrinology Letters*, vol. 27, supplement 2, pp. 134–137, 2006.

[36] A. Krasnodembskaya, Y. Song, X. Fang et al., "Antibacterial effect of human mesenchymal stem cells is mediated in part from secretion of the antimicrobial peptide LL-37," *Stem Cells*, vol. 28, no. 12, pp. 2229–2238, 2010.

[37] M. S. Rao and M. P. Mattson, "Stem cells and aging: expanding the possibilities," *Mechanisms of Ageing and Development*, vol. 122, no. 7, pp. 713–734, 2001.

[38] M. Sasaki, R. Abe, Y. Fujita, S. Ando, D. Inokuma, and H. Shimizu, "Mesenchymal stem cells are recruited into wounded skin and contribute to wound repair by transdifferentiation into multiple skin cell type," *The Journal of Immunology*, vol. 180, no. 4, pp. 2581–2587, 2008.

[39] L. Chen, E. E. Tredget, P. Y. G. Wu, Y. Wu, and Y. Wu, "Paracrine factors of mesenchymal stem cells recruit macrophages and endothelial lineage cells and enhance wound healing," *PLoS ONE*, vol. 3, no. 4, article e1886, 2008.

[40] S. Caspar-Bauguil, B. Cousin, A. Galinier et al., "Adipose tissues as an ancestral immune organ: site-specific change in obesity," *FEBS Letters*, vol. 579, no. 17, pp. 3487–3492, 2005.

[41] W.-S. Kim, B.-S. Park, J.-H. Sung et al., "Wound healing effect of adipose-derived stem cells: a critical role of secretory factors on human dermal fibroblasts," *Journal of Dermatological Science*, vol. 48, no. 1, pp. 15–24, 2007.

[42] E. Y. Lee, Y. Xia, W.-S. Kim et al., "Hypoxia-enhanced wound-healing function of adipose-derived stem cells: increase in stem cell proliferation and up-regulation of VEGF and bFGF," *Wound Repair and Regeneration*, vol. 17, no. 4, pp. 540–547, 2009.

[43] E. A. Jones, S. E. Kinsey, A. English et al., "Isolation and characterization of bone marrow multipotential mesenchymal progenitor cells," *Arthritis and Rheumatism*, vol. 46, no. 12, pp. 3349–3360, 2002.

[44] A. Bentivegna, M. Miloso, G. Riva et al., "DNA methylation changes during *in vitro* propagation of human mesenchymal stem cells: implications for their genomic stability?" *Stem Cells International*, vol. 2013, Article ID 192425, 9 pages, 2013.

[45] N. Liu, R. Zang, S.-T. Yang, and Y. Li, "Stem cell engineering in bioreactors for large-scale bioprocessing," *Engineering in Life Sciences*, vol. 14, no. 1, pp. 4–15, 2014.

[46] V. Falanga, S. Iwamoto, M. Chartier et al., "Autologous bone marrow-derived cultured mesenchymal stem cells delivered in a fibrin spray accelerate healing in murine and human cutaneous wounds," *Tissue Engineering*, vol. 13, no. 6, pp. 1299–1312, 2007.

[47] A. Lafosse, C. Desmet, N. Aouassar et al., "Autologous adipose stromal cells seeded onto a human collagen matrix for dermal regeneration in chronic wounds: clinical proof of concept," *Plastic and Reconstructive Surgery*, vol. 136, no. 2, pp. 279–295, 2015.

[48] A. O'Loughlin, M. Kulkarni, M. Creane et al., "Topical administration of allogeneic mesenchymal stromal cells seeded in a collagen scaffold augments wound healing and increases angiogenesis in the diabetic rabbit ulcer," *Diabetes*, vol. 62, no. 7, pp. 2588–2594, 2013.

[49] K. C. Rustad, V. W. Wong, M. Sorkin et al., "Enhancement of mesenchymal stem cell angiogenic capacity and stemness by a biomimetic hydrogel scaffold," *Biomaterials*, vol. 33, no. 1, pp. 80–90, 2012.

[50] S. E. Navone, L. Pascucci, M. Dossena et al., "Decellularized silk fibroin scaffold primed with adipose mesenchymal stromal cells improves wound healing in diabetic mice," *Stem Cell Research and Therapy*, vol. 5, no. 1, article 7, 2014.

[51] T. J. Kean, P. Lin, A. I. Caplan, and J. E. Dennis, "MSCs: delivery routes and engraftment, cell-targeting strategies, and immune modulation," *Stem Cells International*, vol. 2013, Article ID 732742, 13 pages, 2013.

[52] D. Duscher, J. Barrera, V. W. Wong et al., "Stem cells in wound healing: the future of regenerative medicine a mini-review," *Gerontology*, 2015.

[53] M. J. Lee, J. Kim, K. I. Lee, J. M. Shin, J. I. Chae, and H. M. Chung, "Enhancement of wound healing by secretory factors of endothelial precursor cells derived from human embryonic stem cells," *Cytotherapy*, vol. 13, no. 2, pp. 165–178, 2011.

[54] K. Takahashi and S. Yamanaka, "Induction of pluripotent stem cells from mouse embryonic and adult fibroblast cultures by defined factors," *Cell*, vol. 126, no. 4, pp. 663–676, 2006.

[55] M. Stadtfeld, M. Nagaya, J. Utikal, G. Weir, and K. Hochedlinger, "Induced pluripotent stem cells generated without viral integration," *Science*, vol. 322, no. 5903, pp. 945–949, 2008.

[56] Y. Shamis, K. J. Hewitt, S. E. Bear et al., "IPSC-derived fibroblasts demonstrate augmented production and assembly of extracellular matrix proteins," *In Vitro Cellular and Developmental Biology—Animal*, vol. 48, no. 2, pp. 112–122, 2012.

16

Augmentation Rhinoplasty in Cleft Lip Nasal Deformity: Preliminary Patients' Perspective

William H. C. Tiong, Mohd Ali Mat Zain, and Normala Hj Basiron

Department of Plastic and Reconstructive Surgery, Hospital Kuala Lumpur, Jalan Pahang, 50586 Kuala Lumpur, Malaysia

Correspondence should be addressed to William H. C. Tiong; willhct@yahoo.com

Academic Editor: Selahattin Özmen

The correction of cleft lip nasal deformity is challenging and there have been numerous methods described in the literature with little demonstrated technical superiority of one over another. The common clinical issues associated with cleft lip nasal deformity are its lack of symmetry, alar collapse on the affected side, obtuse nasal labial angle, short nasal length, loss of tip definition, and altered columella show among others. We carried out augmentation of cleft lip rhinoplasties with rib graft in 16 patients over the one-year study period. Each of these patients was reviewed and given questionnaire before and after surgery to evaluate their response on the outcome to the approach. Preoperatively, nasal asymmetry is the main complaint (14/16, 87.5%) among our series of patients. Postoperatively, 12 (75%) patients out of the 16 reported significant improvement in their nasal symmetry with the other four marginal. All patients reported excellent nasal projection postoperatively with good nasal tip definition. Our series of patients reported overall good satisfaction outcome and will recommend this procedure to other patients with cleft lip nasal deformity. In conclusion, augmentation of cleft lip rhinoplasty can be employed to achieve perceivable and satisfactory outcome in patients with cleft lip nasal deformity.

1. Introduction

The nose is one of the most visible organs on the face and its appearance contributes enormously to facial aesthetics [1]. Nasal deformity associated with cleft lip has been viewed as one of the most challenging reconstructive problems in rhinoplasty. The complexity of cleft lip rhinoplasty is demonstrated by the abundance of technique that is available for its correction [2]. Yet, there is no conclusively superior technique among those that were described to date.

The common clinical features associated with cleft lip nasal deformity are its lack of symmetry, alar collapse on the affected side, short nasal length, loss of tip definition, obtuse nasal labial angle, and altered columella show among others [3]. Despite the numerous above features, the typical nose of cleft lip nasal deformity can be summarized as having an asymmetrical, flat dorsum, broad tip, and wide alar base on the cleft side [4, 5]. The horizontally oriented wide nostril on the cleft side is one of the major stigmas of the cleft lip-associated nasal deformity [6].

There have been many anthropometric studies on normal nasal parameter and it is widely accepted that the shape and dimension of nose vary according to different racial and ethnic profiles [7, 8]. Despite numerous descriptions and classifications of Oriental nose, they can be similarly summarized as having a bulbous nasal tip and broad alar bases with lack of tip projection. In a study by Aung et al., it was found that most Oriental patients prefer to have a higher nasal dorsum, increased nasal tip projection, and less flaring of the alar bases [9]. This same, desired nasal feature is also requested among patients with cleft lip nasal deformity [10]. The demand for prominent and narrow nasal profile makes augmentation of the dorsum and tip of nose among the most commonly performed aesthetic rhinoplasty procedures among Orientals [11]. The use of L-shaped nasal strut implant, consisting of a dorsal nasal onlay graft and columellar strut, is a well-established technique in aesthetic Oriental rhinoplasty for combined augmentation of the dorsum and tip of nose, respectively [11]. Yonehara et al. had shown that the appearance of a cleft lip-associated nose can be similarly

TABLE 1: Questionnaire on patients' perception of their cleft lip nasal deformity before and after operation and overall satisfaction of the procedure.

Questionnaire: cleft lip nasal deformity before and after operation and overall satisfaction					
The most undesirable anatomical sites before operation	None	Mild	Moderate	Severe	Unbearable
Nasal symmetry					
Nasal tip					
Dorsum of nose					
Nasal alae					
Nasal apertures					
Rib graft donor site discomfort	None	Mild	Moderate	Severe	Unbearable
The most improved anatomical sites after operation	Worse	Unremarkable	Satisfactory	Good	Excellent
Nasal symmetry					
Nasal tip					
Dorsum of nose					
Nasal alae					
Nasal apertures					
Overall satisfaction of procedure (VAS 0–10)					
VAS score					
Would you recommend it to a friend?	Yes	No			

improved with a well-positioned cantilevered bone graft [10].

There are various materials that can be used to augment nasal dorsum [12–15]. Augmentation of dorsum of the nose can be achieved using alloplastic materials, bone, or cartilage. Although various types of alloplastic materials have been used for dorsal augmentation, they are hampered with long-term complications that make them unattractive for our long-term cleft lip nasal deformity correction [12–15]. As an autogenous tissue, bone graft is a better option but is unsatisfactory due to its variable resorption and difficult handling properties [16, 17]. For most surgeons, an autogenous cartilage graft is the first choice in rhinoplasty because of its resistance to resorption and infection [18]. The common choices of autogenous cartilage graft in rhinoplasty are septal cartilage, auricular cartilage, or rib cartilage [19–21]. In cleft lip nasal deformity among Oriental patients, additional structural support is required to achieve the correction due to weak lower lateral cartilages [22]. Here, we had chosen rib cartilage as a source of graft in our cleft lip rhinoplasty. We described our technique of augmentation using L-shaped cartilage strut implant to improve the appearance of cleft lip-associated nose among Oriental patients and the outcome was evaluated according to patients' own perception. This was based on the premise that aesthetic technique in nasal augmentation with rib cartilage graft can provide perceivable and satisfactory improvement in patients with cleft lip nasal deformity.

2. Materials and Methods

A total of 16 patients, eleven females and five males, with nonsyndromic cleft lip and palate, were identified through retrospective chart review. All patients underwent augmentative open cleft lip rhinoplasty with L-shaped rib cartilage strut implant. Six of the patients were of Chinese ethnicity and 10 Malay. The ages of patients ranged from 14 to 33 years with the median and mean age at 18.5 and 20.4 years, respectively. Nine patients have left unilateral cleft lip and palate (UCLP) deformity, 3 have right UCLP, and 4 with bilateral cleft lip and palate (BCLP) deformity. All patients had clinical follow-up for more than 18 months postoperatively. The patients were interviewed using standard questionnaire in the clinic or by phone (Table 1). The questionnaire was used for the patients to rate their own perceived preoperative appearance and postoperative outcomes and their overall satisfaction with this technique. This is particularly important because it allowed us to assess our technique based on the patients' perception.

2.1. Operative Technique. A marginal (infracartilaginous) incision was made in both nostrils and continued in the columella by a transcolumellar, stair-step incision. This open approach allowed visualization of the cartilaginous and bony vault to facilitate accurate dissection of nasal pocket overlying the lower lateral cartilages, septal cartilage, and nasal bones. The columella and nasal skin flap were raised at supraperichondrial and supraperiosteal level without interfering with the underlying perichondrium and periosteum, respectively. The size of nasal pocket dissection was determined by intraoperative appearance of desired nasal augmentation. It is important to avoid overzealous dissection that can result in unstable cartilage graft position. Care was taken to avoid soft tissue irregularities by judiciously smoothening the undersurface of the soft tissue envelope to prevent overlying irregularities.

Rib cartilage was harvested from the 6th rib through submammary incision in female and subcostal incision in male (Figure 1(a)). The technique in rib cartilage graft harvest

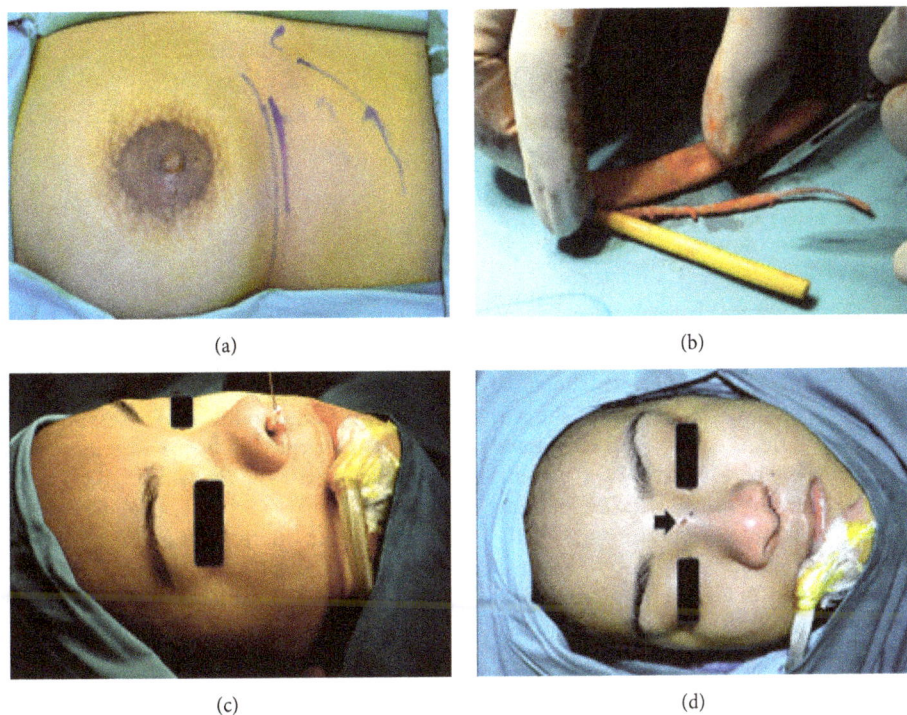

FIGURE 1: (a) Diagram showing the skin marking of the submammary incision. The curved line drawn inferior to the submammary marking represented the inferior margin of the rib cage. (b) The fabrication process of the harvested rib cartilage in which equal portion of the cartilage peripheries was shaved such that only the central most portion of the cartilage was retained for grafting. (c) The columellar component of the L-shaped rib cartilage was secured to the nasal spine, just inferior to the medial crus of lower lateral cartilages with 0.8 mm sized K-wire. (d) The proximal end of the dorsal onlay graft was secured to the nasal bone using K-wire (black arrow).

has been well described by Marin et al. [23]. The harvested rib cartilage was stripped off its peripheral portion such that only the central portion was utilized for fabrication and implant (Figure 1(b)). The 7 cm harvested cartilage graft was carved to appropriate size and shape and contoured with number 10 blade to allow accurate fashioning before implantation. Two components, the dorsal onlay and columellar component of the L-shaped cartilage strut, were obtained from the harvested rib cartilage. The dorsal onlay component is approximately 6 cm in length and columellar component 1 cm. The length of the graft had to be tailored to all individual cases. The grafts were then placed in position to improve cleft lip nose appearance through augmentation of the nasal dorsum and tip support. Finer fabrication proceeded carefully from this point usually by scraping the grafts with the sharp edge of a number 10 blade perpendicular to the graft surface until the exact desired size, shape, and contour were obtained. Note that it is important to tailor the size of the L-shaped cartilage strut to allow nasal augmentation that is proportionate to the facial aesthetic of patient.

After the final position was determined, K-wire was used to anchor the graft in position. The columellar component of the L-shaped rib cartilage was placed just inferior to the medial crus of lower lateral cartilages and secured with 0.8 mm sized smooth K-wire to the nasal spine (Figure 1(c)). The dorsal onlay component of the L-shaped cartilage strut was then inserted to the dorsal nasal pocket with its tip overlying the columellar component at the nasal tip. The position

TABLE 2: The most undesirable anatomical sites before operation as perceived by patients.

The most undesirable anatomical sites before operation	None	Mild	Moderate	Severe	Unbearable
Nasal symmetry			2	14	
Nasal tip		3	8	5	
Dorsum of nose		11	2	2	
Nasal alae		1	3	12	
Nasal apertures		12	4		

of the dorsal onlay graft was secured to the nasal bone using K-wire and covered with rubber tip from syringe plunger (Figure 1(d)). Note that a small pinhole was created only on the undersurface of the dorsal onlay graft over the columellar component to allow the fitting of the K-wire tip from the nasal spine into the pinhole. The percutaneous K-wire over the nasal bone was removed in the office with a wire twister one week postoperatively when the external splint was also removed.

3. Results

In our series of patients with cleft lip nasal deformity, 87.5% (14 out of 16 patients) of patients perceived nasal asymmetry as the most undesirable aspect of a cleft lip nose (Table 2).

TABLE 3: The most improved anatomical sites after operation as perceived by patients.

The most improved anatomical sites after operation	Worse	Unremarkable	Satisfactory	Good	Excellent
Nasal symmetry			4	11	1
Nasal tip				16	
Dorsum of nose					16
Nasal alae		3	7	6	
Nasal apertures		6	8	2	

This was followed by deformity associated with the nasal alae in which 12 out of 16 patients (75%) perceived the alar deformity as severe. Thirteen patients out of the 16 rated nasal tip deformity as moderate to severe. Majority of the patients rated the dorsum of nose deformity as mild and no patients perceived nasal apertures deformity as severe.

After augmentative open cleft lip rhinoplasty, 12 out of 16 (75%) patients reported good or excellent improvement in their nasal symmetry (Table 3). Thirteen patients rated satisfactory or good outcome on the appearance of nasal alae after operation. All patients reported good outcome on nasal tip projection and excellent result for dorsum of nose. The improvement to nasal apertures was unremarkable in 6 patients with 10 others experiencing satisfactory to good outcomes.

There were 3 complications in our series. Two patients with left UCLP experienced L-shaped cartilage graft displacement that required revision surgery. Both cases involved the displacement of the proximal part of the dorsal onlay component due to exceedingly large dorsal nasal pocket. One patient with BCLP had minor wound dehiscence over the columella. The wound dehiscence settled uneventfully with conservative management.

Although there was no rib cartilage graft donor site complication, two patients reported moderate degree of discomfort on the donor site. Majority of the patients (12 patients out of 16) experienced mild discomfort on the donor site during the immediate postoperative period. Other two expressed no discomfort from the donor site. Although a total of 14 patients (87.5%) experienced mild or moderate discomfort during the immediate postoperative period, 93.7% of them scored a visual analogue score (VAS) outcome satisfaction of 5–8 in which 0 represented the worst overall experience and 10 the most pleasant. All patients would recommend the procedure to a friend based on their own experience (Figure 2).

4. Discussion

In clinical practice, there is no universal concept of the "perfect face," and there is not a specific shape of the nose, considered a model of beauty [1]. The definition of nasal aesthetics varies between different cultures and ethnicity in addition to the influence by popular trends of the society [8, 24]. Previous studies comparing the morphology of the Oriental and Caucasian nose noted remarkable differences between them [2, 7]. In Oriental patients, the nasal tip is bulbous with broad alar bases and lacking nasal height and tip projection [9, 11]. Although the deformity in cleft lip nasal deformity varied in its severity, it is characterized by nose that is asymmetrical with a similarly flat dorsum, broad tip, and wide alar base at the cleft side [5, 10]. According to Aung et al., they found that most Oriental patients prefer to have a higher nasal dorsum, increased nasal tip projection, and less flaring of the alar bases [9]. This same, desired nasal feature is also requested among patients with cleft lip nasal deformity [10]. In our group of patients, they rated nasal asymmetry, nasal alae, and tip as the most undesirable anatomical sites of cleft lip-associated nose.

The characteristic cleft lip nose represents a stigma to the cleft lip patient [25]. It is important for these patients to receive not only anthropometric normalization but also aesthetic improvement of the external nose to camouflage the patient's facial deformity [26]. In our series of patients, we used augmentation rhinoplasty technique to correct the nose of patients with cleft lip nasal deformity. We applied L-shaped cartilage strut to augment the nasal profile of our patients with cleft lip nasal deformity. Majority of our patients perceived this as a viable technique to improve their nasal appearance and had rated satisfactory to excellent outcomes for nasal symmetry, nasal alae, and tip of nose appearance after operation. The dorsal onlay component of the L-shaped strut helped to augment the nasal bridge, thus giving the illusion of a narrower and longer nose. There was, however, less improvement noted on the nasal apertures in our series of patients. Six patients rated unremarkable changes on their nasal apertures after operation. This was because augmentative procedure alone only altered the dimension of the nasal apertures and not its size.

In severely deformed, Oriental cleft lip-associated nose, the naturally thick overlying skin, bulbous nasal tip, and weak lower lateral cartilages among Orientals warrant additional structural support to achieve and maintain their correction [11, 27]. Here, we incorporated the columellar strut to enhance the definition and projection of the nasal tip and stabilized the caudal end of the dorsal onlay nasal strut on top of the columellar strut. The overall effect of the augmentation improved nasal symmetry and profile. This was consistent with studies by Yonehara et al. [10], and Jin and Won [24]. It should also be noted that augmentation with both dorsal nasal onlay grafts and columellar struts is not always performed in combination if only one is needed [27]. According to Yonehara et al., cantilever iliac bone graft alone was used but they experienced some loss of nasal tip definition in their patients [10].

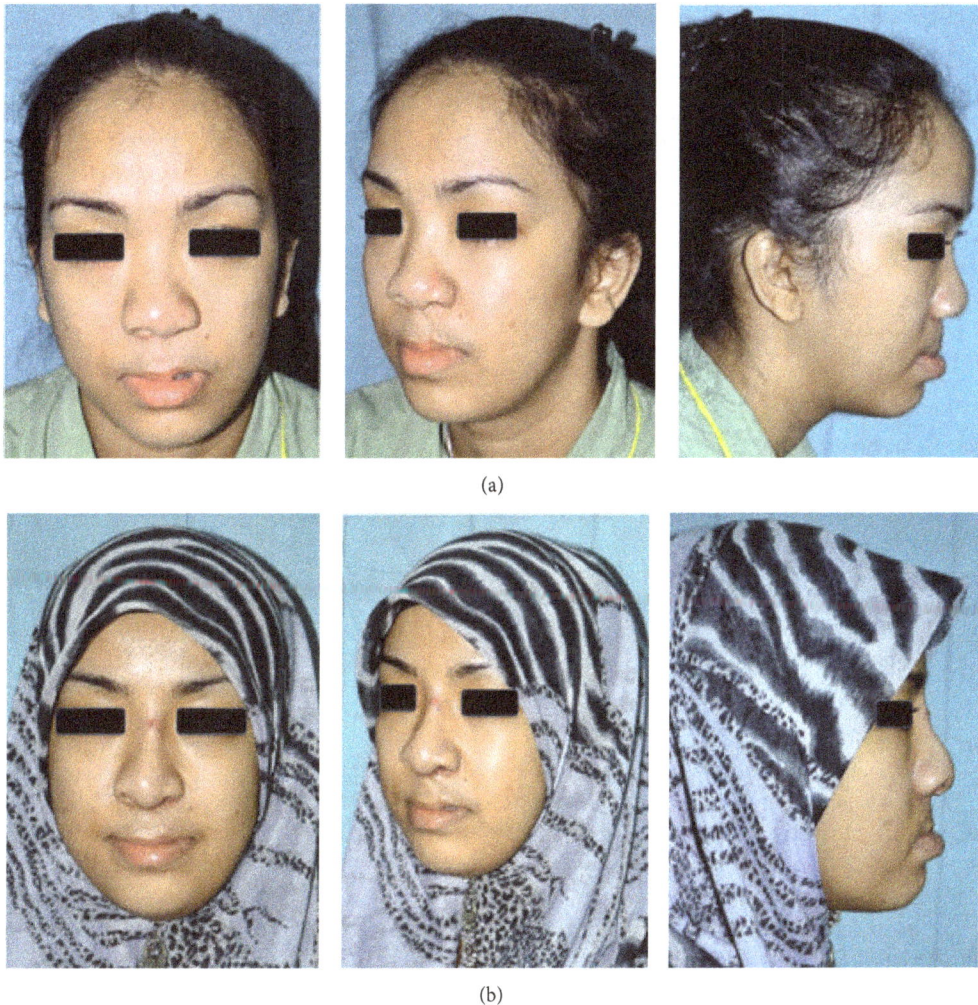

FIGURE 2: A 24-year-old lady with left unilateral cleft lip and palate. The photographs on the top row were taken preoperatively and those on the bottom row postoperatively. Her main complaints were asymmetrical nose with flat dorsum and broad left alar base on the cleft side. Postoperatively, her nasal symmetry had improved with increased dorsal nasal height and tip projection.

In our series of 16 patients, we harvested rib cartilage graft as our cartilage donor. There was no complication with the donor site other than tolerable degree of discomfort in immediate postoperation period. Rib cartilage graft was chosen because it offered abundant supply and the strength needed for our L-shaped strut. Rib cartilage has been recognized to be the most reliable cartilage when structural support is needed in rhinoplasty [20, 21]. It is considerably versatile with respect to shape, length, and width that is important to our fabrication. In augmentation of cleft lip rhinoplasty, it is essential that each fabrication of the L-shaped cartilage strut implant was tailored to the individual needs of the patient [24]. To achieve consistent and satisfactory long-term outcomes, it is important to use rib cartilage graft for its low resorption rate and strength of support [20, 21, 24].

One of the issues associated with cartilage graft is the risk of warping [21, 24]. We did not notice warping among our patients in 18-month follow-up because only the central portion of the rib cartilage was used in our fabrication. It is also important to note that, during cartilage contouring, it has to be carried out in symmetry, meaning that equal portion of the cartilage external surface was discarded (Figure 1(b)). Harris et al. had shown that there was less risk of warping in the central portion of the cartilage [28].

One of our complications was the displacement of dorsal onlay component of the L-shaped strut in two of our patients. In both cases, the pocket that was created for the placement of the dorsal onlay graft was too large. It should be noted that the dorsal nasal pocket dissected should just accommodate the implant. It was possible that, with open rhinoplasty approach, overzealous visualisation and dissection may have resulted in the creation of the excessively large dorsal nasal pocket in both cases.

Another complication was in a patient with BCLP in which she sustained wound dehiscence over the transcolumellar incision site. The wound dehiscence occurred due to inherent short columella in BCLP and was further aggravated by the use of a sturdy columellar component of the L-shaped strut that forced a tight closure.

In our case series, the L-shaped rib cartilage strut continued to show good result at 18-month follow-up. This was consistent with the study by Yilmaz et al., which showed satisfactory nasal profile using rib cartilage grafts for dorsal nasal augmentation [29]. They found that the resorption rates were not high enough to change the shape of their augmented nose at 2-year follow-up. This is particularly important to provide cleft lip nasal deformity patients with a stable and long-term improvement. Our patients continued to be satisfied with the outcome of our cleft lip rhinoplasty that they would recommend their friends to undertake the same procedure.

With the majority of patients who reported good to excellent improvement in their nasal symmetry and profile, L-shaped strut augmentation rhinoplasty with rib cartilage graft presented a viable option in cleft lip rhinoplasty. Using this technique, we were successful in providing our cleft lip nose patients with a perceivable and satisfactory improvement to their nasal deformity.

5. Conclusion

Augmentation rhinoplasty in cleft lip nose can provide patients with a stable and satisfactory nasal appearance. This technique of using L-shaped rib cartilage strut provides many surgeons with added option in their quest to improve the appearance of patients with cleft lip nose. In conclusion, augmentation of cleft lip rhinoplasty can be employed with satisfactory outcome among Oriental patients with cleft lip nasal deformity.

References

[1] P. Szychta, J. Rykała, and J. Kruk-Jeromin, "Individual and ethnic aspects of preoperative planning for posttraumatic rhinoplasty," *European Journal of Plastic Surgery*, vol. 34, no. 4, pp. 245–249, 2011.

[2] B. C. Cho and B. S. Baik, "Correction of cleft lip nasal deformity in Orientals using a refined reverse-U incision and V-Y plasty," *British Journal of Plastic Surgery*, vol. 54, no. 7, pp. 588–596, 2001.

[3] A. L. Van Beek, A. S. Hatfield, and E. Schnepf, "Cleft rhinoplasty," *Plastic and Reconstructive Surgery*, vol. 114, pp. 57e–69e, 2004.

[4] D. G. Dibbell, "Cleft lip nasal reconstruction: correcting the classic unilateral defect," *Plastic and Reconstructive Surgery*, vol. 69, no. 2, pp. 264–271, 1982.

[5] B. van Loon, T. J. Maal, J. M. Plooij et al., "3D Stereophotogrammetric assessment of pre- and postoperative volumetric changes in the cleft lip and palate nose," *International Journal of Oral and Maxillofacial Surgery*, vol. 39, no. 6, pp. 534–540, 2010.

[6] H. M. T. Foda and K. Bassyouni, "Rhinoplasty in unilateral cleft lip nasal deformity," *Journal of Laryngology and Otology*, vol. 114, no. 3, pp. 189–193, 2000.

[7] Y. Dong, Y. Zhao, S. Bai, G. Wu, and B. Wang, "Three-dimensional anthropometric analysis of the Chinese nose," *Journal of Plastic, Reconstructive and Aesthetic Surgery*, vol. 63, no. 11, pp. 1832–1839, 2010.

[8] S. M. Patel and R. K. Daniel, "Indian American rhinoplasty: an emerging ethnic group," *Plastic and Reconstructive Surgery*, vol. 129, no. 3, 2012.

[9] S. C. Aung, C. L. Foo, and S. T. Lee, "Three dimensional laser scan assessment of the Oriental nose with a new classification of Oriental nasal types," *British Journal of Plastic Surgery*, vol. 53, no. 2, pp. 109–116, 2000.

[10] Y. Yonehara, T. Takato, S. Matsumoto, Y. Mori, T. Nakatsuka, and H. Hikiji, "Correction of cleft ltp nasal deformity in orientals with a cantilevered iliac bone graft," *Scandinavian Journal of Plastic and Reconstructive Surgery and Hand Surgery*, vol. 34, no. 2, pp. 137–143, 2000.

[11] H. Jin and T. Won, "Nasal tip augmentation in Asians using autogenous cartilage," *Otolaryngology—Head and Neck Surgery*, vol. 140, no. 4, pp. 526–530, 2009.

[12] Y. Hiraga, "Complications of augmentation rhinoplasty in the Japanese," *Annals of Plastic Surgery*, vol. 4, no. 6, pp. 495–499, 1980.

[13] U. Raghavan, N. S. Jones, and T. Romo III, "Immediate autogenous cartilage grafts in rhinoplasty after alloplastic implant rejection," *Archives of Facial Plastic Surgery*, vol. 6, no. 3, pp. 192–196, 2004.

[14] M. S. Godin, S. R. Waldman, C. M. Johnson Jr., and F. J. Stucker, "The use of expanded polytetrafluoroethylene (Gore-Tex) in rhinoplasty. A 6-year experience," *Archives of Otolaryngology—Head and Neck Surgery*, vol. 121, no. 10, pp. 1131–1136, 1995.

[15] P. K. B. Davis and S. M. Jones, "The complications of silastic implants. Experience with 137 consecutive cases," *British Journal of Plastic Surgery*, vol. 24, pp. 405–411, 1971.

[16] S. W. Chase and C. H. Herndon, "The fate of autogenous and homogenous bone grafts," *The Journal of Bone and Joint Surgery A*, vol. 37, no. 4, pp. 809–841, 1955.

[17] R. Mowlem, "Bone grafting," *British Journal of Plastic Surgery*, vol. 16, pp. 293–304, 1963.

[18] Z. Tosun, F. E. Karabekmez, M. Keskin, A. Duymaz, and N. Savaci, "Allogenous cartilage graft versus autogenous cartilage graft in augmentation rhinoplasty: a decade of clinical experience," *Aesthetic Plastic Surgery*, vol. 32, no. 2, pp. 252–260, 2008.

[19] K. Matsuo and T. Hirose, "Secondary correction of the unilateral cleft lip nose using a conchal composite graft," *Plastic and Reconstructive Surgery*, vol. 86, no. 5, pp. 991–995, 1990.

[20] J. P. Gunter and R. J. Rohrich, "Augmentation rhinoplasty: dorsal onlay grafting using shaped autogenous septal cartilage," *Plastic and Reconstructive Surgery*, vol. 86, no. 1, pp. 39–45, 1990.

[21] J. P. Gunter, C. P. Clark, and R. M. Friedman, "Internal stabilization of autogenous rib cartilage grafts in rhinoplasty: a barrier to cartilage warping," *Plastic and Reconstructive Surgery*, vol. 100, no. 1, pp. 161–169, 1997.

[22] T. Jang, Y. Choi, Y. Jung, K. Kim, K. Kim, and J. Choi, "Effect of nasal tip surgery on Asian noses using the transdomal suture technique," *Aesthetic Plastic Surgery*, vol. 31, no. 2, pp. 174–178, 2007.

[23] V. P. Marin, A. Landecker, and J. P. Gunter, "Harvesting rib cartilage grafts for secondary rhinoplasty," *Plastic and Reconstructive Surgery*, vol. 121, no. 4, pp. 1442–1448, 2008.

[24] H. R. Jin and T. B. Won, "Recent advances in Asian rhinoplasty," *Auris Nasus Larynx*, vol. 38, no. 2, pp. 157–164, 2011.

[25] N. Chaithanyaa, K. K. Rai, H. R. Shivakumar, and A. Upasi, "Evaluation of the outcome of secondary rhinoplasty in cleft lip and palate patients," *Journal of Plastic, Reconstructive and Aesthetic Surgery*, vol. 64, no. 1, pp. 27–33, 2011.

[26] H. Rikimaru, K. Kiyokawa, N. Koga, N. Takahashi, K. Morinaga, and K. Ino, "A new modified forked flap with subcutaneous pedicles for adult cases of bilateral cleft lip nasal deformity: from normalization to aesthetic improvement," *The Journal of Craniofacial Surgery*, vol. 19, no. 5, pp. 1374–1380, 2008.

[27] T. Takato, Y. Yonehara, Y. Mori, and T. Susami, "Use of cantilever iliac bone grafts for reconstruction of cleft lip-associated nasal deformities," *Journal of Oral and Maxillofacial Surgery*, vol. 53, no. 7, pp. 757–762, 1995.

[28] S. Harris, Y. Pan, R. Peterson, S. Stal, and M. Spira, "Cartilage warping: an experimental model," *Plastic and Reconstructive Surgery*, vol. 92, no. 5, pp. 912–915, 1993.

[29] M. Yilmaz, H. Vayvada, A. Menderes, F. Mola, and A. Atabey, "Dorsal nasal augmentation with rib cartilage graft: long-term results and patient satisfaction," *Journal of Craniofacial Surgery*, vol. 18, no. 6, pp. 1457–1462, 2007.

17

Acellular Dermal Matrices and Radiotherapy in Breast Reconstruction

Luigi Valdatta,[1,2] **Anna Giulia Cattaneo,**[1] **Igor Pellegatta,**[2] **Stefano Scamoni,**[2] **Anna Minuti,**[1] **and Mario Cherubino**[1,2]

[1] *Department of Biotechnology & Life Science (DBSV), University of Insubria, 21100 Varese, Italy*
[2] *Plastic and Reconstructive Surgery Division, Ospedale di Circolo di Varese, Viale Borri 57, 21100 Varese, Italy*

Correspondence should be addressed to Igor Pellegatta; igor.pellegatta@me.com

Academic Editor: Georg M. Huemer

The increasing use of commercially available acellular dermis matrices for postmastectomy breast reconstruction seems to have simplified the surgical procedure and enhanced the outcome. These materials, generally considered to be highly safe or with only minor contraindications due to the necessary manipulation in preparatory phases, allow an easier one-phase surgical procedure, in comparison with autologous flaps, offering a high patient satisfaction. Unfortunately, the claim for a higher rate of complications associated with irradiation at the implant site, especially when the radiation therapy was given before the reconstructive surgery, suggested a careful behaviour when this technique is preferred. However, this hypothesis was never submitted to a crucial test, and data supporting it are often discordant or incomplete. To provide a comprehensive analysis of the field, we searched and systematically reviewed papers published after year 2005 and registered clinical trials. On the basis of a meta-analysis of data, we conclude that the negative effect of the radiotherapy on the breast reconstruction seems to be evident even in the case of acellular dermis matrices aided surgery. However, more trials are needed to make solid conclusions and clarify the poor comprehension of all the factors negatively influencing outcome.

1. Introduction

The acellular dermis matrices (ADM) are products derived from the skin, deprived of their cellular component by standardized treatments [1]. They provide a lower-lateral coverage and support of the implants in the immediate expander/implant-based breast reconstruction after mastectomy. Additional main indications for their use are lack of muscular coverage and cancer invasion to the pectoralis major muscle, and skin nipple sparing mastectomy is a relative indication [2].

The customized commercial products mainly differ in their origin and in procedures for processing, storing, and preparing them before usage. A recent paper compared seven customized ADM suitable for the reconstruction of the breast, in order to evaluate their cost/benefit ratios, contraindications, and possible side effects [3]. These authors discuss main contraindications for the use of commercial products, among others, namely, the presence of residues of antibiotics or allergenic substances, the lack of sterility, lower strength and elasticity, and higher cost. The Alloderm (LifeCell Corporation, Branchburg, NJ, USA), a customized derivative of the banked human skin, is the most widely used material, despite a few disadvantages: longer rehydration time, possible presence of antibiotics, and nonsterility of the final product.

We analyzed the data reported in peer-reviewed papers, in which irradiation at the site of ADM implant and its timing are considered as possible interfering factors for surgical outcome. The review includes an exhaustive description

TABLE 1: Inclusion and exclusion criteria for quantitative meta-analysis. Studies marked with asterisk were considered for qualitative analysis.

Inclusion criteria
Primary data from prospective and retrospective observational studies
Human studies
Studies that include data on prophylactic or therapeutic mastectomy for cancer
Studies that stratify results on the basis of delivery of radiotherapy before or after initiation of reconstruction
Studies based on single- or two-stage implant breast reconstruction

Exclusion criteria
Experimental studies performed in laboratory animals or "in vitro"
Review, surgical technique description, or case report; studies with no relevant extractable outcomes*
Studies focused solely on the elderly (>65 years)
Studies not published in English
Papers published before year 2005

of the procedure followed for recording and selecting the published data, followed by their analysis and comment.

2. Materials and Methods

2.1. Search Strategy: Inclusion and Exclusion Criteria. The electronic search was coordinated, according to the Boolean syntax, in the following format: (("acellular dermis" OR "acellular dermal matrix" OR Alloderm OR Strattice OR allomax OR Permacol OR Surgimed) AND ("breast reconstruction" OR mammoplasty OR mammaplasty)). The names of two commercial products (Flex-HD and DermaMatrix) generated ambiguity and therefore were omitted. The additional terms ((radiation) OR irradiation) OR RXT, coordinated with the previous terms by AND, restricted the search to the main aim of this review. A manual refinement rejected duplicate studies (those present in multiple databases), those performed "in vitro" or in animals, and studies not reporting original results or in which radiotherapy (RXT) was not directly investigated. Only the most recently updated studies were used. The reviews were carefully read, and other original reports eventually not found by the electronic procedure were retrieved and considered. The inclusion and exclusion criteria are reported in Table 1.

2.2. Databases. The bibliographic search was performed (final updating: 21st February, 2014) at the PubMed (US National Library of Medicine; http://www.ncbi.nlm.nih.gov/pubmed) and at the Cochrane library (http://www.thecochranelibrary.com/view/0/index.html). The completeness of results was finally checked with a web-based tool, provided by the library of our institution and searching in different databases (Science Citation Index, Medline, Springer Link, Walters Kluwer, Ovid, and Cross Ref).

We also considered the studies registered at the clinical trials (USA, http://www.clinicaltrials.gov/) and at the international clinical trials registry platform (World Health Organisation, http://apps.who.int/trialsearch/Default.aspx) (Table 2).

2.3. Data Collection and Analysis. Data collection included the lead author, publication year, type of acellular dermal matrix, time range of study, total number of patients, and total number of reconstructions, with and without irradiation. The total number and type of complications in each group were recorded, as was the timing of RXT, before or after the reconstruction. Chemotherapy was also considered, when specified. The authors carefully followed the guidelines of the meta-analysis of observational studies in epidemiology [5].

2.4. Statistics. We extracted data from the papers which matched the inclusion criteria to evaluate the excessive risk for complications due to the adjuvant RXT given at the site of breast reconstruction. The forest and funnel plots of the odds ratios with confidence intervals at 95% and log odds ratios versus the standard error were built; the test of null and heterogeneity were calculated under a fixed model. For the necessary calculation we used the comprehensive meta-analysis software version 2.2.064 (released July 27, 2011) [6].

3. Results

3.1. Selected Literature and Main Features. The algorithm for the selection of the literature matching the inclusion criteria is explained in Figure 1. The limited number of studies retrieved at the PubMed ($n = 234$ before the terms "radiation," "radiotherapy," and "RXT" were included) represented no more than 0.04% of all the papers describing different methods of breast reconstruction, in relation with RXT, and present in the same database under the period 2005–2014. This number was reduced to 51 when the terms ((radiation) OR irradiation) OR RXT were added. The search at the Cochrane library and at the institutional web-based tools gave 79 and 36 additional results, respectively. The 97 items remaining after manual revision for duplicates included 29 papers lacking extractable data but with relevant considerations or findings and 17 registered clinical trials (Table 2), one of which with published results [4]. Twenty works added results and were included in the meta-analysis (Table 3). Thirty-two papers (reviews and other publications without extractable data) were excluded.

The level of evidence, according to the rating scale issued by the American Society of Plastic Surgeons [27], was low; 80% of the selected papers scored 3 and the remaining 20% scored 4.

The Alloderm is the most exploited and studied type of ADM (Figure 2); studies on other commercially available products are sporadic, frequently aimed to compare different materials and procedures.

3.2. Meta-Analysis. We extracted the data for statistical analysis from twenty studies matching our inclusion criteria,

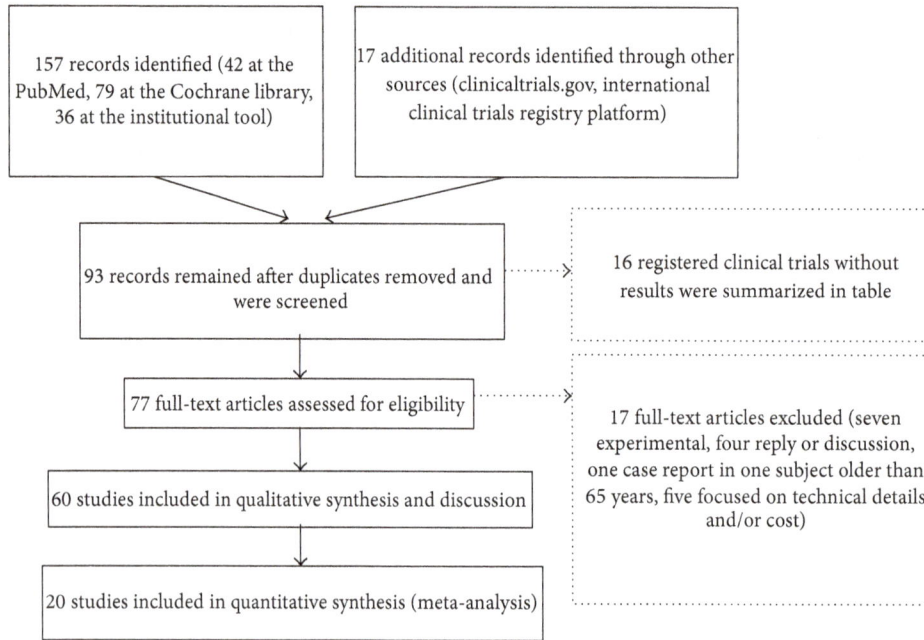

FIGURE 1: The strategy followed for the selection of the literature. All papers were carefully matched with the inclusion/exclusion criteria. Three search engines were used, for a total of 8 independent databases, as explained in the algorithm.

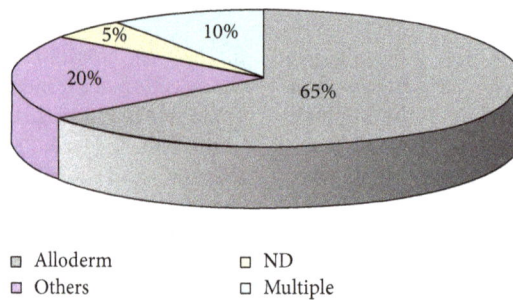

FIGURE 2: The use of different types of acellular dermis matrices in selected studies. Only the 60 papers included in the review were considered. The Alloderm (grey) was used in 65%, 20% used other acellular dermis matrices (fuchsia), 10% multiple ADM (pale blue), and 5% of authors did not specify the type of ADM they used (yellow).

which reported the outcome of 3331 ADM-assisted reconstructions. They were mainly retrospective cohort studies, in which the observation period ranged between the years 2001 and 2012. With the exception of two works, performed in UK [8] and Canada [7], one study reported the results obtained in a private practice in USA [28] and the others were done in departments of hospitals and universities in the USA. Sixteen percent of reconstructions were irradiated before, after, or before and after surgery; in these cases the rate of development for complications was 33%. The percentage of nonirradiated breasts which developed at least one complication was instead lower (6%). The forest plot (Figure 3) shows the odds ratios of each study; the black diamond at the bottom represents the pooled effect. It fell on the left of level 1 and does not cross it; this result means that a significantly higher number of complications occurred

when the ADM-assisted breast reconstruction was combined with RXT. In particular, eight studies found better results in the absence of RXT and only one [21] disagreed. The test of null was significant in both cases (Z value = -8.841, P value < 0.000); the complete results are shown in Tables 4 and 5. The funnel plots (Figure 4) show an acceptable distribution of the log odds ratio.

No more than 11 studies clearly specified the prevalence of implant failure and the most frequent type of complications in the two groups with or without RXT, as shown in Table 6, with higher prevalence of skin necrosis and infection. The prevalence of capsular contracture, reported in seven studies, was low (3%) but increased to 12% in irradiated reconstructions. Others conditions, such as wound dehiscence, haematoma, rippling, or implant migration, were not homogenously reported by all authors; therefore, we have

TABLE 2: Studies registered at the clinical trials registry (http://www.clinicaltrials.gov/) of the United States of America and at the international clinical trials registry platform (World Health Organisation, http://apps.who.int/trialsearch/) concerning the outcome of ADM-assisted breast reconstruction after mastectomy.

NCT	Status	Location	Expected NR	Principal aim	Radiotherapy
NCT 00616824	R	USA	60	D versus B	Exclusion criteria
NCT 00639106	NR	USA	98	A versus B	Exclusion criteria
NCT 00692692	NR	USA	36	E versus D	Not named
NCT 00872859	**NR**	**USA**	**196**	**A or D with/without RXT**	**Principal condition**
NCT 00956384	R	Canada	144	C versus E	Exclusion criteria
NCT 01027637	ND	USA	30	Defining the stretch parameters of A	Exclusion criteria
NCT 01222390	NR	USA	30	F versus E	Not named
NCT 01310075	R	USA	398	A versus SM	Exclusion criteria
NCT 01372917*	NR	USA	39	AM	Exclusion criteria; sterilization with γ-rays
NCT 01561287	R	USA	40	A, neovascularisation	Not named
NCT 01664091	NR	USA	32	ADM versus others, with/without RXT	**Principal condition, postsurgery**
NCT 01679223	NR	USA	60	AM, incorporation	Not named
NCT 1781299	R	UK	50	A RTU versus SM	Anamnestic record
NCT 01823107	R	USA	25	G	Exclusion criteria
NCT 01853436	R	Italy	60	S	Exclusion criteria
NCT 01959867	**NR**	**USA**		**SM versus B**	**Principal condition, prior to surgery**
ISRCTN 67956295	NR	UK	40	S versus SM	Not named

A: alloderm; ADM: acellular dermal matrix; AM: allomax; B: traditional reconstruction; C: 1-stage dermal matrix/implant procedure; D: DermaMatrix; E: 2-stage tissue expander/implant procedure; F: ContourProfile© expander; G: Meso BioMatrix Acellular Peritoneum Matrix; ISCTNR: international standard randomised controlled trial number register; NCT: national clinical trial accession number; R: recruiting; NR: not recruiting; RTU: ready to use; RXT: radiation therapy; S: Strattice; SM: Surgimed; UK: United Kingdom; USA: United States of America. *Published results [4].

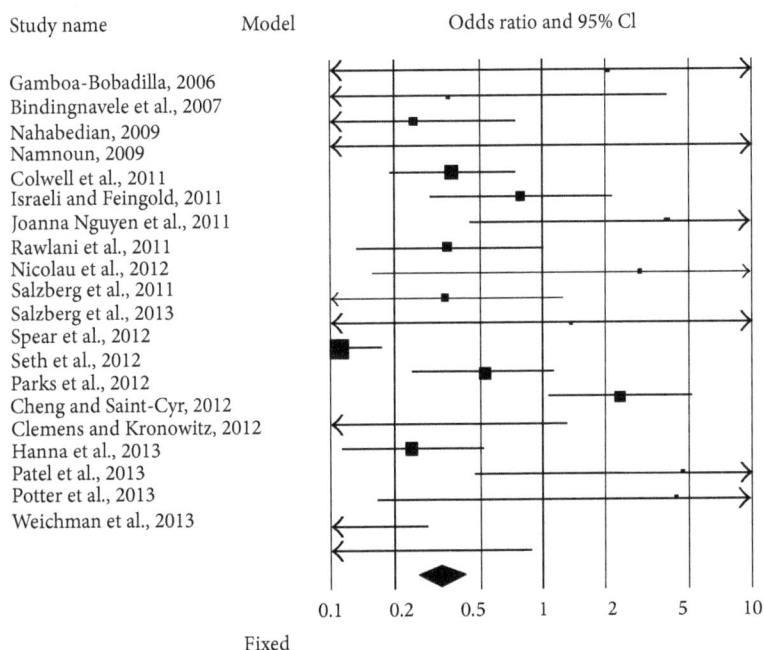

FIGURE 3: Forest plot of 20 studies. The authors reported the complications occurring in ADM-assisted immediate implant breast reconstruction, with or without radiotherapy (RXT). Odds ratios and confidence intervals at 95% are plotted. The black diamond at the bottom is the pooled odds ratio and its CI 95%. It completely falls to the left of 1.0 (<1), meaning that RXT significantly increases the risk of complications.

TABLE 3: List of the published clinical trials in which different types of acellular dermis matrices (ADMs) were used for the implant breast reconstruction. These papers, included in the meta-analysis, analytically reported the rate of complications in patients treated or not with radiotherapy (RXT). All studies but two (Nicolau et al., 2012, Canada, [7], and Potter et al., 2013, UK, [8]) were from groups operating in the USA or cooperating with American institutions. NR: not reported.

Reference	ADM	Period, location	Nr. Of Pts./Reconstr.	Follow-up
Gamboa-Bobadilla, 2006 [9]	Alloderm	2003-2004, Medical College Georgia	11/13	14 months
Bindingnavele et al., 2007 [10]	Alloderm	2004-2005, Univ. South California	41/65	10 months
Nahabedian, 2009 [11]	Alloderm	1997-2008, Georgetown Univ.	76/100	NR
Namnoum, 2009 [12]	Alloderm	NR, Atlanta Plastic Surg.	20/29	21 months
Colwell et al., 2011 [13]	Alloderm versus no ADM	2006-2010, Univ. Massachusetts	211/331 and NR/128	NR
Israeli and Feingold, 2011 [14]	Strattice versus Alloderm	2005-2009, Hofstra Univ.	44/77 versus 72/122	12-22 months
Joanna Nguyen et al., 2011 [15]	Alloderm versus no ADM	1998-2008, Harvard Med. School	NR/75 and 246	NR
Rawlani et al., 2011 [16]	Flex-HD	NR, Northwestern Univ.	84/121	44 weeks
Nicolau et al., 2012 [7]	Alloderm	2008-2010, McGill University Health Centre, Canada	46/73	NR
Salzberg et al., 2011 [17]	Alloderm	2001-2010, NY Med. College	260/466	29 months
Salzberg et al., 2013 [18]	Strattice	2008-2009, NY Med. College	54/105	41 months
Spear et al., 2012 [19]	Alloderm	2004-2010, Georgetown Univ.	289/428	10-14 weeks
Seth et al., 2012 [20]	Alloderm/Flex-HD versus no ADM	2006-2008, Northwestern Univ.	NR/393 and 199	23-24 months
Parks et al., 2012 [21]	Alloderm versus no ADM	2001-2011, private practice, USA	232/346 and 114/165	NR
Cheng et al., 2013 [22]	Alloderm	2008-2012, Univ. of Texas; Emory University and Mayo Clinic.	11/16	9 months
Clemens and Kronowitz, 2012 [23]	Human, porcine, and bovine	2008-2012, Univ. of Texas	364/548	NR
Hanna et al., 2013 [24]	Alloderm versus no ADM	2007-2010, Virginia Univ.	31/38 and 44/62	8-10 months
Patel et al., 2013 [25]	ADM (not specified) versus no ADM	2005-2012, Univ. of California	NR/74 and NR/118	34 and 38 months
Potter et al., 2013 [8]	Protexa	2011-2012, University of Bristol, UK	31/46	3 months
Weichman et al., 2013 [26]	Alloderm	2006-2011, NY University	23/46	19 months

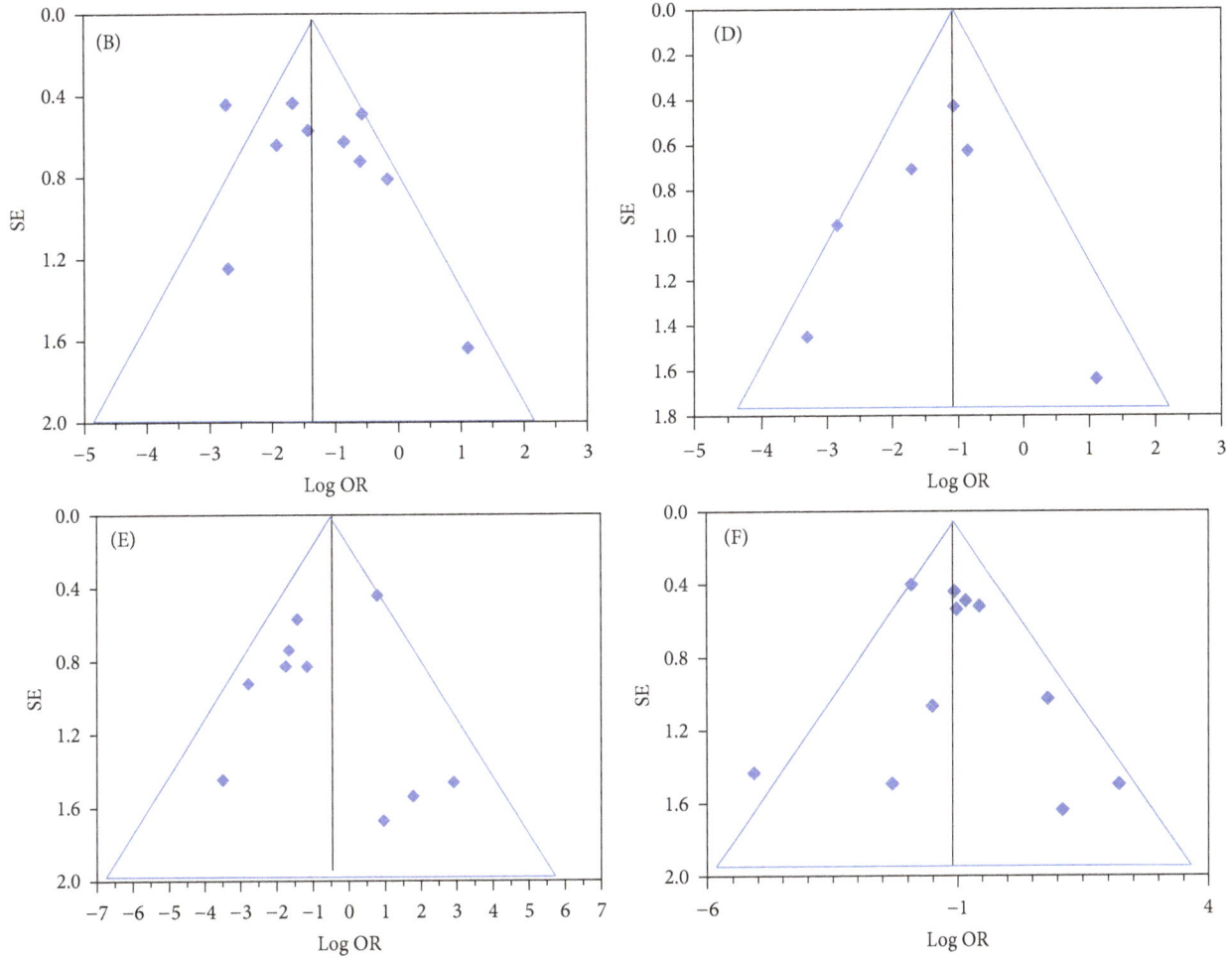

FIGURE 4: Funnel plots of 20 studies. Complications in ADM-assisted immediate implant breast reconstruction with or without RXT, occurring with statistically significant difference. (B) Skin necrosis; (D) capsular contracture; (E) other complications, sparsely described; (F) failure.

grouped them. The RXT significantly enhanced the risk for skin necrosis and capsular contracture, as well as the implant failure due to different conditions.

4. Discussion

The RXT as adjuvant therapy for patients affected by mammary cancer is a trouble for the plastic surgeons as it could cause a tissue insult possibly affecting the final outcome of postmastectomy breast reconstruction. The relatively recent introduction of ADM-assisted implant reconstruction seemed to help a better procedure; however, its safety when RXT is needed is still under debate and experimental data are scanty and not conclusive. In many cases, as in the majority of clinical trials more recently registered at the USA repository, a history of previous irradiation is sufficient to exclude the use of the ADM and prefer an autologous reconstruction instead. In general, the authors of meta-analyses and traditional reviews agreed that the RXT enhances the risk of complications; however, no general agreement was reached, nor all works were conclusive in this aspect. A recent

survey evaluated that at least 25% of patients submitted to postmastectomy breast reconstruction, independently from the use of ADM, and received prereconstruction RXT. The prevalence was large, exceeding 50%, in those which received postmastectomy RXT [29]. The relatively low rate of RXT (16% of all reconstructions considered) in this work could eventually reflect a bias in the choice of the technique, entailing that the autologous reconstruction could be preferred to the use of the ADM when the RXT was performed before surgery or expected to be needed later. While the first case could be confirmed at least in part by the general attitude of considering previous irradiation as an exclusion criteria for the use of expensive ADM (see Table 2), the second remains largely hypothetical.

The rational of these warnings resides in the nature of the ADM. They are generally protein derivatives, mainly composed of collagen, to which elastin, proteoglycans, and glycosaminoglycans may be added. The impact with ionizing radiation to sterilize the dried form of Alloderm affected the 3D structure of the collagen matrix, and different species of free radicals developed [28, 30, 31]. An unsolved issue is how

TABLE 4: Statistics under a fixed model for each study included in the meta-analysis.

Study name	Odds ratio	Lower limit	Upper limit	Z value	P value	Relative weight	Std. residual
Gamboa-Bobadilla, 2006 [9]	0.486	0.018	12.929	−0.431	0.667	0.55	−1.09
Bindingnavele et al. 2007 [10]	2.750	0.256	29.561	0.835	0.404	1.06	−0.08
Nahabedian, 2009 [11]	4.030	1.336	12.159	2.473	1.338	4.89	0.53
Namnoum, 2009 [12]	2.429	0.082	72.046	0.513	0.608	0.52	−0.12
Colwell et al. 2011 [13]	2.654	1.327	5.304	2.761	0.006	12.44	−0.38
Israeli and Feingold, 2011 [14]	1.268	0.474	3.391	0.474	0.636	6.17	−1.78
Joanna Nguyen et al. 2011 [15]	0.253	0.029	2.221	−1.240	0.215	1.27	−2.25
Rawlani et al. 2011 [16]	2.803	1.013	7.757	1.985	0.047	5.76	−0.14
Nicolau et al. 2012 [7]	0.342	0.018	6.468	−0.716	0.474	0.69	−1.46
Salzberg et al. 2011 [17]	2.890	0.791	10.555	1.605	0.108	3.56	−0.06
Salzberg et al. 2013 [18]	0.733	0.038	14.044	−0.206	0.837	0.68	−0.94
Spear et al. 2012 [19]	9.114	5.778	14.377	9.503	0.000	28.74	5.64
Seth et al. 2012 [20]	1.896	0.878	4.094	1.628	0.103	10.07	−1.24
Parks et al. 2012 [21]	0.426	0.191	0.948	−2.091	0.036	9.32	−5.03
Cheng et al. 2013 [22]	29.000	0.780	1077.623	1.826	0.068	0.46	1.23
Clemens and Kronowitz, 2012 [23]	4.126	1.929	8.822	3.655	0.000	10.33	0.86
Hanna et al. 2013 [24]	0.217	0.022	2.131	−1.311	0.190	1.14	−2.27
Patel et al. 2013 [25]	0.231	0.009	6.107	−1.877	0.380	0.56	−1.54
Potter et al. 2013 [8]	36.000	3.453	375.309	2.996	0.003	1.09	2.09
Weichman et al. 2013 [26]	21.364	1.139	400.534	2.047	0.041	0.69	1.31
Model: fixed	**3.010**	**2.358**	**3.844**	**8.841**	**0.000**		

TABLE 5: Statistical evaluation of the results of meta-analysis. The test of null was performed for both the fixed and random models and was significant. The heterogeneity and Tau-squared tests applied to the fixed model are also shown.

Model	Test of null (2-tail)		Heterogeneity				Tau-squared			
	Z value	P value	Q value	df (Q)	P value	I-squared	Tau-squared	SE	Variance	Tau
Fixed	−8.841	0.000	75.243	19	0.000	74.748	1.015	0.603	0.364	1.008

the modalities of irradiation could be modified to reduce the impact on the skin and on the implant. In addition to the timing, which remains a possible additional risk factor (that was, however, not supported by the experimental evidence), the hypofractionation of the total dose of radiation (40 Gy in 15 fractions over 3 weeks) was associated with a higher incidence of severe capsular contracture. A clinical study with similar aim describes the changes of the native capsule architecture in ADM- and non-ADM-assisted reconstructions, before and after RXT [32]. In the presence of ADM and before RXT, the amount of elastin fibers was roughly duplicated and the number of macrophages fivefold reduced. However, when the ADM was used, irradiation did not induce relevant changes in the native capsule, not even excessive neovascularisation. The authors used Alloderm, Strattice, and NeoForm. This work did not report the modalities of irradiation, not even the incidence of complications in no ADM-assisted reconstructions. In 27 reconstructions with ADM, nine capsular contracture (grade III-IV) and nine different complications developed after irradiation. Nine complications exited in implant failure. No capsular contraction nor failure, and only three complications developed in the absence of irradiation.

The results of the meta-analysis presented in this review, in which three previously not reported results have been included [7, 8, 26], supported the thesis that the RXT represents a serious challenge; the influence of its timing in relation with surgery is, however, not noticeable due to the scarcity of data. The general opinion that RXT is a risk for higher rate of complications is, however, a controversial issue. Only few authors of original works lacking extractable data unequivocally concluded that RXT enhanced risk of complications [33–38]. Unfortunately, the only study in the field classified at level 1 of evidence only named RXT among the exclusion criteria [39]. Ibrahim et al., 2013 [40], recently found in a large database (19100 patients identified) the only association of greater risk for postoperative urinary tract infection in the group receiving the ADM and RXT. The authors admitted that unconventional results could be due to a bias derived from the very large number of cases in their analysis. To this, it could be added as an emerging opinion that in the context of greater morbidity due to the additional insult of RXT, the use of ADM seems to be protective and reduces the rate of complications, in particular capsular contracture [41–43]. While a large number of researchers

TABLE 6: Rate of complications by group (no RXT versus RXT).

Complication	Number of studies	No RXT (%)	ES	RXT (%)	ES	P value
Overall	11	15.63	3.59	24.71	5.67	0.000
Infection	10	8.19	2.73	12.04	4.01	0.400
Skin necrosis	10	4.04	1.35	15.50	1.05	0.000
Seroma	9	3.61	1.20	4.60	1.53	0.045
Capsular contracture	6	2.88	1.09	11.90	4.50	0.033
Others	10	4.02	1.34	8.18	2.73	0.000
Failure	11	4.06	1.23	14.05	4.23	0.000

prefer to behave cautiously, as documented by the strategy adopted by the majority of protocols deposited at the clinical trials (Table 2); this suggestion was accepted in some reviews [42, 43] and recently included in the guidelines of the Association of Breast Surgery and the British Association of Plastic, Reconstructive, and Aesthetic Surgeons [44]. This document recognized that the RXT negatively affected the outcome but suggested that the use of ADM could potentially reduce the severity of capsular contracture.

In addition to capsular contracture, infection and implant failure seemed to occur more frequently in irradiated breasts [33]. Data we analysed here confirm this trend for all types of complications and reached the statistical significance in the case of skin necrosis and capsular contracture. The most severe outcome, implant failure, was also significantly enhanced, independently from the causes.

Several biases occur in the analysis. The influence of chemotherapy, in relation with the concomitant need for radiation therapy, was sporadically reported in details in the reviewed papers, as were other recognized risk factors, such as obesity, diabetes, smoking, and breast size [45–47]. The data retrieved from the analysis of the literature did not permit to stratify the observations in relation to the RXT; it is specified by some authors that the risk factors were evenly distributed among groups. Another source of perplexity could rise from the consideration that, for its relatively elevated cost [48], the use of ADM could be addressed to patients with a lower risk for complications, or with a more favourable stage of the cancer. This factor, poorly investigated until now [2, 38], could put the suggested protective effect under a more relative point of view.

5. Conclusions

Radiotherapy is generally considered a concomitant factor negatively influencing the dynamics of breast reconstruction, even when ADM is added. This fact, claimed by many studies published on this argument, seems to emerge from the meta-analysis presented here. The real impact of RXT on the success of breast reconstruction techniques must be better defined by studies falling in the level of evidence I or II, namely, protocols specifically designed to define the importance of the radiotherapy and planned as randomized, single-, or multicenter studies of adequate quality. Better

assessment of anthropometric and behavioural conditions, morbidity, and stage of the cancer in the two groups, with or without RXT, should be added for clarity.

A better definition of histological evolution of the ADM after surgery in sites that were previously irradiated should also be of interest and even more in those undergoing RXT after the surgery, particularly in terms of formation of oxygen reactive species and radicals and collagen integrity.

Acknowledgment

The authors are very grateful to Prof. Douglas Noonan, for kindly reviewing the paper and making substantial improvement of English language.

References

[1] Y. Takami, T. Matsuda, M. Yoshitake, M. Hanumadass, and R. J. Walter, "Dispase/detergent treated dermal matrix as a dermal substitute," *Burns*, vol. 22, no. 3, pp. 182–190, 1996.

[2] K. E. Weichman, S. C. Wilson, P. B. Saadeh et al., "Sterile "ready-to-use" AlloDerm decreases postoperative infectious complications in patients undergoing immediate implant-based breast reconstruction with acellular dermal matrix," *Plastic and Reconstructive Surgery*, vol. 132, no. 4, pp. 725–736, 2013.

[3] A. Cheng and M. Saint-Cyr, "Comparison of different ADM materials in breast surgery," *Clinics in Plastic Surgery*, vol. 39, no. 2, pp. 167–175, 2012.

[4] M. L. Venturi, A. N. Mesbahi, J. H. Boehmler, and A. J. Marrogi, "Evaluating sterile human acellular dermal matrix in immediate expander-based breast reconstruction: a multicenter, prospective, cohort study," *Plastic and Reconstructive Surgery*, vol. 131, no. 1, pp. 9e–18e, 2013.

[5] D. F. Stroup, J. A. Berlin, S. C. Morton et al., "Meta-analysis of observational studies in epidemiology: a proposal for reporting," *The Journal of the American Medical Association*, vol. 283, no. 15, pp. 2008–2012, 2000.

[6] H. Rothstein, A. J. Sutton, and M. Borenstein, *Publication Bias in Meta-Analysis: Prevention, Assessment and Adjustments*, John Wiley & Sons, Chichester, UK, 2005.

[7] I. Nicolau, X. Xie, M. McGregor, and N. Dendukuri, "Evaluation of acellular dermal matrix for breast reconstruction: an update," Tech. Rep. 59, Technology Assessment Unit of the McGill University Health Centre (MUHC), Montreal, Canada,

2012, http://onlinelibrary.wiley.com/o/cochrane/clhta/articles/HTA-32013000290/frame.html.

[8] S. Potter, A. Chambers, S. Govindajulu, A. Sahu, R. Warr, and S. Cawthorn, "Early complications and implant loss in implant-based breast reconstruction with and without acellular dermal matrix (Protexa): a comparative study," *European Journal of Surgical Oncology*, 2013.

[9] G. M. Gamboa-Bobadilla, "Implant breast reconstruction using acellular dermal matrix," *Annals of Plastic Surgery*, vol. 56, no. 1, pp. 22–25, 2006.

[10] V. Bindingnavele, M. Gaon, K. S. Ota, D. A. Kulber, and D.-J. Lee, "Use of acellular cadaveric dermis and tissue expansion in postmastectomy breast reconstruction," *Journal of Plastic, Reconstructive and Aesthetic Surgery*, vol. 60, no. 11, pp. 1214–1218, 2007.

[11] M. Y. Nahabedian, "AlloDerm performance in the setting of prosthetic breast surgery, infection, and irradiation," *Plastic and Reconstructive Surgery*, vol. 124, no. 6, pp. 1743–1753, 2009.

[12] J. D. Namnoum, "Expander/implant reconstruction with Allo-Derm: recent experience," *Plastic and Reconstructive Surgery*, vol. 124, no. 2, pp. 387–394, 2009.

[13] A. S. Colwell, B. Damjanovic, B. Zahedi, L. Medford-Davis, C. Hertl, and W. G. Austen, "Retrospective review of 331 consecutive immediate single-stage implant reconstructions with acellular dermal matrix: indications, complications, trends, and costs," *Plastic and Reconstructive Surgery*, vol. 128, no. 6, pp. 1170–1178, 2011.

[14] R. Israeli and R. S. Feingold, "Acellular dermal matrix in breast reconstruction in the setting of radiotherapy," *Aesthetic Surgery Journal*, vol. 31, no. 7, supplement, pp. 51S–64S, 2011.

[15] T. Joanna Nguyen, J. N. Carey, and A. K. Wong, "Use of human acellular dermal matrix in implant-based breast reconstruction: evaluating the evidence," *Journal of Plastic, Reconstructive and Aesthetic Surgery*, vol. 64, no. 12, pp. 1553–1561, 2011.

[16] V. Rawlani, D. W. Buck, S. A. Johnson, K. S. Heyer, and J. Y. S. Kim, "Tissue expander breast reconstruction using prehydrated human acellular dermis," *Annals of Plastic Surgery*, vol. 66, no. 6, pp. 593–597, 2011.

[17] C. A. Salzberg, A. Y. Ashikari, R. M. Koch, and E. Chabner-Thompson, "An 8-year experience of direct-to-implant immediate breast reconstruction using human acellular dermal matrix (AlloDerm)," *Plastic and Reconstructive Surgery*, vol. 127, no. 2, pp. 514–524, 2011.

[18] C. A. Salzberg, C. Dunavant, and N. Nocera, "Immediate breast reconstruction using porcine acellular dermal matrix (Strattice): long-term outcomes and complications," *Journal of Plastic, Reconstructive & Aesthetic Surgery*, vol. 66, no. 3, pp. 323–328, 2013.

[19] S. L. Spear, M. Seruya, S. S. Rao et al., "Two-stage prosthetic breast reconstruction using AlloDerm including outcomes of different timings of radiotherapy," *Plastic and Reconstructive Surgery*, vol. 130, no. 1, pp. 1–9, 2012.

[20] A. K. Seth, E. M. Hirsch, N. A. Fine, and J. Y. Kim, "Utility of acellular dermis-assisted breast reconstruction in the setting of radiation: a comparative analysis," *Plastic and Reconstructive Surgery*, vol. 130, no. 4, pp. 750–758, 2012.

[21] J. W. Parks, S. E. Hammond, W. A. Walsh et al., "Human Acellular Dermis (ACD) versus No-ACD in tissue expansion breast reconstruction," *Plastic and Reconstructive Surgery*, vol. 130, no. 4, pp. 739–746, 2012.

[22] A. Cheng, C. Lakhiani, and M. Saint-Cyr, "Treatment of capsular contracture using complete implant coverage by acellular dermal matrix: a novel technique," *Plastic and Reconstructive Surgery*, vol. 132, no. 3, pp. 519–529, 2013.

[23] M. W. Clemens and S. Kronowitz, "Acellular dermal matrix in irradiated tissue expander/implant-based breast reconstruction: evidence-based review," *Plastic and Reconstructive Surgery*, vol. 130, no. 5, supplement 2, pp. 27S–34S, 2012.

[24] K. R. Hanna, B. R. DeGeorge Jr., A. F. Mericli, K. Y. Lin, and D. B. Drake, "Comparison study of two types of expander-based breast reconstruction acellular dermal matrix-assisted versus total submuscular placement. Acellular Dermal Matrix-assisted versus total submuscular placement," *Annals of Plastic Surgery*, vol. 70, pp. 10–15, 2013.

[25] K. M. Patel, F. Albino, K. L. Fan, E. Liao, and M. Y. Nahabedian, "Microvascular autologous breast reconstruction in the context of radiation therapy: comparing two reconstructive algorithms," *Plastic and Reconstructive Surgery*, vol. 132, no. 2, pp. 251–257, 2013.

[26] K. E. Weichman, Y. Cemal, C. R. Albornoz et al., "Unilateral preoperative chest wall irradiation in bilateral tissue expander breast reconstruction with acellular dermal matrix: a prospective outcomes analysis," *Plastic and Reconstructive Surgery*, vol. 131, no. 5, pp. 921–927, 2013.

[27] S. C. Haase and K. C. Chung, "An evidence-based approach to treating thumb carpometacarpal joint arthritis," *Plastic and Reconstructive Surgery*, vol. 127, no. 2, pp. 918–925, 2011.

[28] S.-S. Gouk, N. M. Kocherginsky, Y. Y. Kostetski et al., "Synchrotron radiation-induced formation and reactions of free radicals in human acellular dermal matrix," *Radiation Research*, vol. 163, no. 5, pp. 535–543, 2005.

[29] S. A. Chen, C. Hiley, D. Nickleach et al., "Breast reconstruction and post-mastectomy radiation practice," *Radiation Oncology*, vol. 8, article 45, 2013.

[30] S.-S. Gouk, T.-M. Lim, S.-H. Teoh, and W. Q. Sun, "Alterations of human acellular tissue matrix by gamma irradiation: histology, biomechanical property, stability, in vitro cell repopulation, and remodeling," *Journal of Biomedical Materials Research, B: Applied Biomaterials*, vol. 84, no. 1, pp. 205–217, 2008.

[31] N. B. Shah, W. F. Wolkers, M. Morrissey, W. Q. Sun, and J. C. Bischof, "Fourier transform infrared spectroscopy investigation of native tissue matrix modifications using a gamma irradiation process," *Tissue Engineering C: Methods*, vol. 15, no. 1, pp. 33–40, 2009.

[32] H. R. Moyer, X. Pinell-White, and A. Losken, "The effect of radiation on acellular dermal matrix and capsule formation in breast reconstruction: clinical outcomes and histologic analysis," *Plastic and Reconstructive Surgery*, vol. 133, no. 2, pp. 214–221, 2014.

[33] Y. S. Chun, K. Verma, H. Rosen et al., "Implant-based breast reconstruction using acellular dermal matrix and the risk of postoperative complications," *Plastic and Reconstructive Surgery*, vol. 125, no. 2, pp. 429–436, 2010.

[34] A. S. Liu, H.-K. Kao, R. G. Reish, C. A. Hergrueter, J. W. May Jr., and L. Guo, "Postoperative complications in prosthesis-based breast reconstruction using acellular dermal matrix," *Plastic and Reconstructive Surgery*, vol. 127, no. 5, pp. 1755–1762, 2011.

[35] S. L. Spear, M. Seruya, M. W. Clemens, S. Teitelbaum, and M. Y. Nahabedian, "Acellular dermal matrix for the treatment and prevention of implant-associated breast deformities," *Plastic and Reconstructive Surgery*, vol. 127, no. 3, pp. 1047–1058, 2011.

[36] S. Brooke, J. Mesa, M. Uluer et al., "Complications in tissue expander breast reconstruction: a comparison of AlloDerm,

DermaMatrix, and FlexHD acellular inferior pole dermal slings," *Annals of Plastic Surgery*, vol. 69, no. 4, pp. 347–349, 2012.

[37] E. M. Kobraei, J. Nimtz, L. Wong et al., "Risk factors for adverse outcome following skin-sparing mastectomy and immediate prosthetic reconstruction," *Plastic and Reconstructive Surgery*, vol. 129, no. 2, pp. 234e–241e, 2012.

[38] I. A. Pestana, D. C. Campbell, G. Bharti et al., "Factors affecting complications in radiated breast reconstruction," *Annals of Plastic Surgery*, vol. 70, no. 5, pp. 542–545, 2013.

[39] C. M. McCarthy, C. N. Lee, E. G. Halvorson et al., "The use of acellular dermal matrices in two-stage expander/implant reconstruction: a multicenter, blinded, randomized controlled trial," *Plastic and Reconstructive Surgery*, vol. 130, no. 5, supplement 2, pp. 57S–66S, 2012.

[40] A. M. Ibrahim, M. Shuster, P. G. Koolen et al., "Analysis of the national surgical quality improvement program database in 19, 100 patients undergoing implant-based breast reconstruction: complication rates with acellular dermal matrix," *Plastic and Reconstructive Surgery*, vol. 132, no. 5, pp. 1057–1066, 2013.

[41] A. W. Peled, R. D. Foster, E. R. Garwood et al., "The effects of acellular dermal matrix in expander-implant breast reconstruction after total skin-sparing mastectomy: results of a prospective practice improvement study," *Plastic and Reconstructive Surgery*, vol. 129, no. 6, pp. 901e–908e, 2012.

[42] S. L. Spear, S. R. Sher, and A. Al-Attar, "Focus on technique: supporting the soft-tissue envelope in breast reconstruction," *Plastic and Reconstructive Surgery*, vol. 130, no. 5, supplement 2, pp. 89S–94S, 2012.

[43] B. M. Topol, "The use of human acellular dermal matrices in irradiated breast reconstruction," *Clinics in Plastic Surgery*, vol. 39, no. 2, pp. 149–158, 2012.

[44] L. Martin, J. M. O'Donoghue, K. Horgan et al., "Acellular dermal matrix (ADM) assisted breast reconstruction procedures: joint guidelines from the Association of Breast Surgery and the British Association of Plastic, Reconstructive and Aesthetic Surgeons," *European Journal of Surgical Oncology*, vol. 39, no. 5, pp. 425–429, 2013.

[45] G. L. Gunnarsson, M. Børsen-Koch, S. Arffmann et al., "Successful breast reconstruction using acellular dermal matrix can be recommended in healthy non-smoking patients," *Danish Medical Journal*, vol. 60, no. 12, Article ID A4751, 2013.

[46] B. M. Showalter, J. C. Crantford, G. B. Russell et al., "The effect of reusable versus disposable draping material on infection rates in implant-based breast reconstruction: a prospective randomized trial," *Annals of Plastic Surgery*, 2014.

[47] P. T. Thiruchelvam, F. McNeill, N. Jallali et al., "Post-mastectomy breast reconstruction," *British Medical Journal*, vol. 347, Article ID f5903, 2013.

[48] R. K. Johnson, C. K. Wright, A. Gandhi, M. C. Charny, and L. Barr, "Cost minimisation analysis of using acellular dermal matrix (Strattice) for breast reconstruction compared with standard techniques," *European Journal of Surgical Oncology*, vol. 39, no. 3, pp. 242–247, 2013.

18

A Fast-Track Referral System for Skin Lesions Suspicious of Melanoma: Population-Based Cross-Sectional Study from a Plastic Surgery Center

Reem Dina Jarjis, Lone Bak Hansen, and Steen Henrik Matzen

Department of Plastic Surgery & Breast Surgery, Zealand University Hospital, Sygehusvej 10, 4000 Roskilde, Denmark

Correspondence should be addressed to Reem Dina Jarjis; reemdj@outlook.com

Academic Editor: Nicolo Scuderi

Introduction. To minimize delay between presentation, diagnosis, and treatment of cutaneous melanoma (CM), a national fast-track referral system (FTRS) was implemented in Denmark. The aim of this study was to analyze the referral patterns to our department of skin lesions suspicious of melanoma in the FTRS. *Methods.* Patients referred to the Department of Plastic Surgery and Breast Surgery in Zealand University Hospital were registered prospectively over a 1-year period in 2014. A cross-sectional study was performed analyzing referral patterns, including patient and tumor characteristics. *Results.* A total of 556 patients were registered as referred to the center in the FTRS for skin lesions suspicious of melanoma. Among these, a total of 312 patients (56.1%) were diagnosed with CM. Additionally, 41 (7.4%) of the referred patients were diagnosed with in situ melanoma. *Conclusion.* In total, 353 (63.5%) patients had a malignant or premalignant melanocytic skin lesion. When only considering patients who where referred without a biopsy, the diagnostic accuracy for GPs and dermatologists was 29% and 45%, respectively. We suggest that efforts of adequate training for the referring physicians in diagnosing melanocytic skin lesions will increase diagnostic accuracy, leading to larger capacity in secondary care for the required treatment of malignant skin lesions.

1. Introduction

Cutaneous melanoma (CM) is an aggressive tumor of the skin melanocytes. It is a growing health concern with a globally increasing incidence in fair-skinned populations over the last few decades [1]. The cause of CM is probably multifactorial but for the most part attributed to an increase of exposure to UV radiation [1, 2].

To minimize delay between presentation, diagnosis, and treatment of CM, the Danish Health and Medicines Authority implemented a national fast-track referral system (FTRS), which also includes that the surgical management of primary melanoma is according to national clinical guidelines. Other skin malignancies, such as basal cell carcinoma (BCC) and squamous cell carcinoma (SCC), are not intended to be referred through this system. The aim of the national FTRS was *"that cancer patients should experience a well-organized, comprehensive process without undue delay in connection with the clinical evaluation, initial treatment and rehabilitation and palliative care, with the aim to improve the prognosis and quality of life for patients"* [3].

The Department of Plastic Surgery & Breast Surgery, Zealand University Hospital, provides a regional health service to a population base of approximately 820.000 inhabitants in Zealand Region in Denmark, representing nearly 15% of the country's total population. The incidence of melanoma in Zealand Region in a five-year period in 2010 to 2014 increased from 245 to 445 patients, including MIS [4]. In the recent years, this incidence has amounted to approximately 14-15% of the diagnosed CM in the total population, and this regional incidence is slightly increasing correspondingly with the national incidence in Denmark [5].

In the Danish health care system, the general practitioners (GPs) function as gatekeepers for consultant dermatologists, plastic surgeons, and plastic surgery departments, where treatment of CM is performed. The Danish national FTRS

TABLE 1: Results of referrals in the fast-track referral system for skin lesions suspicious of melanoma.

	Females	Males	Total	P value
N (%)	293 (52.7)	263 (47.3)	556	<0.05
Age (mean ± SE)	57 ± 1.0	60 ± 1.0	58 ± 0.7	<0.05
CM	170	142	312	<0.05
In situ (%)	23 (56.1)	18 (43.9)	41	ns
NMSC	13	16	29	ns
Benign	86	85	171	ns

CM: cutaneous melanoma.
NMSC: non-melanoma skin cancer.

for skin lesions suspicious of melanoma implies that a patient who presents with a lesion suspicious of CM is offered an excision biopsy in secondary care within six days. This allows confirmation of the diagnosis within two weeks and permits the second stage of definitive wider excision and sentinel lymph node biopsy (SLNB) to be based on tumor characteristics such as the Breslow thickness, mitotic activity, or presence of ulceration, which is then offered within nine days. If SLNB is positive for metastasis, the patient is offered the third stage comprising radical lymph node dissection within two weeks.

Our plastic surgery department receives referrals regarding lesions suspicious of melanoma from GPs, dermatologists, private plastic surgery clinics, or other specialties for clinical evaluation and treatment. If a biopsy is made prior to the referral, the patients are offered further treatment in the department depending on the histological examination of the biopsy.

The aim of this study was to analyze the referral patterns of suspicious melanocytic skin lesions to our department in the FTRS. We hypothesize that a relatively large proportion of the referrals will present with skin lesions other than CM, leaving room for improving diagnostic accuracy in the primary health care sector. Therefore, the objective was to characterize the referrals in the FTRS of suspected or classified CM, in order to clarify from which health services the referrals originate and how many of the referred patients had in situ melanoma (MIS), invasive cutaneous melanoma (CM), non-melanoma skin cancer (NMSC), or benign lesions.

2. Methods

2.1. Study Design and Setting. Patients referred in the FTRS to the Department of Plastic Surgery and Breast Surgery in Zealand University Hospital, because of a lesion suspicious of CM or with a biopsy-verified CM, were registered prospectively in a population-based cross-sectional study of the Zealand Region consisting of approximately 820.000 inhabitants in Denmark.

2.2. Participants. This study included patients over a 1-year period in 2014, who had undergone surgical biopsy in general practice, by dermatologists, in private plastic surgery clinics or in other medical specialties and who were referred to our department for further treatment. Patients who were referred

by the above health services because of a suspicious lesion without a biopsy prior to the referral were also included. In the first visit to the outpatient clinic, the patient was examined clinically and by manual dermatoscopy, and a total body skin examination was performed. Also, the patient was offered an immediate excision biopsy under local anesthesia, if a biopsy was not performed prior to the referral. The patients were scheduled after two weeks for suture removal and results of histology. Patients who did not show up to the consultation or who did not want to have an excision biopsy performed and patients with metastatic melanoma of unknown primary origin were excluded from the study.

2.3. Variables. Variables are patient age, sex, anatomical location of the lesion, tumor characteristics, and from which health services the referrals originated were registered, along with whether or not a biopsy had been performed prior to referral. All cases were coded as in situ melanoma (MIS), invasive cutaneous melanoma (CM), non-melanoma skin cancer (NMSC), or benign lesions.

The histological examinations of all the tumor biopsies were conducted at the Department of Pathology, Roskilde University Hospital.

2.4. Statistical Methods. All data were tested for distribution of normality and treated statistically accordingly. Comparison between groups was tested by two-tailed t-test and in the case of skewness or few numbers among groups the Mann-Whitney U test for nonparametric data was performed. Statistical significance was set at $P < 0.05$. All data were analyzed using the statistical program PAST (ver. 3.09).

3. Results

3.1. Participants. A total of 565 patients were prospectively registered as referred to the center in the FTRS for skin lesions suspicious of melanoma (Table 1). Of the referred patients, two patients never showed up, one patient did not eventually want a biopsy taken, and seven patients had metastatic melanoma of unknown primary origin demonstrated by PET-CT scan. These nine patients were excluded from the database.

3.2. Data. Most of the patients (393; 70.7%) were referred due to a suspicion of CM and had an excision biopsy taken on

TABLE 2: Origin of the referrals in the fast-track referral system and the proportion of diagnosed CM and diagnostic accuracy.

	GP	Derm.	PS	Other	Total
Referrals	88	441	5	22	556
(i) Without biopsy	55	321	0	17	393
CM diagnosed with biopsy prior to referral	31	106	5	5	113
CM verified with biopsy after referral	16	145	0	4	199
CM in total	47	251	5	9	312

CM: cutaneous melanoma.
Derm.: dermatologist.
PS: plastic surgeon.

TABLE 3: Age, gender, and Breslow thickness (%).

Age	Females			Males		
	≤1 mm	>1–4 mm	>4 mm	≤1 mm	>1–4 mm	>4 mm
20–40	(11.8) 20	(1.8) 3	0	(4.2) 6	(2.8) 4	0
41–55	(26.5) 45	(7.6) 14	0	(11.3) 16	(5.6) 8	(0.7) 1
56–70	(19.4) 33	(5.3) 9	(1.8) 3	(24.6) 35	(12.7) 18	(1.4) 2
>70	(11.2) 19	(8.2) 14	(5.3) 9	(16.9) 24	(13.4) 19	(4.2) 6
Total	(68.8) 117	(22.9) 40	(7.1) 12	(57.0) 81	(34.5) 49	(6.3) 9

TABLE 4: Distribution on Breslow thickness of referrals originating from GPs or dermatologists when biopsy is performed prior to and after referral.

Referrals	Breslow thickness			
	≤1 mm	>1–4 mm	>4 mm	Unclassified
GP				
+ biopsy*	21	7	2	1
÷ biopsy*	9	4	3	0
Dermatologist				
+ biopsy	58	40	4	4
÷ biopsy	89	45	11	0

*+ biopsy: biopsy performed prior to referral.
÷ biopsy: biopsy performed after referral.

the first visit, whereas 159 (28.6%) patients were referred due to a biopsy-verified CM.

A total of 312 patients (56.1%) were eventually diagnosed with CM, significantly more females than males ($P < 0.05$). The rest of the referred patients were diagnosed with MIS (41; 7.4%), NMSC (29; 5.2%), or various benign skin lesions (171; 30.8 %) with no significant difference between males or females (Table 1). Most referrals (441; 79.3%) were from dermatologists and only five from plastic surgeons (Table 2). Of the 393 patients without a biopsy prior to the referral, 55 patients were referred by GPs, 321 patients by dermatologists, and 17 patients by other specialties. Of the patients referred by GPs and dermatologists, a total of 16 and 145 patients, respectively, were diagnosed with CM (Table 2), leading to a diagnostic accuracy of 29% for GPs and 45% for dermatologists.

When Breslow thickness was analyzed according to age groups and sex (Table 3), the largest proportion of both sexes was in the group of thin melanomas (≤1 mm). However, this number was only statistically significant for females ($P = 0.044$ versus males $P = 0.47$). There was a tendency for a relatively larger distribution of males in the middle group of CM thickness, compared to females, but this finding was not statistically significant (Table 3). There were no major differences in distribution on Breslow thickness of the referrals originating from GPs or dermatologists when biopsy is performed prior to and after referral (Table 4). However, there might be a tendency towards a larger proportion of thin melanomas excised by GPs.

All of the included patients were seen after referral within the recommended time period and there was no difference in timing according to who was referring the patient. Furthermore, all patients diagnosed with CM had a definitive wider excision performed based on tumor characteristics in accordance with national guidelines for treatment of melanoma, including SLNB and radical lymph node dissection, if these were indicated.

4. Discussion

This is the first population-based cross-sectional study in Denmark that provides insight into the diagnostic accuracy of referrals of patients with skin lesions suspicious of melanoma, and the referring physicians' ability to differentiate between CM, NMSC, and benign lesions. Of all the referred patients, a total of 312 patients (56.1%) were diagnosed with CM and 41 patients were diagnosed with MIS (7.4%), whereas 200 patients had NMSC or benign lesions (35.9%). The FTRS can improve rapid access for patients with CM, but only when used appropriately due to increased education, clear communication, and improved technology for consistent detection of cancers [6]. A study has demonstrated that physicians can benefit from using dermatoscopy to differentiate between pigmented lesions, and this could possibly reduce the unnecessary referrals [7]. However, this requires proper training and regular use of dermatoscopy in order to improve from its supplementary assessment and therefore it is questionable whether GPs have the time required to gain sufficient experience in using dermatoscopy.

In our presented data, most referrals (441; 79.3%) were from dermatologists and only five from plastic surgeons (Table 2). This fact reflects that in the Zealand Region there are several practitioners in dermatology and none in plastic surgery. Also, this might indicate that most of the patients were referred to a dermatologist by the GPs initially, and these were further referred to our department in the FTRS because of continued clinical suspicion of CM (321; 57.7%) or because a biopsy performed by the dermatologist had verified the diagnosis of CM (106; 19.1%). When evaluating the diagnostic accuracy, the referring GPs had a lower accuracy compared to dermatologists (29% versus 45%), which is not unexpected since most GPs in general do not use dermatoscopy and have a lower experience in diagnosing pigmented skin lesions.

Cutaneous melanoma is still a skin cancer with the highest mortality despite all the preventive and therapeutic efforts, and this is also despite CM being less common than other non-melanoma skin cancers [8]. Breslow thickness, mitotic activity, and ulceration are associated with an increased risk of metastatic potential and mortality. Therefore, early diagnosis of CM at an initial and curable stage is essential for increasing the survival rate of patients [8]. However, waiting list times for dermatologists have increased and several referred lesions, which are a combination of benign and malignant lesions, can result in a puzzling and inefficient situation where early diagnosis can become challenging for patients who actually do have a malignant lesion. Similar fast-track referral systems, as the one described in our study, have also been implemented in the United Kingdom (UK) in 2000 [9]. When an evaluation of the 2-week rule in the UK was made in 2004, it revealed that the referral system was not working as expected in terms of early recognition and skin cancer diagnosis, because only 12% of the referrals had a potentially metastatic tumor such as squamous cell carcinoma (SCC) or melanoma [10]. As presented in our study, the patients with CM amounted to 312 (56.1%) of all the referred patients. Additionally, a total of 41 (7.4%) of the referred patients in our study were diagnosed with MIS. This means that a total of 353 (63.5%) patients had a malignant or premalignant melanocytic lesion, which demonstrates that it is still desirable to improve the diagnostic accuracy of CM in the primary sector, and this is further highlighted when only considering the patients who were referred without a biopsy, where the diagnostic accuracies for GPs and dermatologists were 29% and 45%, respectively.

By using this referral system, it is understandable and appropriate that some referrals will be made on the basis of doubt, especially if the referring physician is less experienced. Also, some physicians may experience pressure from patients

and their concerns of increased waiting times for having routine referrals [11]. In Australia, where there is a high prevalence of skin malignancy, it has been a target to improve awareness and diagnostic skills in Australian GPs for skin malignancies, which has led to improved accuracy and appropriate referral to specialists [12]. In Italy, a formal 4-hour training session on diagnostic and referral accuracy of family doctors in melanoma screening was given to GPs, resulting in improved specificity of suspicious pigmented skin lesion referrals for melanoma from 55% to 73.1% ($P < 0.001$) without significant loss in sensitivity [13]. However, another evaluation in the UK of the 2-week rule after a targeted continuing medical education showed surprisingly that the rate of correctly referred patients with suspected skin malignancies remained low regardless of the education module [14].

Recent evidence has shown that the increase in the incidence of CM is due to a generally higher awareness of skin cancer and the improved strategies for early recognition and diagnosis of suspicious melanocytic lesions. This is resulting in an increasing incidence of early stage melanomas [1]. However, a population-based study presented an increasing incidence of thick CM as well as an increase in incidence of all the other categories of Breslow thickness [15]. Hence, it is essential to ensure that the referrals of patients in FTRS are optimized, to limit unnecessary referrals, in order to gain capacity for the relevant category of patients with CM in the secondary care. Furthermore, distribution of CM over body surface is not only on sun-exposed areas, which indicates the importance of total body skin examination [16]. However, this is rarely performed by the referring physicians, including dermatologists, and thus, it is performed for the first time during patients' visit to the outpatient clinic. Unawareness of the lesion distribution or the time pressure in the clinics may explain why the referring physicians do not perform total body skin examination [16, 17], and this might possibly lead to delayed diagnosis of CM.

A limitation to our study is that this is a single center study based on the figures of one region of the country. However, Denmark is a relatively homogenous country with an even distribution of CM [5], and therefore, the 820.000 inhabitants in Zealand Region are likely representative of the effect and quality of the FTRS. Also, we are aware that we do not have any comparative data from the period before implementation of FTRS. However, since this was a cross-sectional study our objective was to perform a descriptive analysis of the current referral patterns of suspicious skin lesions to our department. Therefore, we conclude that since a definitive screening program for CM does not exist in many countries, it is essential to detect atypical melanocytic skin lesions early and correctly refer these to secondary care, where effective and timely management of CM can be performed. An increase in the level of diagnostic accuracy from the referring physicians is required in order to optimize the precision of the referrals to FTRS. This might be achieved, for example, by formal training sessions or performance of an excision biopsy, leading to an increased diagnostic accuracy and thereby improving and reserving the FTRS to the relevant patients.

Ethical Approval

The study was reported to and approved by the Danish Data Protection Agency (Reference no. 2008-58-0020/15-000241).

Competing Interests

Authors have no conflict of interests to declare.

References

[1] F. Erdmann, J. Lortet-Tieulent, J. Schüz et al., "International trends in the incidence of malignant melanoma 1953–2008- are recent generations at higher or lower risk?" *International Journal of Cancer*, vol. 132, no. 2, pp. 385–400, 2013.

[2] R. M. MacKie, C. A. Bray, D. J. Hole et al., "Incidence of and survival from malignant melanoma in Scotland: an epidemiological study," *The Lancet*, vol. 360, no. 9333, pp. 587–591, 2002.

[3] Sundhedsstyrelsen, "Fast-track referral system for malignant melanoma," 2015, http://sundhedsstyrelsen.dk/~/media/77C35 97F25634DFABCB49F86598ED132.ashx.

[4] Melanoma Sundata, Online database, 2016, https://www.mela- noma.sundata.dk.

[5] Danish Melanoma Group, 2016, http://www.melanoma.dk/.

[6] N. H. Cox, V. Madan, and T. Sanders, "The U.K. skin cancer 'two-week rule' proforma: assessment of potential modifications to improve referral accuracy," *British Journal of Dermatology*, vol. 158, no. 6, pp. 1293–1298, 2008.

[7] S. W. Menzies, J. Emery, M. Staples et al., "Impact of dermoscopy and short-term sequential digital dermoscopy imaging for the management of pigmented lesions in primary care: a sequential intervention trial," *British Journal of Dermatology*, vol. 161, no. 6, pp. 1270–1277, 2009.

[8] F. Brehmer, M. Ulrich, and H. A. Haenssle, "Strategies for early recognition of cutaneous melanoma-present and future," *Dermatology Practical & Conceptual*, vol. 2, no. 3, p. 203a06, 2012.

[9] M. D. Pacifico, R. A. Pearl, and R. Grover, "The UK government two-week rule and its impact on melanoma prognosis: An Evidence-Based Study," *Annals of the Royal College of Surgeons of England*, vol. 89, no. 6, pp. 609–615, 2007.

[10] N. H. Cox, "Evaluation of the U.K. 2-week referral rule for skin cancer," *British Journal of Dermatology*, vol. 150, no. 2, pp. 291–298, 2004.

[11] W. Dodds, M. Morgan, C. Wolfe, and K. S. Raju, "Implementing the 2-week wait rule for cancer referral in the UK: general practitioners' views and practices," *European Journal of Cancer Care*, vol. 13, no. 1, pp. 82–87, 2004.

[12] P. H. Youl, P. D. Baade, M. Janda, C. B. Del Mar, D. C. Whiteman, and J. F. Aitken, "Diagnosing skin cancer in primary care: how do mainstream general practitioners compare with primary care skin cancer clinic doctors?" *Medical Journal of Australia*, vol. 187, no. 4, pp. 215–220, 2007.

[13] P. Carli, V. De Giorgi, E. Crocetti, L. Caldini, C. Ressel, and B. Giannotti, "Diagnostic and referral accuracy of family doctors in melanoma screening: effect of a short formal training," *European Journal of Cancer Prevention*, vol. 14, no. 1, pp. 51–55, 2005.

[14] Z. Shariff, A. Roshan, A. M. Williams, and A. J. Platt, "2-Week wait referrals in suspected skin cancer: does an instructional module for general practitioners improve diagnostic accuracy?" *Surgeon*, vol. 8, no. 5, pp. 247–251, 2010.

[15] E. Linos, S. M. Swetter, M. G. Cockburn, G. A. Colditz, and C. A. Clarke, "Increasing burden of melanoma in the United States," *Journal of Investigative Dermatology*, vol. 129, no. 7, pp. 1666–1674, 2009.

[16] R. B. Aldridge, L. Naysmith, E. T. Ooi, C. S. Murray, and J. L. Rees, "The importance of a full clinical examination: assessment of index lesions referred to a skin cancer clinic without a total body skin examination would miss one in three melanomas," *Acta Dermato-Venereologica*, vol. 93, no. 6, pp. 689–692, 2013.

[17] M. C. J. van Rijsingen, S. C. A. Hanssen, J. M. M. Groenewoud, G. J. van der Wilt, and M.-J. P. Gerritsen, "Referrals by general practitioners for suspicious skin lesions: the urgency of training," *Acta Dermato-Venereologica*, vol. 94, no. 2, pp. 138–141, 2014.

19

Investing in a Surgical Outcomes Auditing System

Luis Bermudez, Kristen Trost, and Ruben Ayala

Research and Outcomes Department, Operation Smile, Inc., Norfolk, VA 23509, USA

Correspondence should be addressed to Kristen Trost; kristen.trost@gmail.com

Academic Editor: Nivaldo Alonso

Background. Humanitarian surgical organizations consider both quantity of patients receiving care and quality of the care provided as a measure of success. However, organizational efficacy is often judged by the percent of resources spent towards direct intervention/surgery, which may discourage investment in an outcomes monitoring system. Operation Smile's established Global Standards of Care mandate minimum patient followup and quality of care. *Purpose.* To determine whether investment of resources in an outcomes monitoring system is necessary and effectively measures success. *Methods.* This paper analyzes the quantity and completeness of data collected over the past four years and compares it against changes in personnel and resources assigned to the program. Operation Smile began investing in multiple resources to obtain the missing data necessary to potentially implement a global Surgical Outcomes Auditing System. Existing personnel resources were restructured to focus on postoperative program implementation, data acquisition and compilation, and training materials used to educate local foundation and international employees. *Results.* An increase in the number of postoperative forms and amount of data being submitted to headquarters occurred. *Conclusions.* Humanitarian surgical organizations would benefit from investment in a surgical outcomes monitoring system in order to demonstrate success and to ameliorate quality of care.

1. Introduction

A strong argument can be made that the success of humanitarian surgical organizations must consider both quantity of patients receiving care and the quality of the care provided. However, the efficacy of a nonprofit organization is often judged by asking what percentage of an organization's resources is spent towards direct intervention; in this case, the percentage that goes directly towards providing surgery. Such scrutiny might discourage humanitarian organizations from investing in adequate review of their outcomes, to the detriment of the patients being served. In order for surgical outcomes to be effectively monitored for both patient followup and measuring success, adequate resources need to be allotted towards the establishment of effective systems.

Operation Smile, an international medical nonprofit providing free surgical care for children with clefts, is striving towards measuring its success both by the quantity and quality of care it provides. In 2006, Operation Smile and representatives from its global medical community established the Global Standards of Care, mandating minimum requirements of practice across 14 aspects of care for cleft

lip and cleft palate patients. Global Standard 12, titled "Minimum Patient Follow-Up," states the following:

> *Effective post-operative care is essential for a good surgical result and effective planning for further treatment. Post-Operative care requires good documentation and extensive education of parents and clinicians to be effective. Post-Operative care from an Operation Smile organized team should review patients at the following intervals:*
>
> *12.1 One week post-surgery (4–7 days post-op). The goal is to recognize and manage immediate surgical complications.*
>
> *12.2 Six months–1 year. Team evaluation for documenting outcomes of surgeries and planning for future treatment [1].*

This global standard established Operation Smile's commitment to evaluate its success, not just by the number of surgeries provided, but the quality of care. A preliminary

Surgical Auditing System was pilot tested in 2008 to determine the effectiveness of evaluating the surgical outcomes of patients [2]. However, In order to implement a large-scale Surgical Outcomes Auditing System, Operation Smile has found that investing in the collection of postoperative data is imperative.

2. Measuring Successful Outcomes

Successful outcomes are often measured by the quantity of services provided to patients. However, the quality of the surgical outcomes should play an equal role in measuring the success of surgery. Good outcomes of primary surgeries reduce the cost spent on secondary revisions as well as ancillary services and procedures. In order to measure success in this manner, a method for evaluating surgical outcomes within a short and a long time frame would be necessary [3].

The widely accepted goal of cleft care is to return patients to a "normal" life with little to no handicaps associated with cleft lip and/or palate, or the surgical repair. However, measuring this success is often considered complex as it requires the consideration of numerous factors such as velopharyngeal function (speech) palate integrity (fistulas), nasolabial appearance, hearing capabilities, dentoskeletal development, quality of life, and the psychosocial adjustment of the patient. Final assessment of surgical outcomes in the areas of hearing, speech, and skeletal growth require a decent amount of time to pass after surgery. However, nasolabial appearance, facial symmetry, and fistula occurrence have been shown to be effective early measures of surgical outcomes [4–7].

3. Background

International humanitarian organizations implement a wide variety of medical mission models. Operation Smile's unique method of utilizing medical missions to build local sustainability has enabled the organization to move from having a mere presence in a country to establishing local foundations and support. There are two main mission methods implemented by Operation Smile. International missions are comprised of team members with at least 50% of volunteers from outside the country in which the mission is occurring and usually lasts 7–10 days, two days of screening, five surgical days, and three days for unpacking and packing of cargo. International missions can take place in both countries that do not have local foundations and countries that do have local foundations. Local missions are comprised of at least 50% local volunteers, volunteers from within the country the mission is occurring. Local missions can last for any length of time, usually between 3 and 10 days and are generally held in countries that have local foundations, which are independently run in-country Operation Smile organization that have the support of Operation Smile International. Occasionally, large unique international missions are implemented for unique projects such as the "World Journey of Smiles," which took place in 2007. The World Journey of Smiles was a culmination event for the organization's 25th Anniversary in which a large international mission was implemented.

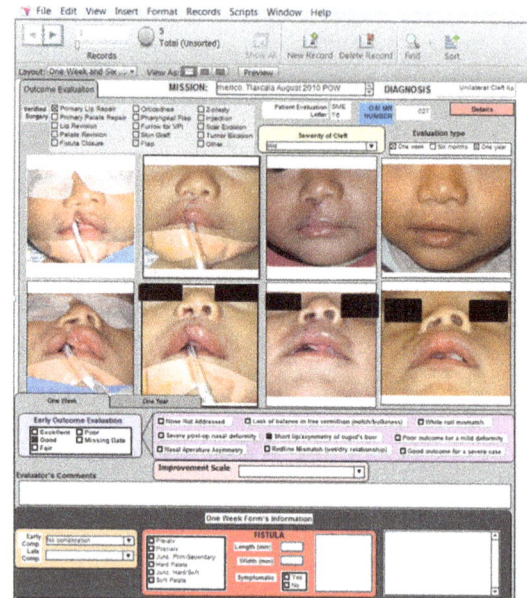

FIGURE 1

During Operation Smiles' "World Journey of Smiles" in 2007, a Surgical Outcomes Auditing System, using digital photography as media, was developed and pilot tested. Four thousand one hundred patients were operated on in 40 different sites, in 25 different countries over 10 days. During these missions, high-quality images were taken for each patient preoperatively and postoperatively. Postoperative evaluations were held one week after the mission and local foundations were encouraged to schedule six-month and one-year postoperative evaluations for patients. During these postoperative evaluations both standardized images as well as post-operative assessment data collected from PostOperative Exam Forms were collected. This data was then returned to Operation Smile Headquarters where six-month and one-year images were matched with patients' preoperative and immediate postoperative images. Standardized angles of the frontal and basal views as well as images of the hard and soft palates were cropped to protect patients' identities, focusing the reviewer on the surgical area, and to eliminate potential bias of the reviewer [8].

After compiling this data and deidentifying patient and surgeon information, the evaluations were sent to unbiased members of the International Outcomes Evaluation Council, a group of trained surgical evaluators, and utilizing a qualitative assessment system a surgical evaluation was completed for each procedure provided [2]. Figure 1 shows the final evaluations that were returned to surgeons in a confidential manner. The Regional Medical Officer, who provides medical oversight and leadership for any medical programs within their particular region, and the Medical Director, who is the medical leader for their particular foundation, also received these evaluations to spur further discussion of outcomes.

During the pilot test of the Surgical Outcomes Auditing System, a series of challenges were identified that needed to be overcome. The first and foremost was the need to socialize

Discrepancy between reported patient
numbers and submitted data

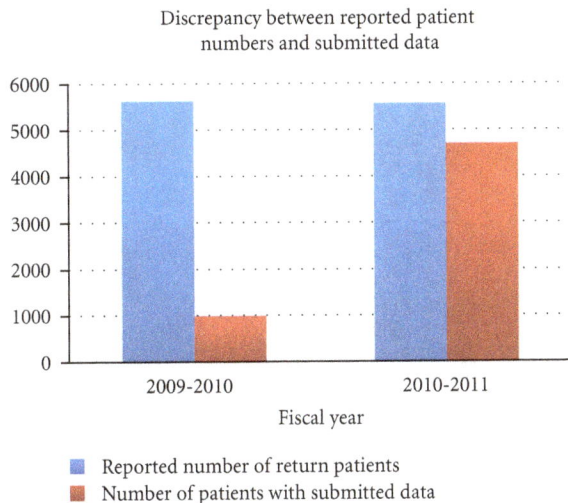

Figure 2

the concept of auditing the results of surgical procedures and the impact it would have on the mission process. It has taken time and the constant education of medical team members to understand new procedures.

After addressing the challenges associated with the capturing of images, the next challenge to overcome was the quality of the photographic data. At the onset, untrained photographers were being used to collect patient images. With little training in the appropriate image capturing techniques and a thorough understanding of the angles needed, the quality of data obtained was of unusable quality.

Once the challenges of acceptance of auditing surgical outcomes and the need for quality trained patient imaging technicians to capture quality standardized images were overcome, the next challenge to overcome was obtaining and analyzing data collected during missions and during postoperative examinations.

4. Method

After the world Journey of Smiles completed in 2007, the postoperative program began to be regularly implemented. Unfortunately, not all of the data from missions were being returned to headquarters. Figure 2 shows the reported number of patients returning for postoperative examinations in comparison with the data returned to headquarters for these patients.

Recognizing the discrepancy between the number of patients attending post-op and the amount of data received, Operation Smile began investing in multiple resources to obtain the missing data necessary to potentially implement a global Surgical Outcomes Auditing System. Existing personnel resources were restructured to focus on post-op program implementation and data acquisition and compilation. Employees responsible for collecting form data and patient image data went from being members of separate teams within different departments to being on the same team within the same department. This enabled team members to

more effectively identify which missions were missing data and initiate the process for obtaining that data.

As part of this restructuring, personnel began increasing the amount of direct contact with local foundations by phone and e-mail to request the submission of postoperative forms and patient images that had not been submitted to headquarters. Training materials used by these team members to educate local foundation employees and international employees were reorganized to focus more on how to implement properly the postoperative program and to submit data rather than concentrating on how the Surgical Outcomes Auditing System would work.

Complete data sets, including both patient images and postoperative information, were also not being received from countries in which more local missions were occurring. An Outcome Data Coordinator role was developed to increase the quality and quantity of data return from countries that implemented more locally run missions. Outcomes Data Coordinators became responsible for training local volunteers in the image and form collections process as well as being responsible for collecting, compiling, and submitting this data to headquarters.

Foreseeing the need to compile the incoming postoperative data and patient images with minimal employee resources, a data entry intern program was established to deal with data compilation. An internship description was created and posted on the headquarters career website. Applicants with interests in medical, nonprofit, or data entry experience were considered and accepted for positions.

To address the increase in one-week postoperative data and the reporting of early complications such as infection and dehiscence, an Early Outcomes Monitoring System was established to identify surgeons with outlying complication rates. Figure 3 shows an anterior fistula after a cleft palate repair. In the immediate postoperative picture, we can see the presence of a fistula, which was a result of the surgical technique as oral flaps were not designed to achieve complete closure of the anterior palate. Because pictures are taken immediately after surgery, it is often possible to identify the cause of the complication as we can see in Figure 3. These images make it easier to address the complication sooner.

Recognizing that such complications could be detected earlier, surgical information and postoperative data were combined in an Access database comprised of over 12,000 surgeries with data from the one-week postoperative evaluations of patients operated on by over 400 surgeons. This database enables Operation Smile to monitor the more immediate postoperative complications by surgeon, mission site, and country. While no acceptable complication rate should ever exist, a high variation of complication rates has been reported from other organizations and studies, between 0% and 33% [9–13].

Operation Smile uses these rates as markers to identify surgeons who have outlying complications rates both high and low. When a surgeon is identified as having an outlying complication rate, one that does not fall within the aforementioned range, Operation Smile's Surgical Council receives a report for this surgeon. The report contains

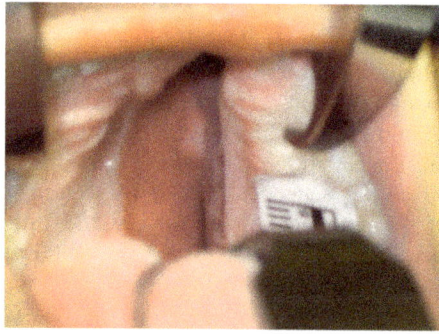

(a) Preoperative picture of the anterior part of a cleft palate

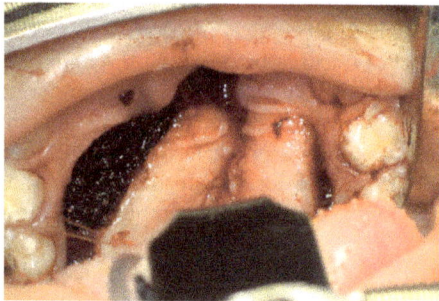

(b) Immediate postoperative picture

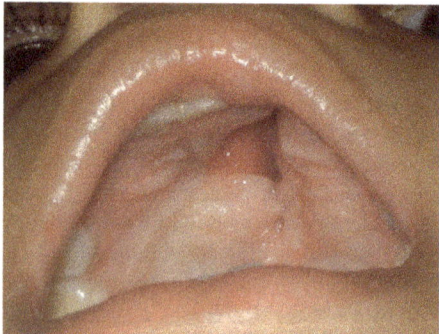

(c) Postoperative picture taken 11 months after surgical repair

FIGURE 3: Clinical Case 1.

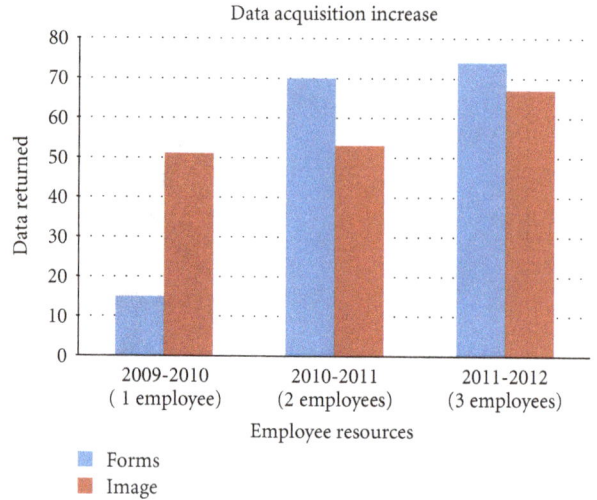

FIGURE 4

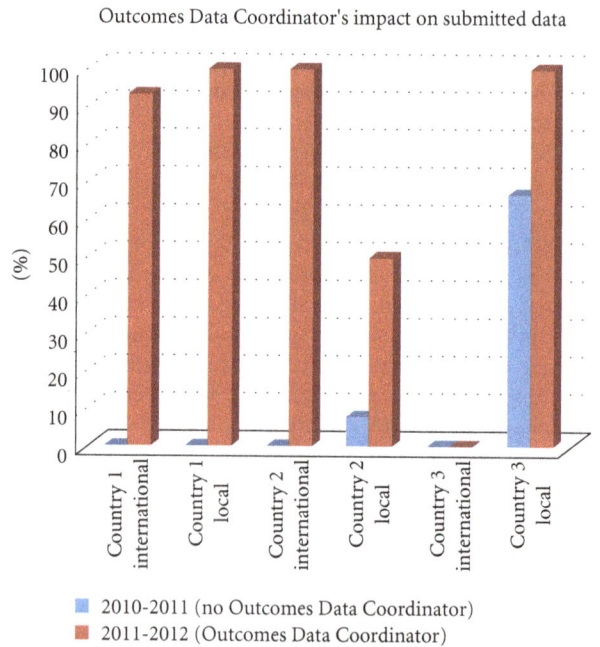

FIGURE 5

information on the cases identified as having complication along with all of the outcomes evaluations on file for the surgeon. This complete report and their surgical cases are then reviewed. The goal is to review and to help in the education of these surgeons, pairing them with mentors and working to enhance their skills.

5. Results

After making direct requests of foundations for specific missing data, an increase in the number of postoperative forms as well as images submitted to headquarters was demonstrated, as seen in Figure 4.

Figure 5, demonstrates the increase in complete data sets submitted to Operation Smile headquarters for both local and international missions by Outcomes Data Coordinators.

As the amount of data being submitted to headquarters increased, the capacity to compile that data was reaching its threshold. Figure 6 shows that by increasing the number of interns more data could be compiled.

6. Discussion

Good surgical outcomes are part of Operation Smile's commitment to the patients receiving surgery during its medical missions and at its cleft care centers. In order to meet this commitment and continue to address the surgical needs of children with cleft lip and palate, implementation of a Surgical Outcomes Auditing System has been initiated. Many

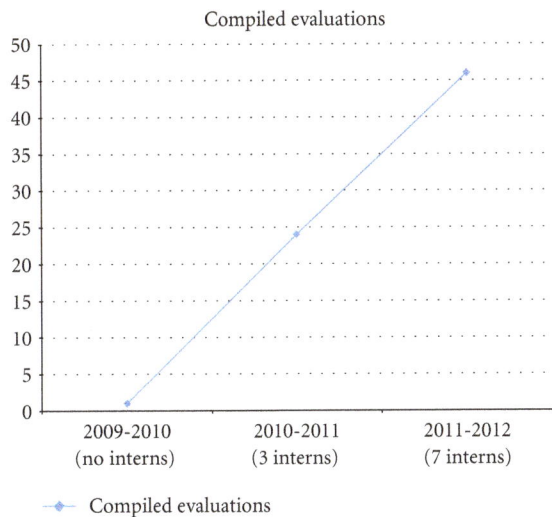

Compiled evaluations

FIGURE 6

7. Conclusion

Operation Smile's investment in resources significantly increased both the amount of data received and the data compiled from both local and international missions. As local foundations become more and more accustomed to the implementation of the postoperative program as well as the submission of data to headquarters, the more realistic the implementation of a Global Surgical Outcomes Auditing System becomes. However, if Operation Smile is to be successful in obtaining its goal to return patients to a normal life, it cannot limit itself to simply evaluating the visual outcomes of the surgeries they perform.

Visual outcomes are only some aspects of evaluation that can be used to measure the success of surgical procedures. Speech evaluations can provide further insight into the success of surgeries provided. A perceptual evaluation system has attempted to be implemented in Spanish speaking countries, but the major obstacle is defining what parameters need to be evaluated and how these parameters can be evaluated in order to achieve a good interobserver reliability [14]. Form and functionality is a large portion of returning patients to a "normal life" but it is also very important to determine how well patients are reintegrated into their communities and how they are managing these psychosocial changes.

As Operation Smile moves forward in the development and implementation of a Global Surgical Auditing System, many other outcomes areas can and should still be measured. With its ever growing global impact through the increasing number of surgeries provided annually, Operation Smile is leading the way in working to ensure that the surgeries they provide are of the best quality.

challenges have played a role in the development and implementation of a global Surgical Outcomes Auditing System, the most impactful of these challenges has been obtaining the necessary data. Recognizing this need, Operation Smile invested in resources to collect and compile the data needed for these evaluations. Through the restructuring and reorganizing of existing personnel, a more cohesive understanding of the specific data needed was gained. This understanding facilitated the direct request of missing postoperative forms and patient images. Figure 2 shows that the investment in personnel resources resulted in an increase of both postoperative data and patient images being returned to headquarters. Initial data collected was primarily images. Restructuring allowed for more focus on collecting missing data from specific missions. This focus brought an increase in the number of postoperative forms submitted to headquarters. Adding a third employee allowed for more direct contact with local foundations and the ability to request more images as well as postoperative forms, resulting in a further increase in data submitted.

Another area of focus was on the three countries where high-volume of surgeries were being provided but no data was being received. After the establishment of the Outcomes Data Coordinator position in these three target countries, the percentage of not only data, but complete data sets comprised of patient images and patient information, increased drastically. Countries 2 and 3 increased the amount of international data submitted from less than 50% to 100% and Countries 1 and 3 increased submitted local mission data to 100%.

Creating a data entry internship program preemptively addressed the challenge of insufficient personnel resources to compile the increase of complete data being submitted to headquarters. As more data arrived due to direct contact and the implementation of the Outcomes Data Coordinator role, more personnel power was needed to compile data into the evaluation templates. Figure 5 demonstrates that as the number of interns doubled so did the amount of compiled evaluations.

References

[1] Operation Smile, "Global standards of care," Operation Smile Inc., 2010, http://www.operationsmile.org/our_work/global-standards-of-care/14-global-standards-of-care.html.

[2] L. Bermudez, V. Carter, W. Magee, R. Sherman, and R. Ayala, "Surgical outcomes auditing systems in humanitarian organizations," *World Journal of Surgery*, vol. 34, no. 3, pp. 403–410, 2010.

[3] L. Bermudez and A. K. Lizarraga, "Operation smile: How to measure its success," *Annals of Plastic Surgery*, vol. 67, no. 3, pp. 205–208, 2012.

[4] V. Brattström, K. Mølsted, B. Prahl-Andersen, G. Semb, and W. C. Shaw, "The Eurocleft study: intercenter study of treatment outcome in patients with complete cleft lip and palate. Part 2: craniofacial form and nasolabial appearance," *Cleft Palate-Craniofacial Journal*, vol. 42, no. 1, pp. 69–77, 2005.

[5] B. A. Coghlan, B. Matthews, and R. W. Pigott, "A computer-based method of measuring facial asymmetry. Results from an assessment of the repair of cleft lip deformities," *British Journal of Plastic Surgery*, vol. 40, no. 4, pp. 371–376, 1987.

[6] S. Kyrkanides, R. Bellohusen, and J. D. Subtelny, "Asymmetries of the upper lip and nose in noncleft and postsurgical unilateral cleft lip and palate individuals," *Cleft Palate-Craniofacial Journal*, vol. 33, no. 4, pp. 306–311, 1996.

[7] K. J. Feragen, G. Semb, and S. Magnussen, "Asymmetry of left versus right unilateral cleft impairments: an experimental study of face perception," *Cleft Palate-Craniofacial Journal*, vol. 36, no. 6, pp. 527–532, 1999.

[8] C. Asher-McDade, C. Roberts, W. C. Shaw, and C. Gallager, "Development of a method for rating nasolabial appearance in patients with clefts of the lip and palate," *Cleft Palate-Craniofacial Journal*, vol. 28, pp. 385–390, 1991.

[9] A. G. A. Assunção, M. A. F. Pinto, S. P. de Barros Almeida Peres, and M. T. Cazal Tristão, "Immediate postoperative evaluation of the surgical wound and nutritional evolution after cheiloplasty," *Cleft Palate-Craniofacial Journal*, vol. 42, no. 4, pp. 434–438, 2005.

[10] S. R. Cohen, J. Kalinowski, D. LaRossa, and P. Randall, "Cleft palate fistulas: a multivariate statistical analysis of prevalence, etiology, and surgical management," *Plastic and Reconstructive Surgery*, vol. 87, no. 6, pp. 1041–1047, 1991.

[11] A. R. Muzaffar, H. S. Byrd, R. J. Rohrich et al., "Incidence of cleft palate fistula: an institutional experience with two-stage palatal repair," *Plastic and Reconstructive Surgery*, vol. 108, no. 6, pp. 1515–1518, 2001.

[12] R. E. Emory, R. P. Clay, U. Bite, and L. T. Jackson, "Fistula formation and repair after palatal closure: an institutional perspective," *Plastic and Reconstructive Surgery*, vol. 99, no. 6, pp. 1535–1538, 1997.

[13] R. A. Hopper, C. Lewis, R. Umbdenstock, M. M. Garrison, and J. R. Starr, "Discharge practices, readmission, and serious medical complications following primary cleft lip repair in 23 U.S. children's hospitals," *Plastic and Reconstructive Surgery*, vol. 123, no. 5, pp. 1553–1559, 2009.

[14] M. Cleves, M. Hanayama, M. C. Tavera et al., "Reliability of the perceptual evaluation of MP3 speech samples," in *Proceedings of the 11th International Congress on Cleft Lip and Palate and Related Craniofacial Anomalies*, Fortaleza, Brazil, 2009.

20

One-Stop Clinic Utilization in Plastic Surgery: Our Local Experience and the Results of a UK-Wide National Survey

Mark Gorman,[1] James Coelho,[2] Sameer Gujral,[2] and Alastair McKay[3]

[1]Castle Hill Plastic Surgery Unit, Hull HU16 5JQ, UK
[2]Department of Plastic Surgery, Royal Devon and Exeter Hospital, UK
[3]Canniesburn Plastic Surgery Unit, Glasgow, UK

Correspondence should be addressed to Mark Gorman; m.gorman@me.com

Academic Editor: Georg M. Huemer

Introduction. "See and treat" one-stop clinics (OSCs) are an advocated NHS initiative to modernise care, reducing cancer treatment waiting times. Little studied in plastic surgery, the existing evidence suggests that though they improve care, they are rarely implemented. We present our experience setting up a plastic surgery OSC for minor skin surgery and survey their use across the UK. *Methods.* The OSC was evaluated by 18-week wait target compliance, measures of departmental capacity, and patient satisfaction. Data was obtained from 32 of the 47 UK plastic surgery departments to investigate the prevalence of OSCs for minor skin cancer surgery. *Results.* The OSC improved 18-week waiting times, from a noncompliant mean of 80% to a compliant 95% average. Department capacity increased 15%. 95% of patients were highly satisfied with and preferred the OSC to a conventional service. Only 25% of UK plastic surgery units run OSCs, offering varying reasons for not doing so, 42% having not considered their use. *Conclusions.* OSCs are underutilised within UK plastic surgery, where a significant proportion of units have not even considered their benefit. This is despite associated improvements in waiting times, department capacity, and levels of high patient satisfaction. We offer our considerations and local experience instituting an OSC service.

1. Introduction

Dating back to the mid-1990s, plastic surgery units have reported issues dealing with growing number of patient referrals in a timely fashion. A significant burden is the diagnosis and treatment of outpatient skin cancer [1, 2]. An internal 2010 audit at the Castle Hill regional UK Plastic Surgery Department identified such a problem, with a failure to manage patient referrals within agreed government time frames. National health care systems employ different waiting time targets. In the UK, it is a legal patient right to receive care (be it surgery or a decision towards conservative management) within 18 weeks of being referred [3, 4]. When struggling to meet the 18-week wait target (18 ww) one strategy has been to streamline care through "see and treat" one-stop clinics (OSCs) [5]. Within UK plastic surgery, the institution of OSCs has been advocated by the National Institute for Health Care and Excellence and the British Association of Plastic Surgery. It was felt to be key to the Department of Health's

modernisation strategies ("action on plastic surgery") [2, 3, 6]. A thorough Medline search indicates that despite such support and evidence of improved service (e.g., cost savings and patient satisfaction) when instituted, OSCs seem to be rarely implemented within plastic surgery [1, 2, 7]. The reasons for this and actual uptake levels across the UK are however unknown. To address these questions, the aims of this study were to conduct a nationwide survey of plastic surgery OSC utilisation and present our local experience setting up an OSC to manage minor outpatient skin cancer surgery. Alongside the primary outcome measure, 18 ww performance, patient satisfaction was also surveyed.

In relation to cancer, the importance of markers such as the 18 ww relates to evidence spanning the surgical specialities (including head and neck, general, breast, gynaecology, and skin/dermatology) indicating that rapid access to diagnosis and treatment decreases patient anxiety and has been associated with improved survival outcomes [8–13]. Previous studies, when measuring waiting time performance in relation to OSCs, have not done so against nationally agreed benchmarks, and whilst believing this is important, we acknowledge the 18 ww to be just one of the many targets instituted by regulatory bodies to promote shorter waiting times and that such thresholds will inevitably change over time [14]. Based upon work by the Cancer Service Collaborative "Improvement Partnership" (CSCIP 2006), surgical departments in the UK should see and treat ≥ 90% of outpatients (≥95% for inpatients) within the 18 ww [14]. The 10% leeway makes allowance for more complex or unforeseen patient scenarios, such that a service operating in a healthy fashion should have the capacity to see and treat the vast majority of patients in the first few weeks, not spread over the 18 ww pathway [15]. Plotted on a graph, an 18 ww curve should thus be shaped like a ski slope (Figure 1(a)) as opposed to a wide spread or bimodal pattern of distribution (Figures 1(b) and 1(c)) [16, 17]. Such patterns, alongside 18 ww target compliance, may aid the assessment of how a department is functioning (further explanation in Figure 1 caption).

Given that a successful OSC delivers care in one clinical session, that before required two or more, an obvious question is why they are not more routinely employed. The answer within UK plastic surgery is unknown and as mentioned before forms part of our motivation to survey OSCs nationwide. It may be that an absence of "lean thinking" elsewhere, as advocated by the NHS and adopted within our department (when planning and conceiving an OSC), may lead to OSCs not being considered or being incorrectly ruled out [18]. Derived from the automotive industry, "lean thinking" is a management philosophy that aims to improve quality by reducing waste and facilitating flow in care processes [19]. Key to its success in healthcare is an open relationship between department managers and senior clinicians, where it is important that senior clinical staff take a leadership role. All staff, especially frontline workers, should be consulted to help map out "current state" processes and identify waste/rate limiting steps in departmental care pathways [20]. Clear outcome measures must be employed to develop and track interventions (i.e., the 18 ww and validated measures of patient satisfaction) [21].

Organisation and Institution of the OSC. The OSC was started in August 2011. An unused clinic space was transformed into an operating room, with adjoining waiting, consultation, and postoperative recovery rooms (Figure 2). The original intention was to conduct five OSCs per week (replacing standard outpatient clinics). The average number was ultimately closer to three per week, operating on as intended a mean average of 6 patients per clinic (clinic duration is three hours).

After referrals were cherry-picked (choosing those most likely to require surgical intervention) by the OSCs respective consultant lead, patients were sent an appointment letter informing them about the possibility of immediate surgery. Patients could alter their appointment date (the NHS choose and book system) to decrease the probability of nonattendance [22].

The layout of the OSC is shown in Figure 2. After assessment by the consultant, if appropriate for surgery (criteria suitable for OSC surgery include skin lesions that once excised would require direct closure, small skin grafts, or simple local flaps; more complicated reconstructions requiring >30 minutes of operating time were not suitable; patients' anticoagulation status was considered on a case by case basis, with an instant skin prick INR test available for those on warfarin (INR < 2.5 preferred)), the patient was admitted and then taken either directly through to the operating room or for a short wait back to the waiting room whilst concurrent procedures finish. The consultant was on hand to assist the operating surgeon (senior house officer or registrar) with marking lesions and advice if required.

Postsurgery patients were taken into an adjoining postoperative space and given instructions by the nursing staff, whilst the next patient was prepped in the operating room. This arrangement minimised time delay. The clinics were staffed by one front desk administrative worker, one consultant, one operating surgeon (senior house officer or registrar), and two nursing staffs. Nursing staff retraining or reallocation (dependent on prior experience) was required to perform roles in the OSC such as circulating and assisting in the operative theatre. The grade and numbers of staff matched those of previous non-OSC clinics and thus, apart from the initial installation to equip the outpatient operating room, the OSC ran without a need to significantly alter resources or staffing.

2. Methods

The patient satisfaction questionnaire and OSC UK survey required local hospital board certification and the experimental methods observed the ethical principles of the Declaration of Helsinki.

2.1. OSC 18-Week Wait Performance and Measures of Departmental Capacity. With established data indicating the unit was struggling with 18 ww compliance, a further one-year analysis (May 2010 to April 2011) of departmental 18 ww performance was undertaken (18 ww referring to the interval between initial patient referral, usually from their family doctor to definitive care). The review commenced four months prior to and continued seven months after the OSCs institution. Additional associated measures of departmental capacity were also recorded, including the weekly totals of patients added to waiting lists.

2.2. Patient Satisfaction Survey. The patient satisfaction survey employed was adapted and validated by Javaid et al. when presenting their 2005 experience instituting a plastic surgery OSC (questions derived from the Newcastle Satisfaction with Nursing Scale) [2, 23]. A random sample of 200 patients was surveyed (from December 2010 to March 2011) at their two-month post-op follow-up visit, divided evenly between those receiving treatment in OSC and those treated in the conventional care pathway (100 OSC and 100 non-OSC conventional pathways). Patient consent was gained at the beginning of clinic, and the self-reported satisfaction survey completed at the end. The survey included four questions, using a 1–10 Likert scale (10 representing the highest degree of satisfaction), enquiring about patient's satisfaction with

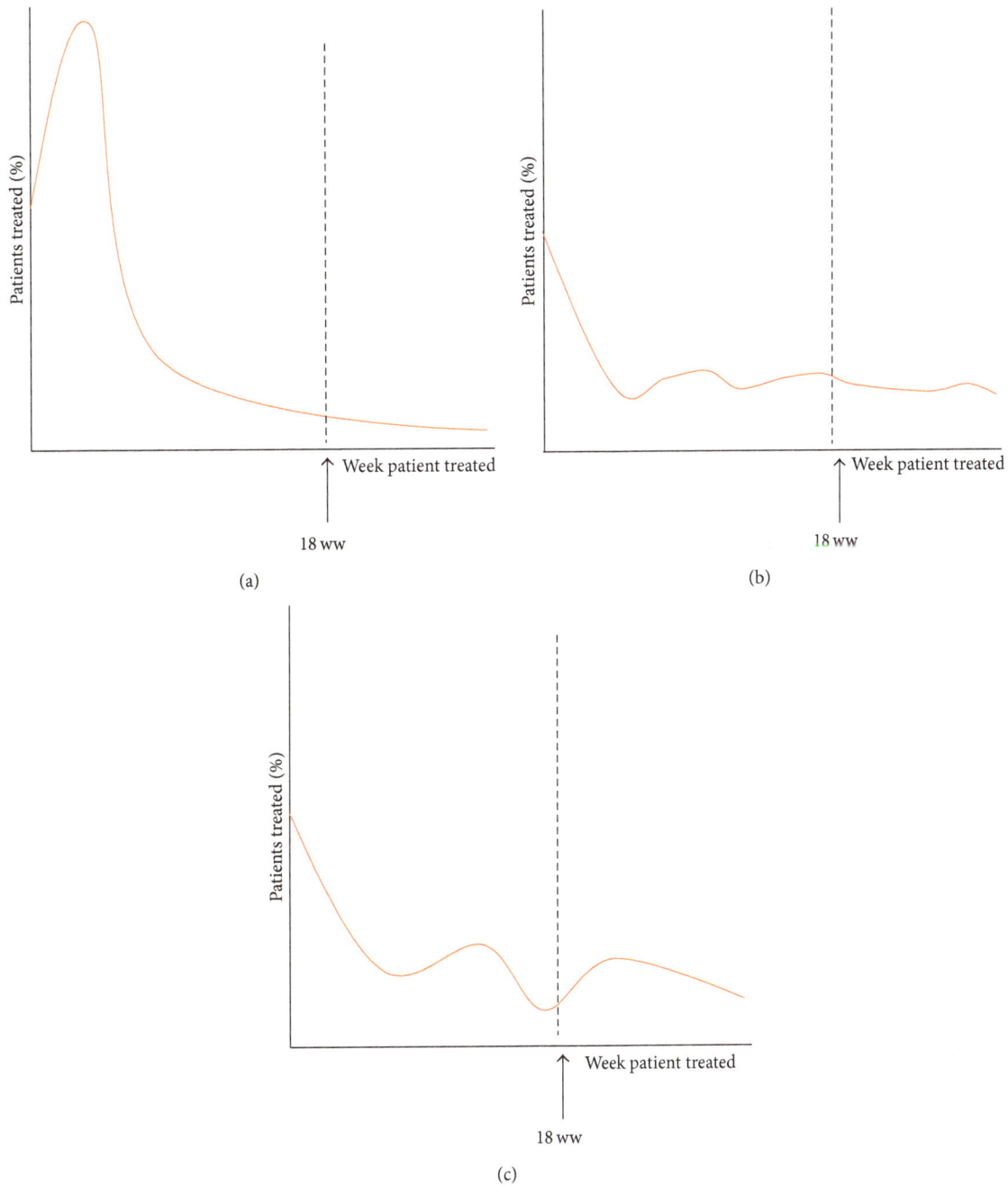

FIGURE 1: Three illustrative figures reflecting how effectively a department delivers care in relation to the 18 ww pathway. The first graph: (a) depicts an ideal negative "ski slope" shape curve, where the majority of referrals are seen and treated at the beginning of the pathway, implying that a department has adequate resource to cope with demand. This is opposed to a wider distribution in (b) or bimodal pattern in (c), with peaks at either side of the 18 ww threshold (or target) implying an unsuccessful attempt to rush through patients at the end of the pathway in order to meet target compliance (avoiding fines imposed by the NHS) rather than improve patient care, as is intended by the 18 ww. *(a) Ideal "ski slope" curve. (b) Wider distribution, and (c) bimodal pattern implying a struggle to meet the demand of referrals.*

consultation, treatment in operation room, the quality/clarity of discharge instructions, and overall ratings of the service.

2.3. UK Survey of Plastic Surgery OSC Utilisation. A list of all adult plastic surgery units in the UK was obtained from the British Association of Plastic, Reconstructive and Aesthetic Surgeons website. A structured telephone interview was conducted with consultants, administration staff, or operational managers. The protocol involved an introductory email followed by two follow-up phone calls with a week's interval. Questions posed included whether the unit offered a "one-stop" or "see and treat" clinic facility. If yes, then what was that unit's experience of it and, if no, was there a reason why not?

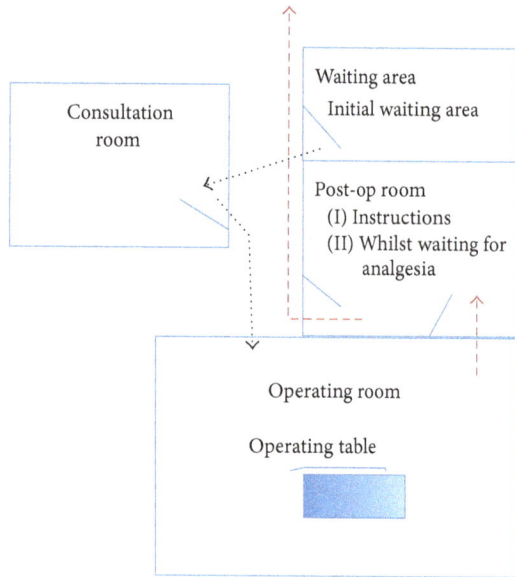

FIGURE 2: Layout and patient flow and though see the one-stop clinic.

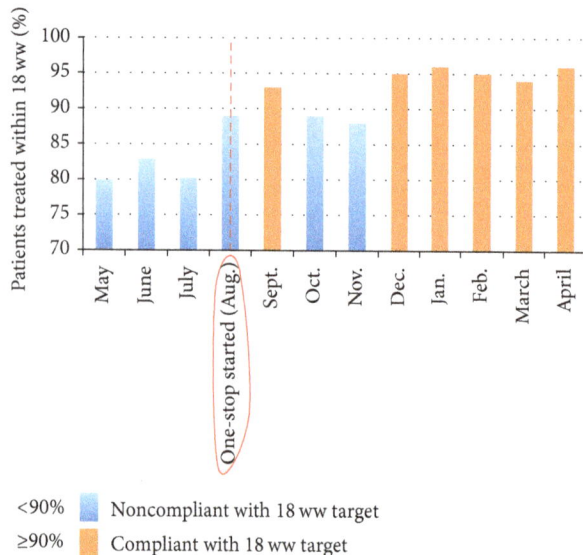

FIGURE 3: 18-week wait compliance before and after institution of the one-stop clinic for minor skin cancer surgery, compliant months (>95%) in orange.

3. Results

3.1. OSC 18-Week Wait Performance and Measures of Departmental Capacity. 18 ww performance improved from a noncompliant pre-OSC mean average of 80% to a compliant mean average of 95% after OSC (compliance ≥ 90% Figure 3). Despite improvement, compliance was however narrowly missed in the months of October and November, when the clinic was first started (88 and 87%, resp.). This was due to improvements required in patient selection (i.e., selecting those more likely to require biopsy) and the fact that the number of OSCs operating per week increased over the first

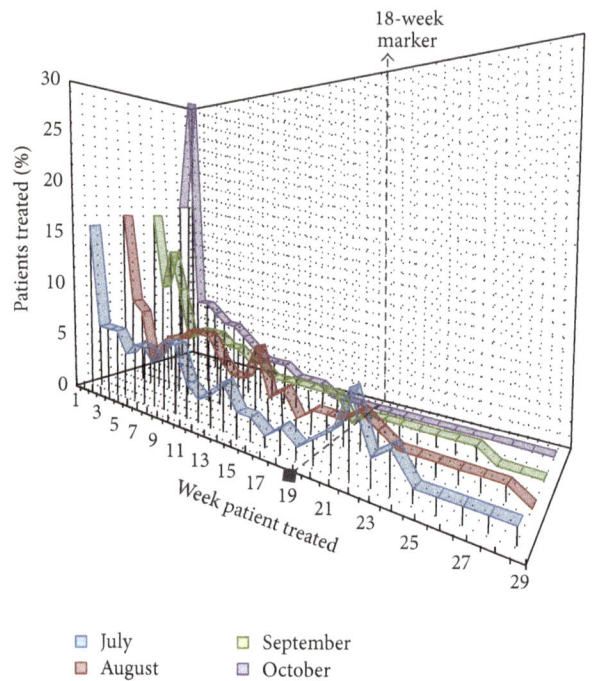

FIGURE 4: Four-month comparison of 18 ww performance, as a percentage distribution pattern of the week patients received treatment after initial referral. The 18 ww threshold is marked as a vertical black dotted line. The comparison commences one month prior to the OSCs institution in August. This figure relates to Figure 1, which provides exemplars to translate changing distributions.

few months. Compliance was consistently achieved after this initial period.

The improvement in 18-week wait compliance was associated with improved measures of department capacity. This can be first illustrated by the changing distribution patterns, regarding which week patients received treatment after referral to the unit. Figure 4 shows a four-month snap shot, illustrating a trend towards a leftward shift of the weekly distribution (after institution of the OSC) indicating that patients received care more consistently in the first few weeks of the 18 ww pathway, as opposed to later, or even after the 18-week threshold. The distribution changes from a wider bimodal (see Figure 1 for further explanation) distribution to the ideal negative ski slope distribution. Note that patients are treated at week "zero" or one, due to a prior backlog, the shortest realistic referral-treatment window being approximately two weeks.

By measuring the number of patients added to departmental waiting lists each week, it was also possible to quantify the number of operating slots that were made available due to the OSC. Figure 5 shows that after the OSC was introduced (~week 40), the median number of additions to the waiting list dropped by approximately 18 patients per week. This means that 18 patients per week were being treated in the OSC that would have normally been added to the standard care pathway waiting list. This translates to the department having an increased capacity of approximately 15% or 72 minor procedural operating slots per month.

TABLE 1: Patients' views on the quality of service in one-stop clinics versus those treated within the standard care pathway[*].

| | Patients who gave a score of 7 or higher | |
Aspect of care	One-stop clinic	Standard pathway
Satisfaction with consultation	85%	70%
Treatment in operation room	82%	72%
Quality and clarity of discharge instructions	80%	64%
Overall rating of quality of service	95%	72%

[*]10 point likert scale (10 best) self-reported survey.

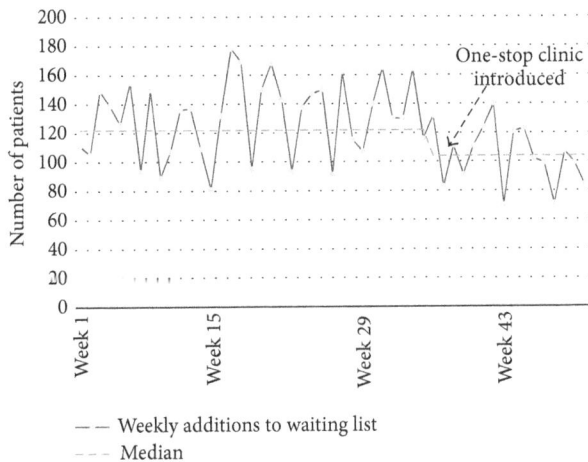

— — Weekly additions to waiting list
- - - Median

FIGURE 5: One-year review of 18 ww performance, showing the number of patients added to the departments' waiting list each week, the median trend represented by the orange dotted line, and weekly fluctuation in purple. The lower the number, the better the performance as patients are being treated in the OSC such that they are not added to the normal waiting list (i.e., standard non-OSC care pathway).

3.2. Patient Satisfaction Survey Results. As patients completed the questionnaire in clinic, the response rate was 100%. 95% of the respondents expressed a high degree of satisfaction (score ≥7, scale 1–10) regarding their overall experience of the OSC, compared with 72% for the conventional pathway. A summary of the results comparing the OSC and conventional pathway is presented in Table 1.

3.3. UK Survey of Plastic Surgery Unit One-Stop Clinic Utilisation. The survey response rate was 68%, data obtained from 32 of the 47 units in the UK (Figure 6).

25% of UK units operate one-stop services for skin cancer; of those who did not, 42% offered no reason, 29% offered alternative services (such as outpatient local anaesthetic lists performed by nurse specialists or combined skin cancer clinics with dermatology), 13% associated the use of such clinics with other specialties, 8% stated they had inadequate facilities, and 8% stated they were developing a one-stop clinic model.

4. Discussion

With the advent of the OSC, waiting times in our department decreased and its 18 ww performance improved from a noncompliant pre-OSC mean average of 80% to a compliant mean average of 95% (target compliance 90%). The department's capacity increased by approximately 15%, equating to 72 minor procedural slots per month. With increased capacity, in addition to becoming target compliant, the unit was also able to respond to the 18 ww in the manner in which the target intends, such that the vast majority of patients were treated in the first few weeks of the pathway instead of later, at the end, or even beyond the 18 ww threshold.

Regarding the UK survey, we obtained responses from 32 (68%) of the 47 UK plastic surgery units. Reviews rationalising the adequacy of survey response rates have concluded that when an entire cohort of interest is surveyed (as opposed to a representative sample), a response rate of one-third is acceptable and two-thirds considered robust [24]. With a respondent rate exceeding two-thirds, we can extrapolate from our survey with confidence, accepting that a degree of responder bias cannot be ruled out (i.e., that respondents may have had a greater or lesser tendency, e.g., to employ OSCs in their units). As was guessed from the paucity of examples in the literature, only 25% of plastic surgery units offered an OSC service. Of the proportion that did not, almost half (42%) had not considered OSCs. This may be, as was our presurvey suspicion, due to a lack of "lean" type managerial thinking principles being employed within those units. Of those that had considered but still did not offer OSCs, half implemented "alternative solutions." Most commonly, this was in the form of surgical nurse practitioner (SNP) led minor skin surgery lists. Otherwise, two units felt they had inadequate facilities, two were working towards an OSC, and three felt the service was already covered by another speciality. The reasons for offering SNP led lists included cost savings (SNP's salary versus a junior surgeon's) and that it maintained staffing continuity. There is little in the literature specific to plastic surgery, but both benefits have been shown with cardiac surgery SNPs [25]. The potential cost savings of SNPs are not well quantified and there have been no comparisons conducted between OSC and SNP led minor skin surgery services. Given that the units that ran SNP plastic surgery lists maintained the routine non-OSC pathway, requiring a minimum of two hospital visits, the other associated benefits of an OSC service are lost. A critique of nurse practitioner led service delivery is that it can lead to junior doctor's roles and learning opportunities being displaced [26]. Given that junior doctors felt that the OSC represents a particularly good training experience, both in our department *and* as cited by previous plastic surgery OSC studies [1, 2], this would be important to consider if SNPs were incorporated into the planning of a new OSC.

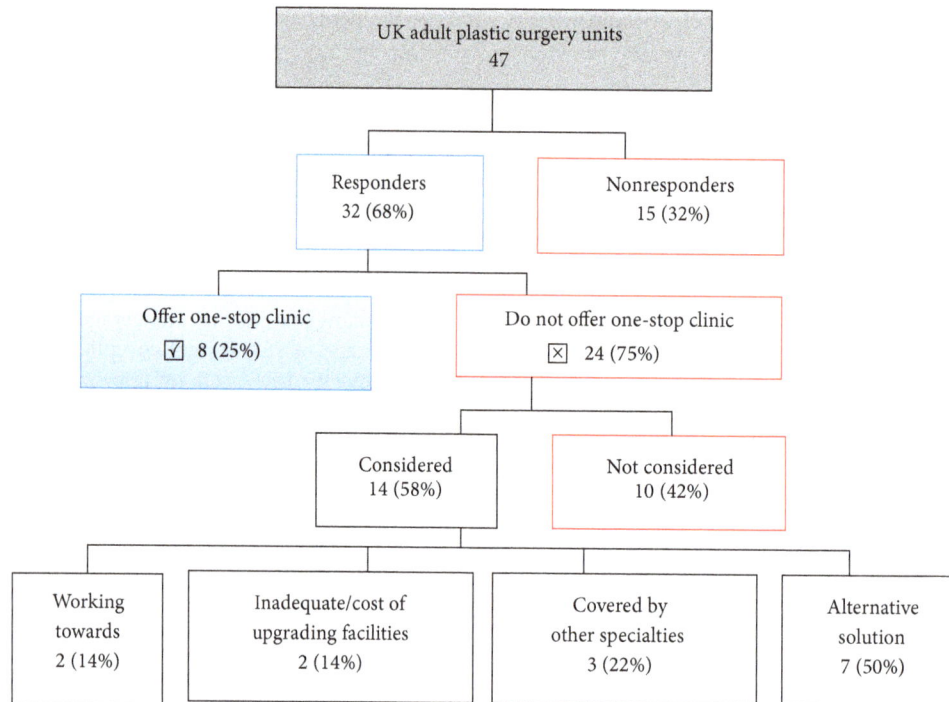

FIGURE 6: A survey of UK plastic surgery departments' utilisation of one-stop minor surgery skin cancer clinics.

Our patient satisfaction questionnaire indicated that patients preferred the OSC compared with the non-OSC service (95% versus 72%). The levels of high satisfaction (≥7 out of 10) were similar to those reported by Javaid et al., in their 2005 plastic surgery OSC experience (93%), though their study did not include a comparison with their local non-OSC service. In our study, in keeping with feelings towards the overall service, patients reported higher satisfaction regarding their OSC consultation, treatment in the operating room, and discharge instructions. The reasons given (free text box questionnaire answers) were that the OSC was more convenient and caused less frustration, anxiety, and general life disruption. Similar feelings have been cited previously regarding OSC experiences in plastic surgery and other surgical specialities [2, 9, 11, 27]. It is likely that patients perceptions of the OSC were not only due to fewer hospital visits, but also as a result of the streamlined, simplified perioperative delivery of care when compared with the standard pathway. Successful examples of this in OSCs have been previously evidenced in an array of conditions (additional to the management of minor skin cancer surgery) treated by plastic surgery, including carpal tunnel syndrome, Dupuytren's contracture, and head and neck and breast cancer [10, 12, 13, 28–30]. In these examples, service adaptations included the use of portable nerve conduction studies for one-stop carpal tunnel clinics (testing carried out by the plastic surgeons as opposed to separate patient visits by neurophysiologists), procedures being carried out under local rather than general anaesthetic and modification to histopathology tests/protocols to reduce the diagnostic turnaround from weeks to hours.

Elements of patients' satisfaction with the OSC, such as patient consultations, were likely to have been influenced by factors not elicited or enquired about explicitly by the survey. For example, it is a reasonable inference that patients may have had more confidence in their OSC consultations due to them being exclusively undertaken by consultants, compared with conventional clinics, staffed by a mixture of junior and senior doctors. A general limitation of the questionnaire was that we did not explore such issues sufficiently and that it was conducted retrospectively, two months after patients perioperative experience. The interval between the OSC and survey completion may have increased the possibility of memory loss and confabulation. We feel that this was more likely to have occurred with reflections regarding clinic consultations and discharge instructions, as opposed to the overall evaluations of OSC/non-OSC services. An example of such bias would be a tendency to adjust ratings of, for example, their operating experience, to match the satisfaction level given to the overall service. This type of responder bias may be as much subconscious as conscious.

Other study design considerations involve our chosen outcome metrics and lack of formal cost analysis. The principle aim of the study was to demonstrate the OSC's efficacy using a national benchmark, the 18 ww, and map out OSC utilisation in UK plastic surgery. Additional outcome metrics that may have been studied include procedural complication and recurrence rates. Reviewing the evidence base, both factors have not been shown to increase significantly, and, employing "lean" thinking principles during our planning of the OSC, it was decided that such factors did not need to be explicitly investigated [1, 12, 13]. We did however take note of significant complications and across the study period no major complications were recorded. Partial local flap failure and post-op bleeds occurred, but not at a rate that significantly deviated from the non-OSC service. In terms of cost analysis, the department saved money by avoiding both fines (incurred by non-compliance to the 18 ww target) and the common prior practice of employing extra operative lists to address patient list backlogs. These were no longer required with the increased capacity afforded by the OSC. The supplementary capacity and operating slots were used by the department with cases that carried a routine NHS tariff. OSCs have already been shown to be cost effective with annual savings in one UK plastic surgery study being estimated to be around £150,000: £355 per OSC patient versus £449 for patients following the conventional pathway [2]. Using these figures to extrapolate for our unit, considering 72 cases per month following the OSC pathway, gives an annual cost saving of over £98,000, on top of which would be added the NHS tariff for the additional 72 cases that could be conducted on standard operating lists. It must be noted that these calculations are based on 2004 data not accounting for inflation so the absolute number value saved in the present day would be greater.

In comparing the OSC and non-OSC services, it should be acknowledged that the criteria applied to include cases appropriate for the OSC (see Section 1) meant that procedures undertaken were on average less complex and of shorter duration than those performed via the conventional pathway. With longer more complex cases, patients may again have felt more anxious and less satisfied with the non-OSC operative experience. However, when cases were matched, the junior surgeons reported that the OSC set-up resulted in a more economical process, such that procedures that would have taken 45–60 minutes were finished within 30 minutes. A more uniform and streamlined approach was achieved through various changes to practice. Information letters were sent to patients prior to clinic detailing the OSC rationale and possible outcomes of the visit. A consultant saw all referrals (as opposed to junior surgeons). Procedural consent and lesion marking was undertaken by the consultants prior to entering the operating room, obviating procedural elements that may delay a more junior surgeon. Nursing staffs' routine roles included the preparation of local anaesthetic, patient draping, pre- and postdebrief of the patient (including post-operative and follow-up instructions), and a general mandate to remove any obstacles to perioperative time. As opposed to in the main operating theatres, disposable instruments were used, trays' modified to contain only the instruments required. Patients skin was cleaned with alchohol (chlorhex-idine) based solution, a sterile field maintained by using a single fenestrated (patient drapes with a predefined lesion window). Operating surgeons dressed in surgical scrubs and sterile gloves only. Template operative notes were devised, doubling up as a discharge letter.

There are of course many considerations that may be expanded upon in more detail with regard to setting up and running an OSC, such as training, staffing, procurement of equipment, and more detailed explanations of "lean" thinking philosophies. We have focused our discussion towards our primary outcome measures, the 18 ww, patient satisfaction, and the national survey of OSC plastic surgery utilisation. However, with regard to training, junior surgeons in our unit (as compared with surgeons coming to the end of their training) reported that the OSC was a good opportunity to operate on simple cases with the potential for consultant supervision as required. As conventional clinics were still being run, there was no impact noted on their ability to undertake outpatient consultations (given this was only performed by consultants in the OSC). OSC set-up and staff training costs could vary significantly, dependent on a department's infrastructure and ability to covert existing facilities. Using "lean" thinking and planning carefully, we were able to utilise preexisting hospital space and adapt available equipment. Examples included using a simple patient trolley as opposed to purchasing a new operative table, procuring disposable instrumentation obviating the need for autoclaves, and retraining staff to perform new/multiple roles (expanded upon in "Organisation and institution of the OSC," Section 2). We have supplied estimates of the cost savings per patient in our department, earlier in the discussion, based upon previous cost analysis in the UK [2]. The overall aim of a OSC should be to improve department performance, in this case in terms of capacity, cost savings, and patient satisfaction, with essentially the same resources. To achieve this is likely to involve changes of practice based upon "Lean" type thinking principles, where care, is streamlined and existing staff often re-trained to perfor new and multiple roles. Procurement of facilities and equipment should be minimised.

5. Conclusion

OSCs are underutilised within UK plastic surgery, where a significant proportion of units acknowledge not having considered their use. This is despite associated improvements in waiting times, department capacity, and being preferred by patients who express high levels of satisfaction. We offer our considerations, planning, and positive local experience instituting an OSC service for minor skin cancer surgery. Our study indicates that the NHS in the UK is right to champion the use of see and treat delivery of care and encourage plastic surgery departments to consider their potential benefit.

Funding

The study was self-funded.

References

[1] J. J. R. Kirkpatrick, I. Taggart, H. S. Rigby, and P. L. G. Townsend, "A pigmented lesion clinic: analysis of the first year's 1055 patients," *British Journal of Plastic Surgery*, vol. 48, no. 4, pp. 247–251, 1995.

[2] M. Javaid, D. Imran, M. Moncrieff, T. J. O'Neill, and E. M. Sassoon, "The see-and-treat clinic in plastic surgery: an efficient, cost-effective, and training-friendly setup," *Plastic and Reconstructive Surgery*, vol. 113, no. 3, pp. 1060–1063, 2004.

[3] NHS, *The National Health Service Commissioning Board and Clinical Commissioning Groups (Responsibilities and Standing Rules) Regulations 2012*, NHS, London, UK, 2012, http://www.nhs.uk/choiceintheNHS/Rightsandpledges/Waitingtimes/Documents/nhs-england-and-ccg-regulations.pdf.

[4] M. Pearson, "Waiting time policies in the health sector—what works?" 2014, http://www.cfhi-fcass.ca/sf-docs/default-source/tq2013/Mark-Pearson-presentation.pdf?sfvrsn=0.

[5] NHS Institute for Innovation & Improvement, *Keep Things Moving—See and Treat Patients in Order*, institute.nhs.uk, 2008, http://www.institute.nhs.uk/quality_and_service_improvement_tools/quality_and_service_improvement_tools/keep_things_moving_-_see_and_treat_patients_in_order.html.

[6] National Collaborating Centre for Cancer, *Guidance on Cancer Services: Improving Outcomes for People with Skin Tumours Including Melanoma*, files.i-md.com, London, UK, 2006, http://files.i-md.com/medinfo/material/77d/4eb14da544ae4ff-e12a8177d/4eb14de744ae4ffe12a81780.pdf.

[7] P. K. Wright, P. M. Geary, R. M. Jose, C. Chou, and R. B. Berry, "See-and-treat plastic surgery: experience at the University Hospital of North Durham," *Plastic and Reconstructive Surgery*, vol. 116, no. 1, pp. 342–344, 2005.

[8] O. Al Hamarneh, L. Liew, and R. J. Shortridge, "Diagnostic yield of a one-stop neck lump clinic," *European Archives of Oto-Rhino-Laryngology*, vol. 270, no. 5, pp. 1711–1714, 2013.

[9] J. A. Moore, C. O'Neil, and D. Fawcett, "A one-stop clinic for men with testicular anxiety," *Annals of the Royal College of Surgeons of England*, vol. 91, no. 1, pp. 23–24, 2009.

[10] D. Kulkarni, T. Irvine, and R. J. Reyes, "The use of core biopsy imprint cytology in the 'one-stop' breast clinic," *European Journal of Surgical Oncology*, vol. 35, no. 10, pp. 1037–1040, 2009.

[11] N. Ratnavelu, I. Biliatis, P. A. Cross, and R. Naik, "Ten-year outcomes of a one-stop colposcopy clinic: a unique service for low grade cytology," *European Journal of Obstetrics & Gynecology and Reproductive Biology*, vol. 169, no. 2, pp. 287–291, 2013.

[12] S. van der Geer, M. Frunt, H. L. Romero et al., "One-stop-shop treatment for basal cell carcinoma, part of a new disease management strategy," *Journal of the European Academy of Dermatology and Venereology*, vol. 26, no. 9, pp. 1154–1157, 2012.

[13] M. A. Salam, V. Matai, M. Salhab, and A. W. Hilger, "The facial skin lesions 'see and treat' clinic: a prospective study," *European Archives of Oto-Rhino-Laryngology*, vol. 263, no. 8, pp. 764–766, 2006.

[14] C. Slade and R. Talbot, "Sustainability of cancer waiting times: the need to focus on pathways relevant to the cancer type," *Journal of the Royal Society of Medicine*, vol. 100, no. 7, pp. 309–313, 2007.

[15] NHS, *Referral to Treatment Pathways: A Guide for Managing Efficient Elective Care*, National Health Service, 2nd edition, 2014, http://www.nhsimas.nhs.uk/fileadmin/Files/Documents/Referral_to_Treatment_Pathways_second_edition_.pdf.

[16] NHS, *Demand and Capacity—A Comprehensive Guide*, NHS Institute for Innovation and Improvement, Institute.nhs.uk, 2014, http://www.institute.nhs.uk/quality_and_service_improvement_tools/quality_and_service_improvement_tools/demand_and_capacity_-_a_comprehensive_guide.html.

[17] J. B. Garfield, D. Ben-Zvi, B. Chance, E. Medina, C. Roseth, and A. Zieffler, *Developing Students' Statistical Reasoning*, Springer, Dordrecht, The Netherlands, 2008.

[18] NHS, *Lean Thinking—NHS Institute for Innovation and Improvement*, National Health Service, 2014, http://www.institute.nhs.uk/quality_and_value/lean_thinking/lean_thinking.html.

[19] R. M. Collar, A. G. Shuman, S. Feiner et al., "Lean management in academic surgery," *Journal of the American College of Surgeons*, vol. 214, no. 6, pp. 928–936, 2012.

[20] P. Mazzocato, C. Savage, M. Brommels, H. Aronsson, and J. Thor, "Lean thinking in healthcare: a realist review of the literature," *Quality and Safety in Health Care*, vol. 19, no. 5, pp. 376–382, 2010.

[21] C. S. Kim, D. A. Spahlinger, J. M. Kin, R. J. Coffey, and J. E. Billi, "Implementation of lean thinking: one health system's journey," *Joint Commission Journal on Quality and Patient Safety*, vol. 35, no. 8, pp. 406–413, 2009.

[22] NHS, *Choose and Book and the 18 Week Wait*, Chooseandbook.nhs.uk, 2009, http://www.chooseandbook.nhs.uk/staff/overview/rtt/cab18wks.pdf.

[23] L. H. Thomas, E. McColl, J. Priest, S. Bond, and R. J. Boys, "Newcastle satisfaction with nursing scales: an instrument for quality assessments of nursing care," *Quality in Health Care*, vol. 5, no. 2, pp. 67–72, 1996.

[24] D. D. Nulty, "The adequacy of response rates to online and paper surveys: what can be done?" *Assessment & Evaluation in Higher Education*, vol. 33, no. 3, pp. 301–314, 2008.

[25] S. S. Foster, "Core competencies required for the cardiac surgical nurse practitioner," *Journal of the American Academy of Nurse Practitioners*, vol. 24, no. 8, pp. 472–475, 2012.

[26] M. Gorman, C. Lochrin, M. A. Khan, and F. Urso-Baiarda, "Waiting times and decision-making behind acute plastic surgery referrals in the UK," *Journal of Hospital Administration*, vol. 2, no. 1, 2013.

[27] C. E. H. Voorbrood, J. P. J. Burgmans, G. J. Clevers et al., "One-stop endoscopic hernia surgery: efficient and satisfactory," *Hernia*, vol. 19, no. 3, pp. 395–400, 2015.

[28] Q. Bismil, M. Bismil, A. Bismil et al., "The development of one-stop wide-awake dupuytren's fasciectomy service: a retrospective review," *JRSM Short Reports*, vol. 3, no. 7, article 48, 2012.

[29] C. Ball, M. Pearse, D. Kennedy, A. Hall, and J. Nanchahal, "Validation of a one-stop carpal tunnel clinic including nerve conduction studies and hand therapy," *Annals of the Royal College of Surgeons of England*, vol. 93, no. 8, pp. 634–638, 2011.

[30] M. J. Reid, L. A. David, and J. E. Nicholl, "A one-stop carpal tunnel clinic," *Annals of the Royal College of Surgeons of England*, vol. 91, no. 4, pp. 301–304, 2009.

21

An Opportunity for Diagonal Development in Global Surgery: Cleft Lip and Palate Care in Resource-Limited Settings

Pratik B. Patel,[1,2] **Marguerite Hoyler,**[1,2] **Rebecca Maine,**[1,2,3]
Christopher D. Hughes,[1,2,4] **Lars Hagander,**[1,2,5] **and John G. Meara**[1,2]

[1] *Program in Global Surgery and Social Change, Department of Global Health and Social Medicine, Harvard Medical School, Boston, MA 02115, USA*

[2] *Department of Plastic and Oral Surgery, Boston Children's Hospital, 300 Longwood Avenue, Enders 1, Boston, MA 02115, USA*

[3] *Department of Surgery, University of California San Francisco Medical Center, San Francisco, CA 94131, USA*

[4] *Department of Surgery, University of Connecticut Health Center, Farmington, CT 06030, USA*

[5] *Department of Pediatric Surgery and International Pediatrics, Faculty of Medicine, Lund University, Lund SE-221 00, Sweden*

Correspondence should be addressed to John G. Meara, john.meara@childrens.harvard.edu

Academic Editor: Renato Da Silva Freitas

Global cleft surgery missions have provided much-needed care to millions of poor patients worldwide. Still, surgical capacity in low- and middle-income countries is generally inadequate. Through surgical missions, global cleft care has largely ascribed to a vertical model of healthcare delivery, which is disease specific, and tends to deliver services parallel to, but not necessarily within, the local healthcare system. The vertical model has been used to address infectious diseases as well as humanitarian emergencies. By contrast, a horizontal model for healthcare delivery tends to focus on long-term investments in public health infrastructure and human capital and has less often been implemented by humanitarian groups for a variety of reasons. As surgical care is an integral component of basic healthcare, the plastic surgery community must challenge itself to address the burden of specific disease entities, such as cleft lip and palate, in a way that sustainably expands and enriches global surgical care as a whole. In this paper, we describe a diagonal care delivery model, whereby cleft missions can enrich surgical capacity through integration into sustainable, local care delivery systems. Furthermore, we examine the applications of diagonal development to cleft care specifically and global surgical care more broadly.

1. Introduction

The inadequacy of surgical and anesthetic capacity in resource-limited settings is well demonstrated [1–5], as is the particular need for more robust pediatric surgical services [6–8]. Total surgical disease burden, estimated at 11–15% of disability-adjusted life years (DALYs) lost worldwide, disproportionately affects low- and middle-income countries (LMICs) [9–11]. Cleft lip and palate (CLP) and other congenital anomalies account for approximately 9% of this burden [9], and the consequences of untreated CLP range from social ostracism to death [12–14]. Although the economic burden of untreated CLP and the value and cost effectiveness of global cleft treatments have been proven [15–17], CLP treatment capacity remains insufficient in LMICs

[18, 19]. Historically plastic surgeons' efforts to address this need have focused on short-term, service-oriented commitments—a vertical approach to healthcare [20].

Narrowly focused, disease-specific, and vertical programs tend to operate outside the existing national and local healthcare structures, supplying their own facilities and delivery mechanisms [21–23]. By contrast, the horizontal approach focuses on developing and strengthening existing public infrastructure, with an emphasis on primary care and broadly applicable health interventions [22, 23].

Although humanitarian cleft care missions have provided crucial treatments for many patients in LMICs who would not otherwise have had access to care, there is an untapped potential in optimally channeling the resources and skills of mission groups into sustainable, local care-delivery systems.

As the plastic surgery community continues to evaluate the ideal role of missions in providing comprehensive cleft care in LMICs, an emphasis should be placed on the concept of diagonal development: an integration of vertical and horizontal approaches in a way that enriches the overall educational and surgical capacity of LMICs. In this paper, we explore the benefits and limitations of the vertical and horizontal approaches to healthcare delivery (Table 1) and apply that framework to global CLP care.

2. Horizontal and Vertical Approaches: Benefits and Limitations

2.1. Vertical Programs. The vertical approach to global health is disease specific and has been a particularly common approach among global infectious disease initiatives [22, 24, 25]. Proponents cite milestones like the eradication of smallpox and dramatic decreases in rates of new HIV infection as evidence of vertical intervention success [22, 26]. Vertical interventions are relatively scalable and are thus ideal for urgent humanitarian responses to disasters or epidemics, which have traditionally garnered significant attention from donors [27]. Additionally, vertical programs efficiently deliver necessary surgical supplies and equipment for disease-specific use in LMICs [28].

However, the vertical approach may also yield parallel and uncoordinated interventions, detract attention from the systemic weakness of national healthcare institutions, compromise countries' autonomy and participation in healthcare initiatives, alienate patients whose healthcare needs exceed the narrow range of provided services, and divert funds from other important causes of morbidity and mortality [22, 29, 30]. The vertical approach has also been criticized for not adequately developing the infrastructure and workforce necessary to address even disease-specific needs, letting alone broader healthcare demands [31–33]. Finally, given the complexity of socioeconomic and environmental disease determinants, narrow vertical efforts, which are not designed to address these issues, may be less effective or even harmful to the populations they aim to serve [22, 24].

2.2. Horizontal Programs. The horizontal approach to healthcare delivery emphasizes long-term investments in healthcare infrastructure and the expansion of publicly funded healthcare systems [20, 34, 35]. Examples include WHO efforts to strengthen primary care systems and World Bank-guided reforms of district-level health administrations [21, 27, 36]. Although the horizontal model of public health interventions preceded the vertical model [20] it has seen renewed emphasis in recent years, particularly as infectious disease treatment groups such as PEPFAR, Human Resources for Health (HRH), and The Global Fund to Fight AIDS, Tuberculosis, and Malaria, transition away from strictly vertical models [21]. Proponents of the horizontal model even argue that disease-specific therapies can be delivered most efficiently through a functional primary healthcare system. Furthermore, horizontal approaches have greater potential to address patients' comorbidities and other health needs, and they intentionally strengthen healthcare systems for the benefit of all current and future patients [21]. As surgery is increasingly acknowledged as an integral part of healthcare worldwide [3], the horizontal model has begun to be applied to surgical disease, through investments in surgical infrastructure and human capital [37].

In surgery and in other domains, however, horizontal development has been hindered by concerns regarding the scope and time frame of horizontal interventions. Horizontal initiatives take extended periods of time to be implemented, may be less suitable to humanitarian emergencies, and depend heavily on governmental legitimacy and functionality in order to be effective [27]. Additionally, defining objective metrics for success in horizontal interventions may be particularly challenging due to larger patient cohorts and diverse causes of morbidity and mortality [21]. For all of these reasons, horizontal development has been of limited appeal to private funding organizations [21]. Lastly, horizontal projects may seem incompatible with the domestic commitments of many global health-oriented physicians in practice in wealthy countries.

2.3. Diagonal Programs. "Diagonal" approaches refer to programs which are neither purely vertical nor purely horizontal [34, 35]. Rather, these programs find synergy between the immediate advantages of vertical inputs and the long-term benefits of horizontal aims, ultimately increasing access and enriching capacity of surgical services (Figure 1).

Diagonal interventions are becoming increasingly common [21], particularly as the horizontal approach is recognized as an effective means of delivering disease-specific care [24, 27]. In addition to infectious disease [38], family planning and maternal and child health are areas in which the integration of vertical and horizontal care has been reported [11, 39, 40]. Although the vertical approach may also yield positive "spill-over," in which focused health initiatives in one disease area or population also benefit the health system as a whole [41]; the diagonal approach embraces these broader impacts as a primary aim instead of as a welcome externality.

3. Building Capacity While Addressing Specific Needs: A Diagonal Approach to Global CLP Care

The traditional "missions" model of cleft care rests partially on the premise that one-time interventions can effectively treat craniofacial anomalies, that they produce a high return for time and resources invested, and that they are feasible commitments for visiting providers [18, 42–44]. However, as cleft palate missions have grown in scale and scope, they have demonstrated a willingness to think critically about their care delivery models. As a result, many cleft treatment groups have begun to integrate vertical and horizontal approaches in order to maximize their positive impact and minimize any negative consequences [42, 43, 45–49]. In the case of Interplast, these changes include an emphasis on local partnerships with the explicit goal of creating self-sufficient,

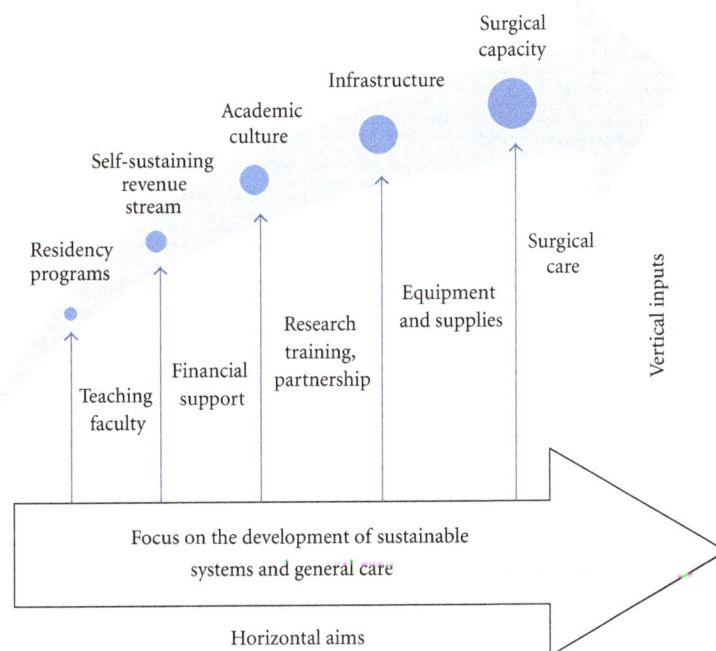

FIGURE 1: A diagonal approach harnesses the power of horizontal aims and vertical inputs.

TABLE 1: The vertical-horizontal debate: benefits and limitations of each approach.

Approach	Description	Examples	Advantages	Disadvantages
Vertical	(i) Disease specific (ii) Narrowly focused (iii) Operates outside the existing healthcare structures and systems (iv) Often privately funded	(i) Polioimmunization program (ii) HIV/AIDS treatment programs (iii) Male circumcision programs (iv) DOTS	(i) Demonstrated effectiveness (HIV/AIDS) (ii) May have a limited, positive impact on other areas of healthcare delivery ("spill over") (iii) Fast implementation (iv) Scalable (v) Donor attractiveness (vi) Efficient delivery of disease, specific equipment and supplies	(i) May not address other diseases, healthcare needs, and health determinants (ii) May yield redundant and poorly coordinated efforts (iii) May divert funds from other diseases and medical priorities
Horizontal	(i) Not disease specific (ii) Focuses on broadly applicable healthcare infrastructure (iii) Long-term interventions and investments	(i) Strengthening primary care systems (ii) Healthcare provider education and training (iii) Human resources for health (HRH)	(i) Strengthens health systems as a whole (ii) Benefits all patients, regardless of disease or diagnosis (iii) May facilitate disease, specific treatments (iv) Builds capacity for long-term change	(i) Long-term interventions (ii) Large, unwieldy projects (iii) Often less attractive to donors, funders (iv) Require functional state and local governments (v) More difficult to measure impact of horizontal interventions

independently functioning local sites [50]. Operation Smile and others have evolved from purely vertical care providers to integrated system creators through a continued emphasis on mindful and reflective practice [18].

We build upon these shifts in global cleft care delivery and argue that a diagonal approach can build on the strengths of the vertical model, while also addressing its weaknesses. In the case of global CLP repair, diagonal programs would retain the focused services and resource inputs of surgical missions, while incorporating efforts to expand surgical capacity, increase human capital, and provide comprehensive care in general. As a result, through diagonal development, surgical care in LMIC can be broadly enriched in several key deliverable areas (Table 2).

TABLE 2: Superior impact of diagonal interventions in global cleft lip and palate care.

	Vertical approach	Diagonal approach
Continuity of care	Short-term interventions	Long-term presence
Interdisciplinary care	Focus on cleft surgery services	Focus on surgical, perioperative, dental, feeding, hearing, speech, and rehabilitation services
Equitable access	Service-driven patient selection	Needs-driven patient selection
Outcomes monitoring	Postoperative	Long term
Local workforce development	Unilateral exchange focusing on cleft surgeons	Bilateral exchange focusing on surgeons, anesthesiologists, surgical intensivists, scrub technicians, perioperative nurses, ward nurses, dentists, feeding specialists, speech therapists, and audiologists
Equitable trainee experiences	Enhanced visiting trainee experience in specialized surgical practice	Enhanced visiting trainee experience in global healthcare delivery; enhanced local trainee experience in surgical practice
Academic culture of investigation and empowerment	Clinical emphasis, transfer of clinical skills, data collection and analysis by visiting providers, research-driven medical missions	Academic emphasis, transfer of research skills, data collection and analysis by local providers, and research-driven local practice
Increased financial sustainability	Dependence on external funding; return on investment may not be optimal	Goal of self-sustained revenue streams; emphasis on increasing ethical, fiscal and systems-wide returns on investments
Implications for local general surgical capacity	"Spill-over" as a welcome positive externality	"Spill-over" as a primary objective

3.1. Integrated, Longitudinal CLP Care. The optimal care of patients with cleft lip and palate patients is complex, longitudinal, and interdisciplinary [51–54]. Children with cleft anomalies benefit from dental and orthodontic services, speech therapy, otologic care, and occasionally revision surgeries [9, 55, 56]. In many wealthy nations, participation in integrated cleft centers allows for parental education and support often from the time of prenatal diagnosis through the postoperative care. Cleft centers provide not only the essential followup to identify and address surgical complications, but also permits tracking of long-term outcomes to support general quality improvement projects. Multidisciplinary services are frequently lacking in LMICs, and often access to long-term followup is limited as well. Unfortunately these same patients in LMICs face increased risk for surgical complications due to higher incidences of malnutrition and concurrent illness [23, 44].

The traditional vertical structure of CLP missions is not well suited to longitudinal, integrated CLP care in LMICs [57], especially because effective delivery of these services may require multiple visits that are beyond the scope of a purely vertical treatment model [14, 58]. Adopting a diagonal approach to cleft palate care would address many of these limitations by transitioning care from fragmented efforts of visiting providers to a more sustained local physician practice over the long term. This could be achieved either by a limited permanent staff complemented by frequent missions or by a constant rotation of visiting teams with no coverage gaps. Additionally, specialized cleft centers, similar to those described in wealthy nations, have been described as feasible

and sustainable delivery models to ensure comprehensive CLP care in LMICs [59]. The diagonal approach takes this concept one step further, by integrating specialized surgical care into the longitudinal services of local healthcare systems and structures. This can foster trust in and utilization of the local healthcare system, both by CLP patients and their families and community members.

The logistical challenges of contacting and locating former patients, varying degrees of patient compliance, especially in the setting of insufficient patient education, and coordinating followup with local professionals [14, 56, 60–63] have been barriers to follow up on vertical missions. Follow-up rates have been correspondingly low: among medical mission groups that do provide postoperative care, rates range from 5% to 35% of patients [58]. Cleft missions groups have made progress in monitoring surgical outcomes, for instance through the development of outcomes databases [18, 43, 49, 62]. However, an increased focus on outcomes is needed. One paper examining the long-term results of palatoplasties, performed by local and visiting surgeons in Ecuador, found a significantly higher rate of fistula formation among Ecuadorian patients than among their counterparts in wealthy countries [56]. Other international researchers have noted that palatal dehiscence and residual or recurrent fistulae were frequently encountered during their studies, even when palate integrity was not an outcome in question [60]. Through its emphasis on longitudinal care, diagonal development provides an optimal framework for outcomes research, which is essential to identify and address the underlying causes of these troubling results.

Furthermore, diagonal approaches can facilitate outcomes monitoring through emphasis on general, not disease-specific, infrastructure improvements, such as electronic medical records, clinical measurement tools, and a culture of medical documentation and outcomes-driven practice. Once in place, these infrastructure improvements could help optimize quality and safety of all clinical care delivery, including CLP treatments.

Improved infrastructure for followup and outcomes monitoring through a diagonal delivery model can also improve access to the variety of specialists needed to provide comprehensive CLP care. While some programs have implemented interdisciplinary, comprehensive services for cleft patients in LMICs [64], for instance by using telemedicine to provide speech therapy [47, 65, 66], this type of care depends on broad manpower and healthcare structure capabilities, neither of which is the focus of a vertical model. By reinforcing the importance of surgical care, a particular strength of the vertical approach, while simultaneously building capacity for other necessary CLP services, the diagonal model has the potential to improve the outcomes of patients in LMICs. Additionally, effective patient education regarding the comprehensive treatment options for CLP would result from utilization of the significant outreach capacity of the existing healthcare system.

An investment and focus on interdisciplinary care would also benefit resource-limited communities at large. Many children and adults without cleft anomalies have need for services like speech therapy and audiologic care, in addition to surgery and anesthesia. If promoted as a component of CLP care in LMICs, these services could be available for patients with and without CLP. In addition, each service would represent a channel by which patients could seek their first contact within the broader healthcare system, promoting a culture of individual health agency.

By providing long-term follow-up of cleft patients, supporting the growth of essential complementary services and developing quality improvement projects through outcomes monitoring, the diagonal model of cleft care delivery would help achieve the ethical goal of providing the same treatment to patients in poor countries which is the standard of care in wealthy countries.

3.2. Equitable Access.

Equitable access results from a focus on patient-centered interventions that are able to prioritize diverse patient needs without the logistical constraints of short-term missions. In wealthy countries, standard of care for patients with cleft anomalies involves careful timing of surgical correction. Patients treated on annual missions have a lower likelihood of being operated on within recommended windows [63], which can impact surgical outcomes, development of facial structures, speech, and hearing [56, 67, 68]. Longitudinally focused, diagonal efforts remove the need to operate based on visiting provider availability, allowing for interventions at the appropriate developmental stage, and enabling more timely and equitable cleft care.

Inadequate physical access—lack of transportation or long travel distances to care facilities—is a significant barrier to care for patients in resource-limited settings [69].

Improved patient transportation and high-quality facilities can help reduce morbidity and mortality attributable to multiple causes in LMICs [70]. A diagonal model could address these barriers, for instance by devoting funds and resources to patient transportation and lodging needs. One might also envision a health-services bus, perhaps integrated with existing local public transport infrastructure, which would travel to remote communities in order to provide regularly-scheduled medical care to patients there. For cleft patients, this service would facilitate initial assessments, transportation to the surgical center, and followup, as needed. For all patients, this service would provide a critical link between communities, clinics, and hospitals, promoting equitable access to care.

3.3. Local Workforce Development.

Cleft missions have been criticized for undermining the efforts and authority of local providers [71]. Importing surgical services may suggest to patients and community members that surgery requires large teams and equipment that may not be accessible locally. This diminishes confidence in local providers, lowers professional morale, and decreases revenue for local facilities as patients with means to pay for local providers to perform their operations rely on visiting surgeons [72].

In response to these criticisms, many cleft missions groups have adopted the training, promotion, and support of local surgeons as a primary objective [58, 73]. However, this method often consists of choppy, "on the spot" intraoperative lectures by the visiting surgeon, with little structure regarding teaching objectives, and even less time for reciprocal teaching by host providers [58]. This unilateral approach to knowledge transfer undermines the important contributions of local surgeons and other healthcare professionals, who are critical to all steps of care delivery and capacity building in resource-limited settings and whose clinical skills are well adapted to the local resource limitations and epidemiology of disease [71]. Additionally, a lack of structure regarding teaching objectives likely impairs the systematic mastering of skills and knowledge for both local and visiting surgeons [74]. Finally, an educational focus on surgeons as providers of cleft care strictly misses the opportunity to train other essential perioperative and interdisciplinary staff—pediatric anesthesiologists, surgical intensivists, scrub technicians, operating room nurses, and speech therapists—in the provision of safe and comprehensive cleft care.

More robust academic partnerships, as fostered by diagonal development, would also promote local academic leaders and would enhance training programs for numerous types of healthcare providers. In particular, greater numbers of well-trained surgeons, scrub technicians, nurses, and anesthesiologists would improve surgical care for all patients in LMIC; cleft patients are included.

3.4. Equitable Trainee Experiences.

It is not uncommon for general or plastic surgery residents from wealthy countries to complete an international rotation in LMICs [75, 76]. Research shows that these experiences enhance the training of the visiting surgical residents [77, 78], but it is less clear that host institutions benefit equally. As institutional partnerships between academic centers in wealthy LMIC become increasingly common [10, 37], the cleft care community, and the surgical community at large, must look beyond the needs of visiting trainees to the needs of students, residents, faculty and staff in host institutions and communities [79].

Diagonal development in cleft care can facilitate equity between visiting and local trainees and providers through its longitudinal view of the surgical care. For instance, the educational objectives for rotating trainees from wealthy countries could perhaps center on tackling systems-based and logistical challenges of surgical care delivery in resource-limited environments, in addition to the acquisition of operative experience. Visiting trainees could be mentored and instructed in these areas by local providers with expertise in local systems and care-delivery challenges. Furthermore, visiting trainees could complement the experiences of local trainees by enabling local residents to spend more time with visiting faculty, learning clinical skills through intraoperative teaching sessions, formal lectures, and skills-based workshops. This approach would benefit local trainees and, ultimately, the patients they will serve in their home communities.

3.5. An Academic Culture of Investigation and Empowerment.
A diagonal approach to cleft care would foster research experience for local trainees and practitioners in countries where its importance may not be emphasized during medical education. Although a majority of plastic surgeons and volunteer pediatric surgeons express their desire to teach clinical skills to colleagues in LMICs, research skills are largely neglected on mission trips. Relatively few (40%) cleft mission organizations regard research as a priority, citing limited funding, manpower, and time [58]. Research is particularly difficult given the heavy operative census and short duration of medical missions. Transitioning away from a strictly vertical model toward a diagonal model could promote research in several ways. For instance, the diagonal goal of increased surgical capacity would reduce the "backlog" of patient need, and lengthier visits and prolonged collaborations between local and visiting providers could alleviate pressure to operate on as many cleft patients as possible during a short mission. As has been suggested by general surgeons and other surgical subspecialists [79], such changes would allow additional time for research planning and execution.

A greater emphasis on global surgery research is important for several reasons. Surgeons in LMICs self-report a need for increased research training and skills, in addition to clinical assistance [80]. Additionally, improving the quality of particular treatments in LMICs, such as cleft surgeries, requires a better understanding of the local needs, barriers to care, outcomes, and predictive factors that define cleft anomalies and other diseases in those countrie, and which may be unique to resource-limited settings. Finally, promoting research partnerships with local providers and investigators could empower local healthcare professionals to take a more active role in determining how best to address the healthcare needs of their populations.

International research partnerships as a component of diagonal development would also challenge researchers in wealthy countries to address previously neglected research topics. For instance, despite the long-accepted model of coordinated care for CLP [51, 53, 81], there is relatively little comparative outcomes research of cleft care in wealthy countries. In order to identify and learn from the weaknesses of current cleft care models, the global cleft community must incorporate research and research capacity building into care delivery models in all settings. Thus, diagonal development can foster research-driven local practice, outcomes-driven quality improvements, and data-driven infrastructure development, for the benefit of all surgical patients.

3.6. Increased Financial Sustainability. Although the cost effectiveness of surgical treatment of cleft palate is well demonstrated by analytic models [15, 16, 82], medical missions may not optimize the return on relatively scarce financial investments in cleft care, in terms of value to individual patients and local communities. The significant financial overhead of medical missions may ultimately detract resources from the patients who need those resources the most. Dupuis [71] estimate that $920 US could be saved, per surgery, if operations were performed by local providers instead of by volunteers from abroad. Additionally, analytic models may not take into account the negative externalities of vertical interventions. While transitioning to a diagonal approach may initially increase some costs, by investing in health systems, infrastructure, human capital, and research capabilities, the diagonal approach can increase the overall value of cleft treatments in LMIC. Indeed, just as domestic programs must justify their value proposition to society [83], the international cleft treatment community must increasingly demonstrate to public and private funders that cleft care investments yield sizable long-term benefits for patients and communities alike. Demonstrating increased capacity could attract funders to global surgery because it offers a superior "return on investment," both financially and ethically. Looking ahead, diagonal approaches can also move local institutions toward the goal of self-sustained revenue streams by promoting increased patient engagement, health systems development, and government involvement in healthcare.

4. Future Directions

4.1. Implications for Global General Surgical Capacity. To reiterate, diagonal development turns attention away from importing clinical resources and services, emphasizing deliverables that not only increase capacity for CLP surgery, but also enrich the surgical ecosystem as a whole. Under the current vertical cleft care mission models, surgeons and trainees make significant contributions, but may not increase local capacity to address those surgical diseases that account for the majority of mortality and morbidity: obstetrical complications, trauma, and acute abdominal emergencies [84]. Just as the capacity to provide cleft lip and palate treatment is necessarily affected by the overall shortages in operating theatres and supplies, the converse holds true: an emphasis on diagonal development would yield infrastructure, manpower, and self-sustaining revenue that could have positive implications for treatment of other surgical diseases. In this way, a diagonal approach makes the "spill-over" effect a primary aim, rather than a welcome positive externality.

4.2. Advocacy and Implementation. The full extent of surgical care needed in resource-limited settings cannot be addressed by global plastic surgeons alone. However, what plastic surgeons can directly do is very powerful—the transformation of a face or the reconstruction of an injury is a metaphor for involvement creating change, which can reach exponentially to more patients [18]. Each specialty must work both within and outside of the global health community both to offer its expertise—whether that is caesarian sections or CLP repair—and also assist in the development of comprehensive surgical care delivery services, not merely concentrate on a specific disease or intervention [9]. Medical mission NGOs have taken the lead in these efforts; it is now incumbent upon academic surgeons, trainees, and researchers to join medical missions groups in further defining and promoting the global surgery agenda.

5. Conclusions

Global surgery is still, in many ways, in its infancy. As we move forward in global CLP care, it is essential to learn from the strengths and limitations of the vertical and horizontal approaches in order to maximize the benefit of these programs to healthcare systems in LMICs. We recognize an ongoing need for vertical humanitarian missions and admire the legacy of many cleft treatment groups. Indeed, it is because of the successes of cleft missions that the cleft care community is now in the position to contribute diagonally to increase surgical capacity and promote quality of care. As funding becomes increasingly available for global surgery interventions, care delivery methods will come to the forefront in terms of achieving optimal outcomes. At this critical juncture, plastic surgeons must serve as thought leaders in global surgery, and a diagonal approach to CLP care is a means of achieving that goal.

Authors' Contribution

Patel and Hoyler contributed equally to the development of the paper.

Acknowledgment

The authors acknowledge P. B. Patel and M. Hoyler as co-first authors.

References

[1] L. M. Funk, T. G. Weiser, W. R. Berry et al., "Global operating theatre distribution and pulse oximetry supply: an estimation from reported data," *The Lancet*, vol. 376, no. 9746, pp. 1055–1061, 2010.

[2] S. C. Hodges, C. Mijumbi, M. Okello, B. A. Mccormick, I. A. Walker, and I. H. Wilson, "Anaesthesia services in developing countries: defining the problems," *Anaesthesia*, vol. 62, no. 1, pp. 4–11, 2007.

[3] P. E. Farmer and J. Y. Kim, "Surgery and global health: a view from beyond the OR," *World Journal of Surgery*, vol. 32, no. 4, pp. 533–536, 2008.

[4] G. Dubowitz, S. Detlefs, and K. A. Kelly McQueen, "Global anesthesia workforce crisis: a preliminary survey revealing shortages contributing to undesirable outcomes and unsafe practices," *World Journal of Surgery*, vol. 34, no. 3, pp. 438–444, 2010.

[5] L. C. Ivers, E. S. Garfein, J. Augustin et al., "Increasing access to surgical services for the poor in rural Haiti: surgery as a public good for public health," *World Journal of Surgery*, vol. 32, no. 4, pp. 537–542, 2008.

[6] S. W. Bickler, J. Kyambi, and H. Rode, "Pediatric surgery in sub-Saharan africa," *Pediatric Surgery International*, vol. 17, no. 5-6, pp. 442–447, 2001.

[7] S. W. Bickler, "Pediatric surgery in the developing world," *Journal of Pediatric Surgery*, vol. 40, no. 12, pp. 1969–1970, 2005.

[8] G. Azzie, S. Bickler, D. Farmer, and S. Beasley, "Partnerships for developing pediatric surgical care in low-income countries," *Journal of Pediatric Surgery*, vol. 43, no. 12, pp. 2273–2274, 2008.

[9] N. B. Semer, S. R. Sullivan, and J. G. Meara, "Plastic surgery and global health: how plastic surgery impacts the global burden of surgical disease," *Journal of Plastic, Reconstructive and Aesthetic Surgery*, vol. 63, no. 8, pp. 1244–1248, 2010.

[10] D. Ozgediz, S. Kijjambu, M. Galukande et al., "Africa's neglected surgical workforce crisis," *The Lancet*, vol. 371, no. 9613, pp. 627–628, 2008.

[11] H. T. Debas, R. Gosselin, C. McCord, and A. Thind, "Surgery," in *Disease Control Priorities in Developing Countries*, D. T. Jamison, J. G. Breman, and A.R. Measham, Eds., The International Bank for Reconstruction and Development/The World Bank Group, Washington, DC, USA, 2006.

[12] S. Mzezewa and F. C. Muchemwa, "Reaction to the birth of a child with cleft lip or cleft palate in Zimbabwe," *Tropical Doctor*, vol. 40, no. 3, pp. 138–140, 2010.

[13] H. O. Nwanze and G. O. Sowemimo, "Maternal stress, superstition and communicative behaviour with Nigerian cleft lip and palate children," *Scandinavian Journal of Plastic and Reconstructive Surgery*, vol. 21, no. 1, pp. 15–18, 1987.

[14] G. A. Moghe, S. Mauli, A. Thomas, and V. A. Obed, "Bridging the gap: addressing challenges towards improvement of cleft teamwork in a tertiary care center in North India-a Pilot Study," *The Cleft Palate-Craniofacial Journal*. In press.

[15] B. Alkire, C. D. Hughes, K. Nash, J. R. Vincent, and J. G. Meara, "Potential economic benefit of cleft lip and palate repair in sub-saharan Africa," *World Journal of Surgery*, vol. 35, no. 6, pp. 1194–1201, 2011.

[16] C. D. Hughes, A. Babigian, S. McCormack et al., "The clinical and economic impact of a sustained program in global plastic surgery: valuing cleft care in resource-poor settings," *Plastic and Reconstructive Surgery*, vol. 130, no. 1, pp. 87e–94e, 2012.

[17] W. P. Magee, R. Vander Burg, and K. W. Hatcher, "Cleft lip and palate as a cost-effective health care treatment in the developing world," *World Journal of Surgery*, vol. 34, no. 3, pp. 420–427, 2010.

[18] W. P. Magee, "Evolution of a sustainable surgical delivery model," *Journal of Craniofacial Surgery*, vol. 21, no. 5, pp. 1321–1326, 2010.

[19] P. Donkor, D. O. Bankas, P. Agbenorku, G. Plange-Rhule, and S. K. Ansah, "Cleft lip and palate surgery in Kumasi, Ghana: 2001–2005," *Journal of Craniofacial Surgery*, vol. 18, no. 6, pp. 1376–1379, 2007.

[20] J. Msuya, *Horizontal and Vertical Delivery of Health Services: What are the Trade-Offs?, in Background Papers for the World Development Report 2004*, World Bank, Washington, DC, USA, 2003.

[21] T. Bärnighausen, D. E. Bloom, and S. Humair, "Health systems and HIV treatment in sub-Saharan Africa: matching intervention and programme evaluation strategies," *Sexually Transmitted Infections*, vol. 88, no. 2, p. e2, 2012.

[22] J. P. Unger, P. De Paepe, and A. Green, "A code of best practice for disease control programmes to avoid damaging health care services in developing countries," *International Journal of Health Planning and Management*, vol. 18, supplement 1, pp. S27–S39, 2003.

[23] C. G. Victora, K. Hanson, J. Bryce, and J. P. Vaughan, "Achieving universal coverage with health interventions," *The Lancet*, vol. 364, no. 9444, pp. 1541–1548, 2004.

[24] M. C. Raviglione and A. Pio, "Evolution of WHO policies for tuberculosis control, 1948–2001," *The Lancet*, vol. 359, no. 9308, pp. 775–780, 2002.

[25] U. K. Griffiths, S. Mounier-Jack, V. Oliveira-Cruz, D. Balabanova, P. Hanvoravongchai, and P. Ongolo, "How can measles eradication strengthen health care systems?" *The Journal of Infectious Diseases*, vol. 204, supplement 1, pp. S78–S81, 2011.

[26] UNAIDS, *UNAIDS World AIDS Day Report 2011*, 2011.

[27] T. Bärnighausen, D. E. Bloom, and S. Humair, "Going horizontal—shifts in funding of global health interventions," *New England Journal of Medicine*, vol. 364, no. 23, pp. 2181–2183, 2011.

[28] A. Patel, I. Sinha, M. McRae, N. Broer, J. Watkins, and J. A. Persing, "The role of academic plastic surgery institutions in addressing the global burden of surgical disease," *Plastic and Reconstructive Surgery*, vol. 127, no. 2, pp. 1019–1020, 2011.

[29] R. G. Biesma, R. Brugha, A. Harmer, A. Walsh, N. Spicer, and G. Walt, "The effects of global health initiatives on country health systems: a review of the evidence from HIV/AIDS control," *Health Policy and Planning*, vol. 24, no. 4, pp. 239–252, 2009.

[30] K. A. Grépin, "Leveraging HIV programs to deliver an integrated package of health services: some words of caution," *Journal of Acquired Immune Deficiency Syndromes*, vol. 57, supplement 2, pp. S77–S79, 2011.

[31] B. D. Fulton, R. M. Scheffler, S. P. Sparkes, E. Y. Auh, M. Vujicic, and A. Soucat, "Health workforce skill mix and task shifting in low income countries: a review of recent evidence," *Human Resources for Health*, vol. 9, article 1, 2011.

[32] A. R. Maddison and W. F. Schlech, "Will universal access to antiretroviral therapy ever be possible? The health care worker challenge," *Canadian Journal of Infectious Diseases and Medical Microbiology*, vol. 21, no. 1, pp. e64–e69, 2010.

[33] J. Price and A. Binagwaho, "From medical rationing to rationalizing the use of human resources for aids care and treatment in africa: a case for task shifting," *Developing World Bioethics*, vol. 10, no. 2, pp. 99–103, 2010.

[34] R. Atun, T. De Jongh, F. Secci, K. Ohiri, and O. Adeyi, "A systematic review of the evidence on integration of targeted health interventions into health systems," *Health Policy and Planning*, vol. 25, no. 1, pp. 1–14, 2010.

[35] R. Atun, T. De Jongh, F. Secci, K. Ohiri, and O. Adeyi, "Integration of targeted health interventions into health systems: a conceptual framework for analysis," *Health Policy and Planning*, vol. 25, no. 2, pp. 104–111, 2010.

[36] *Health Care Reform in Zambia*, The World Bank, 1997.

[37] R. Riviello, D. Ozgediz, R. Y. Hsia, G. Azzie, M. Newton, and J. Tarpley, "Role of collaborative academic partnerships in surgical training, education, and provision," *World Journal of Surgery*, vol. 34, no. 3, pp. 459–465, 2010.

[38] U. V. Amazigo, S. G. A. Leak, H. G. M. Zoure, N. Njepuome, and P.-S. Lusamba-Dikassa, "Community-driven interventions can revolutionise control of neglected tropical diseases," *Trends in Parasitology*, vol. 28, no. 6, pp. 231–238, 2012.

[39] T. Doherty, M. Chopra, M. Tomlinson, N. Oliphant, D. Nsibande, and J. Mason, "Moving from vertical to integrated child health programmes: experiences from a multi-country assessment of the Child Health Days approach in Africa," *Tropical Medicine and International Health*, vol. 15, no. 3, pp. 296–305, 2010.

[40] C. J. Briggs, P. Capdegelle, and P. Garner, "Strategies for integrating primary health services in middle- and low-income countries: effects on performance, costs and patient outcomes," *Cochrane Database of Systematic Reviews*, no. 4, article CD003318, 2001.

[41] F. Rasschaert, M. Pirard, M. P. Philips et al., "Positive spillover effects of ART scale up on wider health systems development: evidence from Ethiopia and Malawi," *Journal of the International AIDS Society*, vol. 14, no. 1, article S3, 2011.

[42] L. H. Hollier, S. E. Sharabi, J. C. Koshy, M. E. Schafer, J. O'Young, and T. W. Flood, "Surgical mission (Not) impossible—now what?" *Journal of Craniofacial Surgery*, vol. 21, no. 5, pp. 1488–1492, 2010.

[43] W. J. Schneider, M. R. Migliori, A. K. Gosain, G. Gregory, and R. Flick, "Volunteers in plastic surgery guidelines for providing surgical care for children in the less developed world: part II. Ethical considerations," *Plastic and Reconstructive Surgery*, vol. 128, no. 3, pp. 216e–222e, 2011.

[44] W. J. Schneider, G. D. Politis, A. K. Gosain et al., "Volunteers in plastic surgery guidelines for providing surgical care for children in the less developed world," *Plastic and Reconstructive Surgery*, vol. 127, no. 6, pp. 2477–2486, 2011.

[45] D. Hunter-Smith, "Equity and participation in outreach surgical aid: interplast ANZ," *ANZ Journal of Surgery*, vol. 79, no. 6, pp. 420–422, 2009.

[46] R. C. W. Goh, R. Wang, P. K. T. Chen, L. J. Lo, and Y. R. Chen, "Strategies for achieving long-term effective outcome in cleft missions: the noordhoff craniofacial foundation and Chang Gung memorial hospital," *Journal of Craniofacial Surgery*, vol. 20, no. 8, supplement 2, pp. 1657–1660, 2009.

[47] M. C. Furr, E. Larkin, R. Blakeley, T. W. Albert, L. Tsugawa, and S. M. Weber, "Extending multidisciplinary management of cleft palate to the developing world," *Journal of Oral and Maxillofacial Surgery*, vol. 69, no. 1, pp. 237–241, 2011.

[48] D. R. Laub Jr. and A. H. Ajar, "A survey of multidisciplinary cleft palate and craniofacial team examination formats," *Journal of Craniofacial Surgery*, vol. 23, no. 4, pp. 1002–1004, 2012.

[49] L. E. Bermudez and A. K. Lizarraga, "Operation smile: how to measure its success," *Annals of Plastic Surgery*, vol. 67, no. 3, pp. 205–208, 2011.

[50] R. I. S. Zbar, S. M. Rai, and D. L. Dingman, "Establishing cleft malformation surgery in developing nations: a model for the new millennium," *Plastic and Reconstructive Surgery*, vol. 106, no. 4, pp. 886–889, 2000.

[51] N. Colburn and R. S. Cherry, "Community-based team approach to the management of children with cleft palate," *Children's Health Care*, vol. 13, no. 3, pp. 122–128, 1985.

[52] P. Mossey and J. Little, "Addressing the challenges of cleft lip and palate research in India," *Indian Journal of Plastic Surgery*, vol. 42, no. 1, supplement, pp. S9–S18, 2009.

[53] J. M. Pascoe, "Team care of the patient with cleft and lip palate," *Current Problems in Pediatric and Adolescent Health Care*, vol. 38, no. 5, pp. 137–158, 2008.

[54] K. Vargervik, S. Oberoi, and W. Y. Hoffman, "Team care for the patient with cleft: UCSF protocols and outcomes," *Journal of Craniofacial Surgery*, vol. 20, no. 8, supplement 2, pp. 1668–1671, 2009.

[55] D. Bearn, S. Mildinhall, T. Murphy et al., "Cleft lip and palate care in the United Kingdom—the Clinical Standards Advisory Group (CSAG) Study. Part 4: outcome comparisons, training, and conclusions," *Cleft Palate-Craniofacial Journal*, vol. 38, no. 1, pp. 38–43, 2001.

[56] R. G. Maine, W. Y. Hoffman, J. H. Palacios-Martinez, D. S. Corlew, and G. A. Gregory, "Comparison of fistula rates after palatoplasty for international and local surgeons on surgical missions in ecuador with rates at a craniofacial center in the United States," *Plastic and Reconstructive Surgery*, vol. 129, no. 2, pp. 319e–326e, 2012.

[57] J. B. Mulliken, "The changing faces of children with cleft lip and palate," *New England Journal of Medicine*, vol. 351, no. 8, pp. 745–747, 2004.

[58] V. K. L. Yeow, S.-T. T. Lee, T. J. Lambrecht et al., "International task force on volunteer cleft missions," *Journal of Craniofacial Surgery*, vol. 13, no. 1, pp. 18–25, 2002.

[59] C. E. Raposo-Amaral and C. A. Raposo-Amaral, "Changing face of cleft care: specialized centers in developing countries," *Journal of Craniofacial Surgery*, vol. 23, no. 1, pp. 206–209, 2012.

[60] H. M. Sharp, J. W. Canady, F. A. C. Ligot, R. A. Hague, J. Gutierrez, and J. Gutierrez, "Caregiver and patient reported outcomes after repair of cleft lip and/or palate in the Philippines," *Cleft Palate-Craniofacial Journal*, vol. 45, no. 2, pp. 163–171, 2008.

[61] D. P. Butler, N. Samman, and J. Gollogly, "A multidisciplinary cleft palate team in the developing world: performance and challenges," *Journal of Plastic, Reconstructive and Aesthetic Surgery*, vol. 64, no. 11, pp. 1540–1541, 2011.

[62] L. Bermudez, V. Carter, W. Magee, R. Sherman, and R. Ayala, "Surgical outcomes auditing systems in humanitarian organizations," *World Journal of Surgery*, vol. 34, no. 3, pp. 403–410, 2010.

[63] O. Adetayo, R. Ford, and M. Martin, "Africa has unique and urgent barriers to cleft care: lessons from practitioners at the Pan-African Congress on Cleft Lip and Palate," *Pan African Medical Journal*, vol. 12, p. 15, 2012.

[64] B. Prathanee, S. Dechongkit, and S. Manochiopinig, "Development of community-based speech therapy model: for children with cleft lip/palate in Northeast Thailand," *Journal of the Medical Association of Thailand*, vol. 89, no. 4, pp. 500–508, 2006.

[65] E. Whitehead, V. Dorfman, G. Tremper, A. Kramer, A. Sigler, and A. Gosman, "Telemedicine as a means of effective speech evaluation for patients with cleft palate," *Annals of Plastic Surgery*, vol. 68, no. 4, pp. 415–417, 2012.

[66] C. A. Glazer, P. J. Bailey, I. L. Icaza et al., "Multidisciplinary care of international patients with cleft palate using telemedicine," *Archives of Facial Plastic Surgery*, vol. 13, no. 6, pp. 436–438, 2011.

[67] R. J. Rohrich, A. R. Rowsell, D. F. Johns et al., "Timing of hard palatal closure: a critical long-term analysis," *Plastic and Reconstructive Surgery*, vol. 98, no. 2, pp. 236–246, 1996.

[68] S. R. Cohen, J. Kalinowski, D. LaRossa, and P. Randall, "Cleft palate fistulas: a multivariate statistical analysis of prevalence, etiology, and surgical management," *Plastic and Reconstructive Surgery*, vol. 87, no. 6, pp. 1041–1047, 1991.

[69] S. Gabrysch, S. Cousens, J. Cox, and O. M. R. Campbell, "The influence of distance and level of care on delivery place in rural Zambia: a study of linked national data in a geographic information system," *PLoS Medicine*, vol. 8, no. 1, Article ID e1000394, 2011.

[70] N. Carvalho, A. S. Salehi, and S. J. Goldie, "National and sub-national analysis of the health benefits and cost-effectiveness of strategies to reduce maternal mortality in Afghanistan," *Health Policy and Planning*. In press.

[71] C. C. Dupuis, "Humanitarian missions in the third world: a polite dissent," *Plastic and Reconstructive Surgery*, vol. 113, no. 1, pp. 433–435, 2004.

[72] T. E. E. Goodacre, "Commentary on "Plastic surgery and global health: how plastic surgery impacts the global burden of surgical disease,"" *Journal of Plastic, Reconstructive and Aesthetic Surgery*, vol. 63, no. 8, pp. 1249–1250, 2010.

[73] F. M. Abenavoli, "A new approach for humanitarian missions," *Plastic and Reconstructive Surgery*, vol. 124, no. 6, pp. 461e–462e, 2009.

[74] J. D. Pollock, T. P. Love, B. C. Steffes, D. C. Thompson, J. Mellinger, and C. Haisch, "Is it possible to train surgeons for rural Africa? A report of a successful international program," *World Journal of Surgery*, vol. 35, no. 3, pp. 493–499, 2011.

[75] A. H. Huang and W. R. Rhodes, "Hospital-based plastic surgery volunteerism: a resident's international experience," *Annals of Plastic Surgery*, vol. 68, no. 4, pp. 396–400, 2012.

[76] A. Campbell, R. Sherman, and W. P. Magee, "The role of humanitarian missions in modern surgical training," *Plastic and Reconstructive Surgery*, vol. 126, no. 1, pp. 295–302, 2010.

[77] A. Campbell, M. Sullivan, R. Sherman, and W. P. Magee, "The medical mission and modern cultural competency training," *Journal of the American College of Surgeons*, vol. 212, no. 1, pp. 124–129, 2011.

[78] S. R. Aziz, V. B. Ziccardi, and S.-K. Chuang, "Survey of residents who have participated in humanitarian medical missions," *Journal of Oral and Maxillofacial Surgery*, vol. 70, no. 2, pp. e147–e157, 2012.

[79] R. Riviello, M. S. Lipnick, and D. Ozgediz, "Medical missions, surgical education, and capacity building," *Journal of the American College of Surgeons*, vol. 213, no. 4, pp. 572–574, 2011.

[80] E. P. Nadler, B. C. Nwomeh, W. A. I. Frederick et al., "Academic needs in developing countries: a survey of the West African College of Surgeons," *Journal of Surgical Research*, vol. 160, no. 1, pp. 14–17, 2010.

[81] R. P. Strauss, "The organization and delivery of craniofacial health services: the state of the art," *Cleft Palate-Craniofacial Journal*, vol. 36, no. 3, pp. 189–195, 1999.

[82] O. Aliu and K. C. Chung, "Discussion: the clinical and economic impact of a sustained program in global plastic surgery: valuing cleft care in resource-poor settings," *Plastic and Reconstructive Surgery*, vol. 130, no. 1, pp. 95e–97e, 2012.

[83] M. M. Abbott and J. G. Meara, "Value-based cleft lip-cleft palate care: a progress report," *Plastic and Reconstructive Surgery*, vol. 126, no. 3, pp. 1020–1025, 2010.

[84] R. A. Gosselin, Y. A. Gyamfi, and S. Contini, "Challenges of meeting surgical needs in the developing world," *World Journal of Surgery*, vol. 35, no. 2, pp. 258–261, 2011.

22

Anatomical Variations in Clefts of the Lip with or without Cleft Palate

K. Carroll and P. A. Mossey

Dental Hospital and School, University of Dundee, 1 Park Place, Dundee DD1 4HR, UK

Correspondence should be addressed to K. Carroll, kris.m.carroll@gmail.com and P. A. Mossey, p.a.mossey@dundee.ac.uk

Academic Editor: Nivaldo Alonso

Objective. Few orofacial cleft (OFC) studies have examined the severity of clefts of the lip or palate. This study examined associations between the severity of cleft of the lip with cleft type, laterality, and sex in four regional British Isles cleft registers whilst also looking for regional variations. *Design*. Retrospective analysis of cleft classification in the data contained in these four cleft registers. *Sample*. Three thousand and twelve patients from cleft registers based in Scotland, East England, Merseyside, and Belfast were sourced from the period 2002–2010. Submucous clefts and syndromic clefts were included whilst stillbirths, abortuses, and atypical orofacial clefts were excluded. *Results*. A cleft of the lip in CLP patients is more likely to be complete in males. A cleft of the lip in isolated CL patients is more likely to be complete in females. Variation in the proportion of cleft types was evident between Scotland and East England. *Conclusions*. Association between severity of cleft of the lip and sex was found in this study with females having a significantly greater proportion of more severe clefts of the lip (CL) and CLP males being more severe ($P < 0.0003$). This finding supports a fundamental difference between cleft aetiology between CL and CLP.

1. Introduction

Maintaining a register of children born with orofacial clefts is recognised as important with regards to audit, research, and the planning and provision of services [1]. The use of a simple classification, such as the LAHSAL system proposed by Kriens in 1989 [2] to describe clefts is recognised as being of prime importance and allows for the accurate recording of cleft types and comparison between locations [3].

The evidence available at a global and European level indicates very significant regional variation in the birth prevalence of orofacial clefts, both cleft palate (CP) and cleft lip and palate (CLP) [4]. It is well known that the aetiology of orofacial clefts is characterised by heterogeneity and that the aetiology is polygenic multifactorial with both environmental and genetic factors contributing to nonsyndromic type [5], which comprises approximately 70% of all orofacial clefts.

The increase in CP seen in some UK studies and in parts of Scandinavia may be as a result of factors associated with their northern position [6]. The proportion of CP in Sweden

was shown to increase with the increase in latitude at which the comparison was carried out [7].

Several studies have shown that females are affected more often than males with regards to isolated CP [6, 8, 9]. Conversely, a predilection for the male sex is observed in clefts involving the lip [9, 10].

With regards to laterality, most studies show a left-sided dominance of clefts involving the lip [11–13]. Contrasting results have been obtained upon examining for a link between sex and laterality. In South-East Scotland, a male dominance for left-sided clefts was recorded [14]. Despite an earlier report in Northern Ireland of a predilection for right-sided clefting in females, a subsequent analysis over a twenty-year period failed to find an association between sex and laterality [15].

Animal studies have shown that during development, the left palatal shelf takes longer to rotate into the horizontal position leaving this side susceptible to developmental interruption for longer [16]. A suggested reason for this is the lower arterial pressure on the left side compared to the internal carotid artery on the right side [13]. Conversely with regard to all other external congenital anomalies, an excess on the right side has been noted [17].

A possible hypothesis for this is revealed in rat embryos where the mitochondrial maturation rate is delayed on the right side making this side more susceptible to prenatal hypoxia [17]. Although this right-sided correlation for most congenital anomalies is not replicated in orofacial clefts, the author goes on to explain that male sex hormones lower mitochondrial respiration rates which could help to explain the male predominance of CL.

Very significant progress has been made in recent years with respect to genetic determinants and a range of environmental risk factors [18]. Current research has resultantly focussed on finding out more about the interactions between genes and environment, the influence of epigenetics, and the targeting of environmental factors that in the presence of genetic polymorphisms become teratogenic.

Research in this field in the past has been hampered by individual population studies, small sample sizes, pooling of a range of different cleft phenotypes in a single analysis, and potentially masking any differences between different subphenotypes of clefts.

One aim of this study was to profile the details of cleft lip ± palate patients from four British Isles cleft registers, recorded in accordance with the LAHSAL system. The majority of papers that have profiled cleft registers do so with regard to the relative proportions of cleft type, sex and laterality. Emphasis has recently been placed on elucidating further subphenotypes associated with orofacial clefts and determining characteristics such as heritability and transmission patterns of orofacial cleft subphenotypes [18]. Research has been carried out to determine further subphenotypes of clefts, including parental features, in order to help unravel the genetic basis for the condition [19].

A further aim of this study was to analyse the registers with regards to the severity of the cleft of the lip and possible associations with laterality and sex. Until recently, the importance of the severity of the cleft of the lip was described only in relation to the optimum timing of surgery and the surgical technique involved [20]. Criticism has recently been apportioned to the recording of cleft type by its presence or absence as being too simplistic which may hamper the genetic determination of orofacial clefts [18]. The identification of subphenotypes within cleft lip could aid recurrence risk estimations and help to refine gene mapping. The profiling of the "severity of cleft" subphenotype in conjunction with the other main variables may present a finding that is relevant as an expression of the genetic and environmental factors underpinning clefts.

2. Method

A retrospective study was undertaken to identify all children born with a cleft of the lip ± cleft palate in the areas covered by the cleft registers in Scotland, East England, Belfast, and Mersey during the period January 2002 to April 2010. The criteria for entering clefts onto the databases were similar in all 4 regions in that abortuses, stillbirths, and atypical orofacial clefts were excluded. Otherwise all typical clefts of the lip and palate were placed on the register, whether or not they were diagnosed at that point with a syndrome, and submucous clefts if detected were also included.

The purpose of selecting these geographical locations was due to the reported differences in prevalence of the various forms of cleft in these areas. Studies report a majority of cleft palate cases in Scotland [5, 13, 21] and Northern Ireland [8].

The databases were downloaded at the commencement of the study in January 2010. The aim was to record information from anonymised data relating to the cleft type, date of birth, sex, side affected, and the severity of the cleft. The registers were compared by interpreting the LAHSAL code assigned to each patient registered with a cleft, where the letters of LAHSAL represent the two sides of the lip and alveolus (the first L and A indicate the right lip and alveolus) and the hard and soft palate. Upper and lower case letters are used to depict "complete" and "incomplete" clefts.

The definition of complete cleft is an area of contrasting explanations in the literature. For the purpose of this study, "complete cleft" relates to a cleft which involves the full height of the lip to the nasal sill (and therefore is the most severe type), whereas "incomplete cleft" relates to those which only involve a portion of the height of the lip (and is less severe). Many articles refer to a complete cleft as one which communicates between the lip and the palate, that is, CLP.

Whilst bilateral cases were included in the totals of clefts for each region, they were excluded from the analysis examining for a link between cleft type and severity, on the basis of the need to record one type of phenotype per case i.e. some bilateral cleft patients had one complete cleft on one side and an incomplete cleft on the contralateral aspect.

3. Results

In this retrospective comparative analysis of cleft classification of populations contained in four British Isles cleft registers, a total of 3012 patients from cleft registers based in Scotland, East England, Mersey, and Belfast were sourced from the period 2002 to 2010. The number of patients in each category is indicated in the Figure 1 and Tables 1, 2, 3, and 4.

4. Discussion

4.1. Cleft Type Proportions in Scotland and East England. The proportion of cleft palate as a percentage of all clefts in Scotland was 50%. The proportion for CLP was 29%. This finding is in keeping with previous results from the west of Scotland [21] which showed a predominance of cleft palate at 52%. The result for CP is also similar to the 53% figure obtained in N. Ireland [15] which is nearby geographically and could be said to have a similar population to Scotland in the genetic sense. The proportion of CP detected in East England was 43%. This is in keeping with the lower prevalence of CP detected in previous English studies in Birmingham [22], Northumberland [9], and the Trent region [23] which recorded CP at 40%, 33%, and 39%, respectively.

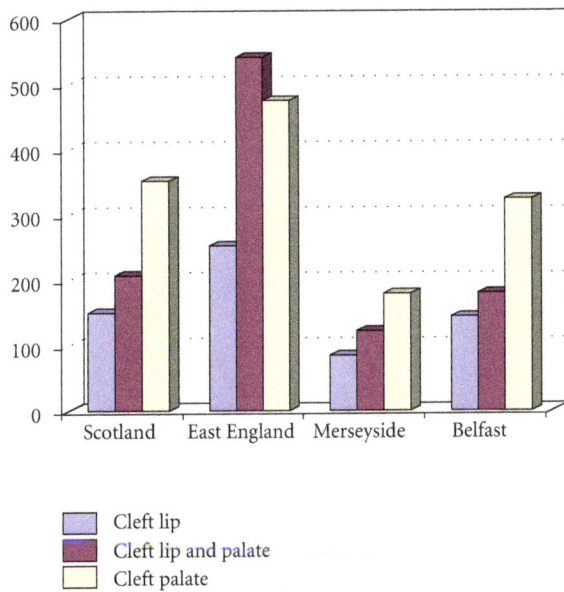

FIGURE 1: The distribution of different types of OFC across 4 UK regions.

TABLE 1: Cleft types in all four UK regions.

	Cleft lip	Cleft lip and palate	Cleft palate
Scotland	150	207	352
East England	253	541	475
Merseyside	85	122	179
Belfast	144	180	324

The prevalence of CLP in Scotland in this study at 29% again compares favourably with the results gained from the west of Scotland [21] in 1987 (34%) and N. Ireland [8] in 1994 (30%). The prevalence obtained from East England in this study was 37%. The same figure of 37% was obtained from Birmingham [22] in 1953 and 36% from Northumberland [9] in 1962. In 1988, Trent region [23] recorded a combined figure for CL and CLP of 61%. The corresponding figure from this study was 57%.

The percentages of cleft type, sex and laterality proportions were found to be very similar between the datasets from Scotland, Merseyside, and Belfast.

4.2. Severity of Cleft—Association with Cleft Type.
In the four registers examined, the cleft in unilateral CL was found to be predominantly incomplete—69%. The opposite was true with unilateral CLP where the cleft of the lip tended to be complete—88%.

Only two previous studies describing the complete versus incomplete proportions of clefts of the lip and palate have been found in the literature in Brazil and Norway. In the Brazilian study from a cleft and craniofacial centre in Bauru, the majority of unilateral cleft lip cases were incomplete [24], while the Norwegian study reported that for CL, 18% were complete clefts of the lip and primary palate, and for CLP 81% of the lips were complete [25]. This represents

consistency in the association between cleft type and the severity of the cleft of the lip. Severity of the cleft of the lip in unilateral CLP was not described in the Brazilian study.

Several studies have shown that comparing congenital anomaly data from different locations can reveal variable characteristics and proportions. A difference in the proportion of cleft types is reported upon in Glasgow in comparison to other locales with the suggestion that this may be due to the interaction of an unidentified environmental teratogen with a susceptible population [21].

An epidemiological study in the UK has shown that true regional variation exists in the prevalence of specific congenital anomalies such as neural tube defects (NTDs), diaphragmatic hernia, and gastroschisis with higher prevalence rates in northern regions such as Glasgow and the north of England [26].

No association could be found regarding the severity of the cleft of the lip and the sex of the patient. Males and females both had a statistically significant level of complete cleft lip in unilateral CLP. While cleft lip is consistently more frequent on the left side, the laterality of the cleft was not associated with the severity of the cleft in either this UK study and the report from Norway. In the Norwegian study it was also reported that in bilateral cleft lip severity was similar on both right and left sides.

4.3. Severity of Cleft—Association with Sex.
Upon combining the data from the four British Isles registers, complete cleft of the lip in CLP patients was found to occur in 90% of males and 85% of females. In isolated CL patients, complete cleft of the lip occurred in 39% of females and 25% of males. Logistic regression analysis of the data revealed that the differences in proportion of complete and incomplete clefts between males and females for these two groups of patients (CL and CLP) were significant ($P < 0.0003$, $\chi^2 = 13.23$).

When CL and CLP patients were considered as one entity, that is, CL $\pm$ P, no association was found between severity of cleft and the sex of the patient ($P < 0.356$, $\chi^2 = 0.852$) or between the severity of cleft and the side affected ($P < 0.530$, $\chi^2 = 0.394$).

This study utilised datasets which excluded atypical lip and facial clefts but did not specifically exclude syndromes which included orofacial clefting as part of the phenotype. The majority of syndromic cleft cases involve patients where the cleft is of the palate only. For example, in Scotland 67% of cases of syndromic clefts where the cleft type was described involved cleft of the palate. This study was concerned with severity of clefts of the lip, and there is evidence of overlap between syndromic and nonsyndromic clefts in terms of aetiology, so for the purposes of this study it was considered acceptable to retain the full data set for the severity analyses.

4.4. The Multifactorial Threshold Model.
The multifactorial threshold (MFT) model is often used to describe the aetiology of orofacial clefting, that is, no one single causative factor accounts for the development of orofacial clefting.

The MFT model does apply to the data in this study when examining the severity of cleft data for cleft lip and

TABLE 2: Cleft lip—severity of cleft according to gender and laterality.

	Scotland		Cambridge		Belfast		Liverpool	
	C	I	C	I	C	I	C	I
Overall	38	95	72	137	39	87	23	53
Males	19	60	36	94	20	57	15	37
Females	19	35	36	43	19	30	8	15
Right side	11	38	24	46	10	35	13	14
Left side	27	57	48	91	29	52	11	38
Males—left	11	34	26	61	13	31	4	28
Females—left	16	23	22	30	16	21	5	10
Males—right	8	26	10	33	7	26	11	9
Females—right	3	12	14	13	3	9	3	5

These figures for CL reveal a reasonable level of consistency across regions in proportions of complete to incomplete clefts with incomplete clefts being consistently more prevalent than complete ones. Also complete clefts of the lip seem to occur more frequently in females. Bilateral clefts were excluded from this analysis.

TABLE 3: Cleft lip and palate—severity of cleft according to gender and laterality.

	Scotland		Cambridge		Belfast		Liverpool	
	C	I	C	I	C	I	C	I
Overall	125	20	273	35	111	17	66	8
Males	81	11	169	17	73	9	55	7
Females	44	9	104	17	38	8	22	2
Right side	52	5	88	16	47	5	23	4
Left side	73	15	185	19	64	12	53	7
Males—left	45	8	115	9	42	6	37	5
Females—left	28	7	70	9	22	6	16	1
Males—right	36	3	54	8	31	3	17	2
Females—right	16	2	34	8	16	2	6	1

These figures for CLP reveal a reasonable level of consistency across regions in proportions of complete to incomplete clefts with complete clefts being consistently more prevalent than incomplete clefts. Bilateral clefts were excluded from this analysis.

TABLE 4: Cleft severity categories for CL and CLP according to sex.

(a)

	Male Cleft lip Incomplete	Female Cleft lip Incomplete	Male Cleft lip Complete	Female Cleft lip Complete
Scotland	60	35	19	19
Cambridge	94	43	36	36
Belfast	57	30	20	19
Liverpool	37	15	15	8

(b)

	Male Cleft lip and palate Incomplete	Female Cleft lip and palate Incomplete	Male Cleft lip and palate Complete	Female Cleft lip and palate Complete
Scotland	11	9	81	44
Cambridge	17	17	169	104
Belfast	9	8	73	38
Liverpool	7	2	55	22

These data reveal that the most common single cleft subphenotype in every region in the UK is a complete cleft of the lip on the left side in a male, with an accompanying cleft of the palate. Bilateral clefts were excluded from this analysis.

palate (CLP) patients. More males than females are affected by CLP as would be predicted by the MFT model; this study shows that more males have a complete cleft of the lip than females. However, for CL the results of this study do not appear to be compatible with the MFT model of aetiology when considering gender and severity combined. The MFT model for isolated cleft lip (CL) would predict more males to be affected by the more severe (complete) cleft of the lip than females. However, the opposite is observed in CL patients, in that females are affected by a complete cleft of the lip more often than males. This points to a different mechanism for the cause or predisposition to CL as opposed to CLP, supporting previous epidemiological findings [27–29] and genetic evidence [30], and thus providing further circumstantial evidence for a different genetic mechanism in these 2 cleft subphenotypes.

5. Conclusion

Cleft lip and cleft lip and palate have traditionally been grouped together epidemiologically as cleft lip ± palate (CL(P)) and considered as one genetic entity in separation from isolated cleft palate (CP), and this has undoubtedly hampered genetic investigations. Based upon the findings in this study relating to severity of cleft and sex, this study provides further evidence that cleft lip may be a distinct genetic entity to cleft lip and palate.

This UK-based study reveals that substantial variation in the proportion of cleft types was evident between Scotland and East England. Furthermore among CLP patients, the cleft of the lip is more severe in males, while the cleft of the lip in isolated CL patients is more severe in females. This association between severity of cleft of the lip and sex was statistically significant ($P < 0.0003$) and supports a fundamental difference between cleft aetiology between CL and CLP.

Further studies are required to determine proportions of cleft severity subphenotypes from centres around the world and to examine possible association with aetiology; more work is also required to standardise and validate the codes in cleft registers to ensure the accuracy and consistency of recording by referring to original clinical photographs and models.

References

[1] M. Hammond and L. Stassen, "Do you care? A national register for cleft lip and palate patients," *British Journal of Orthodontics*, vol. 26, no. 2, pp. 152–157, 1999.

[2] O. Kriens, "LAHSAL—a concise documentation system for cleft lip, alveolus and palate diagnoses," in *What Is Cleft Lip and Palate? A MultidIsciplinary Update*, Thieme, Stuttgart, Germany, 1989.

[3] A. W. Smith, A. K. M. Khoo, and I. T. Jackson, "A modification of the Kernahan 'Y' classification in cleft lip and palate deformities," *Plastic and Reconstructive Surgery*, vol. 102, no. 6, pp. 1842–1847, 1998.

[4] P. A. Mossey and J. Little, "Epidemiology of oral clefts: an international perspective," in *Cleft Lip and Palate: From Origin to Treatment*, D. R. Wyszynski, Ed., pp. 127–158, Oxford University Press, Oxford, UK, 2002.

[5] P. Mossey and J. Little, "Addressing the challenges of cleft lip and palate research in India," *Indian Journal of Plastic Surgery*, vol. 42, no. 1, pp. S9–S18, 2009.

[6] D. R. Fitzpatrick, P. A. M. Raine, and J. G. Boorman, "Facial clefts in the west of Scotland in the period 1980–1984: epidemiology and genetic diagnoses," *Journal of Medical Genetics*, vol. 31, no. 2, pp. 126–129, 1994.

[7] L. Beckman and N. Myrberg, "The incidence of cleft lip and palate in Northern Sweden," *Human Heredity*, vol. 22, no. 5, pp. 417–422, 1972.

[8] T. Gregg, D. Boyd, and A. Richardson, "The incidence of cleft lip and palate in Northern Ireland from 1980–1990," *British Journal of Orthodontics*, vol. 21, no. 4, pp. 387–392, 1994.

[9] G. Knox and F. Braithwaite, "Cleft lips and palates in Northumberland and Durham," *Archives of Disease in Childhood*, vol. 38, pp. 66–70, 1963.

[10] F. Blanco-Davila, "Incidence of cleft lip and palate in the northeast of Mexico: a 10-year study," *The Journal of Craniofacial Surgery*, vol. 14, no. 4, pp. 533–537, 2003.

[11] M. Magdalenić-Meštrović and M. Bagatin, "An epidemiological study of orofacial clefts in Croatia 1988–1998," *Journal of Cranio-Maxillofacial Surgery*, vol. 33, no. 2, pp. 85–90, 2005.

[12] M. M. Elahi, I. T. Jackson, O. Elahi et al., "Epidemiology of cleft lip and cleft palate in Pakistan," *Plastic and Reconstructive Surgery*, vol. 113, no. 6, pp. 1548–1555, 2004.

[13] Y. Shapira, E. Lubit, M. M. Kuftinec, and G. Borell, "The distribution of clefts of the primary and secondary palates by sex, type, and location," *Angle Orthodontist*, vol. 69, no. 6, pp. 523–528, 1999.

[14] T. H. Bellis and B. Wohlgemuth, "The incidence of cleft lip and palate deformities in the south-east of Scotland (1971–1990)," *British Journal of Orthodontics*, vol. 26, no. 2, pp. 121–125, 1999.

[15] T. A. Gregg, A. G. Leonard, C. Hayden, K. E. Howard, and C. F. Coyle, "Birth prevalence of cleft lip and palate in Northern Ireland (1981 to 2000)," *The Cleft Palate-Craniofacial Journal*, vol. 45, no. 2, pp. 141–147, 2008.

[16] A. O. Abubaker and K. J. Benson, *Oral And Maxillofacial Surgery Secrets*, Mosby Elsevier, 2nd edition, 2007.

[17] L. J. Paulozzi and J. M. Lary, "Laterality patterns in infants with external birth defects," *Teratology*, vol. 60, no. 5, pp. 265–271, 1999.

[18] A. Jugessur, P. Farlie, and N. Kilpatrick, "The genetics of isolated orofacial clefts: from genotypes to subphenotypes," *Oral Diseases*, vol. 15, no. 7, pp. 437–453, 2009.

[19] A. Letra, R. Menezes, J. M. Granjeiro, and A. R. Vieira, "Defining subphenotypes for oral clefts based on dental development," *Journal of Dental Research*, vol. 86, no. 10, pp. 986–991, 2007.

[20] S. Yuzuriha, A. K. Oh, and J. B. Mulliken, "Asymmetrical bilateral cleft lip: complete or incomplete and contralateral lesser defect (minor-form, microform, or mini-microform)," *Plastic and Reconstructive Surgery*, vol. 122, no. 5, pp. 1494–1504, 2008.

[21] J. Womersley and D. H. Stone, "Epidemiology of facial clefts," *Archives of Disease in Childhood*, vol. 62, no. 7, pp. 717–720, 1987.

[22] B. McMahon and T. McKeown, "The incidence of harelip and cleft palate related to birth rank and maternal age," *The American Journal of Human Genetics*, vol. 5, pp. 176–183, 1953.

[23] M. A. Coupland and A. I. Coupland, "Seasonality, incidence, and sex distribution of cleft lip and palate births in Trent Region, 1973–1982," *Cleft Palate Journal*, vol. 25, no. 1, pp. 33–37, 1988.

[24] J. A. Freitas, G. S. Dalben, M. Santamaria, and P. Z. Freitas, "Current data on the characterization of oral clefts in Brazil," *Brazilian Oral Research*, vol. 18, no. 2, pp. 128–133, 2004.

[25] A. Sivertsen, A. Wilcox, G. E. Johnson, F. Åbyholm, H. A. Vindenes, and R. T. Lie, "Prevalence of major anatomic variations in oral clefts," *Plastic and Reconstructive Surgery*, vol. 121, no. 2, pp. 587–595, 2008.

[26] J. Rankin, S. Pattenden, L. Abramsky et al., "Prevalence of congenital anomalies in five British regions, 1991–99," *Archives of Disease in Childhood*, vol. 90, no. 5, pp. F374–F379, 2005.

[27] E. W. Harville, A. J. Wilcox, R. T. Lie, H. Vindenes, and F. Åbyholm, "Cleft lip and palate versus cleft lip only: are they distinct defects?" *American Journal of Epidemiology*, vol. 162, no. 5, pp. 448–453, 2005.

[28] O. G. Da Silva Filho, M. Santamaria, G. Da Silva Dalben, and G. Semb, "Prevalence of a Simonart's band in patients with complete cleft lip and alveolus and complete cleft lip and palate," *The Cleft Palate-Craniofacial Journal*, vol. 43, no. 4, pp. 442–445, 2006.

[29] F. Rahimov, M. L. Marazita, A. Visel et al., "Disruption of an AP-2α binding site in an IRF6 enhancer is associated with cleft lip," *Nature Genetics*, vol. 40, no. 11, pp. 1341–1347, 2008.

[30] M. Rittler, J. S. López-Camelo, E. E. Castilla et al., "Preferential associations between oral clefts and other major congenital anomalies," *The Cleft Palate-Craniofacial Journal*, vol. 45, no. 5, pp. 525–532, 2008.

23

The Role of Current Techniques and Concepts in Peripheral Nerve Repair

K. S. Houschyar,[1,2,3] A. Momeni,[1] M. N. Pyles,[1] J. Y. Cha,[1,4] Z. N. Maan,[1] D. Duscher,[5]
O. S. Jew,[1] F. Siemers,[2] and J. van Schoonhoven[3]

[1]Division of Plastic and Reconstructive Surgery, Department of Surgery, Stanford School of Medicine, Stanford, CA 94305, USA
[2]Clinic for Plastic and Reconstructive Surgery, Bergmannstrost Halle, 06112 Halle, Germany
[3]Clinic for Hand Surgery, Rhön-Klinikum AG, 97616 Bad Neustadt an der Saale, Germany
[4]Orthodontic Department, College of Dentistry, Yonsei University, Seoul, Republic of Korea
[5]Section of Plastic and Reconstructive Surgery, Department of Surgery, Johannes Kepler University Linz, 4040 Linz, Austria

Correspondence should be addressed to K. S. Houschyar; khosrow-houschyar@gmx.de

Academic Editor: Georg M. Huemer

Patients with peripheral nerve injuries, especially severe injury, often face poor nerve regeneration and incomplete functional recovery, even after surgical nerve repair. This review summarizes treatment options of peripheral nerve injuries with current techniques and concepts and reviews developments in research and clinical application of these therapies.

1. Introduction

Despite the progress in understanding the pathophysiology of peripheral nervous system injury and regeneration, as well as advancements in microsurgical techniques, peripheral nerve injuries are still a major challenge for reconstructive surgeons. Injuries of the peripheral nerves are common and debilitating, affecting 2.8% of trauma patients and resulting in considerable long-term disability, especially in hand trauma patients [1]. The occurrence of spontaneous axonal regeneration following an insult reflects the tendency of injured peripheral nerves to recover. While their capacity for regeneration is higher than that of the central nervous system, complete recovery is fairly infrequent, misdirected, or associated with debilitating neuropathic pain [1]. In fact, satisfactory outcomes are usually limited to relatively minor injuries and reflect neurapraxia or axonotmesis. A lacerated nerve has no chance of spontaneous recovery, and the discontinuity must be microsurgically repaired. Even patients undergoing immediate nerve repair are subject to a lengthy denervation period of the distal target, given that the rate of regeneration approaches 1 mm/day in humans [2]. The peripheral nervous system (PNS) is also affected by age-related changes. Structural and biochemical changes that result in a slowly progressive loss of neurons and nerve fibers lead to decreased regenerative and reinnervating capabilities of nerve fibers in aged subjects. Achieving better outcomes depends both on the advancements in microsurgical techniques and on the introduction of molecular biology discoveries into clinical practice. The field of peripheral nerve research is dynamically developing and concentrates on more sophisticated approaches tested at the basic science level. In this chapter we review future directions in peripheral nerve reconstruction focusing on tolerance induction and minimal immunosuppression for nerve allografting, cell based supportive therapies, and bioengineering of nerve conduits.

2. Classification of Nerve Injuries

The classification of nerve injuries, originally proposed by Seddon in 1943 (three degrees of injury) and Sunderland in 1951 (five degrees of injury), was subsequently expanded by Mackinnon to include a sixth category representing a mixed injury pattern [3]. The level and degree of injury are important in determining treatment. In the Mackinnon

TABLE 1: Neurosensory impairment classification according to Sunderland and Seddon.

		Classification of nerve injury		
Sunderland	Seddon	Injury	Neurosensory impairment	Recovery potential
I	Neuropraxia	Intrafascicular oedema, conduction block	Neuritis, paresthesia	Full (1 day to 1 week)
		Possible segmental demyelination	Neuritis, paresthesia	Full (1 to 2 months)
II		Axon severed, endoneurial tube intact	Paresthesia, episodic dysesthesia	Full (2 to 4 months)
III	Axonotmesis	Endoneurial tube torn	Paresthesia, dysesthesia	Slow, incomplete (12 months)
IV		Only epineurium intact	Hypoesthesia, dysesthesia, and neuroma formation	Neuroma in continuity
V	Neurotmesis	Loss of continuity	Anaesthetic, intractable pain, and neuroma formation	None
VI		Combination of above	Combination of above	Unpredictable

classification, first-, second-, and third-degree injuries have the potential for recovery and for the most part do not require surgical intervention [3]. With a first-degree injury, the nerve temporarily loses conductive signaling activity but the axonal bundle remains intact. This type of injury recovers function within three months. A second-degree injury recovers slowly at a rate of 1 inch per month. With this injury type, the axon suffers damage but the connective tissue surrounding the nerve remains intact. Because of this, the nerve is able to regenerate completely. Third-degree injuries involve injury to the endoneurium while sparing the epineurium and perineurium. These injuries do not recover well without surgical intervention. Recovery is slow and often incomplete. Fourth- and fifth-degree injuries are more severe and will not recover without surgical intervention. In fourth-degree injury, only the epineurium is intact and in fifth-degree injury, the entire nerve is transected. A sixth degree represents a combination of any of the previous five levels of injury.

The classification of injury type is useful to understand the prognosis and the likelihood of complete recovery. Because of the longitudinal nature of crushing injuries, different levels of nerve injury can be seen at various locations along the nerve. This is the most challenging nerve injury for the surgeon as some fascicles will need to be protected and not "downgraded," whereas others will require surgical reconstruction (Table 1).

3. Pathophysiology of Nerve Degeneration and Regeneration

After a nerve is severed, the distal portion begins to degenerate as a result of protease activity and separation from the metabolic resources of the nerve cell bodies. Wallerian degeneration of the distal stump involves invasion by myelomonocytic cells that destroy myelin and initiate mitosis in Schwann cells. Degeneration of the distal axon ends presumably occurs by autolytic mechanisms (Figure 1(a)). The cytoskeleton begins to breakdown, followed by dissolution of the cell membrane. The proximal end of the nerve stump swells but experiences only minimal damage via retrograde degradation [4]. After the cytoskeleton and membrane degrade, Schwann cells surrounding the distal portion of the axon shed their myelin lipids. Phagocytotic cells, such as macrophages and Schwann cells, clear myelin and axonal debris. In addition to clearing myelin debris, macrophages and Schwann cells also produce cytokines (interleukin-6), which enhance axon growth [5]. Following debris clearance, regeneration begins in the proximal severed end and continues toward the distal stump. New axonal sprouts usually emanate from the nodes of Ranvier, which represent nonmyelinated areas of axon located between Schwann cells. The Schwann cells help to guide the cytoplasmic extensions of the axonal sprout between the basement membrane of two nerve ends [6]. Functional reinnervation requires that axons extend until they reach their distal target. In humans, axon regeneration occurs at a rate of ~1 mm/day; thus, significant injuries can take months to heal [7]. This reinnervation is not without complication or resultant dysfunction. Uncontrolled branching of growing axons at the lesion site and misdirection of axons and target organ reinnervation errors are common complications [8]. The central nervous system's regeneration capacity is not very appreciable compared to the peripheral nervous since. Although astrocytes within the CNS proliferate in a similar manner to that of Schwann cells in the PNS, instead they become "reactive astrocytes" in the CNS, producing glial scars that inhibit regeneration (Figure 1(b)).

4. Nerve Repair

Direct nerve repair with epineural microsutures is still the gold standard surgical treatment for severe axonotmesis and neurotmesis injuries. Epineural repair is performed when a tension-free coaptation can be achieved in a well-vascularized bed which was developed by Millesi. Gross fascicular matching between the proximal and distal nerve ends results from lining up both the internal nerve fascicles and the surface epineural blood vessel patterns.

Other repairs include grouped fascicular repair requiring intranerve dissection and direct matching and suturing of fascicular groups [9]. This is more practical distally in a major peripheral limb nerve. However, the theoretical advantages of better fascicle alignment with this technique are offset by increased trauma and scarring to the healing nerve internally due to the presence of permanent sutures. Despite

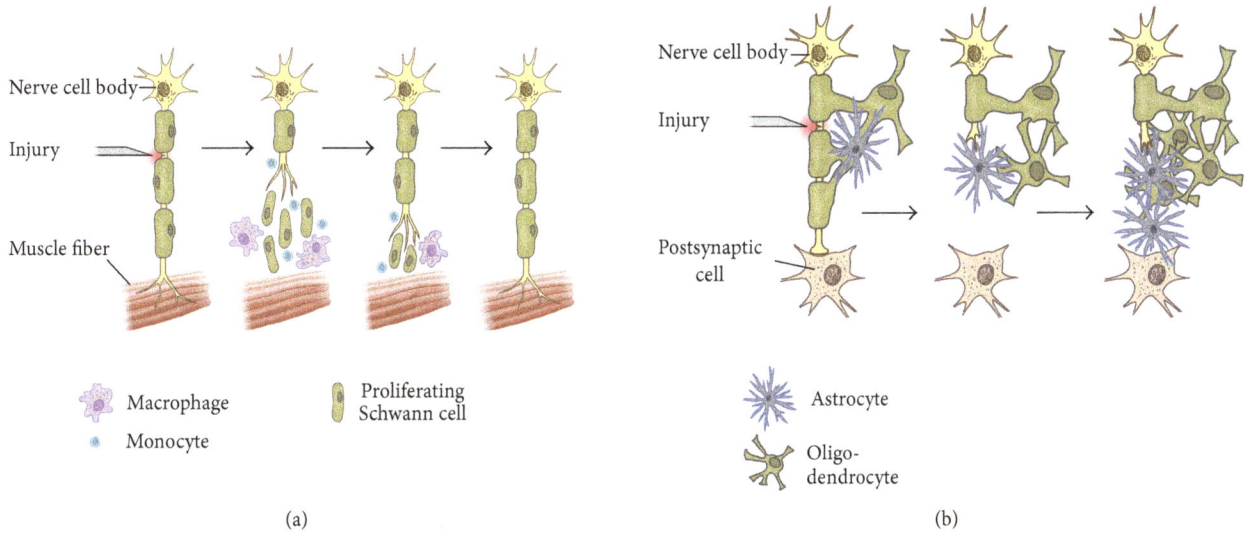

FIGURE 1: (a) In the PNS, support cells aid neuronal regeneration. Proliferating Schwann cells, macrophages, and monocytes work together to remove myelin debris, release neurotrophins, and lead axons toward their synaptic targets, resulting in restored neuronal function. (b) In the CNS, however, the few neurons that survive axotomy attempt regeneration and subsequently meet an impenetrable glial scar composed myelin and cellular debris, as well as astrocytes, oligodendrocytes, and microglia. Fibroblasts, monocytes, and macrophages may also be present in the glial scar. Consequently, regenerating neurons in the spinal cord are blocked from reaching their synaptic target.

its anatomical attractiveness, overall group fascicular repair is no better than epineural repair in functional outcomes [10].

5. Surgical Alternative to Nerve Repair: Nerve Transfers

The definition of nerve transfer is the surgical coaptation of a healthy nerve donor to a denervated nerve. This is usually reserved for important motor nerve reconstruction although it can equally be applied to critical sensory nerves. Nerve transfers use an expendable motor donor nerve to a less important limb muscle [11]. The nerve is cut and then joined to the injured distal end of the prioritized motor nerve.

The benefits of nerve transfers are well described. In most cases there is only one neurorrhaphy site; with nerve grafts, there are two. In addition, nerve transfers minimize the distance over which a nerve has to regenerate because it is closer to the target organ and is more specific [12]. Pure motor donors are joined to motor nerves and sensory donors to sensory nerves, optimizing regeneration potential. As opposed to a tendon transfer, when a nerve transfer is successful, recovered function is similar to the original muscle function because synchronous physiologic motion may be achieved. With quicker nerve recovery, more rapid motor reeducation is also possible. The goal is to maximize functional recovery with fast reinnervation of denervated motor targets. The most common applications of motor nerve transfers include the restoration of elbow flexion, shoulder abduction, ulnar-innervated intrinsic hand function, radial nerve function, and smile reconstruction from facial nerve palsy [13]. Aszmann et al. reported about a case series of three patients who were treated successfully with bionic reconstruction to restore hand function after brachial plexus

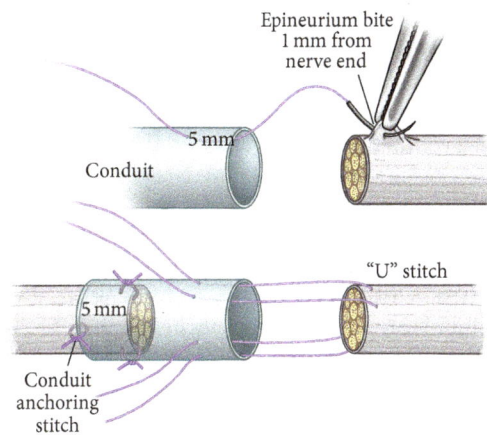

FIGURE 2: Picture showing a vein conduit used to bridge traumatic nerve laceration.

injury [14]. Another publication discussed the role and mechanism of brain plasticity in nerve regeneration [15].

6. Role of Alternative Repair Strategies

6.1. Nerve Conduits. Studies show that nerves will regenerate across a short nerve gap through various conduits, such as veins, pseudosheaths, and bioabsorbable tubes [16]. Figure 2 demonstrates a commonly available vein conduit used to bridge a nerve laceration. When a hollow nerve conduit is used to repair a severed peripheral nerve, an additional step for regeneration is required [17]. After injury, a fibrin bridge is formed through the conduit and across the defect site. This fibrin cable includes macrophages and other cells thought to be involved in debris clearance. The fibrin bridge retracts as Schwann cells and capillaries begin to grow across the gap, and regeneration proceeds as normal [18]. It is not clear if the formation of a fibrin cable also occurs in the absence of a conduit or when a conduit contains an internal matrix.

The characteristics of the ideal nerve conduit include low antigenicity, availability, and biodegradability. The benefits of vein grafts have been used to reconstruct distal sensory nerve defects of less than 3 cm. Sensory results with vein grafts have been acceptable but not as good as conventional grafting [19]. For this reason, vein grafts are recommended only for reconstruction of noncritical nerve gaps of less than 3 cm [20].

Nerve regeneration across a 3 cm gap through a biodegradable polyglycolic nerve tube has been demonstrated in the primate model and in a clinical trial [9]. Clinical recovery was comparable to that across an autologous nerve graft. The insertion of a short piece of nerve graft material into the center of the conduit will enhance regeneration by providing a local source of trophic factors [21]. The ready availability of biodegradable synthetic grafts to span short nerve gaps would eliminate the morbidity associated with nerve graft harvest and would capitalize on the potential benefits of neurotropism in directing nerve regeneration. Synthetic nerve conduits are now available for reconstruction of small diameter nerves with a gap ≤ 3 cm, or with large diameter nerves with gaps ≤ 0.5 cm [22]. Lohmeyer et al. could show that the long-term recovery of sensibility after digital nerve tubulization depends on the nerve gap length with better results in those <10 mm. Nerve regeneration after tubulization seems not to be terminated after 12 months. Manoli et al. demonstrated that muscle-in-vein conduits may be a good alternative solution to autografts for the reconstruction of digital nerves. Siemers et al. presented various tubulization possibilities, including their limitations. In summary, the use of nerve conduits has evolved from an experimental idea to a clinical reality over the last twenty years.

6.2. Nerve Autografts and Allografts. In patients with larger nerve gaps where the injury must be bridged, use of an autograft remains the most reliable repair technique [23]. Whereas nerve conduits rely on fibrin clot stability, a nerve graft provides original internal scaffolding with hundreds to thousands of basal lamina tubes to support Schwann cell and axon migration. The three major types of autografts are cable grafts, trunk grafts, and vascularized nerve grafts [10]. Cable grafts are several sections of small nerve grafts aligned in parallel to connect fascicular groups. Trunk grafts are mixed motor and sensory grafts. Trunk grafts have poor functional results due to their instability and large diameters which inhibits its ability to properly revascularize the center of the graft. Vascularized nerve grafts have the advantage that there is no period of ischemia compared to nonvascularized grafts and the necessity for revascularization is avoided; however there have been conflicting results demonstrating

their clinical superiority over nonvascularized grafts. Sensory donor nerves are most often used, with the sural nerve being the most commonly harvested. Furthermore, it is commonly advised to choose a graft that is 10% to 20% longer than the existing nerve gap to ensure a tension-free repair [23]. Although no large clinical studies exist comparing these techniques, in cases where the diameter is mismatched, the most commonly used approach is the use of cable grafts.

Nerve allografts have demonstrated clinical utility in repairing extensive peripheral nerve injuries where there is a paucity of donor nerve material [23]. Allografts used in peripheral nerve injuries are commercially processed to be cell and protein free. This allows the nerve allograft to serve as a scaffold that is repopulated by host axons and Schwann cells over time. As a result, it challenges the immune system for only a limited period of time. Tacrolimus has been successfully used in patients treated with peripheral nerve allografts, with its beneficial effects being explained by its dual function as an immunosuppressive and neuroregenerative agent [24]. Like autografts, the nerve allograft provides a scaffold for nerve regeneration but has the potential for shorter operative time, abundant supply, and lack of donor site morbidity. Potential candidates for peripheral nerve allotransplantation receive nerve allografts from donors that have been screened for ABO blood typing, HIV, and cytomegalovirus [25]. A recent multicenter retrospective study evaluated seventy-six nerve repairs performed at various centers in a relatively heterogeneous group (forty-nine sensory, eighteen mixed, and nine motor) using processed human nerve allograft [26]. Subgroup analysis was performed to determine the influence of nerve type, gap length, patient age, time to repair, age of injury, and mechanism of injury on outcomes. Griffin et al. reported significant recovery in 87.3% of subjects across subgroups using both qualitative and quantitative outcome measures, with no response to treatment in eight of the subjects [27]. There were no graft-related adverse effects. Additionally, the study showed functional recovery in nerve gaps up to 50 mm.

Immunogenicity has historically been a concern with allografts [28]. Although graft Schwann cells display major histocompatibility complexes that incite a T-cell response, host Schwann cell proliferation and irradiation of the graft improve regeneration and histologic outcome in animal models. Karabekmez et al. retrospectively studied short-term sensory recovery after decellularized cadaveric nerve transplantation in seven patients with ten nerve gaps, eight digital and two ulnar sensory [28]. They examined 2-point discrimination and found that all patients recovered 10 mm or better static 2-point discrimination with five good results and five excellent results with no cases of infection or rejection. Although larger randomized studies are needed, for small gaps up to 3 cm, allograft outcomes may be comparable with that of conduits in sensory outcome. Ray et al. reported success in a mouse model with cold preservation for four weeks to decrease immunogenicity [16]. Whereas most studies have focused on sensory recovery, a recent study design compared motor recovery of autograft to allograft and collagen conduit in rat sciatic nerve gap lesions and found autograft superior to allograft at sixteen weeks postoperatively in terms of

TABLE 2: Various growth factors to promote peripheral nerve regeneration.

Growth factor	Main target
NGF	Sensory neurons and small axons
BDNF	Sensory neurons and large axons
CNTF	Sciatic nerve
IGF-1	Inflammatory cells and sensory and motor neurons
VEGF	Vascular endothelial cells

isometric strength recovery [27]. Allograft and autograft were superior ($p \leq 0.05$) to collagen conduit. Despite this headway, more development is needed prior to recommending allograft use over autograft for longer nerve gaps. In summary, the current gold standard procedure to bridge damaged peripheral nerves is the use of autologous nerve grafts.

6.3. Growth Factors. More recently, studies have demonstrated the efficacy of applying growth factors to the nerve conduit lumen [18]. Studies on the use of various growth factors to promote peripheral nerve regeneration have gradually increased (Table 2), with an improved understanding of neurotrophic components that are released from nerve endings and their effect on nerve growth and differentiation. These neurotrophic factors, expressed at different intervals during nerve regeneration to accelerate axonal growth, include nerve growth factor (NGF), brain derived neurotrophic factor (BDNF), ciliary neurotrophic factor (CNTF), and insulin-like growth factor-1 (IGF-1), all of which are secreted from Schwann cells [29].

Fibroblast growth factors (FGFs) have a significant role in cell growth and regeneration and are released from damaged nerve ending [30]. Subsequent studies have worked on combining FGF with structural components. Midha et al. used synthetic tube bridge material with 10 lg/mL of FGF-1 and collagen matrix in a nerve defect of 10 mm and determined an increase only in regeneration in comparison with the collagen matrix group [31]. After facial nerve decompression surgery, Hato et al. applied basic-FGF-impregnated biodegradable gelatin around the regenerating exposed nerve and found an increased complete recovery rate compared to conventional surgery, demonstrating the efficacy of FGF in enhancing peripheral nerve regeneration [32]. While the mechanism for aFGFs efficacy is unclear, there are various theories, including an increase in the number of Schwann cells in the field of the nerve cut, an enhanced neovascular response, a survival advantage for the injured nerve cells, and a trophic effect for ensuring the continuity of newly occurred axons.

Neuron growth factor (NGF) plays an important role in physiological nerve healing and regeneration [33]. NGF immobilized on gelatin membranes, or PLGL scaffolds, promotes Schwann cell adhesion and survival in vitro and neurite outgrowth from pheochromocytoma cells, indicating this approach is potentially useful for the generation of nerve conduits for clinical nerve repair. Insertion of Schwann cells into the conduit is a relatively simple method that also increases production of NGF [34]. First evidences indicate

that a controlled release of NGF by microspheres, or by adenoviruses expressing this factor, increases the functional recovery of injured peripheral nerves. Although the organic solvent used for the NGF-microspheres production might compromise NGF activity, the possibility of directly adding NGF to nerve conduits has not been studied as an alternative for local treatments.

Glial growth factor (GGF), another epidermal growth factor, is released from neurons that has been shown to induce Schwann cell proliferation [35]. It plays a role in the interaction between neuronal and glial cells with respect to peripheral nerve healing. GGF applied into a conduit for defects of 2–4 cm in a rabbit peroneal nerve model increased the number of newly formed Schwann cells, significantly improved axonal regeneration, and considerably decreased the muscle mass lost in comparison with the control group [36]. Ciliary neurotrophic factor (CNTF) is contained in the cytoplasm of myelin Schwann cells and increases neuron survival following axotomy [37]. It is directly released from the circumference of the neuron. It has been used within silicone conduits in rat sciatic nerve defects of 10 mm and has increased the diameter and number of axons, myelinization, and motor nerve conduction rate, thereby increasing the amplitude of muscle action in comparison with controls [37].

Vascular endothelial growth factor (VEGF) is best described for its influence on endothelial cell biology and its role in neovascularization; however, it has been reported that VEGF also has positive effects on nerve regeneration [38]. Hobson et al. demonstrated that a laminin-based gel (Matrigel) and VEGF (500–700 ng/mL) applied to a silicone conduit in a 1 cm rat sciatic nerve defect enhanced blood vessel penetration around nerve cells and increased Schwann cell migration and axonal regeneration [39]. In summary, impregnation of neurotrophic factors such as NGF or FGF-1 into fabricated collagen/laminin fibrils represents an exciting new therapeutic paradigm in combination with current surgical techniques.

6.4. Neural Tissue Engineering. Advances in bioengineering provide additional biologically stable materials that have the ability to integrate growth-enhancing agents or factors into the lumen of the conduit. One major drawback for current nerve graft techniques is the requirement of a secondary donor site and subsequently injury and repair site. A combination of tissue engineering with cellular seeding could serve as an alternative for nerve grafts without the need for a secondary surgery. An ideal nerve conduit requires a scaffold that is porous, biocompatible, biodegradable, conductive, and resistant to infections [40]. A major challenge is developing a scaffold that can correctly combine all of the required properties. Additionally, cellular and extracellular matrix alignment is critical for adequate function of biological tissues. Within the nervous system, collagen fibers orientate in response to force vectors and also strengthen the ECM. Much of the research in tissue engineering has focused on the development of anisotropic scaffolds that provide the support associated with properly aligned ECM [41]. With a nerve graft, the aligned Schwann cells are able to support and guide the regenerating neurites at the repair site, and the recreation of this anisotropic 3D cellular architecture is the focus of much research in peripheral nerve repair. Current techniques to develop anisotropic cellular substrates conducive to neural regeneration incorporate the use of Schwann cell-seeded aligned fibers made from synthetic polymers [42], collagen based microstructured 3D nerve guide with longitudinal channels seeded with Schwann cells [43], acellular nerve matrix seeded with adipose-derived stem cells [44], and micropatterned conduits comprised of polylactide tubes seeded with neural stem cells [40].

7. Considerations for Optimizing Stem Cell Therapy for Peripheral Nerve Repair

While a variety of strategies have been developed to enhance neuroregeneration in response to trauma, circumstances in which cell loss is extensive, such as following significant injury or in response to degenerative diseases of the nervous system, will likely require complete cell replacement. In the hope of regenerating tissue through cell replacement, many efforts have focused upon the use of stem cells as a source of "replacement" cells [45]. In this case, the stem cells could be harvested before the reconstructive surgery. Neural stem cells have been isolated from rodent brain, spinal cord, skeletal muscle, and bone marrow.

Bone marrow stromal cells, also known as mesenchymal stem cells (MSCs), have been transdifferentiated successfully into neural cells [46]. As MSCs can be isolated relatively easily from bone marrow aspirates and expanded in culture, they provide an interesting alternative to Schwann cell transplantation. Upon implantation of the NC into a rat sciatic nerve gap of 5 mm, functional recovery in terms of conduction velocity and sciatic functional index was significantly improved as compared with MSC-free control NC [47]. Functional recovery was similar to that obtained with a NC loaded with Schwann cells. The similar outcome of the two cell-loaded NC groups is quite remarkable considering that only about 5% of the MSCs transdifferentiated into a Schwann cell-like phenotype, while the major cell population maintained an undifferentiated phenotype, as evidenced by S100 protein staining [47]. The paracrine effects of MSCs likely play a role in the observed phenotype, along with deposition of basal lamina components [48]. Although the mechanism of MSC transdifferentiation and the molecular cross talk between MSCs and peripheral nerves are not fully understood, MSCs may become a promising and abundant therapeutic source for cell based approaches to nerve regeneration [49].

One study compared the neural differentiation capacity between human muscle-derived stem cells and human adipose-derived stem cells (hADSCs) in vitro and found that neural differentiated hADSCs had significantly higher levels of mRNA and protein of neuronal marker β-tubulin III and glial marker GFAP compared to neural differentiated hMDSCs demonstrating that hADSCs have a higher differentiation capacity compared to hMDSCs [50]. In murine models, human muscle-derived stem cells have also shown the potentiation to adopt into neuronal tissues [51]. When adult human skeletal muscle-derived stem cells (hMDSCs) were transplanted into a sciatic nerve injury site, engraftment of hMDSCs promoted axonal regeneration which led to functional recovery without any adverse effects 18 months after the transplant [51]. These data demonstrate the potential to use hMDSCs in the treatment of human neuropathies.

Incidentally, stem cells have also been isolated from hair follicles and have adopted Schwann cell characteristics when placed between the stumps of a transected peripheral nerve [52]. However, extraction of a high number of hair follicle stem cells seems more laborious than harvesting MSC. Interestingly, 2–5 weeks after transplantation, stem cells implanted in injured rat spinal cords have survived; differentiated into neurons, astrocytes, and oligodendrocytes; and migrated up to 8 mm from the lesion. Rats receiving the transplanted stem cells showed improved functional recovery [53]. Similarly, other studies have also found that stem cells implanted into injured spinal cord differentiate into neurons and glial cells [4]. Consequently, it has been suggested that the environment is a greater factor in neural stem cell fate than the intrinsic properties of the cell. Greater control over stem cell differentiation, by in vitro treatments or by using stem cells that are restricted to the neuronal lineage, may allow stem cell transplantation to yield more predictable results. In summary, bone marrow stem cells have been shown to be capable of differentiating into neuronal and glial phenotypes and the clinical use of bone marrow stem cells should be investigated in the future.

8. Electrical Stimulation

There have been limited reports of applying electrical fields/gradients across a repaired peripheral nerve to speed up axonal regeneration. Animal studies demonstrate that as little as one hour of direct nerve electrical stimulation immediately after repair of a transected femoral nerve in the rat promotes a dramatic increase in the kinetics of target muscle reinnervation [54].

In a clinical pilot study, one hour of electrical stimulation was applied after median nerve decompression at the wrist for 21 patients with carpal tunnel syndrome and thenar atrophy [55]. The electrical stimulation group showed evidence of accelerated axonal regeneration and reinnervation evidenced by motor unit number estimation and sensory and motor nerve conduction studies.

9. Conclusions

The requirements for functional nerve regeneration are complex. However, through the combined efforts of scientists and engineers from a variety of disciplines, experimental work in this field has made great progress. While nerve grafting is often the clinical gold standard for larger nerve injuries, recent developments utilizing growth factors, stem cells, and nerve conduits should extend the realm of possibilities of peripheral nerve repair. New potential targets for novel therapies have been discovered through an increased understanding of the molecular biology of neural development and regeneration. Tissue engineering and nanotechnology are suggesting new research therapeutic approaches, potentially orientated to accelerate nerve regeneration and recovery of nerve functionality. As discussed in this review, many significant advances in nerve repair and regeneration have been achieved. Further studies will continue to advance the field of therapeutics in regeneration of the PNS. We are on the verge of a breakthrough in our current understanding that can potentially transform the field of peripheral nerve repair, ultimately offering new options to patients with severe nerve injuries.

References

[1] S. Walsh and R. Midha, "Practical considerations concerning the use of stem cells for peripheral nerve repair," *Neurosurgical focus*, vol. 26, no. 2, p. E2, 2009.

[2] S. Jonsson, R. Wiberg, A. M. McGrath et al., "Effect of delayed peripheral nerve repair on nerve regeneration, Schwann cell function and target muscle recovery," *PLoS ONE*, vol. 8, no. 2, Article ID e56484, 2013.

[3] W. W. Campbell, "Evaluation and management of peripheral nerve injury," *Clinical Neurophysiology*, vol. 119, no. 9, pp. 1951–1965, 2008.

[4] S. Hall, "The response to injury in the peripheral nervous system," *The Journal of Bone and Joint Surgery—British Volume*, vol. 87, no. 10, pp. 1309–1319, 2005.

[5] P. Dubový, I. Klusáková, and I. Hradilová Svíženská, "Inflammatory profiling of Schwann cells in contact with growing axons distal to nerve injury," *BioMed Research International*, vol. 2014, Article ID 691041, 7 pages, 2014.

[6] R. Deumens, A. Bozkurt, M. F. Meek et al., "Repairing injured peripheral nerves: bridging the gap," *Progress in Neurobiology*, vol. 92, no. 3, pp. 245–276, 2010.

[7] M. G. Burnett and E. L. Zager, "Pathophysiology of peripheral nerve injury: a brief review," *Neurosurgical Focus*, vol. 16, no. 5, article E1, 2004.

[8] J. Valls-Sole, C. D. Castillo, J. Casanova-Molla, and J. Costa, "Clinical consequences of reinnervation disorders after focal peripheral nerve lesions," *Clinical Neurophysiology*, vol. 122, no. 2, pp. 219–228, 2011.

[9] L. M. Wolford and E. L. Stevao, "Considerations in nerve repair," *Proceedings/Baylor University Medical Center*, vol. 16, no. 2, pp. 152–156, 2003.

[10] A. Faroni, S. A. Mobasseri, P. J. Kingham, and A. J. Reid, "Peripheral nerve regeneration: experimental strategies and future perspectives," *Advanced Drug Delivery Reviews*, vol. 82-83, pp. 160–167, 2015.

[11] C. P. White, M. J. Cooper, J. R. Bain, and C. M. Levis, "Axon counts of potential nerve transfer donors for peroneal nerve reconstruction," *Canadian Journal of Plastic Surgery*, vol. 20, no. 1, pp. 24–27, 2012.

[12] D. Grinsell and C. P. Keating, "Peripheral nerve reconstruction after injury: a review of clinical and experimental therapies," *BioMed Research International*, vol. 2014, Article ID 698256, 13 pages, 2014.

[13] R. Tse, S. H. Kozin, M. J. Malessy, and H. M. Clarke, "International federation of societies for surgery of the hand committee report: the role of nerve transfers in the treatment of neonatal brachial plexus palsy," *The Journal of Hand Surgery*, vol. 40, no. 6, pp. 1246–1259, 2015.

[14] O. C. Aszmann, A. D. Roche, S. Salminger et al., "Bionic reconstruction to restore hand function after brachial plexus injury: a case series of three patients," *The Lancet*, vol. 385, no. 9983, pp. 2183–2189, 2015.

[15] C. B. Mohanty, D. Bhat, and B. I. Devi, "Role of central plasticity in the outcome of peripheral nerve regeneration," *Neurosurgery*, vol. 77, no. 3, pp. 418–423, 2015.

[16] W. Z. Ray, S. S. Kale, R. Kasukurthi et al., "Effect of cold nerve allograft preservation on antigen presentation and rejection: laboratory investigation," *Journal of Neurosurgery*, vol. 114, no. 1, pp. 256–262, 2011.

[17] E. Karacaolu, F. Yksel, F. Peker, and M. M. Gler, "Nerve regeneration through an epineurial sheath: its functional aspect compared with nerve and vein grafts," *Microsurgery*, vol. 21, no. 5, pp. 196–201, 2001.

[18] X. Gu, F. Ding, Y. Yang, and J. Liu, "Construction of tissue engineered nerve grafts and their application in peripheral nerve regeneration," *Progress in Neurobiology*, vol. 93, no. 2, pp. 204–230, 2011.

[19] M. Y. Lin, G. Manzano, and R. Gupta, "Nerve allografts and conduits in peripheral nerve repair," *Hand Clinics*, vol. 29, no. 3, pp. 331–348, 2013.

[20] F. J. Paprottka, P. Wolf, Y. Harder et al., "Sensory recovery outcome after digital nerve repair in relation to different reconstructive techniques: meta-analysis and systematic review," *Plastic Surgery International*, vol. 2013, Article ID 704589, 17 pages, 2013.

[21] P. Konofaos and J. P. Ver Halen, "Nerve repair by means of tubulization: past, present, future," *Journal of Reconstructive Microsurgery*, vol. 29, no. 3, pp. 149–163, 2013.

[22] G. C. W. de Ruiter, M. J. A. Malessy, M. J. Yaszemski, A. J. Windebank, and R. J. Spinner, "Designing ideal conduits for peripheral nerve repair," *Neurosurgical Focus*, vol. 26, no. 2, article E5, 2009.

[23] W. Z. Ray and S. E. Mackinnon, "Management of nerve gaps: autografts, allografts, nerve transfers, and end-to-side neurorrhaphy," *Experimental Neurology*, vol. 223, no. 1, pp. 77–85, 2010.

[24] D. P. Kuffler, "Chapter 18. Enhancement of nerve regeneration and recovery by immunosuppressive agents," *International Review of Neurobiology*, vol. 87, pp. 347–362, 2009.

[25] L. D. Bozulic, W. C. Breidenbach, and S. T. Ildstad, "Past, present, and future prospects for inducing donor-specific transplantation tolerance for composite tissue allotransplantation," *Seminars in Plastic Surgery*, vol. 21, no. 4, pp. 213–225, 2007.

[26] D. N. Brooks, R. V. Weber, J. D. Chao et al., "Processed nerve allografts for peripheral nerve reconstruction: a multicenter study of utilization and outcomes in sensory, mixed, and motor nerve reconstructions," *Microsurgery*, vol. 32, no. 1, pp. 1–14, 2012.

[27] J. W. Griffin, M. V. Hogan, A. B. Chhabra, and D. N. Deal, "Peripheral nerve repair and reconstruction," *The Journal of Bone & Joint Surgery—American Volume*, vol. 95, no. 23, pp. 2144–2151, 2013.

[28] F. E. Karabekmez, A. Duymaz, and S. L. Moran, "Early clinical outcomes with the use of decellularized nerve allograft for

repair of sensory defects within the hand," *Hand*, vol. 4, no. 3, pp. 245–249, 2009.

[29] S. J. Allen, J. J. Watson, D. K. Shoemark, N. U. Barua, and N. K. Patel, "GDNF, NGF and BDNF as therapeutic options for neurodegeneration," *Pharmacology and Therapeutics*, vol. 138, no. 2, pp. 155–175, 2013.

[30] A. Baird, "Fibroblast growth factors: activities and significance of non-neurotrophin neurotrophic growth factors," *Current Opinion in Neurobiology*, vol. 4, no. 1, pp. 78–86, 1994.

[31] R. Midha, C. A. Munro, P. D. Dalton, C. H. Tator, and M. S. Shoichet, "Growth factor enhancement of peripheral nerve regeneration through a novel synthetic hydrogel tube," *Journal of Neurosurgery*, vol. 99, no. 3, pp. 555–565, 2003.

[32] N. Hato, J. Nota, H. Komobuchi et al., "Facial nerve decompression surgery using bFGF-impregnated biodegradable gelatin hydrogel in patients with bell palsy," *Otolaryngology—Head and Neck Surgery*, vol. 146, no. 4, pp. 641–646, 2012.

[33] F. C. Alsina, F. Ledda, and G. Paratcha, "New insights into the control of neurotrophic growth factor receptor signaling: implications for nervous system development and repair," *Journal of Neurochemistry*, vol. 123, no. 5, pp. 652–661, 2012.

[34] T. Hadlock, C. Sundback, R. Koka, D. Hunter, M. Cheney, and J. Vacanti, "A novel, biodegradable polymer conduit delivers neurotrophins and promotes nerve regeneration," *Laryngoscope*, vol. 109, no. 9, pp. 1412–1416, 1999.

[35] P.-N. Mohanna, R. C. Young, M. Wiberg, and G. Terenghi, "A composite poly-hydroxybutyrate-glial growth factor conduit for long nerve gap repairs," *Journal of Anatomy*, vol. 203, no. 6, pp. 553–565, 2003.

[36] X. Navarro, M. Vivó, and A. Valero-Cabré, "Neural plasticity after peripheral nerve injury and regeneration," *Progress in Neurobiology*, vol. 82, no. 4, pp. 163–201, 2007.

[37] S.-M. Kim, S.-K. Lee, and J.-H. Lee, "Peripheral nerve regeneration using a three dimensionally cultured schwann cell conduit," *Journal of Craniofacial Surgery*, vol. 18, no. 3, pp. 475–488, 2007.

[38] R. Pola, T. R. Aprahamian, M. Bosch-Marcé et al., "Age-dependent VEGF expression and intraneural neovascularization during regeneration of peripheral nerves," *Neurobiology of Aging*, vol. 25, no. 10, pp. 1361–1368, 2004.

[39] M. I. Hobson, C. J. Green, and G. Terenghi, "VEGF enhances intraneural angiogenesis and improves nerve regeneration after axotomy," *Journal of Anatomy*, vol. 197, no. 4, pp. 591–605, 2000.

[40] S.-H. Hsu, C.-H. Su, and I.-M. Chiu, "A novel approach to align adult neural stem cells on micropatterned conduits for peripheral nerve regeneration: a feasibility study," *Artificial Organs*, vol. 33, no. 1, pp. 26–35, 2009.

[41] Y. L. Jung and H. J. Donahue, "Cell sensing and response to micro- and nanostructured surfaces produced by chemical and topographic patterning," *Tissue Engineering*, vol. 13, no. 8, pp. 1879–1891, 2007.

[42] M. Lietz, L. Dreesmann, M. Hoss, S. Oberhoffner, and B. Schlosshauer, "Neuro tissue engineering of glial nerve guides and the impact of different cell types," *Biomaterials*, vol. 27, no. 8, pp. 1425–1436, 2006.

[43] A. Bozkurt, R. Deumens, C. Beckmann et al., "In vitro cell alignment obtained with a Schwann cell enriched microstructured nerve guide with longitudinal guidance channels," *Biomaterials*, vol. 30, no. 2, pp. 169–179, 2009.

[44] Y. Zhang, H. Luo, Z. Zhang et al., "A nerve graft constructed with xenogeneic acellular nerve matrix and autologous adipose-derived mesenchymal stem cells," *Biomaterials*, vol. 31, no. 20, pp. 5312–5324, 2010.

[45] H. Okano, "Identification of neural stem cells in adult human brain: its implication in the strategy for repairing the damaged central nervous system," *Rinsho Shinkeigaku*, vol. 45, no. 11, pp. 871–873, 2005.

[46] U. Galderisi and A. Giordano, "The gap between the physiological and therapeutic roles of mesenchymal stem cells," *Medicinal Research Reviews*, vol. 34, no. 5, pp. 1100–1126, 2014.

[47] M. Karimi, E. Biazar, S. H. Keshel et al., "Rat sciatic nerve reconstruction across a 30 mm defect bridged by an oriented porous PHBV tube with schwann cell as artificial nerve graft," *ASAIO Journal*, vol. 60, no. 2, pp. 224–233, 2014.

[48] K. Menezes, M. A. Nascimento, J. P. Gonçalves et al., "Human mesenchymal cells from adipose tissue deposit laminin and promote regeneration of injured spinal cord in rats," *PLoS ONE*, vol. 9, no. 5, Article ID e96020, 2014.

[49] W. Daly, L. Yao, D. Zeugolis, A. Windebank, and A. Pandit, "A biomaterials approach to peripheral nerve regeneration: bridging the peripheral nerve gap and enhancing functional recovery," *Journal of the Royal Society Interface*, vol. 9, no. 67, pp. 202–221, 2012.

[50] E. B. Kwon, J. Y. Lee, S. Piao, I. G. Kim, J. C. Ra, and J. Y. Lee, "Comparison of human muscle-derived stem cells and human adipose-derived stem cells in neurogenic trans-differentiation," *Korean Journal of Urology*, vol. 52, no. 12, pp. 852–857, 2011.

[51] M. Lavasani, S. D. Thompson, J. B. Pollett et al., "Human muscle-derived stem/progenitor cells promote functional murine peripheral nerve regeneration," *The Journal of Clinical Investigation*, vol. 124, no. 4, pp. 1745–1756, 2014.

[52] P. J. Johnson, M. D. Wood, A. M. Moore, and S. E. MacKinnon, "Tissue engineered constructs for peripheral nerve surgery," *European Surgery*, vol. 45, no. 3, pp. 122–135, 2013.

[53] A. H. All, F. A. Bazley, S. Gupta et al., "Human embryonic stem cell-derived oligodendrocyte progenitors aid in functional recovery of sensory pathways following contusive spinal cord injury," *PLoS ONE*, vol. 7, no. 10, Article ID e47645, 2012.

[54] H. T. Khuong and R. Midha, "Advances in nerve repair," *Current Neurology and Neuroscience Reports*, vol. 13, no. 1, p. 322, 2013.

[55] T. Gordon, N. Amirjani, D. C. Edwards, and K. M. Chan, "Brief post-surgical electrical stimulation accelerates axon regeneration and muscle reinnervation without affecting the functional measures in carpal tunnel syndrome patients," *Experimental Neurology*, vol. 223, no. 1, pp. 192–202, 2010.

24

Treatment of Early-Stage Pressure Ulcers by Using Autologous Adipose Tissue Grafts

Giovanni Francesco Marangi,[1] Tiziano Pallara,[1] Barbara Cagli,[1] Emiliano Schena,[2] Francesco Giurazza,[3] Elio Faiella,[3] Bruno Beomonte Zobel,[3] and Paolo Persichetti[1]

[1] *Department of Plastic and Reconstructive Surgery, "Campus Bio-Medico di Roma" University, Via A. del Portillo 200, 00128 Roma, Italy*
[2] *Laboratory of Research in Biomedical Instrumentation and Measurements, "Campus Bio-Medico di Roma" University, Via A. del Portillo 200, 00128 Roma, Italy*
[3] *Division of Radiology, "Campus Bio-Medico di Roma" University, Via A. del Portillo 200, 00128 Roma, Italy*

Correspondence should be addressed to Barbara Cagli; b.cagli@unicampus.it

Academic Editor: Selahattin Özmen

Assessing pressure ulcers (PUs) in early stages allows patients to receive safer treatment. Up to now, in addition to clinical evaluation, ultrasonography seems to be the most suitable technique to achieve this goal. Several treatments are applied to prevent ulcer progression but none of them is totally effective. Furthermore, the in-depth knowledge of fat regenerative properties has led to a wide use of it. With this study the authors aim at introducing a new approach to cure and prevent the worsening of early-stage PUs by using fat grafts. The authors selected 42 patients who showed clinical and ultrasonographic evidence of early-stage PUs. Values of skin thickness, fascial integrity, and subcutaneous vascularity were recorded both on the PU area and the healthy trochanteric one, used as control region. Fat grafting was performed on all patients. At three months, abnormal ultrasonographic findings, such as reduction of cutaneous and subcutaneous thickness, discontinuous fascia, and decrease in subcutaneous vascularity, all were modified with respect to almost all the corresponding parameters of the control region. Results highlight that the use of fat grafts proved to be an effective treatment for early-stage PUs, especially in the care of neurological and chronic bedridden patients.

1. Introduction

Pressure ulcers (PUs) are necrotic lesions affecting the epidermis, the dermis, and the subcutaneous layers, extending also to the underlying muscles and bones. They are mainly due to the ischemia of both superficial and deep tissues, which is caused by high and/or prolonged capillary compression [1–5]. Studies performed to date have confirmed that the sacral area is the most frequently involved one [6]. PUs prevalence in Europe (stages I–IV) is estimated at 18.1% or 10.5%, when stage I ulcers are excluded [7, 8]; the highest incidence is found to be among the elderly and bedridden patients, especially those who are hospitalized or in long-term care settings [9, 10]. The most widely used staging system was proposed by the National Pressure Ulcer Advisory Panel (NPUAP) in 1989 and then updated in 2007 [11].

Nowadays, a specific landmark for the treatment of PUs does not exist yet. The approaches vary according to the stage of the lesion and any complications that may result. Recent experimental studies have shown that ultrasound (US) examination of subcutaneous deep tissues in high-risk areas is an effective method for early detection of PUs, and it allows the prediction of their deepening towards the underlying tissues. Aoi et al. [12] and Yabunaka et al. [13] reported specific ultrasonographic abnormal findings localized in the subcutaneous fat tissue, both in deep tissue injury and in stage I PU. These signs are reversible with wound healing, unlike tissue necrosis which shows characteristics of irreversibility, as seen in advanced PUs stages. Therefore, the identification of PUs in their early stages would allow physicians to establish an adequate treatment plan at the very beginning of these lesions. Recently, fat grafting has already been performed to treat bedsores; however, its use is restricted to advanced stages [14]. The idea for this study derives from the accredited and established belief that adipose tissue is a great source of adult-derived stem cells (ASCs), capable of differentiating into several cellular lines [15] and regenerating damaged tissues. In this study, the authors aimed at evaluating the potential benefits of autologous adipose tissue grafts in the treatment of early-stage PUs (DTI and stage I). Changes in superficial and deep tissues after fat grafting were also evaluated, in terms of superficial and subcutaneous thickness, tissue vascularization, and integrity of fascia superficialis.

2. Materials and Methods

From January 2011 to December 2012 we performed a longitudinal prospective experimental study at the "Campus Bio-Medico di Roma" University, Italy. In the department of plastic and reconstructive surgery, patients with visible stage I PUs, signs of tissue damage, or at high-risk of developing a bedsore underwent wound assessment. High-resolution US examination was performed by the department of radiology of the same hospital. All patients underwent a preliminary screening, in order to check for strict adherence to inclusion and exclusion criteria. Patients were included according to the following parameters: age between 18 and 65 y and presence of at least one PU at stage I or a deep tissue injury (according to the updated NPUAP staging system), localized on the sacral and/or ischial areas and resistant to common ulcer management (repositioning, nutritional support, appropriate support surfaces, cleansing solutions, and advanced wound care dressings). Patients with a bedsore stage higher than one, with contraindications to surgical procedure, or those who did not sign the informed consent for the study were all excluded. Photographs were taken for evaluating the investigated areas during the follow-up period. The study protocol conformed to the ethical guidelines of the 1975 Declaration of Helsinki was approved by the ethics committee, and the results from this assessment have been documented and stored on authors' database.

2.1. Ultrasonography.
All patients who satisfied all inclusion criteria underwent US examination performed by the same radiologist, familiarly experienced on the use of this technique, for the assessment of skin and subcutaneous tissues. Subjects were investigated in the prone position for PUs analysis and in the lateral one for unaffected great trochanter (homolateral side) scan; the latter was used as a control region. In authors' opinion, in fact, the proximity of the trochanteric zone to the investigated areas and the good ultrasound visualization of its subcutaneous tissue make this area the most suitable element of comparison. Each US examination lasted approximately 15 minutes. Linear-array 7.5–15/13.5 MHz probes (Philips HD11 XE, preset soft tissues) were used. The following parameters have been investigated by US assessment on both sides: skin and subcutaneous thickness, continuity or discontinuity of fascia superficialis, and vascularization ratio between subcutaneous layer and the underlying muscular one. The latter was evaluated using the

TABLE 1: Vascularization ratio between subcutaneous and muscular layers. 0 was considered a normal value.

Grade	Vascularization ratio
+2	Subcutaneous layer $\gg$ muscular layer
+1	Subcutaneous layer $>$ muscular layer
0	Subcutaneous layer $=$ muscular layer
−1	Subcutaneous layer $<$ muscular layer
−2	Subcutaneous layer $\ll$ muscular layer

Doppler technique and it was expressed according to a scale of 5 grades (Table 1); 0 was considered a normal value.

2.2. Fat Grafting.
To ensure consistency, uniformity, quality of results and procedures, and complying with the Good Clinical Practice, the surgical procedure was performed by the same team and with the same technique. After disinfecting with iodopovidone, Klein's modified anesthetic solution was first infiltrated in the donor site (about 1 cc per cc of expected lipoaspirate). To harvest adipose tissue, liposuction from common suitable donor sites (abdomen, hips, or crural region) was performed using a two-holed blunt cannula connected to a 10 mL Luer-Lok syringe. The syringes were then placed into a sterile centrifuge and spun at 3000 rpm for 1 minute. After removing the syringes from the centrifuge, the liquid and oily components were drained leaving only the solid layer, which accounts for the regenerative elements. PU lipofilling was then performed: 1 cc of fat per cm^2 of the recipient area was injected in the deep subcutaneous layer, where ischemic injury originates, using a 3 mm lipostructure cannula connected to the 10 mL Luer-Lok syringe.

The ultrasonographic criteria investigated during the screening visit were reassessed after 3 months. Collecting data was performed with an ad hoc case report form. Data were expressed as mean value ± SD or percentage, where appropriate. Results were analyzed using the paired t-test for parametric values and Fisher's exact test for nonparametric ones. Significance was determined by a P value < 0.05.

3. Results and Discussion

After screening, 42 patients satisfied inclusion criteria, as described in Table 2. After a three-month follow-up, results for the different parameters of investigation are given below.

3.1. Skin and Subcutaneous Thickness.
Following the surgical treatment, the PUs skin thickness values (mean 1.40 ± 0.32 mm), which were lower at baseline than those of the control area in all cases, increased even though not significantly ($P = 0.07$). Ultrasound examination of the subcutaneous tissue, on the other hand, showed a statistically significant increased thickness if compared to preoperative analysis (mean value 8.66 ± 3.42 mm), reaching values close to the control area (mean value 18.67 ± 5.16 mm, $P <$ 0.001) (Figures 1(a), 1(b), and 2). No increase in thickness was observed only in one case.

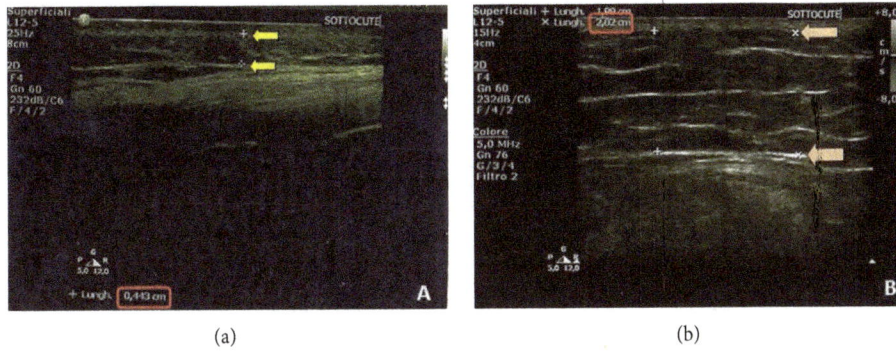

(a)　　　　　　　　　　　　　　　　(b)

FIGURE 1: (a) Preoperative subcutaneous tissue ultrasonography; (b) 3-month postoperative subcutaneous tissue ultrasonography. Shown by the arrows is the increase of the subcutaneous thickness.

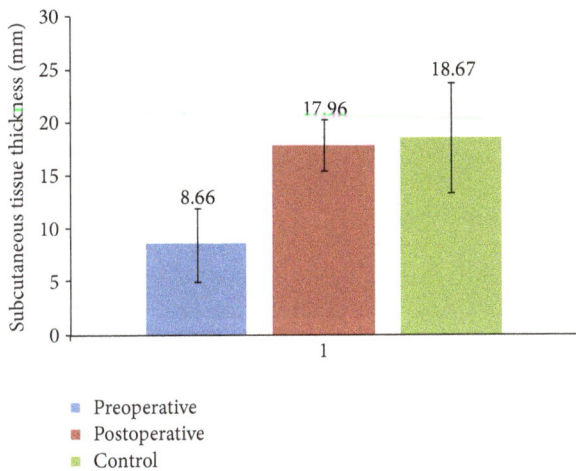

■ Preoperative
■ Postoperative
■ Control

FIGURE 2: Mean values of subcutaneous thickness.

TABLE 2: Patients characteristics.

Patients	42
Mean age	54 ± 10 y
BMI	26 ± 3
Bedsore localization	
Ischium	18
Sacrum	24
Primary disease	
Paraplegia	13
Spina bifida	3
Multiple Sclerosis	8
Poststroke immobilization	5
Tetraplegia	4
Diabetes	9
PU stage	
DTI	14
Stage I	28

3.2. Vascularization Ratio. The evaluation of the vascularization ratio, between the subcutaneous and the underlying muscular layers, confirmed the neovascularization properties of the adipose tissue. At baseline, the subcutaneous tissue presented a decreased vascularization compared to the underlying muscular tissue. After fat grafting, subsequent US and Doppler examination showed an increased vascular spots density (Figures 3(a) and 3(b)) almost in all cases ($P = 0.07$).

3.3. Fascia Superficialis. At screening, discontinuous fascia was found in 79% of patients (Figure 4(a)). This US finding was probably due to the presence of subcutaneous fat edema which prevented its correct visualization. After fat grafting, as the wound healed and inflammation rate decreased, ultrasound images showed an intact continuous fascia superficialis in 85% of patients ($P < 0.001$) (Figure 4(b)).

Furthermore, the skin over the grafted area showed a decrease ($n = 18$) or disappearance ($n = 10$) of fixed erythema, checked by daily photographs and glass plate compression, in the whole stage I PU group [16] and increased elasticity, distensibility, and softness at palpation in all cases (Figures 5(a) and 5(b)). No significant complications were reported.

PUs are a serious medical condition that requires challenging care, especially with regard to the patient management [17]. Moreover, PUs are a cause of discomfort for patients, especially when they occur in an advanced stage [18]. Nowadays, a specific landmark for the treatment of bedsores does not exist yet. Common medical approaches are [19–22] advanced wound care dressings, infusion feeding therapies, antibiotics, and accurate local cleansing (e.g., Vacuum Assisted Closure) [23]; on the other hand, surgical reconstructive techniques, ranging from skin grafts to composite, pedicled, and free flaps, are often the treatment of choice when spontaneous recovery is not possible, especially when wound healing is slow and because superinfections are likely to develop [24, 25]. However, surgical approach is invasive and expensive, requiring long periods for rehabilitation, leading to further deterioration of patients' quality of life, and is not recurrence-free. Therefore, the possibility of treating the earliest stages of PUs and thus preventing their worsening is the most desirable solution to this challenging problem. Recent studies reported the usefulness of US examination in the diagnoses of deep tissue damage and in predicting

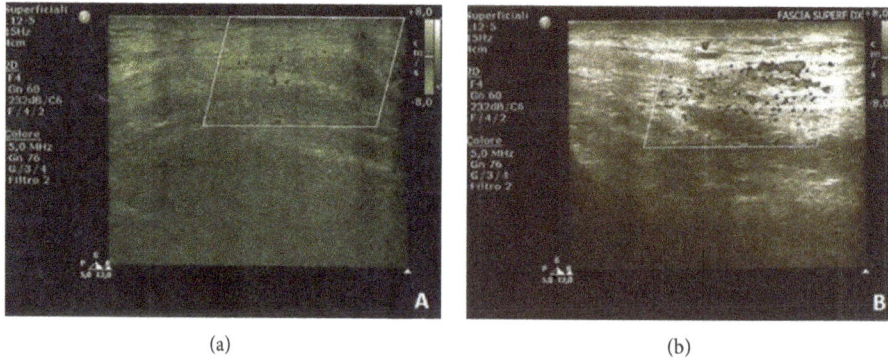

FIGURE 3: (a) Preoperative Doppler ultrasonography (V0); (b) 3-month postoperative Doppler ultrasonography (V1).

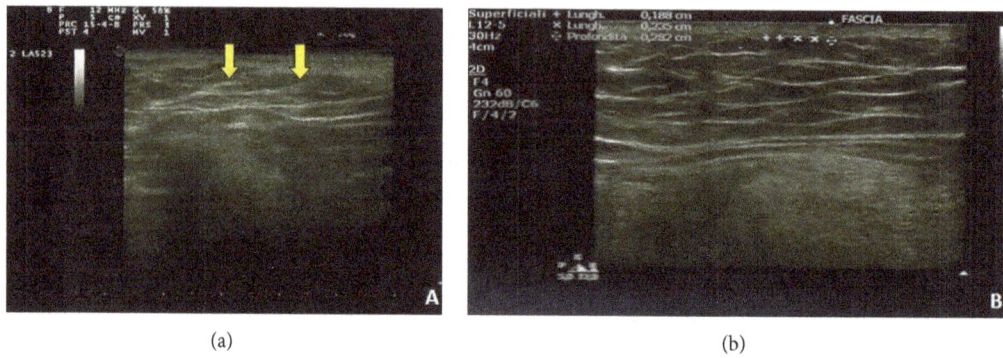

FIGURE 4: (a) Preoperative ultrasonography showed discontinuous fascia; (b) 3-month postoperative ultrasonography showed continuous fascia.

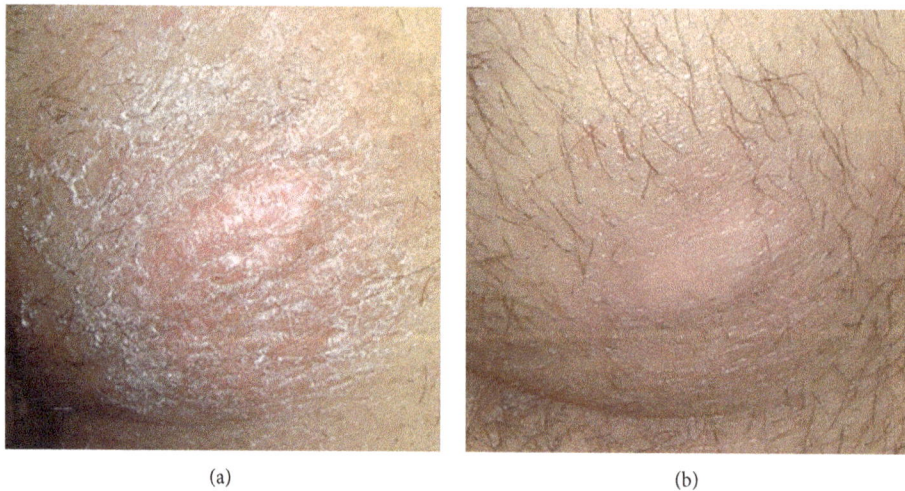

FIGURE 5: (a) Clinical preoperative appearance; (b) clinical postoperative appearance.

the deterioration of bedsores [12, 13, 26, 27]; these results lead us to support the hypothesis above. It is now common to consider fat grafting as a minimally invasive surgical procedure; furthermore not only does it allow correcting volume defects, but also it contributes to local tissue regeneration [28]. The latter is highly dependent on survival, proliferation, and differentiation properties of ASCs, which have proved to be pluripotent stem cells, present in the so-called stromal vascular fraction (SVF) of lipoaspirate, and able to differentiate into several cellular lines (adipocytes, chondrocytes, osteocytes, myocytes, hepatocytes, endothelial, and neuronal cells) [29–34]. Experimental studies have also confirmed the proangiogenetic characteristics of ASCs [35–38]. Therefore, in a condition of decreased adipose tissue and altered architecture of subcutaneous tissues, along with local ischemia, all typical characteristics of early-stage PUs, autologous adipose tissue grafting may be, in authors' opinion, a possible treatment approach. At present, in the literature, no indications are recommended for this purpose. Moreover, the regenerative properties of adipose tissue have been confirmed by the increased thickness of skin and subcutaneous tissue, the repair of the fascia superficialis continuity, and the regeneration and improvement in skin texture, elasticity, and trophism, achieved after treatment. Furthermore, the proangiogenetic properties of fat translated in an increased vascularity of subcutaneous tissue, induced by fat grafts rich in ASCs, as shown by Doppler US examination.

4. Conclusions

According to the authors' statements, the protocol described may be an effective approach for the treatment of early-stage PUs, thanks to the minimally invasive surgical procedure such as fat grafting (which takes advantage of the regenerative properties of adipose tissue) associated with the ultrasonography (cost-effective, reproducible, and easy-to-perform method). Moreover, results reveal the idea that this method may be a multistep treatment in patients chronically subject to a pressure stimulus, without implying a worsening of underlying medical conditions.

This study showed that autologous adipose tissue grafts are an effective treatment in patients with stage I PU or DTI. Furthermore, results achieved with this approach in treated tissues justify the role of prevention from PUs worsening to more advanced stages. Nevertheless, considering the importance of Evidence Based Medicine and the imperative need for more objective methods, further randomized studies with a longer follow-up period are needed to firmly establish the validity of the adopted method and the possibility of including it among the measures of gold standard treatment for certain early-stage PUs.

References

[1] G. M. Yarkony, P. Matthews Kirk, C. Carlson et al., "Classification of pressure ulcers," *Archives of Dermatology*, vol. 126, no. 9, pp. 1218–1219, 1990.

[2] S. M. Dinsdale, "Decubitus ulcers: role of pressure and friction in causation," *Archives of Physical Medicine and Rehabilitation*, vol. 55, no. 4, pp. 147–152, 1974.

[3] S. M. Peirce, T. C. Skalak, and G. T. Rodeheaver, "Ischemia-reperfusion injury in chronic pressure ulcer formation: a skin model in the rat," *Wound Repair and Regeneration*, vol. 8, no. 1, pp. 68–76, 2000.

[4] T. A. Krouskop, "A synthesis of the factors that contribute to pressure sore formation," *Medical Hypotheses*, vol. 11, no. 2, pp. 255–267, 1983.

[5] J. B. Reuler and T. G. Cooney, "The pressure sore: pathophysiology and principles of management," *Annals of Internal Medicine*, vol. 94, no. 5, pp. 661–666, 1981.

[6] J. Thorfinn, F. Sjöberg, and D. Lidman, "Sitting pressure and perfusion of buttock skin in paraplegic and tetraplegic patients, and in healthy subjects: a comparative study," *Scandinavian Journal of Plastic and Reconstructive Surgery and Hand Surgery*, vol. 36, no. 5, pp. 279–283, 2002.

[7] K. Vanderwee, M. Clark, C. Dealey, L. Gunningberg, and T. Defloor, "Pressure ulcer prevalence in Europe: A pilot study," *Journal of Evaluation in Clinical Practice*, vol. 13, no. 2, pp. 227–235, 2007.

[8] T. Defloor, M. Clark, A. Witherow et al., "EPUAP statement on prevalence and incidence monitoring of pressure ulcer occurrence," *Journal of Tissue Viability*, vol. 15, no. 3, pp. 20–27, 2005.

[9] E. Kaltenthaler, M. D. Whitfield, S. J. Walters, R. L. Akehurst, and S. Paisley, "UK, USA and Canada: how do their pressure ulcer prevalence and incidence data compare?" *Journal of Wound Care*, vol. 10, no. 1, pp. 530–535, 2001.

[10] G. Scivoletto, U. Fuoco, B. Morganti, E. Cosentino, and M. Molinari, "Pressure sores and blood and serum dysmetabolism in spinal cord injury patients," *Spinal Cord*, vol. 42, no. 8, pp. 473–476, 2004.

[11] J. Black, M. M. Baharestani, J. Cuddigan et al., "National Pressure Ulcer Advisory Panel's updated pressure ulcer staging system," *Advances in Skin & Wound Care*, vol. 20, no. 5, pp. 269–274, 2007.

[12] N. Aoi, K. Yoshimura, T. Kadono et al., "Ultrasound assessment of deep tissue injury in pressure ulcers: Possible prediction of pressure ulcer progression," *Plastic and Reconstructive Surgery*, vol. 124, no. 2, pp. 540–550, 2009.

[13] K. Yabunaka, S. Iizaka, G. Nakagami et al., "Can ultrasonographic evaluation of subcutaneous fat predict pressure ulceration?" *Journal of Wound Care*, vol. 18, no. 5, pp. 192–196, 2009.

[14] F. Villani, F. Caviggioli, S. Giannasi, M. Klinger, and F. Klinger, "Current applications and safety of autologous fat grafts: a report of the ASPS fat graft task force," *Plastic and Reconstructive Surgery*, vol. 125, no. 2, pp. 758–759, 2010.

[15] K. Yoshimura, H. Suga, and H. Eto, "Adipose-derived stem/progenitor cells: roles in adipose tissue remodeling and potential use for soft tissue augmentation," *Regenerative Medicine*, vol. 4, no. 2, pp. 265–273, 2009.

[16] M. Sato, H. Sanada, C. Konya, J. Sugama, and G. Nakagami, "Prognosis of stage I pressure ulcers and related factors," *International Wound Journal*, vol. 3, no. 4, pp. 318–362, 2006.

[17] C. Giuglea, S. Marinescu, I. P. Florescu, and C. Jecan, "Pressure sores—a constant problem for plegic patients and a permanent challenge for plastic surgery," *Journal of Medicine and Life*, vol. 3, no. 2, pp. 149–153, 2010.

[18] R. M. Allman, P. S. Goode, N. Burst, A. A. Bartolucci, and D. R. Thomas, "Pressure ulcers, hospital complications, and disease severity: impact on hospital costs and length of stay," *Advances in Wound Care*, vol. 12, no. 1, pp. 22–30, 1999.

[19] M. A. Fonder, G. S. Lazarus, D. A. Cowan, B. Aronson-Cook, A. R. Kohli, and A. J. Mamelak, "Treating the chronic wound: a practical approach to the care of nonhealing wounds and wound care dressings," *Journal of the American Academy of Dermatology*, vol. 58, no. 2, pp. 185–206, 2008.

[20] T. A. Mustoe, K. O'Shaughnessy, and O. Kloeters, "Chronic wound pathogenesis and current treatment strategies: a unifying hypothesis," *Plastic and Reconstructive Surgery*, vol. 117, no. 7, pp. S35–S41, 2006.

[21] G. Langer, G. Schloemer, A. Knerr, O. Kuss, and J. Behrens, "Nutritional interventions for preventing and treating pressure ulcers," *Cochrane Database of Systematic Reviews*, vol. 4, Article ID CD003216, 2003.

[22] M. Clark, J. Black, P. Alves et al., "Systematic review of the use of prophylactic dressings in the prevention of pressure ulcers," *International Wound Journal*, 2014.

[23] L. C. Argenta and M. J. Morykwas, "Vacuum-assisted closure: a new method for wound control and treatment: clinical experience," *Annals of Plastic Surgery*, vol. 38, no. 6, pp. 563–577, 1997.

[24] C. N. Tchanque-Fossuo and W. M. Kuzon, "An evidence-based approach to pressure sores," *Plastic and Reconstructive Surgery*, vol. 127, no. 2, pp. 932–939, 2011.

[25] O. I. Schryvers, M. F. Stranc, and P. W. Nance, "Surgical treatment of pressure ulcers: 20-year experience," *Archives of Physical Medicine and Rehabilitation*, vol. 81, no. 12, pp. 1556–1562, 2000.

[26] P. R. Quintavalle, C. H. Lyder, P. J. Mertz, C. Phillips-Jones, and M. Dyson, "Use of high-resolution, high-frequency diagnostic ultrasound to investigate the pathogenesis of pressure ulcer development," *Advances in Skin & Wound Care*, vol. 19, no. 9, pp. 498–505, 2006.

[27] C. Konya, H. Sanada, and J. Sugama, "Assessing the effectiveness of ultrasound for pressure ulcer staging," *Japanese Journal of Pressure Ulcers*, vol. 1, no. 2, pp. 249–243, 1999.

[28] A. Mojallal, C. Lequeux, C. Shipkov et al., "Improvement of skin quality after fat grafting: clinical observation and an animal study," *Plastic and Reconstructive Surgery*, vol. 124, no. 3, pp. 765–774, 2009.

[29] N. Pallua, A. K. Pulsfort, C. Suschek, and T. P. Wolter, "Content of the growth factors bFGF, IGF-1, VEGF, and PDGF-BB in freshly harvested lipoaspirate after centrifugation and incubation," *Plastic and Reconstructive Surgery*, vol. 123, no. 3, pp. 826–833, 2009.

[30] L. P. Bucky and I. Percec, "The science of autologous fat grafting: views on current and future approaches to neoadipogenesis," *Aesthetic Surgery Journal*, vol. 28, no. 3, pp. 313–321, 2008.

[31] K. Yoshimura, T. Shigeura, D. Matsumoto et al., "Characterization of freshly isolated and cultured cells derived from the fatty and fluid portions of liposuction aspirates," *Journal of Cellular Physiology*, vol. 208, no. 1, pp. 64–76, 2006.

[32] H. Suga, D. Matsumoto, K. Inoue et al., "Numerical measurement of viable and nonviable adipocytes and other cellular components in aspirated fat tissue," *Plastic and Reconstructive Surgery*, vol. 122, no. 1, pp. 103–113, 2008.

[33] S. A. Brown, B. Levi, C. Lequex, V. W. Wong, A. Mojallal, and M. T. Longaker, "Basic science review on adipose tissue for clinicians," *Plastic and Reconstructive Surgery*, vol. 126, no. 6, pp. 1936–1946, 2010.

[34] H. Thangarajah, I. N. Vial, E. Chang et al., "IFATS collection: adipose stromal cells adopt a proangiogenic phenotype under the influence of hypoxia," *Stem Cells*, vol. 27, no. 1, pp. 266–274, 2009.

[35] A. Miranville, C. Heeschen, C. Sengenès, C. A. Curat, R. Busse, and A. Bouloumié, "Improvement of postnatal neovascularization by human adipose tissue-derived stem cells," *Circulation*, vol. 110, no. 3, pp. 349–355, 2004.

[36] M. Cherubino and K. G. Marra, "Adipose-derived stem cells for soft tissue reconstruction," *Regenerative Medicine*, vol. 4, no. 1, pp. 109–117, 2009.

[37] J. A. de Villiers, N. Houreld, and H. Abrahamse, "Adipose derived stem cells and smooth muscle cells: implications for rsegenerative medicine," *Stem Cell Reviews and Reports*, vol. 5, no. 3, pp. 256–265, 2009.

[38] C. Tremolada, G. Palmieri, and C. Ricordi, "Adipocyte transplantation and stem cells: plastic surgery meets regenerative medicine," *Cell Transplantation*, vol. 19, no. 10, pp. 1217–1223, 2010.

25

Growth Hormone-Releasing Peptide 6 Enhances the Healing Process and Improves the Esthetic Outcome of the Wounds

Yssel Mendoza Marí,[1] Maday Fernández Mayola,[1] Ana Aguilera Barreto,[2] Ariana García Ojalvo,[1] Yilian Bermúdez Alvarez,[2] Ana Janet Mir Benítez,[3] and Jorge Berlanga Acosta[1]

[1] Wound Healing and Cytoprotection Group, Biomedical Research Direction, Center for Genetic Engineering and Biotechnology, Avenue 31/158 and 190, P.O. Box 6162, Playa, 10600 Havana, Cuba
[2] Formulation Department, Technological Development Direction, Center for Genetic Engineering and Biotechnology, Avenue 31/158 and 190, P.O. Box 6162, Playa, 10600 Havana, Cuba
[3] Esthetic Surgery Department, "Joaquín Albarrán" Hospital, Avenue 26 and Boyeros, Plaza de la Revolución, 10600 Havana, Cuba

Correspondence should be addressed to Yssel Mendoza Marí; yssel.mendoza@cigb.edu.cu

Academic Editor: Selahattin Özmen

In addition to its cytoprotective effects, growth hormone-releasing peptide 6 (GHRP-6) proved to reduce liver fibrotic induration. CD36 as one of the GHRP-6 receptors appears abundantly represented in cutaneous wounds granulation tissue. The healing response in a scenario of CD36 agonistic stimulation had not been previously investigated. Excisional full-thickness wounds (6 mmØ) were created in the dorsum of Wistar rats and topically treated twice a day for 5 days. The universal model of rabbit's ears hypertrophic scars was implemented and the animals were treated daily for 30 days. Treatments for both species were based on a CMC jelly composition containing GHRP-6 400 μg/mL. Wounds response characterization included closure dynamic, RT-PCR transcriptional profile, histology, and histomorphometric procedures. The rats experiment indicated that GHRP-6 pharmacodynamics involves attenuation of immunoinflammatory mediators, their effector cells, and the reduction of the expression of fibrotic cytokines. Importantly, in the hypertrophic scars rabbit's model, GHRP-6 intervention dramatically reduced the onset of exuberant scars by activating PPARγ and reducing the expression of fibrogenic cytokines. GHRP-6 showed no effect on the reversion of consolidated lesions. This evidence supports the notion that CD36 is an active and pharmacologically approachable receptor to attenuate wound inflammation and accelerate its closure so as to improve wound esthetic.

1. Introduction

Hypertrophic scarring is a form of abnormal, exuberant healing, locally aggressive, and recurrent cutaneous fibroproliferative condition, characterized by excessive extracellular matrix (ECM) accumulation during the cutaneous healing process. Including keloids and hypertrophic scars (HTS), these aberrant processes lead to esthetically disfiguring scars, patients' psychological stress, and functional impairment [1]. The cellular and molecular mechanisms underlying the formation of these raised dermal scars are poorly understood. Recent whole genome profiling and proteomic studies have led to the identification of regulatory elements with different expression profiles in HTS and keloid tissues [2]. The limited understanding of the pathophysiology of these processes has led to investigating a broad spectrum of potential antihypertrophic scarring candidates [3].

Triamcinolone acetonide (TA) has long been the steroid of choice for the treatment of skin fibrotic disorders, providing the best relief of local symptoms such as scars flattening. Nevertheless, TA is associated with adverse events such as dermal atrophy, telangiectasia, and immunosuppression [4, 5]. Despite the multitude of therapeutic strategies to prevent or reduce keloid and HTS formation, these conditions remain as orphan clinical niches of ultimately effective interventions [6].

Our group recently demonstrated the antifibrotic effects of the growth hormone-releasing peptide 6 (GHRP-6) in a rat model of liver cirrhosis. GHRP-6 prevented parenchymal fibrotic induration in more than 85% and removed in about 75% the accumulated fibrotic material in both preventive and therapeutic administration schemes. Differentially expressed genes in a microarray experiment indicated that GHRP-6 modulates the expression of genes involved in the redox metabolism, as in the mesenchymal cells response to injury [7].

During the last 15 years, a plethora of experimental evidence supports the pharmacological benefits of the exogenous administration of synthetic growth hormone-releasing peptides (GHRPs). In parallel to their growth hormone-releasing action, these agents exert cytoprotective effects encompassing cardiac and extracardiac organs [8]. GHRP-6 is a class of peptidyl GH secretagogue, similar to met-enkephalin, that has reproducibly shown antinecrogenic and antiapoptotic properties in multiple experimental scenarios, including ischemia/reperfusion [9–11]. Globally speaking, exogenously administered GHRP-6 has broadly been shown to act as a prosurvival factor for cells and tissues threatened by otherwise lethal insults.

More than a decade ago, CD36 was identified as one of the GHRP-6 receptors [12]. This is a scavenger receptor endowed with multiligand and multifunctional capabilities and is expressed by a broad constellation of mammalian cells [13]. Granulation tissue neovascularization is perhaps the most renowned physiological role of CD36 in wound healing [14]. Serendipitous observations of our laboratory indicated that CD36 mRNA transcript appeared abundantly represented in clinical samples of granulation tissue of either acute (deep burn injuries) or chronic (pressure ulcers) wounds, as in laboratory rat's controlled full-thickness wounds. This finding incited us to speculate on the effects associated with CD36 agonistic stimulation beyond that of the angiostatic action via thrombospondin binding [15]. Here we provide the first experimental evidence on the favorable impact of the topical administration of GHRP-6, as a candidate to qualitatively improve the healing process.

2. Materials and Methods

2.1. Ethics. The experiments were conducted following the approval by the institutional Animal Welfare Committee. All the procedures were conducted following the internal standards of animal care and protection established by the Animal Facility Core of the Center for Genetic Engineering and Biotechnology, Havana, Cuba.

2.2. GHRP-6 Formulation and Treatments. The hexapeptide GHRP-6 (His-d-Trp-Ala-Trp-d-Phe-Lys-NH2) was purchased from BCN Peptides (Barcelona, Spain). Fresh preparations were obtained by diluting the peptide in sterile 1% sodium carboxymethylcellulose- (CMC-) based jelly formulation to a final concentration of 400 μg/mL.

2.3. Wound Healing in Rats. Healthy male Wistar rats (250–270 g) were purchased from the National Center for Animal Breeding (CENPALAB, Havana, Cuba). Animals were individually housed at the animals' facility of the Center for Genetic Engineering and Biotechnology, Havana, Cuba, and maintained under controlled environmental conditions and light cycles (12/12 hrs). Rats were fed with standard laboratory rodent's chow under no restriction. Following an acclimation week, the dorsum of the rats was conditioned to receive two controlled full-thickness wounds, under sodium pentobarbital (30 mg/kg) anesthesia. The cuts were generated with disposable 6 mm diameter punch biotomes (Acuderm, Ft. Lauderdale, USA). Two independent experiments were performed using the above described wound model. Thus, 10 rats ($n = 20$ wounds) were used for either GHRP-6 formulation or vehicle (1% CMC) groups in each experiment. Upon wounds induction the rats were randomly assigned to either group. The wounds were cleansed daily with saline, their contours traced on transparent plastic sheets and treated accordingly. Treatments were topically applied twice a day at the same hours during four days. Wounds closure dynamic was measured by planimetric analysis as described previously [16] using the ImageJ software, version 1.46r. Since the GHRP-6 intervention increased the rate of closure, the animals were terminated by anesthesia overdose on day five after wounding. Ulcers and a surrounding margin of intact skin (~5 mm) were collected and hemisectioned. One hemisection was preserved in RNA Later solution for further gene expression studies. The other hemisection was fixed in 10% buffered formalin, paraffin embedded, and 5-μm sectioned. The specimens were stained with hematoxylin/eosin (H/E) and Mallory trichrome to examine collagen deposit. Other slides were destined for immunohistochemistry (as described below).

The impact of the treatment on the neodermal matrix reconstitution was qualitatively graded as described [17, 18]:

(0) Immature granulation tissue with a null or incipient formation of collagen fibrils, focally distributed with no alignment and not organized meshwork. Fibrin material prevails in the field. Mallory staining is detected in scarce foci.

(1) Scarce collagen fibrils suggestive of a primitive degree of organization, focally distributed, without horizontal alignment along the wound bed. Yet, fibrin occupies more than 50% of the field. Limited number of primitive neoformed vessels with empty lumen. Relative increase of positivity to Mallory staining.

(2) A general but coarse image of ECM granulation tissue accumulation, containing intermixed vertically and horizontally oriented collagen fibrils. Full replacement of fibrin by collagen. Fibrin has been fully replaced by collagen. Affinity to Mallory staining is observed.

(3) Complete ECM reconstitution, with mature and finely organized collagen fibrils horizontally deposited in the neodermis. The whole matrix appears positive to Mallory staining.

The number of infiltrating immunoinflammatory cells and neoformed vessels was determined within the granulation tissue of each wound. For this purpose, images of at least 10 microscopic fields (10–20x magnification) were captured and photographed so that mature vascular structures and infiltrated mononuclear cells were counted along with the assistance of the ImageJ processing system, version 1.46r.

2.4. CD31 Immunohistochemistry. Immunohistochemical determination of CD31 expression (platelet endothelial cell adhesion molecule-1, PECAM-1) was conducted as this is a marker protein of mature vascular endothelium [19]. Sections (5 μm) were mounted on chromalum-coated slides, dewaxed, rehydrated, rinsed, and washed in PBS 1x solution for 30 min. Once endogenous peroxidase was quenched, the specimens were treated with target retrieval solution (Dako) equilibrated at 99°C. Tissue samples were then incubated for 40 min with 1/50 dilution of anti-CD31 antibody (Abcam 28364, USA) in background reducing solution (Dako). The immunohistochemical reactions were carried out using the labelled streptavidin/biotin-horseradish peroxidase conjugate method, according to the manufacturer's instructions (Dako). The peroxidase reaction was developed with diaminobenzidine and counterstained with hematoxylin.

2.5. Hypertrophic Scars Induction in Rabbit Ears. White male New Zealand rabbits (4.3–4.5 kg) were used in four independent and extemporaneous experiments. Three to four wounds were created on the ventral side of each ear, down to the surface of the cartilage, using a 6 mm diameter punch biotome (Acuderm) as described [20]. For the surgical procedures, rabbits were anesthetized with intramuscular ketamine (60 mg/kg) and xylazine (5 mg/kg). In order to ensure an exuberant scarring, the perichondrium was carefully scrapped with the surgical blade. The wounds were made on each side of the midline, avoiding the central ear artery and the marginal ear veins. In three experiments, rabbits were randomly assigned to either GHRP-6 (400 μg/mL) treatment or 1% CMC placebo gel. The jelly solutions were administered using 1 mL sterile disposable syringes; 250 μL was applied to each wound, which for the group of GHRP-6 represented an actual dose of 100 μg per wound. Treatments were initiated immediately after surgery and continued thereafter until day 30, when most of the wounds had already completed reepithelialization.

The wounds were monitored and followed from day 14 until day 30 after wounding so as to detect the nodular firm consistency that precedes the clinical exuberance. The animals remained in observation for another 20 days after GHRP-6 administration had been completed. The incidence of firm, protruded nodules with nipple-like appearance arising in resurfaced wounds was registered weekly until day 50. After euthanasia (anesthesia overdose), the samples were collected in block, longitudinally bisected along the largest point of nodular growth. One hemisection was nitrogen frozen for additional studies and the other one was fixed in 10% neutral buffered formaldehyde and processed for

histology. Five-micrometer sections were stained with H/E staining. Scar overgrowth was measured using the previously described scar elevation index (SEI) based on the cross-sectional scar area to the area of tissue excised to induce the wound [21]. Blinded researchers measured the sections using the ImageJ software package, version 1.46r.

2.6. Gene Expression Analysis. Total RNA was purified according to TRI Reagent standard procedure (Sigma, USA), following digestion with RQ1 DNase I (Promega, USA) to remove contaminating genomic DNA. Afterward, 500 ng of DNA-free RNA was reverse transcribed using Omniscript RT kit (Qiagen, Germany) with oligo-dT primer. The RT reaction was performed at 42°C for 60 min. PCR mixtures contained 1 μL cDNA, 1 μL of each primer (10 μM), and 12.5 μL 2x Taq MasterMix (Qiagen, Germany) in a final volume of 25 μL. Specific sense and antisense primers, annealing temperatures, and number of repeating cycles for both studies are referred to in Table 1. Amplifying conditions were performed as follows: a first step of 95°C for 5 minutes, thereafter repeating cycles comprised of 95°C for 30 seconds, specific annealing temperature for 30 seconds and 72°C for 30 seconds, and a final extension step of 5 minutes at 72°C. PCR bands (8 μL of PCR product plus 2 μL of gel loading buffer) were resolved on 1.5% (w/v) agarose gel electrophoresis and visualized under ultraviolet light subsequent to being stained with ethidium bromide. PCR products were quantified using the Kodak ID 3.6 software package (Kodak Inc, USA). Beta-2 microglobulin was used as housekeeping gene for normalization.

2.7. Statistical Analysis. Statistical analyses were carried out using GraphPad Prism 6 for Windows, version 6.01. For clinical response, histomorphometric parameters, and gene expression data, normal distribution (Kolmogorov-Smirnov) and variance homogeneity (Brown-Forsythe) tests were performed. Once normality was demonstrated, differences between GHRP-6-treated and placebo-treated animals were determined using two-tailed unpaired Student's t-test. For non-Gaussian distributed data, Mann-Whitney U test was performed. For analyzing closure kinetics of rat wounds, two-way ANOVA was performed, followed by Sidak's multiple comparisons test. In all cases, values of $p < 0.05$ were considered statistically significant. The values shown represent mean ± SD (error bars).

3. Results

3.1. GHRP-6 Reduced Inflammation Markers and the Expression of Profibrogenic Cytokines in Normal Wounds. As shown in Figure 1, GHRP-6 administration significantly enhanced wound closure as compared to 1% CMC placebo solution. Differences were noted after the first 24 hours ($p = 0.016$) following the initial administrations, which continued thereafter until the end of the experiment ($p < 0.001$).

At the histological analysis, and from a qualitative perspective, these wounds appeared less inflamed and with a higher degree of ECM organization, given by far less fibrin accumulation and thinner and horizontally distributed

TABLE 1: Genes in study and PCR amplification data.

Symbol	Name	Gene Bank accession number		Sequence	Annealing temp. (°C)	Number of cycles	Product length (bp)
Rat oligonucleotides							
Col1a1	Collagen, type I, alpha 1	NM_053304	Sense	CCCTCTGTGCCTCAGAAGAACT	58	30	234
			antisense	GCCAGTCTGTTGGTCCATGTAG			
Col3a1	Collagen, type III, alpha 1	NM_032085	Sense	AAGAGCGGAGAATACTGGGTTG	58	30	214
			antisense	CAGGATTGCCATAGCTGAACTG			
Tgfb1	Transforming growth factor, beta 1	NM_021578	Sense	TGCCAGAACCCCATTGCTG	70	35	700
			antisense	TCCACCTTGGGCTTGCGACC			
Ctgf	Connective tissue growth factor	NM_022266	Sense	AGAGCTGGGTGTGTGTCCTCC	70	30	547
			antisense	GCAGCAAACACTTCCTCGTGG			
Acta2	Actin, alpha 2, smooth muscle, aorta	NM_031004	Sense	GTGCCTATCTATGAGGGCTATGCTCTGC	68	35	601
			antisense	CATACTCCTGTTTGCTGATCCACATCTGC			
Tnf	Tumor necrosis factor	NM_012675	Sense	ATGGCATGGATCTCAAAGACAA	58	40	150
			antisense	TCTCCTGGTATGAAGTGGCAAA			
Adam17	ADAM metallopeptidase domain 17	AJ012603	Sense	TGGACAAGAATGCTGAAAGGAA	55	40	172
			antisense	GTGTATGGTGTGCTGGACATT			
Cd36	CD36 molecule (thrombospondin receptor)	NM_031561	Sense	TGGCTTGACCAGTATGTTGACC	62	35	217
			antisense	GGATTTCTCTGCCTCTTCCAAA			
Vim	Vimentin	NM_031140	Sense	GTCATCGTGGTGCTGAGAAGTC	62	35	164
			antisense	TCCGTGCTCAGTATGAGACCAT			
Des	Desmin	NM_022531	Sense	GCATCAATCTCGCAGGTGTAGG	62	35	181
			antisense	AACATGACCCGAGCACATTCT			
Pdgfb	Platelet-derived growth factor beta polypeptide	NM_031524	Sense	TGGCTTCTTTCTCACAATTTCG	62	35	303
			antisense	GTGGTCATTTCAGATGCGATTC			
Fn1	Fibronectin 1	NM_019143	Sense	GGCTCCGAGATACTCTTTCTGC	62	35	227
			antisense	CGGTGACCGTGATCTTTCTGGT			
B2m	Beta-2 microglobulin	NM_12512	Sense	GGTGACGGGTTTTGGGCTCCTT	58	30	332
			antisense				
Rabbit oligonucleotides							
TGFB1	Transforming growth factor, beta 1	XM_008249704	Sense	TCATTTACCGTCACCTGGATTG	72	40	229
			antisense	TGTGTAGATGTTGAGCCCGTTC			
PDGFB	Platelet-derived growth factor beta polypeptide	XM_008257019	Sense	GGTGAGAAAGATCGAGATTGTGC	62	40	231
			antisense	GTGTGCTTGAACTTGTGGTGCT			
CTGF	Connective tissue growth factor	XM_008263527	Sense	GGGCTAAGTTCTGCGGAGTATG	62	30	162
			antisense	CATTGTCCCCAGGACAGTTGTA			

Growth Hormone-Releasing Peptide 6 Enhances the Healing Process and Improves the Esthetic Outcome...

167

TABLE 1: Continued.

Symbol	Name	Gene Bank accession number		Sequence	Annealing temp. (°C)	Number of cycles	Product length (bp)
MMP3	Matrix metallopeptidase 3 (stromelysin 1, progelatinase)	NM_001082280	Sense	TCTCTTCCTTCAGCAGTGGATG	58	40	186
			antisense	TTCCTTATCAGAAATGGCAGCA			
COL1A1	Collagen, type I, alpha 1	XM_008271783	Sense	CCTGGGCAGAGAGGAGAAAGAG	62	30	157
			antisense	CCTCACGTCCAGATTCACCAG			
IGFBP3	Insulin-like growth factor binding protein 3	NM_000598 (human)	Sense	TGCCGTAGAGAAATGGAAGACA	72	40	172
			antisense	GCCCATACTTATCCACACACCA			
PPARG	Peroxisome proliferator-activated receptor gamma 1	AY166780	Sense	TGATGAATAAAGACGGGGTCCT	62	40	187
			antisense	CCACTGAGAATGATGACGGCTA			
P4HB	Prolyl 4-hydroxylase, beta polypeptide	NM_001171047	Sense	ATGACCAAGTACAAGCCCGAGT	62	30	212
			antisense	GCGTAGAACTCCACGAAGACG			
COL3A1	Collagen, type III, alpha 1	XM_002712333	Sense	AAAGAAAGCCCTGAAGCTGATG	62	30	195
			antisense	CCACCAATATCATAGGGTGCAA			
B2M	Beta-2 microglobulin	XM_002717921	Sense	CGCCCCAGATTGATATTGAGTT	62	30	195
			antisense	GATCCCATTTCACTGTCATAGGC			

TABLE 2: Impact of GHRP-6 topical administration on inflammation and fibroangiogenesis.

	Inflammatory cells	Active vessels	Dermal matrix reconstitution
GHRP-6	$7.86 \pm 2.41^*$	8.34 ± 3.02	$1.9 \pm 0.36^*$
Placebo	15.74 ± 3.91	8.38 ± 2.89	2.49 ± 0.38

$^*p = 0.001$. Two-tailed unpaired Student's t-test.

TABLE 3: Effect of GHRP-6 in HTS prevention.

Group	Total # wounds	Hypertrophic phenotype	Normal phenotype	SEI	SEI$^\&$
GHRP-6	84	8 (9.5%)	76 (90.5%)	$1.12 \pm 0.11^*$	1.63 ± 0.44
Placebo	80	70 (87.5%)	10 (12.5%)	1.67 ± 0.15	1.66 ± 0.36

$^\&$SEI: scar elevation index measured in 8 nonresponsive wounds of the GHRP-6 treated group. $^*p = 0.001$; two-tailed unpaired Student's t-test.

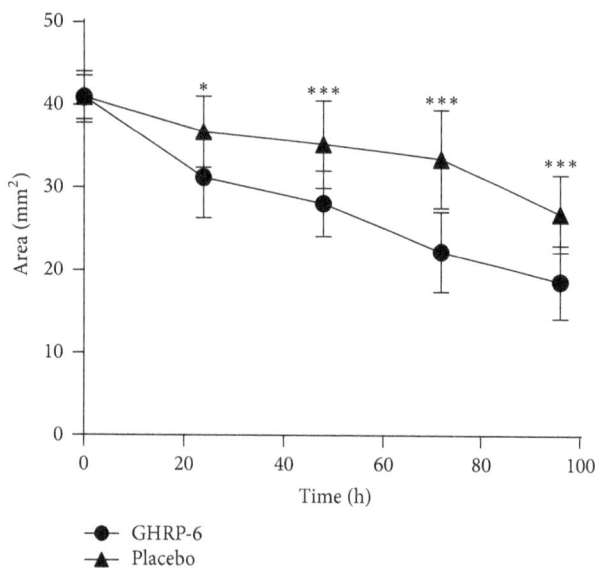

FIGURE 1: GHRP-6 accelerated wound closure. Differences in wounded area reduction appeared since the first 24 hours of postinjury. GHRP-6-induced contraction remained stable until hour 96, when the animals were terminated. Two-way ANOVA ($^*p = 0.016$, $^{***}p < 0.001$).

collagen bundles. Vessels were also aligned with the collagen fibers. Thus, the treatment not only reduced the wound area but also appeared to be associated with differences in the quality of the ECM as the inflammatory infiltrate. Figure 2(a) is representative of the GHRP-6 effect on the inflammatory response, illustrating the reduction of infiltrated cells as compared to placebo-treated wounds (Figure 2(b)).

Since CD36 is implicated in angiogenesis regulation, special attention was addressed to the population of neovessels as to their general morphology. By routine staining, we ascertained that GHRP-6 treatment did not reduce the number of vessels, which also exhibited normal structure, organization, and distribution. Furthermore, CD31 expression was detected in all these vascular structures suggesting mature angiogenesis. Conclusively, GHRP-6 administration did not hinder wound angiogenesis in any respect (Figure 3(a)), as compared to placebo-treated wounds (Figure 3(b)). These histological

findings support the scoring on the ECM maturation and the quantification of inflammatory cells across the wounds (Table 2).

Following the preliminary histological data, suggesting a reduction of wound inflammation and a far more organized ECM, we addressed the gene expression study toward inflammatory and profibrogenic markers. We primarily examined Cd36 expression following topical GHRP-6 application and found that peptide reduced its receptor expression ($p = 0.004$) (Figure 4). Furthermore, the treatment significantly reduced Adam17 expression ($p = 0.0306$) and approached to significantly reduce Tnf ($p = 0.07$), which may partially contribute to explaining the substantial reduction of infiltrated inflammatory cells within the wound bed (Figure 4).

Furthermore, the most potent profibrogenic growth factors: Tgfb1, Pdgfb, and Ctgf also appeared significantly underexpressed in the GHRP-6-treated wounds (all $p < 0.05$) (Figure 4). In line with this, we observed a significant reduction in the expression levels of Col1a1 and Col3a1 (Figure 4, both $p < 0.01$). Concomitantly, we addressed the attention to filamentous and contractile proteins associated with fibroblasts and other differentiated mesenchyme-derived cells. Acta2 appeared close to a significant reduction ($p = 0.06$), whereas Des, Vim, and Fn transcriptional expression appeared significantly reduced (all $p < 0.05$), as compared to placebo-treated wounds.

3.2. GHRP-6 Prevented the Onset of HTS in Rabbits. According to pilot studies, our group determined that $400 \mu g/mL$ represented an optimal dose level by reducing inflammation, promoting collagen fibers alignment, while aborting the onset of HTS in rabbit ears. A lower dose ($200 \mu g/mL$) did not prevent the exuberant phenotype whereas a higher dose ($800 \mu g/mL$) delayed reepithelialization in rats and rabbits (data not shown).

Placebo-treated wounds appeared hypertrophied and proved a firm consistency by day 17 onward. For the three experiments, day 30 following injury established a clear definition on the wounds evolution. The most remarkable effect of GHRP-6 intervention can be ascribed to HTS prevention. As shown in Table 3, GHRP-6 administration aborted the debut of HTS in 90.5% of the treated wounds. These wounds

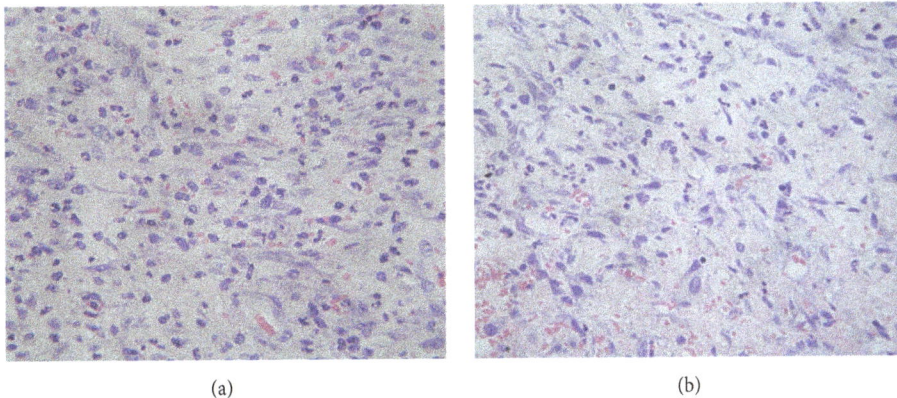

(a)

(b)

FIGURE 2: GHRP-6-mediated response to inflammation. Images are representative of (a) wounds topically treated with vehicle (1% CMC); (b) wounds topically treated with GHRP-6. GHRP-6 treatment reduced the inflammatory infiltration of mononuclear basophilic round cells. In contrast, CMC-treated wounds exhibit a physiologically normal infiltration, which matches the biological stage of the wound. 5 μm section, H/E, 20x magnification.

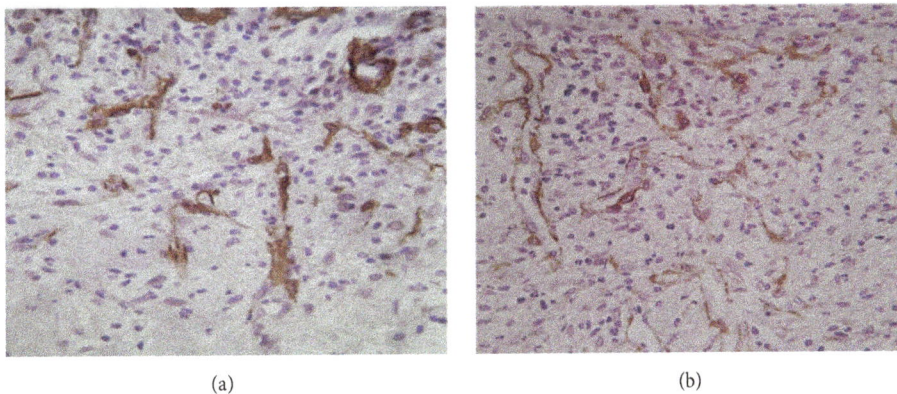

(a)

(b)

FIGURE 3: Impact of GHRP-6 treatment on wound angiogenesis. Anti-CD31 immunolabeling for mature endothelial cells. Images are representative of (a) vehicle (1% CMC)-treated wounds; (b) GHRP-6-treated wounds. No histological differences were detected between the groups in relation to the number of neovessels, their structure, distribution, organization, or CD31 positivity.

were also negative to palpation. On the contrary, 87.5% of the wounds receiving the jelly CMC solution evolved to HTS with nipple-like, reddish appearance and a firm consistency nodule at palpation (Figures 5(a) and 5(b)).

The qualitative microscopic analysis of the GHRP-6 responsive wounds indicated that the peptide seems to primarily reduce both local hypercellularity associated with the cartilage perichondrium cells and the resulting ECM accumulation (Figures 6(a) and 6(b)). Accordingly, their SEI (1.12 ± 0.11) appeared largely different ($p = 0.001$) as compared to the placebo samples group (1.62 ± 0.15). It is notorious, however, that those GHRP-6 nonresponsive wounds ($n = 8$) that evolved to HTS exhibited similar microscopic appearance (not shown) and SEI values as compared to placebo control wounds (Table 3).

RT-PCR experiments shed light on the molecular mechanisms by which GHRP-6 appeared to modulate the fibrotic response. Among the genes studied (Table 1), GHRP-6 proved to significantly reduce TGFB1 and CTGF ($p < 0.05$) expression, with no effect on PDGFB gene expression. An unexpected finding was that MMP3 appeared significantly

reduced in the GHRP-6-treated wounds ($p = 0.02$). Most meaningfully is that PPARG expression became significantly elevated with GHRP-6 treatment ($p = 0.016$), as compared to placebo-treated wounds (Figure 7).

4. Discussion

The evidence derived from these experiments supports the notion that CD36 is an active and approachable receptor to modulate the healing process. Here we have observed that CD36 occupation by GHRP-6 attenuates wound inflammation, accelerates wound closure, and above all improved wound's esthetic outcome by impacting ECM proteins accumulation. To our knowledge these findings are unprecedented for GHRP-6 within the context of cutaneous healing.

The experiment in rats, based on clean full-thickness controlled wounds, indicated that GHRP-6 pharmacodynamics has likely involved attenuation of immunoinflammatory mediators, their effector cells, and the reduction of fibrosis-inducing cytokines. The concerted action of these two elemental mechanisms may have theoretically translated

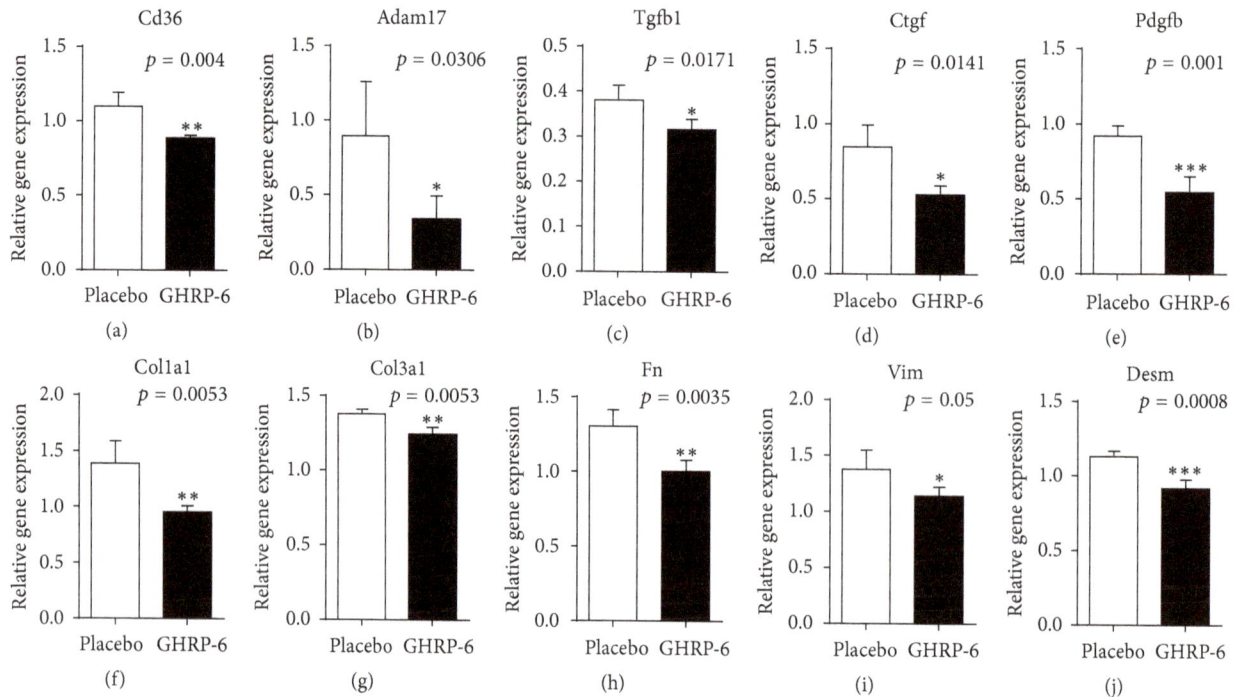

FIGURE 4: Influence of GHRP-6 on the expression of different gene families. RT-PCR experiments demonstrate the GHRP-6-induced reduction of the expression of its own receptor (Cd36). Concurrently, the peptide significantly reduced proinflammatory and profibrogenic cytokines. It is likely that the attenuation of these fibrogenic growth factors accounted for a reduction of extracellular matrix proteins and mesenchymal cells cytoskeleton proteins. Unpaired t-test ($^*p < 0.05$, $^{**}p < 0.01$, and $^{***}p < 0.001$).

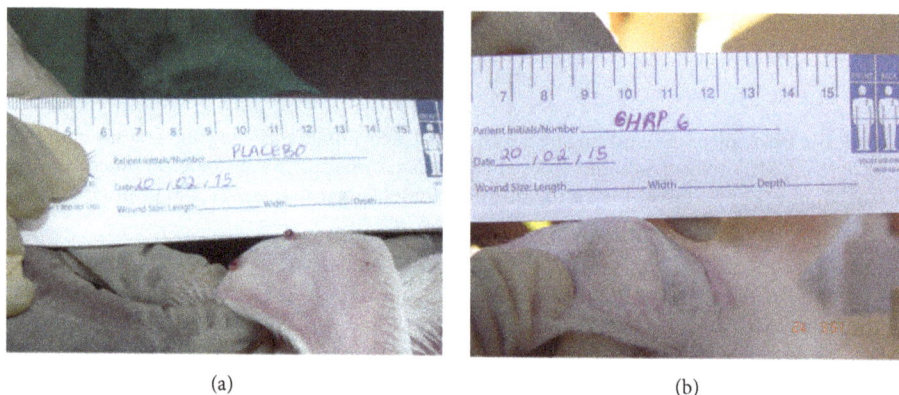

FIGURE 5: Topical GHRP-6 improved the macroscopic aspect of the wounds. (a) Representative wounds that evolved to hypertrophic scars (HTS). (b) Representative image of the effect of GHRP-6 administration.

into a particular modulation of fibroblasts response to injury, leading to precocious closure with a reduced scarring. Outstandingly, the mechanisms underlying this pattern of healing do not appear to interfere with the angiogenic repopulation nor with the reepithelialization process.

The response of these wounds reminds us of the pattern of healing described for MG53 protein (a membrane repair machinery member), so that the treatment facilitated wound healing along with a reduced scarring in rodent models. This antiscar effect was explained by interfering with TGF-β-dependent activation of myofibroblasts differentiation and reduction of ECM proteins accumulation [22]. Similarly,

antiscarring healing properties are described for plants' principles that downregulate the expression of fibrogenic-related molecules such as TGF-β1 and the downstream events, leading to fibrosis and scar formation [23]. In addition to a direct action of GHRP-6 on TGFB1 gene expression, we deem that the reduction of inflammatory effectors could have also contributed to enhancing the healing process and to reducing fibrosis. In an animal model of liver ischemia/reperfusion, we previously demonstrated that GHRP-6 prevented internal organs parenchymal activation and the onset of a systemic inflammatory response syndrome by downregulating proinflammatory cytokines [24]. Subsequent studies have

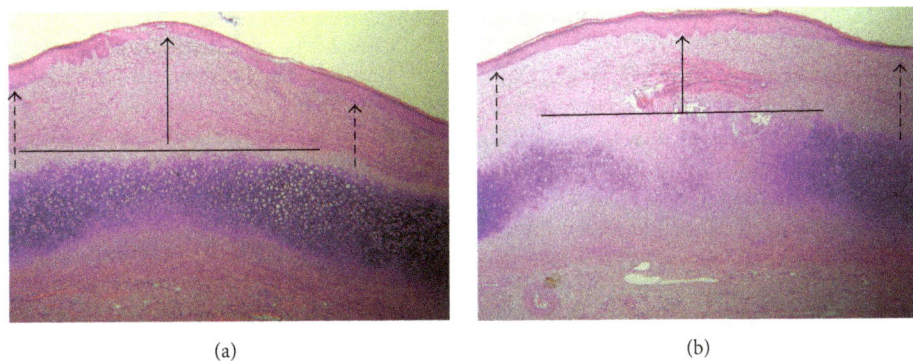

(a)   (b)

FIGURE 6: Microscopic aspect of the rabbits' ears wounds. (a) Representative image of "nipple" in which, above the cartilage and the perichondrium, there is a prominent accumulation of extracellular matrix. (b) Representative image of the effect induced by the GHRP-6 intervention. Note the reduction of extracellular matrix accumulation within the injured area. The "flattening" aspect is indicated by the solid line arrow. The dotted arrows indicate that the elevation within the center of the scar is similar to the adjacent intact skin. Images suggest that GHRP-6 reduced the local hypercellularity associated with the cartilage cells response. H/E 10x magnification.

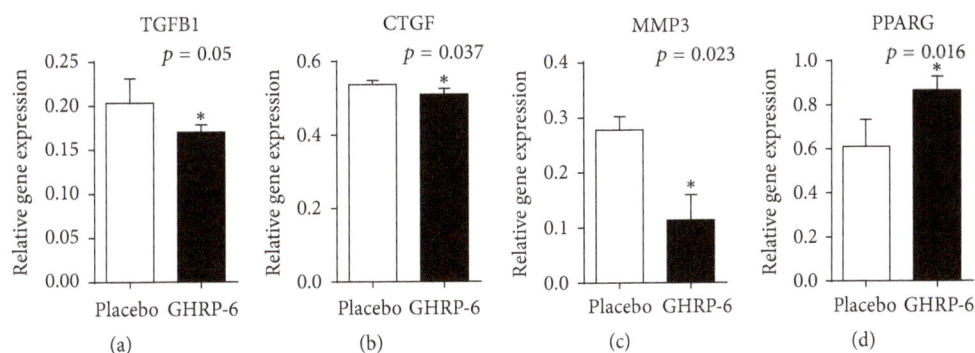

(a)   (b)   (c)   (d)

FIGURE 7: Potential bases of GHRP-6-mediated antifibrotic effect. Among these four genes significantly modulated by GHRP-6 of biological relevance within this realm are TGFB1 reduction and PPARG increase. Mann-Whitney U test. $^*p < 0.05$.

demonstrated the ability of different GHRPs to ameliorate local and systemic inflammatory processes in a variety of experimental scenarios by suppressing the activation of NF-κB, the consequent expression of proinflammatory cytokines, and acting as chemokine receptor antagonist [25–27]. Differentiation to myofibroblasts, collagen fibrillogenesis, and matrix accumulation are controlled by opposing forces: proinflammatory and profibrogenic, that require a fine tuning to ensure a proper esthetic healing and effective mechanical properties of the ECM [28, 29]. The overall interpretation of the data from (i) the rate of closure, (ii) microscopic appearance of the collagen fibrils alignment/organization, (iii) impact of the treatment on the transcriptional expression of cytoskeleton filamentous proteins (smooth muscle α-actin (α-SMA), desmin, and vimentin) supports the hypothesis that, in this context, GHRP-6 has shifted the balance toward "a more regenerative" rather than a reparative phenotype.

Aside from the limitations of this work to fully elucidate the underlying mechanism by which GHRP-6 mediated the refinement of the wounds fibrogenesis in the rats experiment, an important contribution is the unprecedented evidence that the peptide reduced the onset of HTS in the rabbit's ear model. This represents an extension of the GHRP-6 antifibrotic potential demonstrated years ago by our group

in an animal model of liver fibrosis [7]. Nevertheless, and in contrast to the liver fibrosis data, we have no evidence that GHRP-6 is able to revert the consolidated HTS following repeated experimental attempts. Thus, the reproducible findings regarding GHRP-6-mediated HTS prevention are based on the immediate and consecutive administration of the molecule once the injury is induced.

The mechanisms supporting the GHRP-6-mediated HTS prevention may be related to a potential modulation of the fibrogenic response, especially by TGF-β1 transcriptional deactivation and its downstream effector CTGF, as has been previously described [30]. Nevertheless, we have not elucidated the pathways involved in the GHRP-6-mediated TGFB1 gene expression reduction. Under these circumstances, we have reproducibly observed [7] that GHRP-6 increases PPARG expression which may have counteracted TGF-β1-associated fibrogenic input. The fact that CD36 occupation by GHRP-6 upregulates PPARG gene expression is noteworthy in this context and represents an additional pharmacologic property for this peptide. Although the molecular pathways underlying the antifibrotic effects of PPARγ remain elusive, an antagonistic relationship is proposed between PPARγ and TGF-β1 signaling in fibrosis. For more than a decade ago, PPARγ has been reputed as a fibrosis-response regulating factor and its activation represents an innovative pathway to control fibrotic diseases [31, 32].

Taking into account the broad spectrum of TGF-β1 physiology in the fibroblasts/myofibroblasts differentiation events [33], we deem that the reduction of the local scar cellularity and perichondrial matrix accumulation in those animals receiving GHRP-6 could be attributable to TGFB1 transcriptional and functional switch-off. Since the predominant microscopic aspect of the GHRP-6-treated wounds was characterized by meagre cartilage scars, slimmer perichondrium membranes, and far less active cells, we hypothesize that the peptide somehow attenuates the perichondrial activation response to the trauma and/or a possible mesenchyme-to-mesenchyme redifferentiation process, thus lessening the surge of fibroblast and myofibroblasts. In line with this notion, we had documented that GHRP6 prevented hepatic stellate cells activation by reducing CD68, α-SMA, and vimentin local expressions. All these events could be primarily presided by the GHRP-6-related reduction of TGFB1 and CTGF expression in both parenchymal and nonparenchymal cells [7].

5. Conclusions

The evidence described here presupposes the existence of a GHRP-6/CD36-mediated anti-inflammatory and antifibrotic loop that appears to improve wound closure and esthetic. The activity of this binomium may represent a novel and attractive avenue toward the timely prevention of dismal cutaneous processes such as keloids and HTS.

Competing Interests

The authors declare that they have no competing interests.

References

[1] N. Jumper, R. Paus, and A. Bayat, "Functional histopathology of keloid disease," *Histology and Histopathology*, vol. 30, no. 9, pp. 1033–1057, 2015.

[2] G. P. Sidgwick and A. Bayat, "Extracellular matrix molecules implicated in hypertrophic and keloid scarring," *Journal of the European Academy of Dermatology and Venereology*, vol. 26, no. 2, pp. 141–152, 2012.

[3] Q. Ye, S.-J. Wang, J.-Y. Chen, K. Rahman, H.-L. Xin, and H. Zhang, "Medicinal plants for the treatment of hypertrophic scars," *Evidence-Based Complementary and Alternative Medicine*, vol. 2015, Article ID 101340, 15 pages, 2015.

[4] W. S. Jang, J. Park, K. H. Yoo et al., "Branch-shaped cutaneous hypopigmentation and atrophy after intralesional triamcinolone injection," *Annals of Dermatology*, vol. 23, no. 1, pp. 111–114, 2011.

[5] A. Asilian, A. Darougheh, and F. Shariati, "New combination of triamcinolone, 5-fluorouracil, and pulsed-dye laser for treatment of keloid and hypertrophic scars," *Dermatologic Surgery*, vol. 32, no. 7, pp. 907–915, 2006.

[6] N. N. Goyal and M. H. Gold, "A novel triple medicine combination injection for the resolution of keloids and hypertrophic scars," *Journal of Clinical and Aesthetic Dermatology*, vol. 7, no. 11, pp. 31–34, 2014.

[7] J. Berlanga-Acosta, D. Vázquez-Blomquist, D. Cibrín et al., "Growth Hormone Releasing Peptide 6 (GHRP6) reduces liver fibrosis in CCl4 chronically intoxicated rats," *Biotecnologia Aplicada*, vol. 29, no. 2, pp. 60–72, 2012.

[8] D. Cibrián, J. Berlanga, L. Guevara et al., "Cardiac and extracardiac cytoprotective effects of GHRP6 peptide," *Biotecnología Aplicada*, vol. 25, no. 3, pp. 276–281, 2008.

[9] J. Berlanga, D. Cibrian, L. Guevara et al., "Growth-hormone-releasing peptide 6 (GHRP6) prevents oxidant cytotoxicity and reduces myocardial necrosis in a model of acute myocardial infarction," *Clinical Science*, vol. 112, no. 3-4, pp. 241–250, 2007.

[10] A. Delgado-Rubín De Célix, J. A. Chowen, J. Argente, and L. M. Frago, "Growth hormone releasing peptide-6 acts as a survival factor in glutamate-induced excitotoxicity," *Journal of Neurochemistry*, vol. 99, no. 3, pp. 839–849, 2006.

[11] Y.-T. Shen, J. J. Lynch, R. J. Hargreaves, and R. J. Gould, "A growth hormone secretagogue prevents-ischemic-induced mortality independently of the growth hormone pathway in dogs with chronic dilated cardiomyopathy," *Journal of Pharmacology and Experimental Therapeutics*, vol. 306, no. 2, pp. 815–820, 2003.

[12] A. Demers, N. McNicoll, M. Febbraio et al., "Identification of the growth hormone-releasing peptide binding site in CD36: a photoaffinity cross-linking study," *Biochemical Journal*, vol. 382, no. 2, pp. 417–424, 2004.

[13] S. Cho, "CD36 as a therapeutic target for endothelial dysfunction in stroke," *Current Pharmaceutical Design*, vol. 18, no. 25, pp. 3721–3730, 2012.

[14] J. E. Nor, L. Dipietro, J. E. Murphy-Ullrich, R. O. Hynes, J. Lawler, and P. J. Polverini, "Activation of latent TGF-beta1 by thrombospondin-1 is a major component of wound repair," *Oral Biosciences & Medicine*, vol. 2, no. 2, pp. 153–161, 2005.

[15] P. R. Lawler and J. Lawler, "Molecular basis for the regulation of angiogenesis by thrombospondin-1 and -2," *Cold Spring Harbor Perspectives in Medicine*, vol. 2, no. 5, Article ID a006627, 2012.

[16] S. O. Canapp Jr., J. P. Farese, G. S. Schultz et al., "The effect of topical tripeptide-copper complex on healing of ischemic open wounds," *Veterinary Surgery*, vol. 32, no. 6, pp. 515–523, 2003.

[17] J. Berlanga, J. Lodos, and V. P. Labarta, "The effect of epidermal growth factor treatment schedule on the healing of full-thickness wounds in pigs," *Biotecnología Aplicada*, vol. 14, no. 3, pp. 163–168, 1997.

[18] J. Berlanga, E. Moreira, L. C. Pérez, E. Boix, T. González, and P. López-Saura, "Wound healing promotion in rats is EGF dose dependent," *Biotecnología Aplicada*, vol. 13, no. 3, pp. 181–185, 1996.

[19] J. R. Privratsky and P. J. Newman, "PECAM-1: regulator of endothelial junctional integrity," *Cell and Tissue Research*, vol. 355, no. 3, pp. 607–619, 2014.

[20] D. E. Morris, L. Wu, L. L. Zhao et al., "Acute and chronic animal models for excessive dermal scarring: quantitative studies," *Plastic and Reconstructive Surgery*, vol. 100, no. 3, pp. 674–681, 1997.

[21] S. Jia, Y. Zhao, M. Law, R. Galiano, and T. A. Mustoe, "The effects of collagenase ointment on the prevention of hypertrophic scarring in a rabbit ear scarring model: a pilot study," *Wounds*, vol. 23, no. 6, pp. 160–165, 2011.

[22] H. Li, P. Duann, P.-H. Lin et al., "Modulation of wound healing and scar formation by MG53 protein-mediated cell membrane repair," *Journal of Biological Chemistry*, vol. 290, no. 40, pp. 24592–24603, 2015.

[23] X. Bai, T. He, J. Liu et al., "Loureirin B inhibits fibroblast prolif-eration and extracellular matrix deposition in hypertrophic scar via TGF-β/Smad pathway," *Experimental Dermatology*, vol. 24, no. 5, pp. 355–360, 2015.

[24] D. Cibrián, H. Ajamieh, J. Berlanga et al., "Use of growth-hormone-releasing peptide-6 (GHRP-6) for the prevention of multiple organ failure," *Clinical Science*, vol. 110, no. 5, pp. 563–573, 2006.

[25] M. Granado, A. I. Martin, M. Lopez-Menduina, A. Lopez-Calderon, and M. A. Villanua, "GH-releasing peptide-2 admin-istration prevents liver inflammatory response in endotoxemia," *American Journal of Physiology–Endocrinology and Metabolism*, vol. 294, no. 1, pp. E131–E141, 2007.

[26] K. Patel, V. D. Dixit, J. H. Lee et al., "The GHS-R blocker D-[Lys3] GHRP-6 serves as CCR5 Chemokine receptor antago-nist," *International Journal of Medical Sciences*, vol. 9, no. 1, pp. 51–58, 2012.

[27] G. Li, J. Li, Q. Zhou, X. Song, H. Liang, and L. Huang, "Growth hormone releasing peptide-2, a ghrelin agonist, attenuates lipopolysaccharide-induced acute lung injury in rats," *Tohoku Journal of Experimental Medicine*, vol. 222, no. 1, pp. 7–13, 2010.

[28] B. S. Herrera, A. Kantarci, A. Zarrough, H. Hasturk, K. P. Leung, and T. E. Van Dyke, "LXA$_4$ actions direct fibroblast function and wound closure," *Biochemical and Biophysical Research Communications*, vol. 464, no. 4, pp. 1072–1077, 2015.

[29] H.-M. Zhou, J. Wang, C. Elliott, W. Wen, D. W. Hamilton, and S. J. Conway, "Spatiotemporal expression of periostin during skin development and incisional wound healing: lessons for human fibrotic scar formation," *Journal of Cell Communication and Signaling*, vol. 4, no. 2, pp. 99–107, 2010.

[30] M. Sisco, Z. B. Kryger, K. D. O'Shaughnessy et al., "Antisense inhibition of connective tissue growth factor (CTGF/CCN2) mRNA limits hypertrophic scarring without affecting wound healing in vivo," *Wound Repair and Regeneration*, vol. 16, no. 5, pp. 661–673, 2008.

[31] A. T. Dantas, M. C. Pereira, M. J. B. de Melo Rego et al., "The role of PPAR gamma in systemic sclerosis," *PPAR Research*, vol. 2015, Article ID 124624, 12 pages, 2015.

[32] S. M. Ferrari, A. Antonelli, A. Di Domenicantonio, A. Man-fredi, C. Ferri, and P. Fallahi, "Modulatory effects of peroxi-some proliferator-activated receptor-γ on CXCR3 chemokines," *Recent Patents on Inflammation and Allergy Drug Discovery*, vol. 8, no. 2, pp. 132–138, 2014.

[33] R. Vivar, C. Humeres, C. Muñoz et al., "FoxO1 mediates TGF-betal-dependent cardiac myofibroblast differentiation," *Bio-chimica et Biophysica Acta (BBA)—Molecular Cell Research*, vol. 1863, no. 1, pp. 128–138, 2016.

26

The Versatility of Autologous Fat Transplantation in Correction of Facial Deformities: A Single-Center Experience

Niels Hammer-Hansen, Javed Akram, and Tine Engberg Damsgaard

Plastic Surgical Research Unit, Department of Plastic Surgery, Aarhus University Hospital, 8000 Aarhus, Denmark

Correspondence should be addressed to Niels Hammer-Hansen; nielhamm@rm.dk

Academic Editor: Francesco Carinci

Deformities in the craniofacial region are of great social and functional importance. Several surgical techniques have been used to treat such pathologies often with high morbidity and lacking the ability to address smaller contour defects. The minimally invasive technique of fat transplantation has evolved rapidly within the last few decades. The objective of this paper is to present the versatility and applicability of fat transplantation in a wide range of contour deformities in the craniofacial region. We share our experiences in treating 13 patients with autoimmune disorders, congenital malformations, and acquired defects. Future perspectives of fat transplantation in the field of craniofacial reconstruction are discussed.

1. Introduction

Gustav Neuber performed the first autologous fat transfer in 1893 for treatment of adhesive scars due to childhood tuberculous osteitis. He transferred fat parcels from the upper extremity to the infraorbital margin [1]. Since then refinements have improved the technique of fat transfer, primarily due to Coleman's systemization of fat transfer techniques in the 1990s, focusing on atraumatic fat transfer [2]. Initially autologous fat transplantation was considered an aesthetic procedure. However, autologous fat transfer is now considered a valid option in reconstructive surgery as well as in correction of scars [3–11]. The purpose of this study is to describe our experiences and the versatility of autologous fat tissue transfer in patients with a wide variety of facial disfigurations caused by trauma, inflammatory, infectious, or congenital conditions as well as after excision of tumors.

2. Materials and Methods

Medical records of 13 treated patients from August 2012 to July 2014 at the Department of Plastic Surgery at Aarhus University Hospital were reviewed. All patients who received fat transplantation to the head and neck area were included.

Preoperative and postoperative standardized photographs were used to evaluate outcome at postoperative follow-up.

2.1. Surgical Technique. One patient was treated under sedation and local anesthesia, while all other procedures were performed under general anesthesia. Fat harvest was performed as described by Coleman [2]. A Sattlers or Khouris 3 mm extraction cannula connected to a 10 mL Luer-Lock syringe was used to harvest fat. Manual vacuum was created progressively to minimize destruction of adipocytes. Fat was harvested from the flanks, abdomen, breast, and thigh. The harvested fat was then centrifuged at 1800 rpm for 3 minutes and the supernatant oil and liposuction fluid were removed. In patients with scar tissue, rigottomy with 3-dimensional micromeshing was performed using a 12- to 18-gauge needle. The prepared adipose tissue was evenly distributed subcutaneously, fan-shaped, dropwise and evenly with a 21/20 G PIXL- or Coleman-cannula with a 3 mL syringe. Injection sites were closed with resorbable sutures and steristrips. Postoperative regimen was standardized with elevated headrest to 30 degrees and patients were instructed in avoiding pressure on the recipient site for 7 days. During the first 3 postoperative days the patients wore a protective

TABLE 1: Demographics and treatments of patients.

Age	Sex	Diagnosis	Number of procedures	Donor site Abdomen (A) Thigh (T) Breast (B)	Months since initial surgery	Further transplantations needed	Transplanted volume (mL)
19	Female	Hemifacial microsomia	3	T, T, T	12	Yes	19, 23, 14.5
57	Male	Treacher Collins	1	B	8	Yes	17
49	Female	Necrotizing fasciitis	2	A, A	13	No	20, 19
44	Male	Gunshot	1	A	7	To be decided	5
20	Male	Hemifacial microsomia	1	A	1	Yes	13
16	Female	Hemangioma	1	A	6.5	Yes	15.5
11	Female	Mesenchymal chondrosarcoma	3	A, A, A	15	To be decided	13, 15, 17.5
21	Male	Neurofibroma (Figures 3(a) and 3(b))	1	A	16	No	31
62	Female	Systemic lupus erythematosis	1	A	4	To be decided	8.2
9	Male	Scleroderma (Figures 1(a) and 1(b))	3	T, T, T	22	To be decided	14, 22, 36
36	Female	Abscess	1	T	7	Yes	12
31	Male	Hemifacial microsomia (Figures 2(a) and 2(b))	2	A, A	17	Yes	12, 12
41	Male	Hemifacial microsomia	2	A, A	9.5	To be decided	39, 49.5

nonadhesive dressing. Most of the patients at our department have a clinical follow-up 3 months postoperatively.

3. Results

The study population consisted of 13 patients as follows: 7 males and 6 females. The mean age was 32 years (range 9–62). No complications were observed in the 22 procedures performed. The mean number of series of fat transplantations, the patients had, was 1.69 (range 1–3). The mean volume of injected fat was 19.41 mL. (range 5–49.5). Ten patients had undergone previous surgical procedures, such as a Le Fort 1-osteotomy and a paramedian forehead flap. Mean follow-up was 10.6 months (range 1–22). Table 1 summarizes the demographics and treatments of patients.

3.1. Autoimmune Disorders

3.1.1. Scleroderma. Scleroderma is an autoimmune systemic disorder of unknown etiology characterized by microvasculature damage and fibrotic changes of involved tissue. Scleroderma is classified as either diffuse with involvement of internal organs or limited when internal organs are not affected. Both limited and diffuse types can involve the skin of the face and may cause aesthetic disfiguration and disability in eating, drinking, and orthodontic care [4]. We treated a 9-year-old patient with localized scleroderma (Figures 1(a) and 1(b)). The skin of the chin and right side of the mandible were affected with atrophy and hyperpigmentation. The patient had undergone treatment with methotrexate. Due to slender stature, donor sites were limited and fat was therefore harvested from the gluteal and thigh

regions. Three series of transplantations were done. Clinical controls have thus far shown good results with regard to volume retention. Unfortunately pigmentation of the skin has remained unchanged. However, the bony atrophy of the right side of the mandible has not progressed indicating a beneficial effect.

3.1.2. Systemic Lupus Erythematosis. Lupus erythematosis is an autoimmune connective tissue disease with a variety of clinical presentations and can affect different organ systems. Women are more often affected than men, with peak presentation being from late teens to the 40s [12]. Facial involvement is often in the form of a malar rash (butterfly rash). A 62-year-old patient with systemic lupus erythematosus was treated for thinning of the subcutaneous tissue in the area of the classical malar rash and defects of the sternum and both breasts. The procedure was done under sedation supplemented with local anesthesia. Additional series of fat transplantations were planned in sedation with local anesthesia.

3.2. Acquired Defects

3.2.1. Necrotizing Fasciitis. Necrotizing fasciitis is an uncommon condition characterized by infection of the fascia and may involve the subcutaneous tissue. It can rapidly progress to systemic toxicity and even death. All parts of the body can be involved. Management consists of immediate debridement and administration of antibiotics [13]. Autologous fat transplantation is a common treatment for scar correction, yet very little literature exists on the use of fat transplantations in the correction of scars after necrotizing fasciitis. We used the technique in a patient with necrotizing fasciitis of

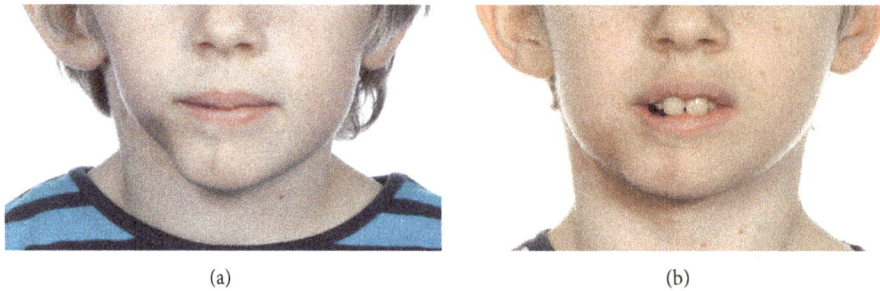

(a)   (b)

FIGURE 1: (a) Before fat transplantation. (b) Three months after third series of fat transplantation.

the epiglottis and involvement of the anterior part of the neck a year after infection. Following primary surgical intervention the patient had extension deficit of the neck, because of adherence of the scars to underlying tissue. After only two series of fat transplantation with rigottomy of adherent scars and a V-Y advancement flap from the left side of the neck, the patient experienced increased symmetry and mobility of the neck. Further treatment was therefore unnecessary.

3.2.2. Abscess. A 36-year-old patient was treated for a contour deformity of her left cheek, which she sustained more than three decades earlier following drainage of an abscess of the cheek. The first series of treatment had modest effect and further treatments were scheduled.

3.2.3. Gunshot. A study by Arcuri et al. investigated 19 patients who underwent posttraumatic reconstruction of maxillofacial deformities with fat transplantation. They achieved excellent results with adequate facial balance after clinical and software analysis [6]. We treated a 44-year-old patient, who had suffered a gunshot wound to the face two decades ago, resulting in enucleation of the right eye and the need for reconstruction of the right lower eyelid with a paramedian forehead flap. The patient presented with lack of filling in the right zygomatic region. 5 mL autologous fat was injected. There was no follow-up on this patient.

3.3. Congenital Malformations

3.3.1. Hemangioma. Hemangiomas are congenital vascular tumors of rapidly dividing endothelial cells. They frequently occur as solitary lesions of the head and neck. Hemangiomas are considered the most common tumor in infancy, the majority of which regress spontaneously. Esthetic sequelae however frequently persist, leaving fibro-fatty residual scars. Treatment options include surgery, laser, nonselective beta-blockers, systemic or intralesional corticosteroids, chemotherapy, or combinations [14]. We treated a 16-year-old patient with sequelae after regression of a hemangioma affecting the right half of the face. The patient had undergone CO_2 laser treatment with modest effects on scar development. Fat transplantation was performed without any excessive bleeding or hematoma. Clinical follow-up of 6.5 months has been without recurrence of the hemangioma. Softening of the skin was achieved after the first series of fat transplantation.

Further treatments were planned to restore the natural contours of the face.

3.3.2. Mesenchymal Chondrosarcoma. Mesenchymal chondrosarcoma is a very rare tumor accounting for 1% of sarcomas, with potential of highly aggressive behavior. Peak incidence is in the second decade of life, most commonly affecting the axial skeleton [15]. We performed three series of fat transplantations in an 11-year-old patient 9 months after surgical removal of a chondrosarcoma involving the right orbit, frontal, and temporal regions. Removal of the chondrosarcoma with osseous involvement resulted in enucleation of the right eye and resection of the right temporal muscle with contour defect and scar formation. Furthermore the patient underwent proton radiation of the involved area and chemotherapy prior to fat transplantation. After three fat transplantations the patient's facial contour defects were corrected to such a degree that fitting of a prosthetic right eye was possible. After 15 months of clinical follow-up there was no sign of recurrence.

3.3.3. Treacher Collins Syndrome. Treacher Collins syndrome (mandibulofacial dysostosis) is a rare autosomal dominant congenital disorder. Characteristic abnormalities include hypoplasia of the facial bones, particularly the maxilla, mandible, and zygoma. Teeth may be widely spaced, with a high palate often with cleft. Abnormal position and shape of the auricle are common, often accompanied by conductive hearing loss as well as ophthalmic abnormalities such as downward slanting of palpebral fissures. Mental retardation and psychomotor delay may also occur [16]. There are several studies on fat transplantation in patients with Treacher Collins syndrome [3, 7]. Guibert et al. performed a three-dimensional evaluation of transplanted children for objectively quantifying graft survival. The study found a 40% survival rate of the graft in line with prior MRI studies [3]. Lim et al. found that there was a 7.67% increase in symmetry in patients treated with fat transplantations [7]. Patients in these studies were typically treated in adolescence. We treated a 57-year-old patient who had undergone multiple reconstructive operations due to Treacher Collins syndrome, including a left side Tessier 7 facial cleft. The patient had pronounced adherence to the underlying tissue at the scar after the cleft repair. The patient wished a reduction of breast volume and two series of fat transplantations were

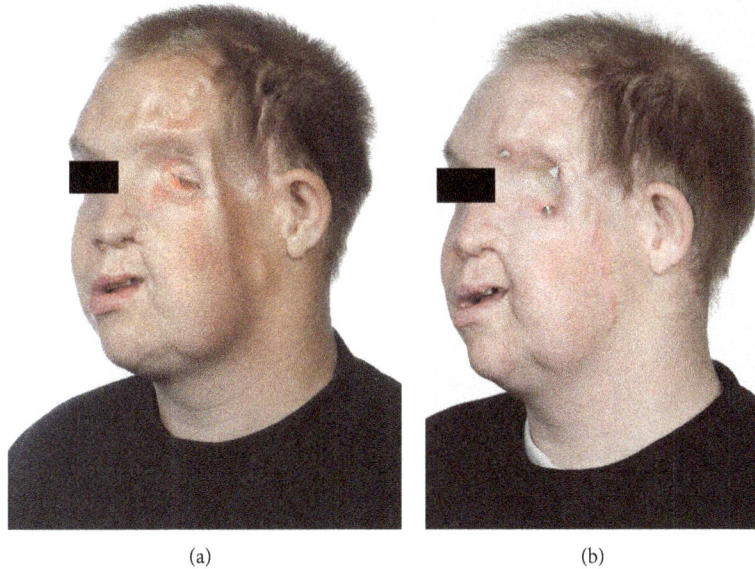

(a)   (b)

FIGURE 2: (a) Before fat transplantation. (b) Three months after two series of fat transplantation. The increased volume surrounding the orbita allowed better adaptation of the patient's prosthetic eye.

planned using donor fat transplanted from the breasts. Good clinical results were achieved after the first transplantation and the engraftment of fat was clinically evident; still further corrections were necessary.

3.3.4. Hemifacial Microsomia. Hemifacial microsomia is the second most common facial birth defect after clefts and is the result of dysmorphogenesis and hypoplasia of the first and second branchial arch. There is great phenotypical variation but in particular mandibular, maxillary, and zygomatic hypoplasia is seen. Ear malformations, abnormal tooth development, and abnormal orbita size and position as well as facial nerve involvement may be present in a varying degree [17]. We treated four patients with hemifacial microsomia, aged 19, 20, 31, and 41 years. All had undergone extensive reconstructive surgery. The primary goal of treatment for the youngest two patients was to increase facial symmetry and soften facial clefts. Softening of the scars was achieved after the initial treatments, whereas volume retention and facial symmetry were more demanding, requiring several series of treatment. The older patients had prostheses, one orbital (Figures 2(a) and 2(b)) and the other auricular. These patients had fat transplantations with good result to contour defects in proximity of the prostheses, thus minimizing focus on the prostheses.

3.3.5. Neurofibromatosis Recklinghausen. Neurofibromatosis is an autosomal dominant disorder in which patients have a high risk of tumor development. Neurofibromas manifest as benign focal cutaneous, subcutaneous, or plexiform lesions derived from peripheral nerve sheaths, nerves, and nerve roots [18]. Craniofacial neurofibromas are very stigmatizing and are most often located at the orbital-temporal region [19].

We treated a 21-year-old patient with neurofibromatosis Recklinghausen with autologous fat transplantation into a cranial contour deformity of the right temporal region (Figures 3(a) and 3(b)). The elasticity of the overlying skin allowed the transplantation of a large amount, 31 mL of fat, which had a lasting effect; further treatments were therefore not indicated.

4. Discussion

It is well accepted that survival of fat grafts depends on the fat drops having a maximum radius of 2 mm, so the transplant can survive by plasmatic imbibition until revascularization establishes a recipient capillary network. In addition, it is theorized that an increase in volume to a recipient site decreases the compliance of the tissue. This decrease in compliance results in an increase in interstitial fluid pressure which in turn decreases capillary circulation and subsequently graft survival [20]. It is consequently imperative that one considers every transplantation unique as a delicate balance between graft volume and recipient site.

Autologous fat transplantation shows its elegance when detailed modulation is needed for small contour defects that attract the eye. The primary challenge when conducting procedures with need for such high detail is the large variation in graft take, ranging from 25 to 80% [21]. Fortunately a recent randomized control study has shown that adipose-derived stem cells have a much larger and more consistent graft take. Thus, this allows surgeons to perform fewer procedures with less overcompensation and increasing the level of detail [21]. There is, though, an ongoing debate on the use of adipose-derived stem cells in cancer patients. It has been hypothesized that adipose-derived stem cells could reactivate or increase activity of malignant cells [22]. Thus far several large studies

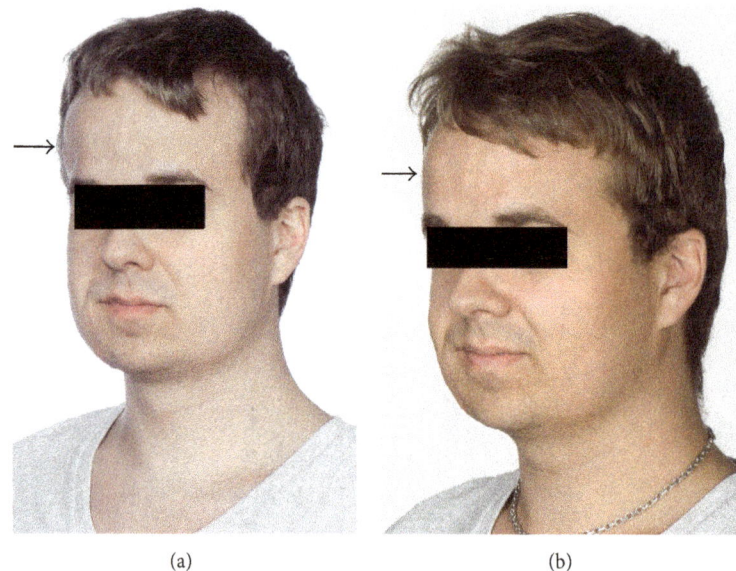

(a)   (b)

FIGURE 3: (a) Before fat transplantation contour defect on the right frontal region in the location of the black arrow. (b) Three months after one fat transplantation with a decreased contour defect on the right frontal region of the head in the location of the black arrow.

have shown that autologous fat transplantation does not increase the risk of breast cancer recurrence in patients [23].

In our experience, fat transplantation into radiated areas requires multiple treatments due to increased adherence to underlying structures and is hence clinically demanding. It is therefore of clinical interest that Rigotti et al. found promising results using adipose-derived stem cells to treat radiation induced skin lesions [24].

We believe that the role of fat transplantation in the correction of craniofacial deformities *currently* lies after major reconstructive surgery. Autologous fat transplantation is ideal in settings which require modulations of contour defects, which cannot be addressed during primary surgical intervention. Regarding the future of craniofacial reconstruction, we are convinced that fat transplantation, possibly with the use of stem cells, will play an increasingly important role. In the future and with the rapid ongoing evolution of fat transplantation, the need for larger reconstructive surgical procedures will diminish. This will undoubtedly reduce the associated morbidity and donor site morbidity. Hopefully in the near future a safe and less invasive approach to craniofacial reconstruction will allow reconstruction of patients earlier in life, limiting the psychological impact of aforementioned deformities. Continued development in the field of fat transplantation requires further research in fat and stem cell transplantation, including documentation of clinical experience.

5. Conclusion

The present report has highlighted the multiple utilities of fat transplantation in patients with various deformities of the craniofacial region. In our experience, autologous fat transplantation to the face, head, and neck with rigottomy, when

deemed necessary, is a safe procedure, and we observed no complications in 13 patients who in total had 22 procedures. Improvement of contours and softening of the skin were achieved. Fat transplantation has a wide range of application in contour deficits, scar adherence and disfiguration caused by trauma, inflammatory, infectious, or congenital conditions and after tumor removals. Although multiple procedures are usually required, the procedures are minimally invasive and hospitalization is short. We also found that sedation and local anesthesia can be sufficient when transplanting fat into the head and neck area, as has been described in prior studies [6, 25, 26].

We hope that our experiences will help other surgeons when contemplation surgical techniques in similar clinical cases. Hopefully this report will also contribute to the design of further studies in which the survival of transplanted fat into craniofacial deformities can be verified by, for example, MRI. We also believe that patient's satisfaction should be registered in such studies as we found that fat transplantation in addition to volume formation may influence softness and compliancy of the surrounding skin.

References

[1] Raaf ROCVANDEG, Orteweg STFSK. G a n (1850–1932) - 1893. 2010;1:7–11.

[2] S. R. Coleman, "Structural fat grafting: more than a permanent filler," *Plastic and Reconstructive Surgery*, vol. 118, no. 3, supplement, pp. 108S–120S, 2006, http://www.ncbi.nlm.nih.gov/pubmed/16936550.

[3] M. Guibert, G. Franchi, E. Ansari et al., "Fat graft transfer in children's facial malformations: a prospective three-dimensional evaluation," *Journal of Plastic, Reconstructive & Aesthetic Surgery*, vol. 66, no. 6, pp. 799–804, 2013.

[4] N. del Papa, F. Caviggioli, D. Sambataro et al., "Autologous fat grafting in the treatment of fibrotic perioral changes in patients with systemic sclerosis," *Cell Transplantation*, 2013.

[5] L. C. Clauser, R. Tieghi, M. Galiè, and F. Carinci, "Structural fat grafting: facial volumetric restoration in complex reconstructive surgery," *Journal of Craniofacial Surgery*, vol. 22, no. 5, pp. 1695–1701, 2011.

[6] F. Arcuri, M. Brucoli, N. Baragiotta, L. Stellin, M. Giarda, and A. Benech, "The role of fat grafting in the treatment of posttraumatic maxillofacial deformities," *Craniomaxillofacial Trauma & Reconstruction*, vol. 6, no. 2, pp. 121–126, 2013.

[7] A. A. Lim, K. Fan, K. A. Allam et al., "Autologous fat transplantation in the craniofacial patient: the UCLA experience," *Journal of Craniofacial Surgery*, vol. 23, pp. 1061–1066, 2012.

[8] D. Masden and S. Baker, "A novel approach for correcting mandibular asymmetry with a combination of autologous fat and alloplastic implants," *Aesthetic Surgery Journal*, vol. 30, no. 4, pp. 513–515, 2010.

[9] O. Reiche-Fischel, L. M. Wolford, and M. Pitta, "Facial contour reconstruction using an autologous free fat graft: a case report with 18-year follow-up," *Journal of Oral and Maxillofacial Surgery*, vol. 58, no. 1, pp. 103–106, 2000.

[10] N. Tanna, P. N. Broer, J. Roostaeian, J. P. Bradley, J. P. Levine, and P. B. Saadeh, "Soft tissue correction of craniofacial microsomia and progressive hemifacial atrophy," *Journal of Craniofacial Surgery*, vol. 23, no. 7, supplement 1, pp. 2024–2027, 2012.

[11] R. F. Mazzola, G. Cantarella, S. Torretta, A. Sbarbati, L. Lazzari, and L. Pignataro, "Autologous fat injection to face and neck: from soft tissue augmentation to regenerative medicine," *Acta Otorhinolaryngologica Italica*, vol. 31, no. 2, pp. 59–69, 2011.

[12] D. P. D'Cruz, M. A. Khamashta, and G. R. V. Hughes, "Systemic lupus erythematosus," *The Lancet*, vol. 369, no. 9561, pp. 587–596, 2007.

[13] S. Hasham, P. Matteucci, P. R. W. Stanley, and N. B. Hart, "Necrotising fasciitis," *The British Medical Journal*, vol. 330, no. 7495, pp. 830–833, 2005.

[14] L. M. Buckmiller, G. T. Richter, and J. Y. Suen, "Diagnosis and management of hemangiomas and vascular malformations of the head and neck," *Oral Diseases*, vol. 16, no. 5, pp. 405–418, 2010.

[15] P. K. Pellitteri, A. Ferlito, J. J. Fagan, C. Suárez, K. O. Devaney, and A. Rinaldo, "Mesenchymal chondrosarcoma of the head and neck," *Oral Oncology*, vol. 43, no. 10, pp. 970–975, 2007.

[16] P. A. Trainor, "Craniofacial birth defects: the role of neural crest cells in the etiology and pathogenesis of Treacher Collins syndrome and the potential for prevention," *American Journal of Medical Genetics A*, vol. 152, no. 12, pp. 2984–2994, 2010.

[17] R. R. Cousley, "A comparison of two classification systems for hemifacial microsomia," *The British Journal of Oral & Maxillofacial Surgery*, vol. 31, no. 2, pp. 78–82, 1993, http://www.ncbi.nlm.nih.gov/pubmed/8471584.

[18] R. E. Ferner, "Neurofibromatosis 1 and neurofibromatosis 2: a twenty first century perspective," *The Lancet Neurology*, vol. 6, no. 4, pp. 340–351, 2007.

[19] D. Singhal, Y.-C. Chen, Y.-J. Tsai et al., "Craniofacial neurofibromatosis: treatment of the midface deformity," *Journal of Cranio-Maxillofacial Surgery*, vol. 42, pp. 595–600, 2014.

[20] R. K. Khouri, G. Rigotti, E. Cardoso, and T. M. Biggs, "Megavolume autologous fat transfer: part I. Theory and principles," *Plastic and Reconstructive Surgery*, vol. 133, pp. 550–557, 2014.

[21] S.-F. T. Kølle, A. Fischer-Nielsen, A. B. Mathiasen et al., "Enrichment of autologous fat grafts with ex-vivo expanded adipose tissue-derived stem cells for graft survival: a randomised placebo-controlled trial," *The Lancet*, vol. 382, no. 9898, pp. 1113–1120, 2013.

[22] L. Zimmerlin, T. S. Park, E. T. Zambidis, V. S. Donnenberg, and A. D. Donnenberg, "Mesenchymal stem cell secretome and regenerative therapy after cancer," *Biochimie*, vol. 95, no. 12, pp. 2235–2245, 2013.

[23] J. K. Fraser, M. H. Hedrick, and S. R. Cohen, "Oncologic risks of autologous fat grafting to the breast," *Aesthetic Surgery Journal*, vol. 31, no. 1, pp. 68–75, 2011.

[24] G. Rigotti, A. Marchi, M. Galiè et al., "Clinical treatment of radiotherapy tissue damage by lipoaspirate transplant: a healing process mediated by adipose-derived adult stem cells," *Plastic and Reconstructive Surgery*, vol. 119, no. 5, pp. 1409–1424, 2007, http://www.ncbi.nlm.nih.gov/pubmed/17415234.

[25] E. Guisantes, J. Fontdevila, and G. Rodríguez, "Autologous fat grafting for correction of unaesthetic scars," *Annals of Plastic Surgery*, vol. 69, no. 5, pp. 550–554, 2012.

[26] I. C. Mazzola, G. Cantarella, and R. F. Mazzola, "Management of tracheostomy scar by autologous fat transplantation: a minimally invasive new approach," *The Journal of Craniofacial Surgery*, vol. 24, no. 4, pp. 1361–1364, 2013.

27

Complex Biological Reconstruction after Wide Excision of Osteogenic Sarcoma in Lower Extremities

Kashif Abbas,[1,2] **Masood Umer,**[3] **and Haroon ur Rashid**[3]

[1] *Islam Medical College, Sialkot, Pakistan*
[2] *H No. 88 K-1, Wapda Town, Lahore, Pakistan*
[3] *Aga Khan University Hospital, Karachi, Pakistan*

Correspondence should be addressed to Kashif Abbas; kashah_pk@yahoo.com

Academic Editor: G. L. Robb

Wide margin resection of extremity tumor sometimes leaves a huge soft tissue and bony defects in limb salvage surgery. Adequate management of these defects is an absolute requirement when aiming for functional limb. Multidisciplinary management in such cases is an answer when complex biologic reconstruction is desired. We aim to present cases of osteogenic sarcoma of lower extremity requiring combined surgical approach to achieve effective musculoskeletal reconstruction. *Patients and Methods.* From 2006 to 2010 ten patients were operated on for osteogenic sarcoma of lower extremity requiring complex musculoskeletal reconstruction. *Results.* Six patients had pathology around knee joint, whereas one each with mid tibia, mid femur, proximal femur, and heel bone. Locking compression plate was used in 7 patients including six with periarticular disease. Eight out of ten patients underwent biologic reconstruction using autograft; endoprosthetic reconstruction and hindquarter amputation were done in the remaining two patients. Vascularized fibula was done in five patients, sural artery flap which was primarily done in three patients, spare part fillet flap, free iliac crest flap, and Gastrocnemius flap was done in one patient each. Secondary hemorrhage, infection, nonunion, wound dehiscence, and flap failure were notable complications in four patients. The Average Musculoskeletal Tumor Society score was 89%. *Conclusion.* Combined surgical approach results in cosmetically acceptable and functional limb.

1. Introduction

Osteogenic sarcoma is the most common primary malignant bone tumor in children and adolescents. Historically, more radical treatment options were employed in the management of these tumors in the form of amputation or disarticulations. With advances in multidisciplinary approach toward management, over 90% are limb preserving surgeries. Options for limb salvage reconstruction after wide resection include osteoarticular allograft, allograft prosthetic composite, recycled autograft, and modular or custom made endoprosthesis [1–3].

Due to financial constraints, biologic reconstruction with recycled autograft is common in our part of the world. The long-term result in terms of joint range of motion (ROM) is as good as endoprosthetic reconstruction. However, it requires immobilization during immediate postoperatively till the time of union.

Conventionally, wide margin resection is an absolute requirement to ensure adequate resection in order to decrease the risk of disease recurrence. However with recent advances in surgical oncology, more conservative resections have been proposed near vital regions [4, 5].

The most heroic and beautifully performed vascular and bony reconstructions are wasted without concomitant soft tissue coverage of these repairs. Suboptimal coverage can lead to prosthesis infection, subsequent hardware exposure, or loss with eventual amputation. The strategy of meticulous resection as well as reconstruction of bone and soft tissue works together for optimum results. This strategy may require additional microvascular skills on part of a single surgeon or two surgeons can work together as a team.

The aim of the current study is to present our cases of osteogenic sarcoma of lower limb requiring combined surgical approach to achieve effective musculoskeletal reconstruction.

2. Materials and Methods

This is a retrospective review of ten patients who underwent reconstruction of oncologic defects at our institution from 2006 to 2010. All patients with osteogenic sarcoma of lower extremities requiring combined musculoskeletal and soft tissue reconstruction for wound closure in index surgery were included. We excluded cases that required split or full thickness skin grafting as a sole means of wound coverage. Any patients who underwent flap surgery as a result of initial wound related complications were also excluded. Medical record number is retrieved through surgical team database and demographics and further details were reviewed through confidential files and hospital based software called Patient Care Inquiry (PCI), containing patient records of hospital visits. The tumor length, width, and depth were measured based on sagittal, coronal, and axial magnetic resonance imaging (MRI). Primary outcomes, that is, uptakes of the flap, were evaluated. Perioperative complications were also noted including donor as well as recipient sites. Functional outcome was assessed using Musculoskeletal Society Tumor Score.

3. Surgery

Our surgery team comprises two surgeons; each specialized in tumor surgery and soft tissue reconstruction. All surgical, metastatic workup and baseline investigations were done in outpatient setting. In nine, tissue diagnosis is confirmed by biopsies done in outpatient setting under local anesthesia. In one of our patients with recurrent disease biopsy was done in operating room from proximal femur in general anesthesia; rest of the work up was on the same lines. Multidisciplinary care structure was followed in all patients. All patients received neoadjuvant chemotherapy. For surgery, patients got admitted a day prior to surgery for final preoperative assessment by anesthetist as well as surgical team.

All surgeries were done under general anesthesia. Preoperative dose of Tranexamic acid 1 g and cefazolin 1 gm is a routine at the time of induction. Most resections were done under tourniquet. We routinely send frozen section of tissue or bone marrow from all margins after wide margin resection before embarking on final reconstructive procedure, bony as well as soft tissue. Reconstruction following tumor resection is done with new sets of instrument. Microsurgical aids were used where required. In few cases of vascularized fibula, the procedure (tumor resection and reconstruction) was started simultaneously with two different teams and different set of instruments to minimize surgical timing.

As a part of our protocol, the patient stays in the recovery room until becoming hemodynamically stable for two consecutive hours. Flap monitoring protocol includes assessment for capillary refill and color and warmth which is done on hourly basis for the initial 12 hours followed by 4 hourly monitoring. First dressing is usually done after 3 days. Followup is weekly for the first 3 weeks followed by monthly visit for the next 3 months. Patients are then followed up according to need. Patients living in remote cities are followed on phone and mail.

4. Results

During this period 10 patients underwent wide margin resection for osteogenic sarcoma followed by reconstruction. Seven patients were female. Mean age of patient was 18 yrs (12–40 yrs). Mean followup of 18 months is available. Six out of ten had pathology around knee joint, one with mid tibia, mid femur, proximal femur and calcaneum each. Skeletal reconstruction in periarticular tumor is relatively more challenging than diaphyseal tumor. We used locking compression plate in skeletal reconstruction of 7 patients including six with periarticular disease. Eight out of ten patients underwent biologic reconstruction using autograft; in addition three had autoclaved bone whereas the rest had fibula from the other leg mixed with corticocancellous graft. Synthetic bone granules of beta tricalcium phosphate were used in three patients. Endoprosthetic reconstruction and hindquarter amputation were done in the remaining two patients. Vascularized fibula was done in five patients to augment biologic reconstruction; out of this, one had this in addition to sural artery flap which was primarily done in three patients. Spare part fillet flap was done in a patient with proximal femur osteosarcoma after hind quarter amputation. Free iliac crest flap was done to reconstruct heel after tumor resection. gastrocnemius muscle flap was done in patients with extra-articular resection of knee joint to provide soft tissue cushion and vascularity (Table 1).

Complications included flap failure, reactive hemorrhage, and infection and wound dehiscence in each patient.

Bony union was noticed in all except one, who had undergone vascularized fibula and rigid fixation with longer plate.

All patients with tumor around knee joint showed no instability of the knee in the followup. All patients had no evidence of disease until the last followup. The MSTS functional outcome score was 89%.

5. Discussion

Advances in the management of bone sarcoma have resulted in significant improvements in survival and quality of life [6, 7]. Several factors have likely contributed to these advances, including improved surgical technique and the development of referral centers for sarcoma treatment that have embraced a multidisciplinary approach [6]. The goal is to optimize oncologic outcome and maximize functional restoration. Reconstructive surgery after musculoskeletal sarcoma resection provides adequate coverage of wound, preserves function, and optimizes the cosmetic outcome.

There are many methods that can be used to close excision defect. Primary closure is best for smaller defect. For slightly larger defects that are not amenable to primary closure, split thickness skin graft can be done if fascia or muscle is preserved [8]. In the case of long bone sarcoma resection, the resulting defect is usually large and complex and the traditional reconstruction is based on avascular allografts and local tissue flaps. However, allografts are associated with high rates of infection, nonunion, and fracture, leading to failure in about 50% of cases. Microvascular free flaps that contain bone

TABLE 1

	Gender	Age (yrs)	Site	Biopsy	Surgery	Flap	Followup (months)	Status at last followup	Complication	MSTS functional score (%)
1	Male	40	Right neck of femur	Osteosarcoma	Hindquarter amputation	Fillet flap	30 months	NED	Secondary hemorrhage	70
2	Female	13	Left proximal tibia	Osteosarcoma	Wide margin excision	Sural artery flap	24 months	NED	Nil	95
3	Female	19	Right proximal tibia	Osteosarcoma	Wide margin excision	Tibialization + sural artery flap	24 months	NED	Nil	95
4	Female	20	Calcaneum mass	Osteosarcoma	WME	Free iliac crest flap	32	NED	Flap failure	88
5	Male	17	Right proximal tibia	Osteosarcoma	Wide margin excision	Sural artery flap	14	NED	Infection/nonunion	95
6	Female	20	Left distal femur mass	Osteosarcoma	Extra-articular resection of knee mass	Gastrocnemius flap/free latissimus dorsi flap	20	NED	Initial wound dehiscence	92
7	Female	14	Distal femur mass	Osteosarcoma	Wide margin excision	Vascularized fibula	14	NED	Nil	90
8	Female	15	Right mid tibia	Osteosarcoma	Wide margin resection	Vascularized fibula	12	NED	Nil	85
9	Female	13	Right mid femur mass	Osteosarcoma	Wide margin resection	Vascularized fibula	10	NED	Nil	92
10	Male	12	Distal femur lesion	Osteosarcoma	Wide margin resection	Vascularized fibula	10	NED	Nil	90

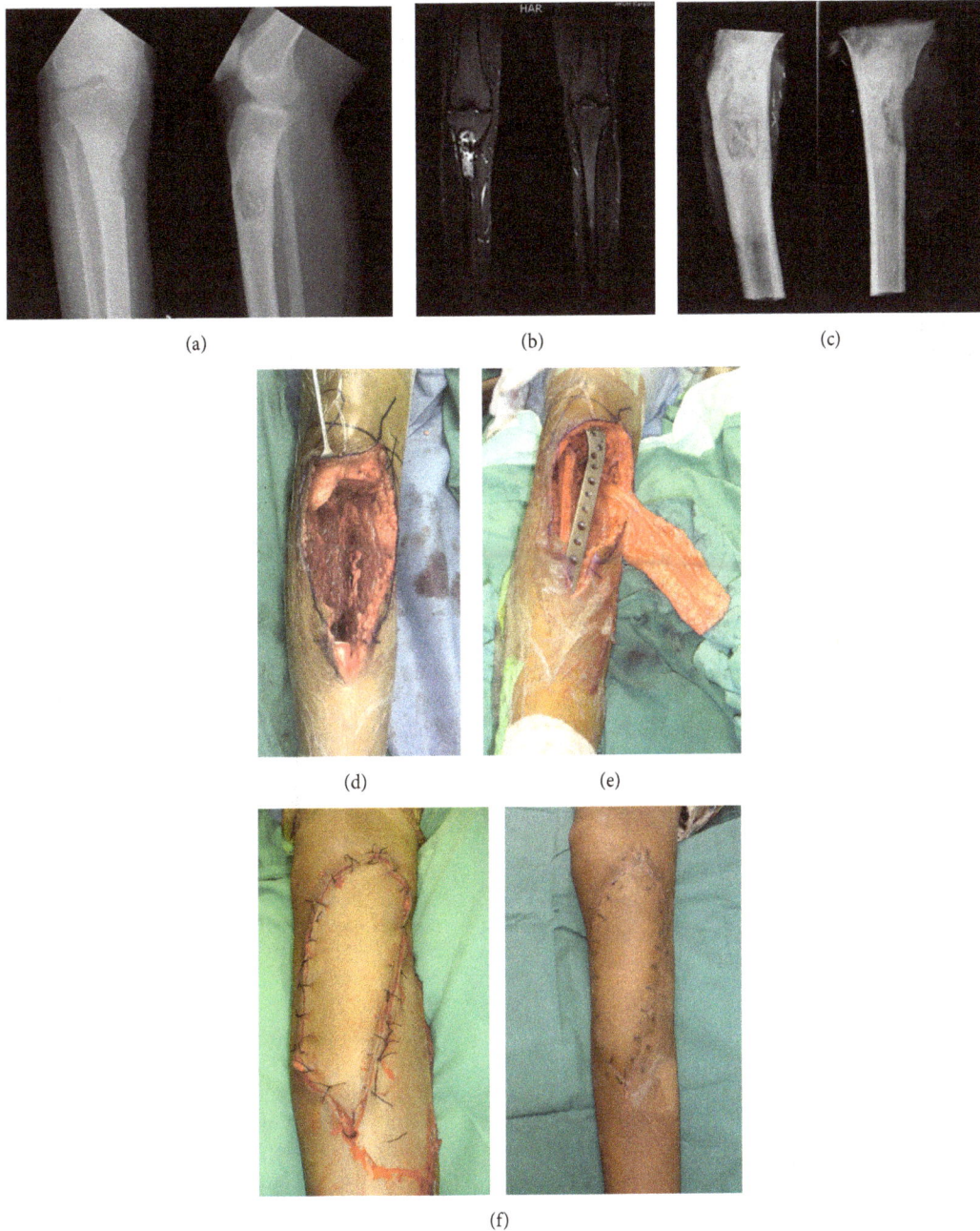

FIGURE 1: (a) Preoperative radiograph showing lesion in proximal tibia, (b) MRI showing exact dimension of signal changes in proximal tibia, (c) specimen radiograph taken intraoperatively, (d) Intraoperative picture showing defect after tumor excision, (e) reconstruction of defect with vascularized fibula and Locking compression plate and sural artery based myocutaneous flap, (f) immediate postoperative picture comparison with 2-week postoperative picture, (g) postoperative X-rays, (h) picture at 2 yrs of followup showing flap and donor site.

such as free fibula flaps have been used instead of allografts with good success rates.

Defects of proximal third of the leg can usually be covered with medial or lateral gastrocnemius muscle or myocutaneous flap or a combination of the two. In our series we have done this flap to cover implants used for knee reconstruction. Wound dehiscence was noted within two weeks of surgery but fortunately implant was not directly exposed to the external environment. To overcome the feared complication

of infection, free latissimus dorsi flap was done to cover the defects produced after wound dehiscence. Subsequent recovery of the patient was uneventful.

Sural flap coverage is classically done for defects around mid or distal tibia but in our series it was done for three cases of proximal tibia osteosarcoma (Figure 1). With slight modification in the technique and selection of donor site more proximally in the calf it is possible to extend the pedicle for proximal tibia defect coverage without additional flap related morbidities [9]. Bony reconstruction was done with the help of autograft nonvascularized fibula with corticocancellous graft. In one case vascularized fibula was done in addition to sural artery flap.

Salvage of a nonfunctional limb is of little value for the patient. Likewise, patients with severe medical problems may not be good candidates for limb salvage procedures. In those situations, amputation of the lower extremity is indicated. Coverage should be enough to provide a good stump to fit an external prosthesis. Fillet flaps are harvested immediately and converted to flaps transferred to defect site. Studies show that they are oncologically safe and reliable [10]. In our series one patient had undergone hindquarter amputation for recurrent tumor. Fillet flap was done successfully without additional donor site morbidity. On the 4th postoperative day excessive drop in hemoglobin and expanding hematoma was noticed underneath the flap; thus he was rushed to the operating room for exploration where only generalized ooze was found without any gross evidence of infection; thus the wound closed again over drain. Subsequent recovery was uneventful without disease recurrence in 30 months of followup.

The use of free fibular flap has been widespread since it was first described by Taylor in 1975 [11]. The presence of a free fibular flap to augment the construct does not provide strength to the overall construct. However it does appear to hasten the time to full weight bearing. Presence of free fibular flap appears to reduce the number of secondary procedures required.

In series using free fibular flaps as the sole modality, fibular union occurs in 74%–100% of cases reported. The incidence of delayed union is 16.7%–45%. The infection rates are 10%–15.4%. The stress fracture rates with free fibular flaps alone are 7.7%–22.2%. The overall complication rate with free fibular flaps alone is of the order 50%–54% [12].

In our series four patients had undergone vascularized fibula as an adjunct in the primary procedure to expedite biological reconstruction. One patient had delayed union in which 24 cm of ipsilateral vascularized fibula was used along with nonvascularized contralateral fibula, to fill the diaphyseal defect of tibia. Initial fixation device was removed and limb was put in cast for 2 months following healing. Full weight bearing is not yet allowed as the tibialization of fibulas is not complete in this case. In the rest of the cases vascularized fibula was used as onlay graft; thus good healing was evident with return to previous weight bearing status in an average of 11 months.

In one of the patients, heel defect was reconstructed with vascularized iliac crest flap which failed gradually. Her wound was managed with secondary intention with local control of infection with antibiotics and resection of sequestrum. She is now ambulating with a heel minus foot and has a well-adapted gait.

6. Conclusion

Combined surgical approach is an essential need especially when aiming for limb salvage. It gives an opportunity to ensure adequate surgical margins without fear of resultant wound defects and their coverage. Close liaison with histopathologist is also required to have margins status intraoperatively so that one stage reconstruction is carried out.

References

[1] T. H. Chen, W. M. Chen, and C. K. Huang, "Reconstruction after intercalary resection of malignant bone tumours: comparison between segmental allograft and extracorporeally-irradiated autograft," *The Bone and Joint Journal*, vol. 87, no. 5, pp. 704–709, 2005.

[2] M. J. Khattak, M. Umer, H. ur Rasheed, and M. Umar, "Autoclaved tumor bone for reconstruction: an alternative in developing countries," *Clinical Orthopaedics and Related Research*, no. 447, pp. 138–144, 2006.

[3] W. M. Chen, T. H. Chen, C. K. Huang, C. C. Chiang, and W. H. Lo, "Treatment of malignant bone tumours by extracorporeally irradiated autograft-prosthetic composite arthroplasty," *Journal of Bone and Joint Surgery*, vol. 84, no. 8, pp. 1156–1161, 2002.

[4] K. Hayashi, H. Tsuchiya, N. Yamamoto, A. Takeuchi, and K. Tomita, "Functional outcome in patients with osteosarcoma around the knee joint treated by minimised surgery," *International Orthopaedics*, vol. 32, no. 1, pp. 63–68, 2008.

[5] Y. Kanazawa, H. Tsuchiya, A. Nonomura, K. Takazawa, N. Yamamoto, and K. Tomita, "Intentional marginal excision of osteosarcoma of the proximal fibula to preserve limb function," *Journal of Orthopaedic Science*, vol. 8, no. 6, pp. 757–761, 2003.

[6] T. Morii, K. Mochizuki, A. Takushima, M. Okazaki, and K. Satomi, "Soft tissue reconstruction using vascularized tissue transplantation following resection of musculoskeletal sarcoma: evaluation of oncologic and functional outcomes in 55 cases," *Annals of Plastic Surgery*, vol. 62, no. 3, pp. 252–257, 2009.

[7] L. Heller and S. J. Kronowitz, "Lower extremity reconstruction," *Journal of Surgical Oncology*, vol. 94, no. 6, pp. 479–489, 2006.

[8] E. Tukiainen, T. Böhling, and R. Huuhtanen, "Soft tissue sarcoma of the trunk and extremities," *Scandinavian Journal of Surgery*, vol. 92, no. 4, pp. 257–263, 2003.

[9] A. D. Shaw, S. J. Ghosh, and A. A. Quaba, "The island posterior calf fasciocutaneous flap: an alternative to the gastrocnemius muscle for cover of knee and tibial defects," *Plastic and Reconstructive Surgery*, vol. 101, no. 6, pp. 1529–1536, 1998.

[10] Y. C. Chiang, F. C. Wei, J. W. Wang, and W. S. Chen, "Reconstruction of below-knee stump using the salvaged foot fillet flap," *Plastic and Reconstructive Surgery*, vol. 96, no. 3, pp. 731–738, 1995.

[11] G. I. Taylor, G. D. H. Miller, and F. J. Ham, "The free vascularized bone graft. A clinical extension of microvascular techniques," *Plastic and Reconstructive Surgery*, vol. 55, no. 5, pp. 533–544, 1975.

[12] R. W. W. Hsu, M. B. Wood, F. H. Sim, and E. Y. S. Chao, "Free vascularised fibular grafting for reconstruction after tumour resection," *The Journal of Bone and Joint Surgery B*, vol. 79, no. 1, pp. 36–42, 1997.

28

Predictors of Nasal Obstruction: Quantification and Assessment Using Multiple Grading Scales

Macario Camacho,[1,2] **Soroush Zaghi,**[3,4] **Victor Certal,**[5,6] **Jose Abdullatif,**[7] **Rahul Modi,**[3,8] **Shankar Sridhara,**[9] **Anthony M. Tolisano,**[1] **Edward T. Chang,**[1] **Benjamin B. Cable,**[1] **and Robson Capasso**[3]

[1]*Otolaryngology-Head and Neck Surgery, Tripler Army Medical Center, Honolulu, HI 96859, USA*
[2]*Department of Psychiatry and Behavioral Sciences, Sleep Medicine Division, Stanford Hospital and Clinics, Stanford, CA 94063, USA*
[3]*Otolaryngology-Head and Neck Surgery, Division of Sleep Surgery and Medicine, Stanford Hospitals and Clinics, Stanford, CA 94304, USA*
[4]*Department of Head and Neck Surgery, David Geffen School of Medicine at UCLA, Los Angeles, CA 90095, USA*
[5]*Department of Otorhinolaryngology, Sleep Medicine Centre, Hospital CUF, 4100-180 Porto, Portugal*
[6]*Centre for Research in Health Technologies and Information Systems (CINTESIS), University of Porto, 4200-450 Porto, Portugal*
[7]*Department of Otorhinolaryngology, Hospital Bernardino Rivadavia, C1425ASQ Buenos Aires, Argentina*
[8]*Department of Otolaryngology-Head and Neck Surgery, Dr. L. H. Hiranandani Hospital Mumbai, Maharashtra 400076, India*
[9]*Otolaryngology-Head and Neck Surgery, Dwight D. Eisenhower Army Medical Center, Fort Gordon, GA 30905, USA*

Correspondence should be addressed to Macario Camacho; drcamachoent@yahoo.com

Academic Editor: Selahattin Özmen

Objective. To evaluate the association between nasal obstruction and (1) demographic factors, (2) medical history, (3) physical tests, and (4) nasal exam findings. *Study Design.* Case series. *Methods.* Chart review at a tertiary medical center. *Results.* Two hundred-forty consecutive patients (52.1 ± 17.5 years old, with a Nasal Obstruction Symptom Evaluation (NOSE) score of 32.0 ± 24.1) were included. Demographic factors and inferior turbinate sizes were not associated with NOSE score or Nasal Obstruction Visual Analog Scale (NO-VAS). A significant association was found between higher NOSE score on univariate analysis and positive history of nasal trauma ($p = 0.0136$), allergic rhinitis ($p < 0.0001$), use of nasal steroids ($p = 0.0108$), higher grade of external nasal deformity ($p = 0.0149$), higher internal nasal septal deviation grade ($p = 0.0024$), and narrow internal nasal valve angle ($p < 0.0001$). Multivariate analysis identified the following as independent predictors of high NOSE score: NO-VAS: ≥50 (Odds Ratio (OR) = 17.6 (95% CI 5.83–61.6), $p < 0.0001$), external nasal deformity: grades 2–4 (OR = 4.63 (95% CI 1.14–19.9), $p = 0.0339$), and allergic rhinitis: yes (OR = 5.5 (95% CI 1.77–18.7), $p = 0.0041$). *Conclusion.* Allergic rhinitis, NO-VAS score ≥ 50, and external nasal deformity (grades 2–4) were statistically significant independent predictors of high NOSE scores on multivariate analysis. Inferior turbinate size was not associated with NOSE scores or NO-VAS.

1. Introduction

Nasal obstruction is a frequent complaint, which affects breathing during wakefulness and sleep [1]. Systematic evaluation of nasal obstruction remains challenging due to the high number of variables and factors that can contribute to nasal obstruction. These can be grouped into four major categories: (1) demographic factors, (2) medical history, (3) physical tests, and (4) nasal exam findings. Notably, nasal exam findings do not always correlate with patient symptoms. For example, some patients with internal nasal septal deviations, narrow internal nasal valve angles, and/or large inferior turbinates may have no or few complaints of nasal obstruction, while other patients may complain of nasal obstruction despite the presence of minimal objective anatomical abnormalities. These observations are well known to otolaryngologists, but the efforts to quantify obstruction in a way that allows for systematic study have been a long term challenge. Several grading scales and classification systems (for nasal physical exam findings) and questionnaires (for nasal obstruction) have been developed over the years to assist in the quantification and assessment of nasal obstruction.

The Nasal Obstruction Symptom Evaluation (NOSE) scale [3] developed by Stewart et al. is a validated quality of life instrument which quantifies nasal obstruction and is commonly used in the international literature. The NOSE scale questionnaire is composed of five questions. Each question is graded on a Likert scale from 0 (not a problem) to 4 (severe problem), and the final summed score is multiplied by 5 so that the total score ranges from 0 to 100 (0 = no obstruction, 100 = severe obstruction) [3]. Additionally, the Nasal Obstruction Visual Analog Scale (NO-VAS) is another reliable tool to quantify nasal obstruction in the absence of rhinomanometry and has a very strong direct relationship with nasal airflow resistance [4]. NO-VAS is generally performed by having patients quantify their perceived nasal obstruction using a continuous scale from 0 to 10 in which 0 corresponds to no obstruction and 10 corresponds to complete obstruction [4]. Additionally, the nasal anatomy can be evaluated by using grading scales, such as the inferior turbinate classification system, in which there are 4 grades that correspond to the space occupied by the anterior aspect of the inferior turbinate relative to the total airway space at that location [2].

The objective of this study was to evaluate the association of demographic factors, medical history, physical tests, and nasal exam findings with nasal obstruction using the NOSE score and the NO-VAS.

2. Materials and Methods

The Stanford University Institutional Review Board provided written approval for the protocol. This study is a retrospective case series of 240 consecutive patients evaluated in the Stanford Sleep Clinic between February 1st and June 30th, 2014, by a single board certified otolaryngologist (M.C.) specializing in sleep surgery and sleep medicine. History and physical examination data were cataloged using Microsoft® Excel® 2013 (Redmond, WA, USA). JMP 11.2 Pro (SAS Institute Inc., Cary, NC) was used for statistical analysis. The age, gender, body mass index (BMI), and ethnicity of the patients were recorded. The following items were assessed on a yes or no scale for medical history: history of nasal trauma, prior nasal surgery, history of allergic rhinitis, use of nasal steroids, use of nasal antihistamines, and use of oral antihistamines.

A detailed physical examination of the nasal passages was performed via anterior rhinoscopy using a simple handheld otoscope without distorting the patients' anatomy. Assessment was performed of external nasal deformity, internal nasal septal deviation, internal nasal valve angle, internal nasal valve collapse, and inferior turbinate size using ordinal scales ranging from 1 to 4. Inferior turbinate size was based on the degree of obstruction caused by the anterior aspect of the inferior turbinate relative to the total airway space and was graded as 0–25%, 26–50%, 51–75%, and 76–100%; see Figure 1 [2]. External nasal deformity was graded as none, mild, moderate, and severe. Internal nasal septal deviation was graded as 0–25% deflection, 26–50% deflection, 51–75% deflection, and 76–100% deflection (based on deflection from midline toward the lateral wall). Internal nasal valve angle was graded as <5 degrees, 5 to <10 degrees, 10 to <15 degrees, and 15 or more degrees. Internal nasal valve collapse was graded as no collapse, mild collapse (<33%), moderate collapse (33–66%), and severe collapse (>66%) [5].

Additionally, patients were asked to rate the degree of nasal obstruction at the time of the physical exam using a modified Nasal Obstruction Visual Analog Scale (NO-VAS) from 0 to 10 in which 0 corresponds to no obstruction and 10 corresponds to complete obstruction (converted to 0 to 100% obstruction) in each of three conditions: both nostrils open, left nostril open (cover right), and right nostril open (cover left) [4]. The Cottle sign (Cottle maneuver) was performed to assess the subjective effect on nasal airflow and graded 1–4 as no improvement, mild improvement, moderate improvement, and significant improvement [6]. The external nasal deformities, cephalocaudal internal nasal septal deviations, and anteroposterior internal nasal septal deviations were classified as C-shaped, reverse C-shaped, S-shaped, or reverse S-shaped if a deviation was present [7].

Distribution of patients' characteristics, medical history, and nasal exam findings are reported using the percent total for nominal and ordinal data and mean ± standard deviation (M ± SD) for continuous data. Univariate analysis was performed to assess an association with the NOSE score [3] using Pearson correlation for continuous variables, ANOVA for multinomial and ordinal data, and Student's t-test for binomial data. Multivariate analysis was performed with a nominal logistic model to include each of the variables found to have a significant association on univariate analysis: NO-VAS score, internal nasal valve angle, external nasal deformity, history of allergic rhinitis, effect of the Cottle maneuver, positive nasal septal deviation, and history of nasal trauma. Continuous and ordinal data were transformed into binomial data using cut-offs and were guided by using the Connecting Letters Report of ANOVA, Compare Means, Each Pair function of JMP. Statistical significance was defined as a p value < 0.05.

3. Results

There were 240 patients included in this study. The M ± SD for age was 52.1 ± 17.5 years and for BMI was 29.0 ± 6.8 kg/m^2. There were 159 males (66.3%) and 81 females (33.7%). See Table 1 for summary of patient demographic characteristics. The inferior turbinate sizes were averaged for all 240 patients (480 inferior turbinates) and the M ± SD were 2.37 ± 1.03.

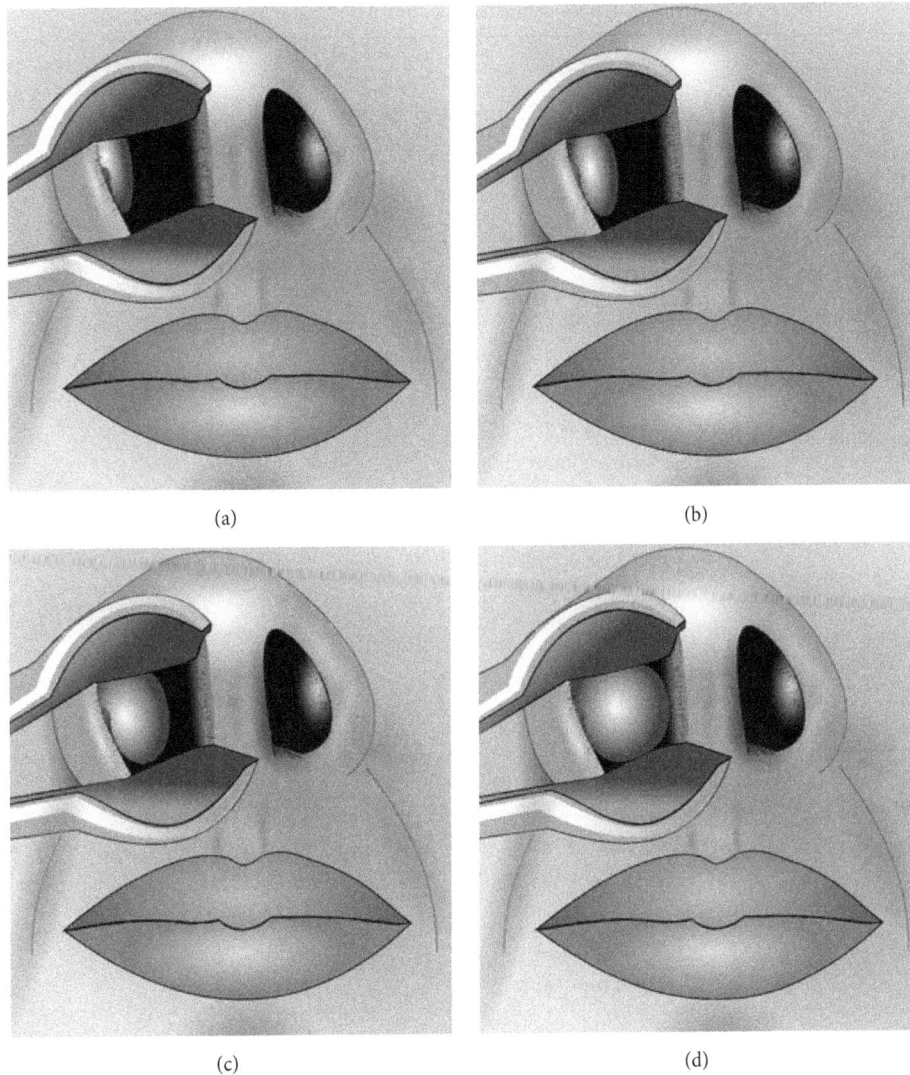

FIGURE 1: Inferior turbinate sizes. (a) Grade 1 (0%–25% of total airway space). (b) Grade 2 (26%–50% of total airway space). (c) Grade 3 (51%–75% of total airway space). (d) Grade 4 (76%–100% of total airway space). Reproduced with permission [2].

These were subcategorized by race, Asian: 2.78 ± 0.81 ($n = 94$ turbinates), Black: 3.00 ± 0.66 ($n = 20$ turbinates), Caucasian: 2.19 ± 0.89 ($n = 332$ turbinates), and Latino: 2.53 ± 0.97 ($n = 34$ turbinates).

The mean NOSE score for this population was 32.0 ± 24.1 (range: 0/100 to 92.5/100) corresponding to overall mild to moderate complaints of symptomatic nasal obstruction. None of the demographic factors were found to have a significant association with NOSE scores. For medical history, a positive history of nasal trauma ($p = 0.0136$), allergic rhinitis ($p < 0.0001$), and use of nasal steroids ($p = 0.0108$) were significantly associated with higher NOSE scores on univariate analysis. The following nasal physical exam findings were also associated with higher NOSE scores on univariate analysis: higher grade of external nasal deformity (Odds Ratio (OR) $= 3.59$, $p = 0.0002$), higher grade of internal nasal septal deviation (OR $= 2.05$, $p = 0.0168$), and narrow internal nasal valve angle (OR $= 4.34$, $p < 0.0001$). In addition, the clinical test findings associated with high NOSE scores were NO-VAS patient subjective sensation of nasal obstruction (OR $= 11.1$, $p < 0.0001$) and significant improvement with the Cottle maneuver on subjective sensation of nasal airflow (OR $= 2.28$ (95% CI $= 1.03$), $p = 0.0399$). There was no significant relationship between the classification of external nasal deformity and internal septal deviation on NOSE scores. See Tables 2(a) and 2(b).

Multivariate analysis was used to develop a nominal logistic model with seven variables in which three clinical factors were identified as statistically significant independent predictors of high NOSE scores: NO-VAS: ≥ 50 (OR $= 17.6$ (95% CI 5.83–61.6), $p < 0.0001$), external nasal deformity: grades 2–4 (OR $= 4.63$ (95% CI 1.14–19.9), $p = 0.0339$), and allergic rhinitis: yes (OR $= 5.5$ (95% CI 1.77–18.7), $p = 0.0041$); see Table 3. Exploratory analysis with backward elimination revealed that the variable "internal nasal valve angle" was significant on multivariate analysis only when external nasal

TABLE 1: Summary of patient characteristics and association with NOSE score.

	Percent total or mean ± SD (n = number of patients)	NOSE score mean ± SD or Pearson's R	p value, statistical test ‡ (one-way ANOVA) † (Student's t-test) ¶ (Pearson correlation) * = statistical significance
Demographics			
Age (years)	52.1 ± 17.5 years (n = 240)	$R^2 = 8.5 \times 10^{-5}$ No or negligible relationship	p = 0.8843, ¶
Gender (%)			
Male	66.3% (n = 159)	30.4 ± 22.5	p = 0.1486, †
Female	33.7% (n = 81)	35.2 ± 26.8	
BMI (kg/m²)	29.0 ± 6.8 kg/m² (n = 240)	$R^2 = 0.0007$ No or negligible relationship	p = 0.6815, ¶
Ethnicity (%)			
Caucasian	69.1% (n = 166)	33.4 ± 24.5	
Asian	12.5% (n = 30)	26.8 ± 23.5	
Hispanic	7.1% (n = 17)	25.2 ± 20.3	p = 0.2572, ‡
Indian	6.3% (n = 15)	27.1 ± 19.0	
Black	4.1% (n = 10)	44.3 ± 29.9	
Pacific Islander	0.83% (n = 2)	27.5 ± 3.5	
Medical history			
History of nasal trauma (%)			
Yes	18.7% (n = 45)	**40.0 ± 23.6**	**p = 0.0136, †***
No	81.3% (n = 195)	**30.2 ± 23.9**	
Prior nasal surgery (%)			
Yes	22.5% (n = 54)	36.3 ± 23.6	p = 0.1421, †
No	77.5% (n = 186)	30.8 ± 24.2	
Allergic rhinitis (%)			
Yes	33.8% (n = 81)	**41.2 ± 25.8**	**p < 0.0001, †***
No	66.3% (n = 159)	**27.3 ± 21.8**	
Nasal steroids (%)			
Yes	14.6% (n = 35)	**41.5 ± 24.9**	**p = 0.0108, †***
No	85.4% (n = 205)	**30.4 ± 23.7**	
Nasal antihistamines (%)			
Yes	10.8% (n = 26)	38.0 ± 25.0	p = 0.1820, †
No	89.1% (n = 214)	31.3 ± 23.9	
Oral antihistamines (%)			
Yes	5.0% (n = 12)	31.5 ± 23.8	p = 0.1379, †
No	95.0% (n = 228)	42.0 ± 28.8	

deformity was excluded, suggesting that the two variables overlap to a significant degree. Pearson chi square analysis demonstrated a significant association between external nasal deformity (grades 2–4) and internal nasal valve angle < 10 degrees (either <5 degrees or 5 to <10 degrees) (OR = 3.33 (95% CI 1.67–6.64), p = 0.0004). Univariate analysis with one-way ANOVA showed that external nasal deformity and internal nasal valve angles were significantly associated with NO-VAS scores; see Table 4. Inferior turbinate size was not associated with NOSE scores or any of the NO-VAS measures.

4. Discussion

There are four main findings in this study. First, physical exam tests were significantly associated with nasal obstruction. This study demonstrated that the presence of an external nasal deformity and a narrow internal nasal valve angle are associated with higher NO-VAS scores. In some cases, especially when nasal steroids do not improve nasal breathing, a referral to an otolaryngologist may be warranted, as some patients may have fixed anatomical obstructions

TABLE 2: (a) Distribution of nasal physical exam findings and association with NOSE scores. (b) Additional nasal physical exam findings and association with NOSE scores.

(a)

	Percent total (n = number of patients)		NOSE score by subgroup (mean ± SD)		p value (one-way ANOVA) ∗ = statistical significance	
External nasal deformity						
Grade 1: none	82.5% (n = 198)		30.1 ± 22.8			
Grade 2: mild	9.2% (n = 22)		34.5 ± 25.3		**p = 0.0149∗**	
Grade 3: moderate	7.9% (n = 19)		48.5 ± 30.2			
Grade 4: severe	0.4% (n = 1)		35.0			
Nasal septum deviation						
Grade 1: 0 to 25% deflection	53.3% (n = 128)		27.7 ± 22.0			
Grade 2: 26–50% deflection	31.6% (n = 76)		33.5 ± 22.9		**p = 0.0024∗**	
Grade 3: 51–75% deflection	8.3% (n = 20)		43.3 ± 32.8			
Grade 4: 76–100% deflection	6.7% (n = 16)		45.9 ± 25.4			
Internal nasal valve angle	*Right*	*Left*	*Right*	*Left*	*Right*	*Left*
Grade 1: <5 degrees	3.8% (n = 9)	4.2% (n = 10)	66.1 ± 18.3	58.0 ± 27.4		
Grade 2: 5 to <10 degrees	18.1% (n = 43)	18.1% (n = 43)	44.3 ± 25.5	44.1 ± 24.8	**p < 0.0001**	**p < 0.0001**
Grade 3: 10 to <15 degrees	51.9% (n = 123)	53.6% (n = 127)	29.1 ± 21.9	28.9 ± 21.5		
Grade 4: 15 or more degrees	26.2% (n = 62)	24.1% (n = 57)	24.8 ± 21.6	25.7 ± 22.6		
Internal nasal valve collapse	*Right*	*Left*	*Right*	*Left*	*Right*	*Left*
Grade 1: no collapse	74.1% (n = 178)	74.2% (n = 178)	No significant difference between groups		p = 0.4210	p = 0.1053
Grade 2: mild collapse ≤ 33%	17.9% (n = 43)	18.3% (n = 44)				
Grade 3: moderate collapse = 34–66%	7.5% (n = 18)	6.7% (n = 16)				
Grade 4: severe collapse ≥ 67%	0.4% (n = 1)	8.3% (n = 2)				
Inferior turbinate size	*Right*	*Left*	*Right*	*Left*	*Right*	*Left*
Grade 1: 0–25% AP nasal airway space	27.9% (n = 67)	25.0% (n = 60)	No significant difference between groups		p = 0.9472	p = 0.1618
Grade 2: 26–50% AP nasal airway space	24.1% (n = 58)	27.1% (n = 65)				
Grade 3: 51–75% AP nasal airway space	30.0% (n = 72)	32.9% (n = 79)				
Grade 4: 76–100% AP nasal airway space	17.9% (n = 43)	15.0% (n = 36)				

(b)

	Subgroup % total or mean ± SD (n = number)	NOSE score mean ± SD or Pearson's R	p value, statistical test ‡ (one-way ANOVA) ¶ (Pearson correlation) ∗ = statistical significance
Nasal obstruction visual analog scale (NO-VAS): 0–100			
Bilateral (both nostrils open)	22.3 ± 23.8	R^2 = 0.38; moderate positive relationship	p < 0.0001, ¶∗
Left nostril (cover right)	27.6 ± 28.0	R^2 = 0.37; moderate positive relationship	p < 0.0001, ¶∗
Right nostril (cover left)	23.0 ± 25.7	R^2 = 0.21; weak positive relationship	p < 0.0001, ¶∗

(b) Continued.

	Subgroup % total or mean ± SD (n = number)	NOSE score mean ± SD or Pearson's R	p value, statistical test ‡ (one-way ANOVA) ¶ (Pearson correlation) * = statistical significance
Cottle maneuver effect on nasal airflow			
Grade 1: no improvement	11.1% (n = 16)	15.0 ± 17.9	
Grade 2: mild improvement	39.6% (n = 57)	30.3 ± 22.9	p = 0.0087, ‡*
Grade 3: moderate improvement	25.7% (n = 37)	37.4 ± 24.1	
Grade 4: significant improvement	23.6% (n = 34)	37.4 ± 27.2	
Classification of external nasal deformities			
C-shaped	26.7% (n = 4)		
Reverse C-shaped	60.0% (n = 9)	No significant difference between groups	p = 0.8352, ‡
S-shaped	13.3% (n = 2)		
Reverse S-shaped	0% (n = 0)		
Classification of septal deviations: cephalocaudal dimension			
C-shaped	51.4% (n = 35)		
Reverse C-shaped	36.8% (n = 25)	No significant difference between groups	p = 0.5270, ‡
S-shaped	7.4% (n = 5)		
Reverse S-shaped	4.4% (n = 3)		
Classification of septal deviations: anteroposterior dimension			
C-shaped	50.0% (n = 32)		
Reverse C-shaped	36.0% (n = 23)	No significant difference between groups	p = 0.6841, ‡
S-shaped	10.9% (n = 7)		
Reverse S-shaped	3.1% (n = 2)		

TABLE 3: Clinical factors related to high NOSE score (≥50, "moderate to severe problem"): results of univariate and multivariate analysis.

Prognostic factor	Univariate analysis			Multivariate analysis		
	Odds ratio	95% confidence interval	p value (Pearson's chi square)	Odds ratio	95% confidence interval	p value (Pearson's chi square)
Nasal obstruction visual analog scale: ≥50	11.1	4.40–28.11	p < 0.0001*	17.6	5.83–61.6	p < 0.0001*
Internal nasal valve angle: <10 degrees (grade 1 or 2)‡	4.34	2.31–8.12	p < 0.0001*	NS	NS	p = 0.2433
External nasal deformity: mild to severe (grades 2–4)	3.59	1.79–7.22	p = 0.0002*	4.63	1.14–19.9	p = 0.0339*
Allergic rhinitis: yes	3.36	1.83–6.16	p < 0.0001*	5.5	1.77–18.7	p = 0.0041*
Use of nasal steroids: yes	2.30	1.08–4.89	p = 0.0266*	NS	NS	p = 0.2262
Cottle maneuver: moderate to significant improvement (grade 3 or 4)	2.28	1.03–5.07	p = 0.0399*	NS	NS	p = 0.2862
Nasal septal deviation: mild to severe (grades 2–4)	2.05	1.13–3.72	p = 0.0168*	NS	NS	p = 0.1906
History of nasal trauma: yes	1.89	0.94–3.80	p = 0.0697	NS	NS	p = 0.6106

‡ At least one nasal valve (right or left) with angle < 10 degrees.
* Statistical significance.

TABLE 4: Association of nasal physical exam findings with NO-VAS scores at time of exam.

	Percent total (n = number of patients)		NO-VAS score by subgroup (mean ± SD)		p value (one-way ANOVA) * = statistical significance	
External nasal deformity			*NO-VAS: bilateral*			
Grade 1: none	88.6% (n = 132)		20.6 ± 23.9			
Grade 2: mild	0%		N/A		**p = 0.0099***	
Grade 3: moderate	11.4% (n = 17)		36.3 ± 18.2			
Grade 4: severe	0%		N/A			
Nasal septum deviation						
Grade 1: 0 to 25% deflection	60.4% (n = 90)		No significant difference between groups		p = 0.0612	
Grade 2: 26–50% deflection	21.4% (n = 32)					
Grade 3: 51–75% deflection	12.1% (n = 18)					
Grade 4: 76–100% deflection	6.0% (n = 9)					
Internal nasal valve angle	*Right*	*Left*	*NO-VAS: right*	*NO-VAS: left*	*Right*	*Left*
Grade 1: <5 degrees	4.1% (n = 6)	6.1% (n = 9)	54.8 ± 29.9	48.2 ± 34.2		
Grade 2: 5 to <10 degrees	17.8% (n = 26)	17.8% (n = 26)	24.9 ± 20.1	39.7 ± 24.5	**p = 0.0023***	**p = 0.0014***
Grade 3: 10 to <15 degrees	43.8% (n = 64)	45.8% (n = 67)	23.8 ± 26.1	25.6 ± 26.1		
Grade 4: 15 or more degrees	34.2% (n = 50)	30.1% (n = 44)	15.6 ± 23.0	18.3 ± 27.2		
Internal nasal valve collapse	*Right*	*Left*	*Right*	*Left*	*Right*	*Left*
Grade 1: no collapse	86.5% (n = 128)	86.6% (n = 129)	No significant difference between groups		p = 0.6166	p = 0.2666
Grade 2: mild collapse ≤ 33%	4.0% (n = 6)	3.4% (n = 5)				
Grade 3: moderate collapse = 34–66%	10.0% (n = 15)	9.4% (n = 14)				
Grade 4: severe collapse ≥ 67%	0%	0.7% (n = 1)				
Inferior turbinate size	*Right*	*Left*	*Right*	*Left*	*Right*	*Left*
Grade 1: 0–25% AP nasal airway space	26.8% (n = 40)	22.1% (n = 33)	No significant difference between groups		p = 0.1487	p = 0.9494
Grade 2: 26–50% AP nasal airway space	24.8% (n = 37)	22.8% (n = 34)				
Grade 3: 51–75% AP nasal airway space	30.2% (n = 45)	40.9% (n = 61)				
Grade 4: 76–100% AP nasal airway space	18.1% (n = 27)	14.0% (n = 21)				

which could be improved with surgery. Examples include a narrow internal nasal valve angle and/or internal nasal septal deviation. We found that 89% of patients reported at least mild improvement in nasal breathing and nearly half of all patients reported moderate or significant improvement with the Cottle maneuver. For patients with no improvement in breathing with the Cottle maneuver, the NOSE score was very low (15.0±17.9), while those with mild (30.3±22.9), moderate (37.4 ± 24.1), or significant (37.4 ± 27.2) improvement with the Cottle maneuver had higher NOSE scores. Given that the Cottle maneuver improved the subjective sensation of nasal airflow in 89% of patients in this study, this test may not be as helpful in determining the site of nasal obstruction, especially with regard to trying to determine if a specific nasal surgery would benefit the patient. However, it potentially could assist with determining who might benefit from surgery, generally.

Second, there are several different anatomical variables that may contribute to nasal obstruction. By using grading scales, this study was able to determine the specific grades of nasal anatomical variables that were associated with

nasal obstruction. For example, we demonstrated that internal nasal septal deviations contribute significantly to nasal obstruction. More importantly, we identified a "severity-dependent" relationship, such that the average NOSE score increased with higher grade deflections. In contrast, the shape of the internal nasal septal deviations (in either the cephalo-caudal or anteroposterior dimensions) was not associated with nasal obstruction, demonstrating that the severity of the septal deviation is most important. Furthermore, patients with an external nasal deformity were found to be highly likely to also have narrowing of the internal nasal valve, and narrow angles were associated with higher NOSE scores in a similar severity-dependent relationship. This underscores the importance of examination of the internal nasal valve angle during evaluation of the upper airway, particularly if an external nasal deformity is present.

Third, although the inferior turbinates seemingly contribute significantly to the overall nasal cavity airway space at the level of the internal nasal valve, the size of the inferior turbinates was not associated with either the NOSE score or NO-VAS measures. This study demonstrated that inferior turbinates are generally of larger sizes for Asians (2.78 ± 0.81) and Blacks (3.00 ± 0.66), while they tend to be smaller in Caucasians (2.19 ± 0.89) and are in between for Latinos (2.53 ± 0.97). Caution, therefore, should always be exercised in evaluating a patient with isolated turbinate hypertrophy, particularly if they do not have an elevated NOSE or NO-VAS score. Moreover, additional anatomic contributors to nasal obstruction should be sought in the patient with presumed isolated turbinate hypertrophy as the sole cause for nasal obstruction. In a systematic review, Rhee et al. identified several studies reporting a significant decrease in the NOSE score after inferior turbinoplasties were performed [8]. Therefore, inferior turbinoplasties alone may benefit patients with nasal obstruction and the isolated nasal exam finding of inferior turbinate hypertrophy. Inferior turbinoplasties are commonly performed at the time of septoplasties, septorhinoplasties, or sinus surgeries in order to increase the size of the nasal airway, which provides the additional benefit of increasing continuous positive airway pressure (CPAP) device use and decreasing therapeutic CPAP treatment pressures [9].

Lastly, we would encourage the use of questionnaires, grading scales, and classification systems as a means to help identify specific factors (demographics, medical history, physical tests, and nasal exam findings) that contribute to nasal obstruction. The use of these tools allows for the treatment (medical or surgical) to be evaluated in a systematic fashion before and after the intervention. The use of grading scales and the reporting of outcomes (with means and standard deviations) based on grades can also facilitate future research to include meta-analyses. Currently, there are several grading scales and classification systems in the published literature. In the head and neck, it is common to use four grades per subsite and this promotes high intra- and interrater reliability during validation testing [2]. Some head and neck subsites such as tonsil sizes [10] are commonly incorporated into the medical record. In this study, we referenced questionnaires and nasal exam classification systems based on a 1 to 4 grading scale, which have easily been incorporated into the standard physical examination. Future research could be aimed at evaluating the general population (especially in patients with no complaints of nasal obstruction) in order to help establish normative data.

5. Limitations

This study was a retrospective review, and, like any retrospective review, the authors are limited to what has been documented previously. However, because the first author incorporated a detailed upper airway exam to include the use of grading scales for nasal examinations, these were consistently documented into the medical record in a standardized way. The findings from this study are based on a single institution; the goal of the authors is to perform future multi-institutional studies evaluating the effect of multiple variables on nasal obstruction.

6. Conclusion

Allergic rhinitis, NO-VAS score ≥ 50, and external nasal deformity were statistically significant independent predictors of high NOSE scores on multivariate analysis. Inferior turbinate size was not associated with NOSE scores or NO-VAS.

Disclosure

Authors have no financial interests in any companies or other entities that have an interest in the information in the contribution (e.g., grants, advisory boards, employment, consultancies, contracts, honoraria, royalties, expert testimony, partnerships, or stock ownership in medically related fields). Institution where the work was primarily performed is Stanford Hospital. The views herein are the private views of the authors and do not reflect the official views of the Department of the Army or the Department of Defense.

Competing Interests

The authors declare that they have no competing interests.

Authors' Contributions

All authors met the criteria for authorship established by the International Committee of Medical Journal Editors; specifically Macario Camacho and Soroush Zaghi were responsible for substantial contribution to the conception, design, statistical analysis, and drafting the work, revising the work, and reviewing the paper. Victor Certal, Jose Abdullatif, Rahul Modi, and Shankar Sridhara were responsible for substantial contribution to the conception, design, revising the work, and reviewing the paper. Anthony M. Tolisano, Edward T. Chang, Benjamin B. Cable, and Robson Capasso had substantial contributions to the nonstatistical analysis and interpretation of data for the work and revising the work critically for important intellectual content. Additionally, all authors provided final approval of the version to be published and agreed to be accountable for all aspects of the work in ensuring the accuracy and/or integrity of the work.

References

[1] J. C. Hsia, M. Camacho, and R. Capasso, "Snoring exclusively during nasal breathing: a newly described respiratory pattern during sleep," *Sleep & Breathing*, vol. 18, no. 1, pp. 159–164, 2014.

[2] M. Camacho, S. Zaghi, V. Certal et al., "Inferior turbinate classification system, grades 1 to 4: development and validation study," *The Laryngoscope*, vol. 125, pp. 296–302, 2015.

[3] M. G. Stewart, D. L. Witsell, T. L. Smith, E. M. Weaver, B. Yueh, and M. T. Hannley, "Development and validation of the Nasal Obstruction Symptom Evaluation (NOSE) Scale," *Otolaryngology—Head and Neck Surgery*, vol. 130, no. 2, pp. 157–163, 2004.

[4] G. Ciprandi, F. Mora, M. Cassano, A. M. Gallina, and R. Mora, "Visual analog scale (VAS) and nasal obstruction in persistent

allergic rhinitis," *Otolaryngology-Head and Neck Surgery*, vol. 141, no. 4, pp. 527–529, 2009.

[5] G. J. Tsao, N. Fijalkowski, and S. P. Most, "Validation of a grading system for lateral nasal wall insufficiency," *Allergy & Rhinology*, vol. 4, no. 2, pp. e66–e68, 2013.

[6] C. E. Heinberg and E. B. Kern, "The Cottle sign: an aid in the physical diagnose of nasal airflow disturbances," *Rhinology*, vol. 11, no. 3, pp. 89–94, 1973.

[7] R. J. Rohrich, J. P. Gunter, M. A. Deuber, and W. P. Adams Jr., "The deviated nose: optimizing results using a simplified classification and algorithmic approach," *Plastic and Reconstructive Surgery*, vol. 110, no. 6, pp. 1509–1524, 2002.

[8] J. S. Rhee, C. D. Sullivan, D. O. Frank, J. S. Kimbell, and G. J. M. Garcia, "A systematic review of patient-reported nasal obstruction scores: defining normative and symptomatic ranges in surgical patients," *JAMA Facial Plastic Surgery*, vol. 16, no. 3, pp. 219–225, 2014.

[9] M. Camacho, M. Riaz, R. Capasso et al., "The effect of nasal surgery on continuous positive airway pressure device use and therapeutic treatment pressures. a systematic review and meta-analysis," *SLEEP*, vol. 38, no. 2, pp. 279–286, 2015.

[10] M. Friedman, H. Tanyeri, M. La Rosa et al., "Clinical predictors of obstructive sleep apnea," *The Laryngoscope*, vol. 109, no. 12, pp. 1901–1907, 1999.

29

Clinical Outcomes for Breast Cancer Patients Undergoing Mastectomy and Reconstruction with Use of DermACELL, a Sterile, Room Temperature Acellular Dermal Matrix

Christopher Vashi[1,2]

[1] The Plastic Surgery Group, Chapel Place II, 340 Thomas More Parkway, Crestview Hills, KY 41017, USA
[2] The Plastic Surgery Group of Greater Cincinnati, 4850 Red Bank Expressway, Cincinnati, OH 45227, USA

Correspondence should be addressed to Christopher Vashi; christopher.vashi@gmail.com

Academic Editor: Francesco Carinci

Background. Decellularized human skin has been used in a variety of medical applications, primarily involving soft tissue reconstruction, wound healing, and tendon augmentation. Theoretically, decellularization removes potentially immunogenic material and provides a clean scaffold for cellular and vascular in growth. The use of acellular dermal matrix in two-stage postmastectomy breast reconstruction is described. *Methods*. Ten consecutive breast cancer patients were treated with mastectomies and immediate reconstruction from August to November 2011. There were 8 bilateral and 1 unilateral mastectomies for a total of 17 breasts, with one exclusion for chronic tobacco use. Reconstruction included the use of a new 6 × 16 cm sterile, room temperature acellular dermal matrix patch (DermACELL) soaked in a cefazolin bath. *Results*. Of the 17 breasts, 15 reconstructions were completed; 14 of them with expander to implant sequence and acellular dermal matrix. Histological analysis of biopsies obtained during trimming of the matrix at the second stage appeared nonremarkable with evidence of normal healing, cellularity, and vascular infiltration. *Conclusion*. Postoperative observations showed that this cellular dermal matrix appears to be an appropriate adjunct to reconstruction with expanders. This acellular dermal matrix appeared to work well with all patients, even those receiving postoperative chemotherapy, postoperative radiation, prednisone, or warfarin sodium.

1. Introduction

For breast cancer patients, the use of expanders and/or implants is the most common method of breast reconstruction following mastectomy [1]. This typically involves a two-stage process where tissue expanders are placed postmastectomy and filled gradually for a period of several months. Once the desired expander volume is reached, the second reconstructive stage involves replacing the expanders with silicone implants. Another reconstruction option is the use of autologous tissue from a separate patient site to supply needed skin for wound closure at the mastectomy site. However, the cosmetic issues of this method remain negative for patients due to scarring and differences in skin coloration between the autologous and surrounding tissues. Donor site morbidity also remains a concern for many patients. When postmastectomy implantation is feasible and desired,

structural support of the breast can provide ideal shape and implant positioning. Such support can be accomplished by introducing biocompatible mesh, but there have been some complications observed with this procedure [2].

As an alternative, acellular dermal matrices (ADMs) are produced by the removal of the epidermal layer from thin slices of skin, leaving the dermal layer and extracellular matrix followed by a decellularization process. The removal of donor cellular material including major histocompatibility complex (MHC) proteins is performed to theoretically minimize immunological response in ADM recipients [3] and promote revascularization and cellular infiltration [4], thus yielding clinically promising materials for soft tissue reconstruction, wound healing, and tendon augmentation [5–24]. However, there exists a nascent complication rate with ADMs in breast reconstruction procedures, including seromas and reports of "red breast syndrome," an apparent inflammatory response to residual components in the ADM [16, 25–27]. A new ADM, DermACELL, (here referred to as D-ADM) is manufactured using a proprietary decellularization process [28] that removes at least 97% of nucleic acid material, is not freeze-dried, and is provided hydrated with a Sterility Assurance Level (SAL) of 10^{-6}. This unique process yields a material that has demonstrated rapid *in vivo* cellular infiltration and vascularization [4] with both properties being advantageous in healing [29]. At the time of this writing, there were no known published reports of the use of this material in breast reconstruction. Here, we report the postmastectomy outcome of D-ADM used in two-stage breast reconstructions.

2. Materials and Methods

2.1. Study Overview.
Ten consecutive female breast cancer patients between the ages of 28 and 60 years old were scheduled to undergo mastectomies from August to November 2011. All eligible patients were included with criteria for exclusion being tobacco use (smoking) or a known planned course of postoperative radiation after mastectomy. One patient was excluded prior to beginning the study under the criteria of smoking and two patients did have previously unplanned radiation treatments following ADM implantation due to unanticipated laboratory results and were still included in the series. Procedures for the 9 remaining patients included 8 bilateral mastectomies and 1 unilateral mastectomy for a total of 17 breasts in the study. The final filling volumes of their tissue expanders ranged between 450 and 800 cc. Eight patients totaling 14 breasts advanced to the 2nd stage operation which involved removing the tissue expanders to be replaced with silicone implants. One of the eight patients lost the right expander, presumably due to smoking. Subsequently, this patient received an autologous Transverse Rectus Abdominis Myocutaneous (TRAM) flap on the right and completed the expander to implant exchange on the left. The ninth patient opted for bilateral expander removal after metastatic disease was diagnosed.

2.2. Clinical Procedure and Implant Description.
The mastectomies were performed by a total of 4 general surgeons. The D-ADM (DermACELL, LifeNet Health, Virginia Beach, VA) is manufactured [28] using a combination of nondenaturing anionic detergent (N-Lauroyl sarcosinate), recombinant endonuclease (Benzonase), and antibiotics (Polymixin B, Vancomycin, and Lincomycin) and then terminally sterilized with a low dosage of gamma irradiation at low temperatures to a SAL of 10^{-6}. The material is never freeze-dried and is stored at room temperature, ready to use. The 6 × 16 cm D-ADM patches were soaked in a Cefazolin (ANCEF, GlaxoSmithKline, Philadelphia, PA) bath and split along a hypotenuse. When possible, intraoperative expansion was performed to the point of light tension on closure. Two drains were placed, one in the superior/axilla area and one in the inframammary fold at the D-ADM application site. Expansion began at 3 weeks postop. at a rate of 30–60 cc per week even if drains remained in place. An example of the surgical procedure is shown in Figure 1.

2.3. Case Descriptions and Course of Treatment

2.3.1. Patient 1.
A 46-year-old patient received bilateral mastectomies on September 9, 2011 and advanced to the 2nd stage on February 28, 2012. She underwent chemotherapy during expansion and developed DVT in the left leg during this period, which was treated with warfarin sodium (Coumadin, Bristol-Myers Squibb Company, New York, NY). Her expanders were filled to the full 550 cc and replaced with 700 cc silicone implants. She has completed nipple areolar reconstruction.

2.3.2. Patient 2.
A 55-year-old patient received a unilateral mastectomy of the right breast and required evacuation of a hematoma on the first postoperative day after placement of the D-ADM. At that time, the D-ADM was intact and was not removed. She advanced to the 2nd stage at 6 weeks and to a 3rd stage nipple reconstruction at 16 weeks. She was expanded to 450 cc and received a 500 cc implant. Her areolar micropigmentation was completed several months later.

2.3.3. Patient 3.
A 60-year-old patient received bilateral mastectomies on September 26, 2011, was expanded to 450 cc, and advanced to the 2nd stage on January 24, 2012 with 533 cc implants. She opted not to proceed with nipple areolar reconstruction.

2.3.4. Patient 4.
A 52-year-old patient received bilateral mastectomies on October 11, 2011, was expanded to 510 cc, and advanced to the 2nd stage at 19 wks with 600 cc implants. She has completed nipple and areolar reconstruction.

2.3.5. Patient 5.
A 43-year-old patient received bilateral mastectomies on October 20, 2011. She received unanticipated radiation therapy to the left side and was eventually expanded to 510 cc after radiation. She advanced to the 2nd stage on April 17, 2012 with 600 cc implants. She has completed nipple and areolar reconstruction.

2.3.6. Patient 6.
A 28-year-old patient, former smoker, relapsed postoperatively after receiving bilateral mastectomies. She experienced right expander extrusion at 4 wks, and reconstruction was put on hold until smoking cessation. Her left side was fully expanded to 510 cc, and she was reconstructed with a 533 cc implant on the left and a TRAM flap on the right. She has completed nipple reconstruction and remained nicotine free.

2.3.7. Patient 7.
A 54-year-old patient received bilateral mastectomies on August 5, 2011. Her drains fell out 4 days postoperatively and she experienced seromas with incisional dehiscence, which required irrigation and drain replacement. She experienced recurrent incisional reopening in the left breast which required left expander removal and replacement after cultures of the excision showed negative gram stains. She was expanded to 800 cc and successfully underwent stage two on March 6, 2012 with 800 cc implants. She has completed nipple and areolar reconstruction.

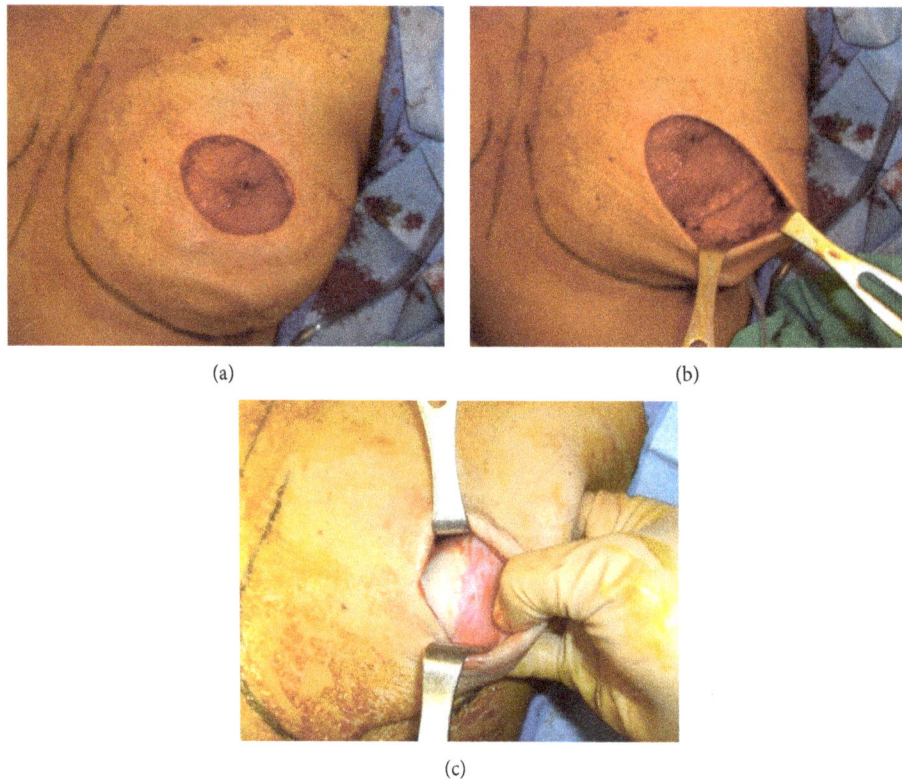

(a)

(b)

(c)

FIGURE 1: (a) Showing placement of expander. (b) Showing D-ADM and intraoperative expansion. (c) Showing D-ADM incorporation at second stage reconstruction.

2.3.8. Patient 8. A 43-year-old patient received bilateral mastectomies on November 7, 2011 and was expanded to 800 cc, and the 2nd stage was completed on February 23, 2012 with 800 cc implants. She has completed nipple and areolar reconstruction.

2.3.9. Patient 9. A 48-year-old patient received bilateral mastectomies on November 4, 2011 and had shown complete response to neoadjuvant chemotherapy by preoperative imaging. She had a positive margin to the chest wall and received postoperative radiation therapy. Despite complete resolution of radiation dermatitis and expansion, she elected to have her expanders removed and abort reconstruction when she was found to have hepatic metastases.

3. Results

3.1. Clinical Performance. Of the 9 implant patients, most had acceptable results (Table 1). The healthy patients and those with post-ADM placement chemotherapy, hematomas, or warfarin sodium treatment all did well with full recoveries and without further complications, capsule contracture, or need of reoperation. The ADM was 100% adhered and revascularized in all of the patients. Although a demarcation line between the matrix and native capsule was noted (e.g., see Figure 1), the matrix was incorporated at this line. Also, one notable seroma was recorded. Two patients had radiated expanders, and one patient, a smoker, lost a unilateral

expander. D-ADM seemed to work well with those patients who received unanticipated postmastectomy radiation treatments. These were scheduled to start three weeks after the mastectomies. Observation, quality, and incorporation of the radiated D-ADM were seen at the second stage of expander to implant exchange and found to be comparable to the nonradiated side in the same patients. Typical patients are shown in Figures 2, 3, and 4. Of particular note was the absence of "red breast syndrome" in all patients, although the limited number of patients in this series precludes any generalizable conclusions.

3.2. Histological Analysis. Biopsy specimens were obtained from 8 of the 9 patients and submitted in formalin to Dominion Pathology Laborator (Norfolk, VA) for sectioning and staining. Stains included hematoxylin and eosin (H&E) to assess cellularity and general ultrastructure, immuno-histochemical stain CD34, an endothelial cell marker, to assess vascularity, and Verhoeff-Van Gieson (VVG) to assess elastic fibers. Histological assessments were made by dermatopathologists Kevaghn Fair, DO (Dominion Pathology Laboratory) and Antoinette Hood, MD (Eastern Virginia Medical School, Norfolk, VA).

General histological observations for all biopsied patients included presence of fibroblasts, vasculature, and intact ultrastructure, including elastin. Occasional foreign body response was noted, localized to polarizable material which

TABLE 1: Patient overview and results.

Patient number	Age (yrs)	Postop. chemotherapy	Post-ADM implant radiation	Uni- or bilateral	Duration of implant prior to 2nd stage (wks)	Expander size	Implant size	Nipple/Areola reconstruction	Surgical site infection	Seroma
1	46	Yes	No	Bilateral	16	550 cc	700 cc	Yes	No	—
2	55	No	No	R only	6	450 cc	500 cc	Yes	No	—
3	60	No	No	Bilateral	16	450 cc	533 cc	No	No	—
4	52	No	No	Bilateral	19	510 cc	600 cc	Yes	No	—
5	43	No	Yes	Bilateral	16	510 cc	600 cc	Yes	No	—
6	28	No	No	Bilateral	Right side TRAM* and left implant	510 cc	533 cc	Yes	No	—
7	54	No	No	Bilateral	7 weeks	800 cc	800 cc	Yes	Yes	Yes
8	43	No	No	Bilateral	14 weeks	800 cc	800 cc	Yes	No	—
9	48	Neo-adj.	Yes	Bilateral	11/4/2011 stage 1	Aborted	Aborted	Aborted	No	—
10	Excluded due to smoking	—	—	—	—	—	—	—	—	—

*Transverse Rectus Abdominis Myocutaneous.

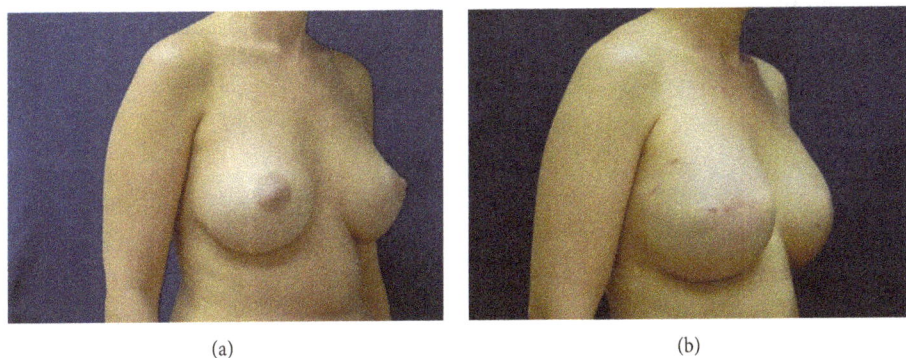

FIGURE 2: (a) Preoperative before mastectomy. (b) Postoperative after 700 cc silicone implant placed.

was present in a regular pattern consistent with suture material. Little inflammation was noted except in conjunction with this foreign body response. In general, the side of the implant facing the expander exhibited pseudocapsule formation as a benign response to the expander material. When observed, the opposite interface between the implant and the host tissue demonstrated some level of tissue integration with minimal inflammation consistent with normal healing. Compared to the host tissue, the implant material appeared more organized with fewer living cells and less vasculature, a finding expected for a stable material slowly being incorporated and remodeled after a few weeks to a few months following surgery when the specimens were collected. Specific histology samples from patient number 1 are shown in Figure 5.

4. Discussion

Two-stage breast reconstruction procedures can be facilitated by the use of a sling under the expander for both support and cosmetic benefits. Among many other factors,

the choice of this material is key in ensuring a good outcome. Decellularized human skin (ADM) is often used for these procedures. It is hypothesized that certain complications may arise from these materials as a function of successful cellular removal. One of these materials (D-ADM) is validated to remove ≥97% DNA while maintaining structural integrity. Here, we used this material and assessed its performance through patient follow-up and histological analysis of biopsies taken upon expander removal. Overall results were good. One observation of note is that there were no observed drug effects of warfarin sodium and prednisone on the outcome of the procedure. Warfarin sodium use presents a concern for uncontrolled hemorrhaging in these patients, and this was not noted. Prednisone is a corticosteroid drug used in patients with low steroid levels and also used as an anti-inflammatory medication. Clotting and generating an immune response are key biological processes that stimulate wound healing, which are affected to some degree in the patients taking warfarin sodium and prednisone. These patients had no adverse effects postoperatively. One patient exhibited a hematoma that required evacuation on

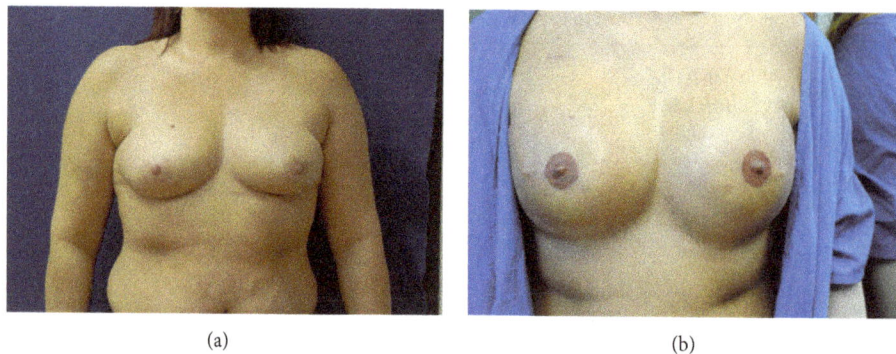

(a)

(b)

FIGURE 3: (a) Preoperative before mastectomy. (b) Postoperative after 800 cc silicone implant placed.

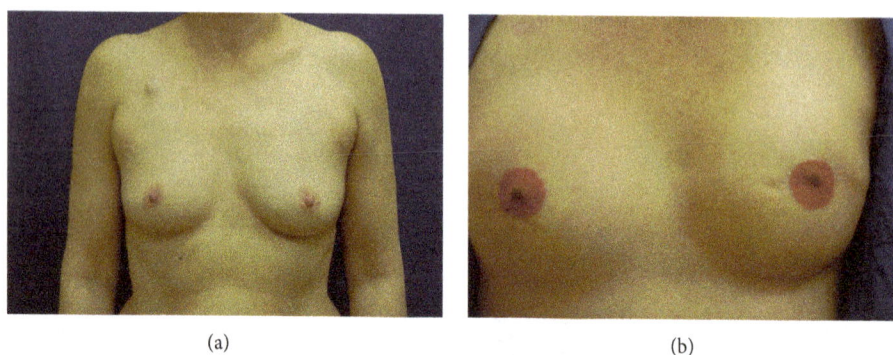

(a)

(b)

FIGURE 4: (a) Preoperative before mastectomy. (b) Postoperative after left radiation and reconstruction.

postoperative day one after placement of the D-ADM. At that time, the D-ADM was intact and was not removed. She went on to complete successful expansion. There are several concerns with postoperative hematomas, one of which being the inherent risk of surgery when needed to correct them. Also, the accumulation of blood from hematomas can lead to increased tension on the surgical area causing local infection that prevents proper wound healing [27]. This did not appear to be a factor in the patient with the hematoma in this study. In addition, the absence of "red breast syndrome" in these patients is especially noteworthy. This complication is commonly noted in breast reconstruction procedures using HADM [25, 26]. The factors leading to red breast syndrome are not fully understood, but inflammation in response to the foreign material is thought to be the leading cause. The cause of the absence of red breast syndrome in these patients is unclear, but the complete decellularization of this particular ADM may be a key factor, although the limited sample size prevents firm conclusions. Finally, the patient who relapsed into a previous smoking habit experienced the most complications postoperatively.

5. Conclusions

D-ADM appears to be an appropriate adjunct to reconstruction with expanders. D-ADM worked well with patients receiving chemotherapy for further cancer treatment and

seemed to work well with those who had received postoperative radiation treatments while the D-ADM was in place. As far as other drug effects on the procedure, there appeared to be none with patients in this study taking warfarin sodium and prednisone as they both responded favorably postoperatively. Additionally, the patient experiencing hematoma responded well with D-ADM despite this complication. Overall, healthy patients had the most favorable results, while those with unhealthy lifestyles, particularly smokers, experienced the most complications.

Acknowledgments

The author would like to acknowledge Antoinette Hood, MD (Eastern Virginia Medical School, Norfolk, VA) and Kevaghn Fair, DO (Dominion Pathology Laboratory, Norfolk, VA) for histological assessments of biopsies and interpretation of findings.

References

[1] American Society of Plastic Surgeons, "Reconstructive Plastic Surgery Trends," 2011, http://www.plasticsurgery.org/ Documents/news-resources/statistics/2011-statistics/2011-ms-reconstructive-surgery-trends.pdf.

(a)

(b)

(c)

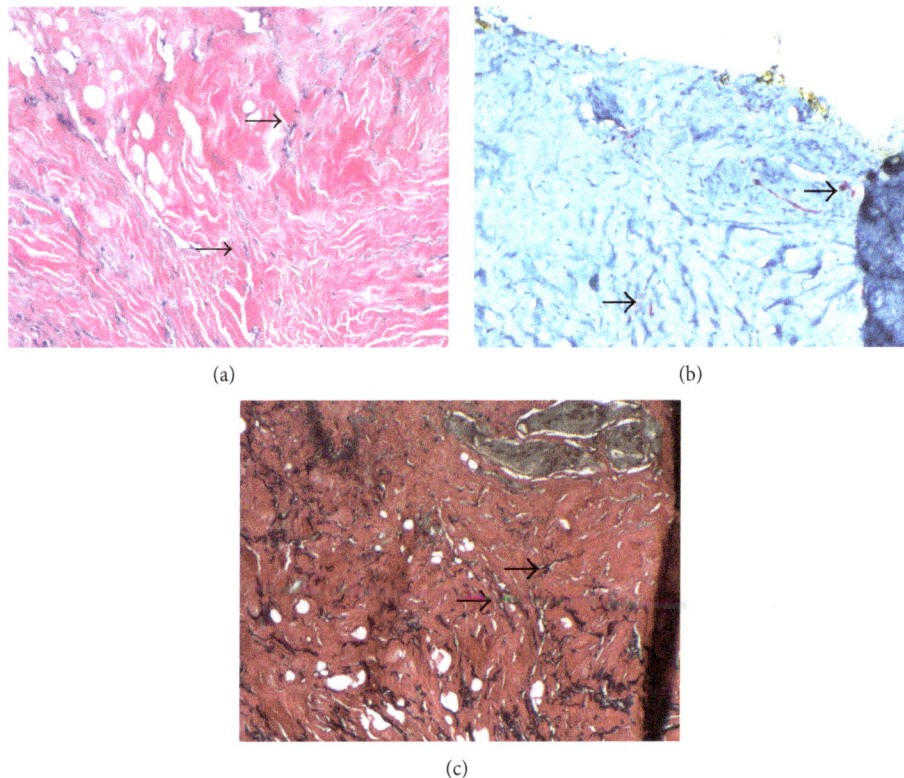

FIGURE 5: (a) Hematoxylin and eosin staining of biopsy specimen from patient number 1 following 16 weeks *in situ* placement of ADM. Note the intact ultrastructure and also evidence of cellular in growth as apparent fibroblasts (arrows) at 10x magnification. (b) CD34 staining of biopsy from patient number 1 following 16 weeks *in situ* placement of ADM. Evidence of robust vascularization is noted by reddish-brown stains apparently associated with blood vessels (arrows) at 10x magnification. (c) Verhoeff-Van Geisen staining of biopsy from patient number 1 following 16 weeks *in situ* placement of ADM. Note abundance of elastin (arrows) in this 10x magnification.

[2] M. Y. Koo, S. K. Lee, S. M. Hur et al., "Results from over one year of follow-up for absorbable mesh insertion in partial mastectomy," *Yonsei Medical Journal*, vol. 52, no. 5, pp. 803–808, 2011.

[3] D. J. Wainwright and S. B. Bury, "Acellular dermal matrix in the management of the burn patient," *Aesthetic Surgery Journal*, vol. 31, no. 7, pp. 13S–23S, 2011.

[4] A. E. Capito, S. S. Tholpady, H. Agrawal, D. B. Drake, and A. J. Katz, "Evaluation of host tissue integration, revascularization, and cellular infiltration within various dermal substrates," *Annals of Plastic Surgery*, vol. 68, no. 5, pp. 495–500, 2012.

[5] I. Wong, J. Burns, and S. Snyder, "Arthroscopic GraftJacket repair of rotator cuff tears," *Journal of Shoulder and Elbow Surgery*, vol. 19, no. 2, pp. 104–109, 2010.

[6] S. J. Snyder and J. L. Bond, "Technique for arthroscopic replacement of severely damaged rotator cuff using "graftjacket" allograft," *Operative Techniques in Sports Medicine*, vol. 15, no. 2, pp. 86–94, 2007.

[7] F. A. Barber, M. A. Herbert, and M. H. Boothby, "Ultimate tensile failure loads of a human dermal allograft rotator cuff augmentation," *Arthroscopy*, vol. 24, no. 1, pp. 20–24, 2008.

[8] W. Z. Burkhead Jr., S. C. Schiffern, and S. G. Krishnan, "Use of graft jacket as an augmentation for massive rotator cuff tears," *Seminars in Arthroplasty*, vol. 18, no. 1, pp. 11–18, 2007.

[9] J. L. Bond, R. M. Dopirak, J. Higgins, J. Burns, and S. J. Snyder, "Arthroscopic replacement of massive, irreparable rotator cuff tears using a graftjacket allograft: technique and preliminary results," *Arthroscopy*, vol. 24, no. 4, pp. 403.e1–403.e8, 2008.

[10] R. Dopirak, J. L. Bond, and S. J. Snyder, "Arthroscopic total rotator cuff replacement with an acellular human dermal allograft matrix," *International Journal of Shoulder Surgery*, vol. 1, pp. 7–15, 2007.

[11] R. M. Wilkins, "Acellular dermal graft augmentation in quadriceps tendon rupture repair," *Current Orthopaedic Practice*, vol. 21, no. 3, pp. 315–319, 2010.

[12] D. K. Lee, "Achilles tendon repair with acellular tissue graft augmentation in neglected ruptures," *Journal of Foot and Ankle Surgery*, vol. 46, no. 6, pp. 451–455, 2007.

[13] D. K. Lee, "A preliminary study on the effects of acellular tissue graft augmentation in acute achilles tendon ruptures," *Journal of Foot and Ankle Surgery*, vol. 47, no. 1, pp. 8–12, 2008.

[14] F. A. Barber, M. A. Herbert, and D. A. Coons, "Tendon augmentation grafts: biomechanical failure loads and failure patterns," *Arthroscopy*, vol. 22, no. 5, pp. 534–538, 2006.

[15] H. Sbitany, S. N. Sandeen, A. N. Amalfi, M. S. Davenport, and H. N. Langstein, "Acellular dermis-assisted prosthetic breast

reconstruction versus complete submuscular coverage: a head-to-head comparison of outcomes," *Plastic and Reconstructive Surgery*, vol. 124, no. 6, pp. 1735–1740, 2009.

[16] M. Y. Nahabedian, "AlloDerm performance in the setting of prosthetic breast surgery, infection, and irradiation," *Plastic and Reconstructive Surgery*, vol. 124, no. 6, pp. 1743–1753, 2009.

[17] C. A. Salzberg, "Nonexpansive immediate breast reconstruction using human acellular tissue matrix graft (AlloDerm)," *Annals of Plastic Surgery*, vol. 57, no. 1, pp. 1–5, 2006.

[18] S. A. Kapfer and T. H. Keshen, "The use of human acellular dermis in the operative management of giant omphalocele," *Journal of Pediatric Surgery*, vol. 41, no. 1, pp. 216–220, 2006.

[19] D. Albo, S. S. Awad, D. H. Berger, and C. F. Bellows, "Decellularized human cadaveric dermis provides a safe alternative for primary inguinal hernia repair in contaminated surgical fields," *American Journal of Surgery*, vol. 192, no. 5, pp. e12–e17, 2006.

[20] R. Candage, K. Jones, F. A. Luchette, J. M. Sinacore, D. Vandevender, and R. L. Reed II, "Use of human acellular dermal matrix for hernia repair: friend or foe?" *Surgery*, vol. 144, no. 4, pp. 703–711, 2008.

[21] C. R. Mitchell and R. R. Cima, "A novel technique for the repair of urostomal hernias using human acellular dermal matrix," *Urology*, vol. 77, no. 3, pp. 746–750, 2011.

[22] C. L. Winters, S. A. Brigido, B. A. Liden, M. Simmons, J. F. Hartman, and M. L. Wright, "A multicenter study involving the use of a human acellular dermal regenerative tissue matrix for the treatment of diabetic lower extremity wounds," *Advances in Skin & Wound Care*, vol. 21, no. 8, pp. 375–381, 2008.

[23] K. L. Randall, B. A. Booth, A. J. Miller, C. B. Russell, and R. T. Laughlin, "Use of an acellular regenerative tissue matrix in combination with vacuum-assisted closure therapy for treatment of a diabetic foot wound," *Journal of Foot and Ankle Surgery*, vol. 47, no. 5, pp. 430–433, 2008.

[24] S. A. Brigido, S. F. Boc, and R. C. Lopez, "Effective management of major lower extremity wounds using an acellular regenerative tissue matrix: a pilot study," *Orthopedics*, vol. 27, no. 1, pp. s145–s149, 2004.

[25] G. Onelio, "Managing complications including red breast syndrome," in *Proceedings of the Plastic Surgery Symposium*, Chicago, Ill, USA, June 2012.

[26] J. Y. S. Kim, A. A. Davila, S. Persing et al., "A meta-analysis of human acellular dermis and submuscular tissue expander breast reconstruction," *Plastic and Reconstructive Surgery*, vol. 129, no. 1, pp. 28–41, 2012.

[27] J. Bullocks, B. Basu, P. Hsu, and R. Singer, "Prevention of hemotomas and seromas," *Seminars in Plastic Surgery*, vol. 20, no. 4, pp. 233–240, 2006.

[28] US Patents 7, 338, 757, 6, 743, 574, 6, 734, 018.

[29] International Consensus, *Acellular Matrices for the Treatment of Wounds. An Expert Working Group Review*, Wounds International, London, UK, 2010.

30

Combined Liposuction and Excision of Lipomas: Long-Term Evaluation of a Large Sample of Patients

Libby R. Copeland-Halperin,[1] Vincenza Pimpinella,[2] and Michelle Copeland[3]

[1]Department of Surgery, Inova Fairfax Hospital, 3300 Gallows Road, Falls Church, VA 22042, USA
[2]Division of Nursing, Mount Sinai Beth Israel Medical Center, 245 5th Avenue, New York, NY 10016, USA
[3]Division of Plastic and Reconstructive Surgery, Icahn School of Medicine at Mount Sinai, 1001 5th Avenue, New York, NY 10028, USA

Correspondence should be addressed to Michelle Copeland; mcopeland@drcopeland.com

Academic Editor: Nicolo Scuderi

Background. Lipomas are benign tumors of mature fat cells. They can be removed by liposuction, yet this technique is seldom employed because of concerns that removal may be incomplete and recurrence may be more frequent than after conventional excision. *Objectives.* We assessed the short- and long-term clinical outcomes and recurrence of combined liposuction and limited surgical excision of subcutaneous lipomas. *Methods.* From 2003 to 2012, 25 patients with 48 lipomas were treated with liposuction followed by direct excision through the same incision to remove residual lipomatous tissue. Initial postoperative follow-up ranged from 1 week to 3 months, and long-term outcomes, complications, and recurrence were surveyed 1 to 10 years postoperatively. *Results.* Lipomas on the head, neck, trunk, and extremities ranged from 1 to 15 cm in diameter. Early postoperative hematoma and seromas were managed by aspiration. Among 23 survey respondents (92%), patients were uniformly pleased with the cosmetic results; none reported recurrent lipoma. *Conclusions.* The combination of liposuction and excision is a safe alternative for lipoma removal; malignancy and recurrence are uncommon. Liposuction performed through a small incision provides satisfactory aesthetic results in most cases. Once reduced in size, residual lipomatous and capsular tissue can be removed without expanding the incision. These favorable outcomes support wider application of this technique in appropriate cases.

1. Introduction

Lipomas are common, benign soft tissue tumors that occur on the body surface either sporadically or in association with inherited disorders of fat metabolism. They are typically painless and mobile and enlarge slowly. Histologically, they consist of enlarged adipocytes with uniform nuclei and are usually surrounded by a fibrous capsule [1]. They are aesthetically unpleasing and can become irritated or infected. Surgical intervention is typically performed when the lipoma is uncomfortable, limits function, or otherwise bothers the patient. Several methods have been described for removal, including direct excision, excision through a remote incision [2], liposuction [3, 4], endoscopic excision [5], and laser extirpation [6]. Although small lipomas (up to 3 cm in diameter) can usually be excised directly, excision of large lipomas can be associated with more extensive scarring. Suctioning prior to excision to debulk the lipoma reduces the size of the incision and resulting scar. For lipomas of intermediate (4–10 cm) or large (>10 cm) size [7], liposuction can improve the early cosmetic result, minimize operative time, and reduce the risk of postoperative hematoma and seroma formation [4, 8].

Although there have been multiple reports of successful liposuction for lipoma removal, the technique is not widely embraced. Objectors argue that liposuction limits visualization of the tumor, fragments the specimen confounding histopathological examination for features of malignancy, and leaves residual lipomatous or capsular tissue that predisposes to recurrence [5, 7, 9].

We describe the largest series of lipomas removed through a combination of liposuction and direct excision and report patient outcomes over a decade to address concerns about recurrence and malignancy.

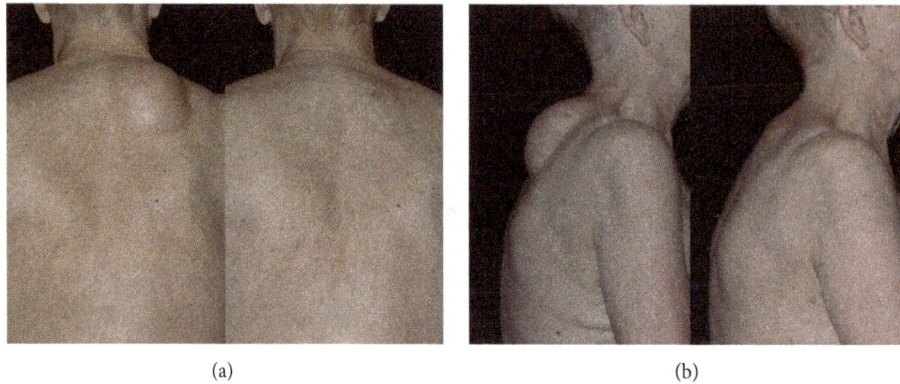

(a)   (b)

FIGURE 1: Pre- and 1-month postoperative photographs of an 80-year-old woman with 15 × 13 cm lipoma. (a) Back view and (b) right lateral view.

2. Methods

For 25 consecutive patients with superficial fat tumors typical of lipomas seeking excision, we offered two alternative techniques for removal: direct excision alone or a combination of liposuction and direct excision. Patients were advised that, should fluid accumulate following excision, serial aspiration might be required with either method. After discussion of the potential benefits, limitations, and risks of each technique, all patients chose the liposuction and excision combination approach.

2.1. Technique of Removal.
The lipomatous mass was outlined in its entirety and infiltrated with a solution 1% xylocaine with epinephrine, 1 : 100,000 for local anesthesia and to promote hemostasis. A 3 mm sharp liposuction cannula was then inserted through a 1 cm incision made in the midportion of the surface of the mass with a #15 scalpel blade. The bulk of the lipoma was removed by aspiration before removing residual tissue and capsule by direct, sharp, and step-wide excision. All extracted specimens were submitted for histopathological examination to exclude liposarcoma or atypical cells. The wound was then irrigated and assessed for hemostasis. Closure was achieved with subcutaneous 5-0 Vicryl and Monocryl sutures without drain placement, Steri-strips were applied, and a bulky dressing was secured. After suctioning of lipomas from the back or abdomen, compressive garments were used to secure the bulkier dressings.

2.2. Postprocedural Management.
While drain insertion after removal of large lipomas is reasonable, serial aspiration avoids the need for additive drainage scars or elongation of the incision and is preferred to control postoperative fluid accumulation. The dressing was changed 1 week postoperatively and topical silicone gel and pigment-reducing cream were applied for several weeks to reduce scar thickening, retraction, or discoloration. The incision was evaluated postoperatively by the senior surgeon to assess healing and the aesthetic result.

2.3. Late Follow-Up.
Follow-up questionnaires were sent to all patients in 2013 (1–10 years postoperatively) to collect retrospective data about the quality and durability of the result, late complications, further treatment, or development of additional lipomas (see appendix).

3. Results

Between 2003 and 2012, 48 lipomas were removed by combined liposuction and excision from 25 patients (17 women and 8 men), ranging in age from 19 to 77 years (mean 49.8 years). Six had multiple lipomas and 19 had solitary masses. Lipomas ranged in diameter from 1 to 15 cm (mean 5.4 cm); 7 were smaller than 3 cm. Two were located on the head or neck, 11 on the back, 2 on the abdomen, 31 on the extremities, and 2 on the groin (see Table 1). In one case, liposuction was used to reduce the volume of a diffuse lipoma following which the capsule was removed by direct excision.

3.1. Pathological Examination.
All extracted and excised specimens submitted for histopathological evaluation were sufficient for analysis and had characteristics of benign lipomas; none contained morphologically dysplastic or malignant cells.

3.2. Early Postoperative Follow-Up.
During early follow-up 1 to 12 weeks postoperatively, repeated aspiration was required in 18 cases with eventual resolution, including one hematoma after removal of a 10 cm abdominal lipoma and one seroma after removal of a 15 cm lipoma from the back (see Figure 1).

3.3. Long-Term Outcomes.
Later outcomes were assessed by written responses to a survey, to which 23 patients responded (92%) 4 months to 10 years postoperatively (mean 7 years; median 6.5 years); two patients did not respond. None of the respondents identified complications of the procedure or recurrence of lipoma, appearance of new lipomas, hyperpigmentation, scarring, or clinical evidence of malignant transformation.

TABLE 1: Summary of patients and lipomas.

Patient	Age (years)	Lesion diameter (cm)	Location	Initial follow-up (weeks)	Long-term follow-up (years)
(1) S. R.	44	5 cm; 7 cm	RT shoulder; LT flank	3	10
(2) M. S.	50	7 cm	LT shoulder	1	10
(3) C. T.	55	5 cm	LT arm	1	10
(4) C. K.	40	10 cm	RT back	4	9
(5) G. G.	77	15 cm	Upper back	8	8
(6) A. C.	65	10 cm	RT posterior knee	1	8
(7) P. T.	24	6 cm	Back	1	7
(8) H. F.	49	10 cm	Upper back	3	7
(9) A. T.	19	10 cm	RT ankle	52	7
(10) D. S.	52	7 cm	RT back	4	7
(11) R. M.	46	7 cm	Upper back	none noted	N/A
(12) S. A.	54	10 cm	Upper back	2	7
(13) R. T.	59	2 cm	RT temple	4	6
(14) A. K.	52	4 cm	LT mid back	1	5
(15) A. I.	42	3 cm; 4 cm; 5 cm	RT upper back; RT lower back; LT jawline	2	N/A
(16) C. L.	53	2–5 cm	RT lower lateral thigh; RT midlateral thigh; RT upper medial thigh; RT middle medial thigh; RT lower medial thigh; HIP; RT upper buttock; RT lower buttock; RT outer thigh	6	5
(17) N. P.	46	13 cm	Upper back	8	5
(18) C. L.	53	2–5 cm	LT buttock; LT infragluteal fold; LT midlateral exterior thigh; LT interior thigh; LT arm	6	5
(19) C. L.	53	2–5 cm	LT upper forearm; LT lower forearm; LT inner thigh; LT upper outer thigh; LT medial thigh, LT lower thigh; LT upper anterior thigh; LT medial thigh; LT lower anterior thigh	6	5
(20) L. Q.	42	10 cm	LT lower abdomen	12	5
(21) A. S.	50	10 cm	RT rectal-vaginal	5	5
(22) J. Z.	62	10 cm	RT arm	1	3
(23) S. I.	60	7 cm	RT shoulder	12	1
(24) M. A.	47	1.5 cm; 3 cm	RT upper elbow; LT groin	1	1
(25) A. D.	80	15 cm	RT upper back	4	1

4. Discussion

Since its introduction in 1975 by Fischer, followed by Illouz's "wet technique" in 1977 [9], the indications for liposuction have expanded to include lipodystrophy, gynecomastia, and evacuation of lipomas [10–14]. Removal of lipomas by this technique to decrease incision size and scarring was described in 1990. Al-Basti and El-Khatib [15] followed liposuction by capsular excision through the cannula incision, and Choi et al. [16] used tumescent liposuction to remove lipomas. Despite reports of favorable experiences, surgeons often forego liposuction out of concern that incomplete removal or recurrence might compromise outcomes or that

cellular disruption might impede histopathological examination or mask malignant features.

The combined liposuction and excision technique facilitates complete removal of lipomas through small incisions. Fibrous lipomas and angiolipomas are less amenable to liposuction; others have indistinct borders or transitions to nonlipomatous adipose tissue. While these require greater direct excision of the fibrous components, initial liposuction aided debulking and facilitated removal through smaller incisions. Early postoperative fluid accumulation developed in over a third of cases (incidence 37.5%) but responded to percutaneous aspiration without residua. Postoperative hematoma or seroma might have been avoided by placement of conventional drains, which would entail additional scarring, as discussed with patients preoperatively. There was no clinical recurrence among the 23 patients we queried after a median postoperative interval of 6.5 years. The local recurrence rate of lipomas after surgical excision has been reported as 1-2% over an indefinite period [17]; hence while a larger sample of patients is required to establish more precisely the rate when liposuction is initially employed, the long-term durability of the procedures appears comparable. Caution is appropriate in applying this technique in patients with single or multiple small lipomas in the same body region, as occurs in cases of multiple familial lipomatosis, because disrupting the individual capsules of these lipomas can be ultimately more traumatic to surrounding tissue than conventional excision.

None of the lesions in this series had clinical features suggestive of liposarcoma, hibernoma, or lipoblastoma. Liposarcomas typically occur between the 5th and 7th decades of life in the deeper soft tissues of the extremities [18]. Several studies have demonstrated preservation of adipocyte integrity after liposuction [19, 20]. Histopathologic examination of the specimens in this series was not hampered, and none identified malignancy. A particular concern with the combined liposuction/excision method is the potential risk of disseminating malignant cells upon capsular disruption. Although liposarcomas account for approximately 20% of all soft tissue sarcomas in adults [17], their population incidence is relatively low (approximately 2.5 cases per million annually) [21]. Before utilizing liposuction for lipoma, therefore, the surgeon should assure the absence of clinical features associated with liposarcoma, including rapid growth, pain, or immobility of the soft tissue tumor. When liposarcoma is suspected, biopsy is essential, coupled with ultrasound examination prior to complete excision.

This study is limited by sample size, which is insufficient to identify recurrence rates less than about 2 percent. None of the lipomas had malignant features, and we caution clinicians to carefully assess soft tissue tumors for atypical clinical features before employing the intervention we describe. Despite these limitations, our observations suggest that the combination of liposuction and excision is a safe option for removal of subcutaneous lipomas that yields successful results. Outcomes could differ for submuscular lipomas. While a questionnaire is not entirely sufficient for evaluating recurrence, it provides a subjective method of assessing whether the patient detects recurrence. The outcomes in the two patients who failed to respond to the survey could not be determined.

Since the management of lipomas is inherently conservative, excision is recommended only when the tumors are symptomatic because of their size or location, have suspicious clinical features, or are cosmetically unacceptable to the patient, and the incidence of malignancy is low; we believe that removal by combined liposuction and direct excision is a reasonable alternative to direct, open excision.

The use of liposuction permits a smaller incision and favorable aesthetic results, without exposing patients to recurrence or compromising pathological analysis in the vast majority of cases. A randomized trial comparing liposuction with conventional direct excision is necessary to more conclusively compare the outcomes of these techniques.

Appendix

Lipoma Follow-Up Questionnaire

(1) Did your lipoma return or did you need to seek further treatment for your lipoma? yes or no
If so, what year?

(2) Did you have any postoperative bruising or skin dimpling at the surgical site? yes or no

(3) Have you had other lipomas removed before or after this one? yes or no
If so, what year and how did your postoperative recovery compare (pain, bruising, etc.)?

(4) Do you have a history of cancer? yes or no

(5) Do you have any other concerns about the procedure or your recovery?

References

[1] T. Brenn, "Neoplasms of subcutaneous fat," in *Fitzpatrick's Dermatology in General Medicine*, L. A. Goldsmith, S. I. Katz, B. A. Gilchrest, A. S. Paller, D. J. Leffell, and N. A. Dallas, Eds., McGraw-Hill, New York, NY, USA, 8th edition, 2012.

[2] J. A. Pereira and F. Schonauer, "Lipoma extraction via small remote incisions," *British Journal of Plastic Surgery*, vol. 54, no. 1, pp. 25–27, 2001.

[3] A. L. Spinowitz, "Liposuction surgery: an effective alternative for treatment of lipomas," *Plastic and Reconstructive Surgery*, vol. 86, no. 3, p. 606, 1990.

[4] K. S. Pinski and H. H. Roenigk Jr., "Liposuction of lipomas," *Dermatologic Clinics*, vol. 8, no. 3, pp. 483–492, 1990.

[5] G. G. Hallock, "Endoscope-assisted suction extraction of lipomas," *Annals of Plastic Surgery*, vol. 34, no. 1, pp. 32–34, 1995.

[6] S. H. Lee, J. Y. Jung, M. R. Roh, and K. Y. Chung, "Treatment of lipomas using a subdermal 1,444-nm micropulsed neodymium-doped yttrium aluminum garnet laser," *Dermatologic Surgery*, vol. 37, no. 9, pp. 1375–1376, 2011.

[7] Ö. K. Silistreli, E. Ü. Durmuş, B. G. Ulusal, Y. Öztan, and M. Görgü, "What should be the treatment modality in giant cutaneous lipomas? Review of the literature and report of 4 cases," *British Journal of Plastic Surgery*, vol. 58, no. 3, pp. 394–398, 2005.

[8] H. Ilhan and B. Tokar, "Liposuction of a pediatric giant superficial lipoma," *Journal of Pediatric Surgery*, vol. 37, no. 5, pp. 796–798, 2002.

[9] W. P. Coleman III, "The history of liposuction and fat transplantation in America," *Dermatologic Clinics*, vol. 17, no. 4, pp. 723–727, 1999.

[10] J. Apesos and R. Chami, "Functional applications of suction-assisted lipectomy: a new treatment for old disorders," *Aesthetic Plastic Surgery*, vol. 15, no. 1, pp. 73–79, 1991.

[11] K. H. Calhoun, J. J. Bradfield, and C. Thompson, "Liposuction-assisted excision of cervicofacial lipomas," *Otolaryngology—Head and Neck Surgery*, vol. 113, no. 4, pp. 401–403, 1995.

[12] T. Kaneko, H. Tokushige, N. Kimura, S. Moriya, and K. Toda, "The treatment of multiple angiolipomas by liposuction surgery," *The Journal of Dermatologic Surgery and Oncology*, vol. 20, no. 10, pp. 690–692, 1994.

[13] L. S. Nichter and B. R. Gupta, "Liposuction of giant lipoma," *Annals of Plastic Surgery*, vol. 24, no. 4, pp. 362–365, 1990.

[14] P. K. Sharma, C. K. Janniger, R. A. Schwartz, G. E. Rauscher, and W. C. Lambert, "The treatment of atypical lipoma with liposuction," *Journal of Dermatologic Surgery and Oncology*, vol. 17, no. 4, pp. 332–334, 1991.

[15] H. A. Al-Basti and H. A. El-Khatib, "The use of suction-assisted surgical extraction of moderate and large lipomas: long-term follow-up," *Aesthetic Plastic Surgery*, vol. 26, no. 2, pp. 114–117, 2002.

[16] C. W. Choi, B. J. Kim, S. E. Moon, S. W. Youn, K. C. Park, and C. H. Huh, "Treatment of lipomas assisted with tumescent liposuction," *Journal of the European Academy of Dermatology and Venereology*, vol. 21, no. 2, pp. 243–246, 2007.

[17] K. M. Dalal, C. R. Antonescu, and S. Singer, "Diagnosis and management of lipomatous tumors," *Journal of Surgical Oncology*, vol. 97, no. 4, pp. 298–313, 2008.

[18] T. Mentzel, "Cutaneous lipomatous neoplasms," *Seminars in Diagnostic Pathology*, vol. 18, no. 4, pp. 250–257, 2001.

[19] G. L. M. Campbell, N. Laudenslager, and J. Newman, "The effect of mechanical stress on adipocyte morphology and metabolism," *The American Journal of Cosmetic Surgery*, vol. 4, pp. 89–94, 1987.

[20] M. A. Shiffman and S. Mirrafati, "Fat transfer techniques: the effect of harvest and transfer methods on adipocyte viability and review of the literature," *Dermatologic Surgery*, vol. 27, no. 9, pp. 819–826, 2001.

[21] L. G. Kindblom, L. Angervall, and P. Svendsen, "Liposarcoma a clinicopathologic, radiographic and prognostic study," *Acta Pathologica et Microbiologica Scandinavica. Supplement*, no. 253, pp. 1–71, 1975.

31

Helping Hands: A Cost-Effectiveness Study of a Humanitarian Hand Surgery Mission

Kashyap K. Tadisina,[1] Karan Chopra,[2] John Tangredi,[3] J. Grant Thomson,[3] and Devinder P. Singh[4]

[1] College of Medicine, University of Illinois at Chicago, Chicago, IL 60612, USA

[2] Department of Plastic and Reconstructive Surgery, Johns Hopkins University, Baltimore, MD 21287, USA

[3] Section of Plastic and Reconstructive Surgery, Yale University School of Medicine, New Haven, CT 06511, USA

[4] Division of Plastic Surgery, University of Maryland Medical Center, Wing S8D, 22 South Greene Street, Baltimore, MD 21201, USA

Correspondence should be addressed to Devinder P. Singh; dsingh@smail.umaryland.edu

Academic Editor: Bishara S. Atiyeh

Purpose. Congenital anomalies and injuries of the hand are often undertreated in low-middle income countries (LMICs). Humanitarian missions to LMICs are commonplace, but few exclusively hand surgery missions have been reported and none have attempted to demonstrate their cost-effectiveness. We present the first study evaluating the cost-effectiveness of a humanitarian hand surgery mission to Honduras as a method of reducing the global burden of surgically treatable disease. *Methods.* Data were collected from a hand surgery mission to San Pedro Sula, Honduras. Costs were estimated for local and volunteer services. The total burden of disease averted from patients receiving surgical reconstruction was derived using the previously described disability-adjusted life years (DALYs) system. *Results.* After adjusting for likelihood of disability associated with the diagnosis and likelihood of the surgery's success, DALYs averted totaled 104.6. The total cost for the mission was $45,779 (USD). The cost per DALY averted was calculated to be $437.80 (USD), which is significantly below the accepted threshold of two times the per capita gross national income of Honduras. *Conclusions.* This hand surgery humanitarian mission trip to Honduras was found to be cost-effective. This model and analysis should help in guiding healthcare professionals to organize future plastic surgery humanitarian missions.

1. Introduction

Humanitarian missions to low-middle income countries (LMICs) have become a major source of medical care for underserved populations, particularly in plastic surgery. Teams consist of a variety of healthcare professionals who travel to the country in need, with all required supplies and equipment. On location, surgeons perform life-changing procedures for patients with congenital deformities, trauma, or burns, all of which cause significant disease burden on the local population [1, 2]. This service is provided free of charge to the patients. All expenses are paid by charitable donations, usually without religious, financial, cultural, or political agendas [3].

Honduras is a democratic nation in Central America with a population of approximately 7.5 million. Over half of the population lives below the poverty line and an estimated 30% are unemployed [4]. Like many LMICs, Honduras lacks both resources and an adequate health care infrastructure to provide the care for its citizens. According to the World Health Organization, "roughly 30.1% of the population receives no healthcare, 83% are uninsured, and there is marked exclusion of ethnic minorities and rural populations." Further, there are only 8.8 physicians and 3 nurses per 10,000 citizens, compared to 26 physicians and 94 nurses per 10,000 in the United States [5]. In 2005, the per capita total expenditure on healthcare in Honduras was $91 versus $6,350 in the United States [4]. Furthermore, patients' access to hospitals can be limited geographically and by a lack of transportation means. At the same time, medical technology and surgical techniques in developed countries continue to advance rapidly. This has created a growing dichotomy in healthcare between rich and poor countries [6, 7]. In particular, areas of subspecialty surgery, such as reconstructive plastic surgery and hand surgery, which are increasingly specialized in countries like the United States, are all but absent in some developing nations [8, 9]. Because of this, humanitarian missions to the developing world are becoming more and more relevant as a way to provide direct aid and training to local surgeons. Many medical and surgical mission trips throughout the world have been reported in the literature with plastic surgery volunteer trips being especially common, and the majority of which involve cleft lip and palate repair [10]. Some reported mission trips involve treatment of both hand anomalies and craniofacial defects. However, very few of the reported humanitarian mission trips have focused solely on hand surgery. Further, the cost-effectiveness of such trips has not been previously reported. In the present paper, we present a report on the cost-effectiveness of a mission trip to Honduras in May 2006 that exclusively focused on hand surgery.

2. Methods

2.1. Study Population. In May 2006, our group of 20 health-care professionals traveled to San Pedro Sula, Honduras. Our local sponsor, the Ruth Paz Foundation, a nonprofit charitable group, assisted on site with organization, logistics, and advertising. We worked out of a local public hospital called Leonardo Martinez, which hosts a variety of medical and surgical humanitarian mission trips. Team personnel consisted of 3 hand/microsurgery trained surgeons, 1 plastic surgery trained surgeon, 1 hand/microsurgery fellow, 1 plastic surgery resident, 3 anesthesiologists, 1 pediatrician, 1 nurse anesthetist, 5 operating room nurses, 1 recovery room nurse, 1 hand therapist, 1 team administrator, and 1 photographer. All surgical supplies (including gowns, drapes, sponges, sutures, dressings, and plaster) and surgical instruments were brought with the team for the trip.

Members of the Ruth Paz Foundation set up the screening clinic and organized the follow-up visits. Potential patients were alerted about the available services, through radio announcements and fliers. The majority of the patients were screened for surgery on the primary screening day with additional patients, who missed the main screening day, screened each day. The operating schedule for the next five days was created based on the patients seen on the main screening day. Those screened for surgery were then immediately referred to waiting anesthesiologists and pediatrician for same day medical clearance. Patients were then instructed when to return for surgery before they left.

Many minor procedures were performed with local surgeons present in order to provide training for their future practice. Ganglion cysts and masses were removed for extreme size, intractable pain, or functional limitation. Because of the team's yearly trip to Honduras, we were also able to perform more complex two-staged procedures.

All surgeries were performed by either a board certified plastic surgeon or orthopedic surgeon. Each day, the team would round on all postoperative patients in the morning and in the evening. The patients were seen in follow-up clinic by local physicians, who removed splints, dressings, sutures, and k-wires, as necessary. Patients were also seen by local physical and occupational therapists that provided assistance with splints as well as therapy.

2.2. Costs. The team's costs for the trip were calculated by adding the team's travel expenses, which included transportation, lodging, and donated supplies that were brought with them (Table 1(a)). The team's 2006 costs were then adjusted for inflation to present day based on data obtained from World Bank's data [4]. Weekly hospital personnel salaries and preoperative, intraoperative, and postoperative medication costs were obtained from the Ruth Paz Foundation (Tables 1(b) and 1(c)). We were unable to obtain operative room cost or daily hospital stay costs. Other fixed costs, such as utilities and building costs, were not included as we were not able to obtain this information. Patients were charged a symbolic fee based on their household income by the local hospital for services, but due to the nominal nature of the fee (ranging from $0 to $50), this was not included for analysis.

2.3. Outcome. The total burden of musculoskeletal disease was calculated for each patient that underwent surgery using disability-adjusted life years (DALYs) format. As no surgery performed was life-saving, all of the DALYs attributed were from years lost to disability (YLD) and none from years of life lost (YLL). YLD is calculated using disability weight and the remaining life expectancy. In previous calculations of YLD, age weighting factors and discount rate were also incorporated in the calculation; however, the recently published Global Burden of Disease 2010 study has moved away from those adjustments [11]. Every patient's diagnosis and associated disability was matched as closely as possible to a health state based on each state's lay description as described in Global Burden of Disease 2010 study. Each patient was then assigned a disability weight based on the closest available health state (Table 2). For each patient, the potential years lived with disability value was calculated using the patient's age and life expectancy chart found in the Global Burden of Disease 2010 study. For each patient, the DALY value represents the burden of an untreated condition. This value has been subsequently adjusted for likelihood of permanent disability and likelihood of treatment success as described in the literature by McCord and Chowdry and modified by Gosselin et al. [12–16] and represents the DALYs averted with surgery (Table 3). To err on side of overestimating cost per DALY averted, we chose conservative weights for disability, likelihood of permanent disability, and effectiveness of treatment. The scoring system used in assigning likelihood of permanent disability and likelihood of treatment success is shown in Table 4.

TABLE 1: Mission costs.

(a) Team costs

	Value (USD) in 2006	Cumulative inflation rate (2006 to 2013)	Inflation adjusted value (USD) in 2013	% of total costs
Transportation and lodging	$23,000	15.90%	$26,650.34	62.2%
Donated supplies	$14,000	15.90%	$16,226.00	37.8%
Total cost	**$37,000**	**15.90%**	**$42,876.34**	

(b) Local personnel salary

	Weekly salary (USD) in 2013	Number	Weekly cost (USD)	% of total costs
Local surgeon	$345	2	$690	45.3%
Surgical tech.	$185	2	$370	24.3%
Nurse	$185	2	$370	24.3%
Cleaning	$92	1	$92	6.0%
Total cost			**$1,522**	

(c) Hospital costs

	Weekly cost (USD) in 2013
Pre- and postoperative medications	$448.84
Intraoperative medications	$932
Total costs	**$1,380.84**

(d) Overall mission cost

	Cost (USD)	% of total costs
Team costs	$42,876.34	93.7%
Local personnel costs	$1,522.00	3.3%
Hospital costs	$1,380.84	3.0%
Total overall costs	**$45,779.18**	

(e) Cost-effectiveness metrics

		If 2 × TC (i.e., doubled)	If 5 × TC
Total cost (TC)	$45,779.18	**$91,558.36**	**$228,895.90**
Cost per patient	$572.24	$1,144.48	$2,861.20
Cost per DALY averted	$437.80	$875.32	$2,188.30*
			*Still below $3,890 (2 × PCGNI)

*PCGNI: per capita gross national income.

3. Results

In total, 120 patients were screened and 80 patients were found to be candidates for surgery. Over the week, 128 total procedures were performed on 54 adults (68%) and 26 children (32%). The average age of the patient undergoing surgery was 31 years with ages ranging from 10 months to 68 years. Of these patients, 27 were female (34%) and 53 were male (66%). Table 4 includes the procedures performed on each patient, as well as their age and gender. Operative time for the entire trip totaled 93 hours and 50 minutes over 5 days. Average operative time was 18 hours and 46 minutes per day and 6 hours and 15 minutes per operative table per day. Most of the procedures were very short in duration, with 43 cases (53%) lasting less than 1 hour. 25 cases (31%) took 1-2 hours, 9 cases (11%) lasted 2-3 hours, and only 4 cases (5%) were longer than 3 hours in duration. No immediate complications, such as ischemic loss or early wound infection,

were noted. There were no anesthetic complications and no mortalities.

As shown in Table 4, the total number of DALYs potentially avertable totaled 220.5. Adjusting for likelihood of disability associated with the diagnosis and likelihood of the surgery's success, DALYs averted totaled 104.6. The total cost (in current USD) for the volunteer trip including the team's travel and lodging cost of $45,779.18 and local hospital's cost of $2,903 (USD) is detailed in Table 1. On average, it costs $572.24 (USD) per patient that was surgically treated. Cost-effectiveness was measured using cost per DALY averted and, for this trip, the cost for each DALY averted was conservatively estimated to be $437.80 (USD), which is significantly less than the accepted threshold of two times the per capita gross national income of Honduras, $3,890 (USD). Further, a brief sensitivity analysis provided in Table 1(e) displays that even if total costs were to increase by 500%, the cost per DALY averted would still be below the threshold of $3,890 (USD).

TABLE 2: Patient characteristics.

Age	Sex	Diagnosis	Available disability weight	Disability weight
9	F	Tendon adhesion	Musculoskeletal problems: arms, mild	0.024
16	M	Finger flexor tendon injury	Musculoskeletal problems: arms, mild	0.024
26	M	Finger flexor tendon injury and nerve laceration	Injured nerves: long term	0.136
60	M	Posttraumatic joint contracture	Musculoskeletal problems: arms, mild	0.024
68	F	Trigger finger	Musculoskeletal problems: arms, mild	0.024
3	F	Finger flexor tendon injury	Musculoskeletal problems: arms, mild	0.024
13	M	Cubitus varus	Disfigurement: level 1	0.013
14	M	Polydactyly	Disfigurement: level 1	0.013
47	M	Lipoma	Disfigurement: level 1, with itch or pain	0.029
57	F	Trigger finger	Musculoskeletal problems: arms, mild	0.024
11	M	Burn scar contracture	Burns of <20% total surface area or <10% total surface area if head or neck or hands or wrist involved: long term, with or without treatment	0.018
12	M	Burn scar contracture	Musculoskeletal problems: arms, mild	0.024
21	F	Partial traumatic amputation	Amputation of finger(s), excluding thumb: long term, with treatment	0.03
30	F	Nerve laceration	Injured nerves: long term	0.136
34	M	Skin contracture	Musculoskeletal problems: arms, mild	0.024
47	M	Radius and ulna fracture	Fracture of radius or ulna: short term, with or without treatment	0.065
8	M	Metacarpal fracture	Musculoskeletal problems: arms, mild	0.024
11	M	Cubitus varus	Disfigurement: level 1	0.013
21	M	Burn scar contracture	Burns of <20% total surface area or <10% total surface area if head or neck or hands or wrist involved: long term, with or without treatment	0.018
45	M	Posttraumatic joint contracture	Musculoskeletal problems: arms, mild	0.024
48	M	Carpal tunnel syndrome	Injured nerves: short term	0.065
51	F	Ganglion cyst	Disfigurement: level 1, with itch or pain	0.029
67	M	Dupuytren's contracture	Musculoskeletal problems: arms, moderate	0.114
5	M	Burn scar contracture	Burns of <20% total surface area or <10% total surface area if head or neck or hands or wrist involved: long term, with or without treatment	0.018
7	M	Polydactyly	Disfigurement: level 1	0.013
19	F	Tumor	Disfigurement: level 1, with itch or pain	0.029
21	M	Tumor	Disfigurement: level 1, with itch or pain	0.029
31	M	Dorsal ganglion cyst	Disfigurement: level 1, with itch or pain	0.029
42	F	Nonunion radius	Fracture of radius or ulna: long term, without treatment	0.05
56	F	De Quervain's syndrome	Musculoskeletal problems: arms, moderate	0.114
11 mo	M	Thumb hypoplasia	Amputation of thumb: long term	0.013
23	M	Burn scar contracture	Musculoskeletal problems: arms, mild	0.024
33	M	Burn scar contracture	Musculoskeletal problems: arms, moderate	0.114
37	F	Hook nail deformity	Disfigurement: level 1	0.013
48	M	Dupuytren's contracture	Musculoskeletal problems: arms, mild	0.024
8	M	Flexor tendon injury	Musculoskeletal problems: arms, mild	0.024
10	F	Scar contracture	Musculoskeletal problems: arms, mild	0.024
20	M	Flexor tendon injury with nerve laceration	Injured nerves: long term	0.136
55	M	Carpal tunnel syndrome	Injured nerve: short term	0.065
5	M	Syndactyly	Musculoskeletal problems: arms, mild	0.024
17	M	Thumb hypoplasia	Musculoskeletal problems: arms, moderate	0.114
18	M	Foreign body with ulnar neuropathy	Injured nerves: short term	0.065
23	M	Foreign body	Musculoskeletal problems: arms, mild	0.024
34	M	Radial head fracture	Fracture of radius or ulna: short term, with or without treatment	0.065

TABLE 2: Continued.

Age	Sex	Diagnosis	Available disability weight	Disability weight
44	M	Posttraumatic joint contracture	Musculoskeletal problems: arms, mild	0.024
49	M	Extensor tendon laceration	Musculoskeletal problems: arms, mild	0.024
20	M	Flexor tendon injury	Musculoskeletal problems: arms, moderate	0.114
22	F	Posttraumatic joint contracture	Musculoskeletal problems: arms, mild	0.024
22	M	Posttraumatic joint contracture	Musculoskeletal problems: arms, mild	0.024
47	M	Shoulder lipoma	Disfigurement: level 1, with itch or pain	0.029
61	F	Ganglion cyst and ulnocarpal abutment	Musculoskeletal problems: arms, moderate	0.114
5	M	Burn scar contracture	Burns of <20% total surface area or <10% total surface area if head or neck or hands or wrist involved: long term, with or without treatment	0.018
32	M	Flexor tendon injury	Musculoskeletal problems: arms, moderate	0.114
60	F	Ganglion cyst	Disfigurement: level 1, with itch or pain	0.029
61	M	Finger flexor tendon injury	Musculoskeletal problems: arms, moderate	0.114
65	F	L ulna nonunion	Fracture of radius or ulna: long term, without treatment	0.05
10	M	Syndactyly	Musculoskeletal problems: arms, mild	0.024
24	M	Malunion	Musculoskeletal problems: arms, moderate	0.114
35	F	Nerve laceration	Injured nerves: long term	0.136
38	M	Nerve laceration	Injured nerves: long term	0.136
10 mo	M	L MF-RF syndactyly	Musculoskeletal problems: arms, mild	0.024
17	M	Malunion	Fracture of hand: long term, without treatment	0.016
18	M	Flexor tendon injury	Musculoskeletal problems: arms, moderate	0.114
28	M	Radial nerve laceration	Injured nerves: long term	0.136
42	F	Carpal tunnel syndrome	Injured nerve: short term	0.065
14	M	Flexor tendon injury with nerve laceration	Musculoskeletal problems: arms, moderate	0.114
23	F	Burn scar contracture	Burns of <20% total surface area or <10% total surface area if head or neck or hands or wrist involved: long term, with or without treatment	0.018
50	M	Radial nerve laceration	Injured nerves: long term	0.136
9	F	Burn scar contracture	Burns of <20% total surface area or <10% total surface area if head or neck or hands or wrist involved: long term, with or without treatment	0.018
16	F	Malunion	Musculoskeletal problems: arms, mild	0.024
31	F	Ganglion cyst	Disfigurement: level 1, with itch or pain	0.029
47	F	Ulnocarpal abutment	Musculoskeletal problems: arms, moderate	0.114
55	F	Carpal tunnel syndrome	Injured nerve: short term	0.065
14	F	Burn scar contracture	Musculoskeletal problems: arms, moderate	0.114
39	F	Ganglion cyst	Disfigurement: level 1, with itch or pain	0.029
42	M	Posttraumatic joint contracture	Musculoskeletal problems: arms, mild	0.024
46	M	Posttraumatic joint contracture	Musculoskeletal problems: arms, mild	0.024
57	F	Carpal tunnel syndrome	Injured nerve: short term	0.065
23	M	Finger mass	Disfigurement: level 1, with itch or pain	0.029
62	M	Skin lesion	Disfigurement: level 1, with itch or pain	0.029

4. Discussion

This study demonstrates that hand surgery mission trips are a cost-effective means of providing surgical care at HNQCP in San Pedro Sula, Honduras, using an established economic evaluation model. We also inherently validate the effectiveness of the DALY system as a useful and versatile method of evaluating surgical mission trips. While it is one

of the first quantitative systems of evaluating such trips, it is also only one of the many possible ways to analyze mission trips. However, this analysis also represents an important step in standardizing the evaluation of such trips to better optimize foreign intervention by surgical teams, as proposed by McCord [13].

The $437.80 per DALY averted for this week long surgical mission trip is similar to those previously reported in

TABLE 3: DALY averted.

Case #	Age	Remaining life expectancy	Sex	Diagnosis	Procedure	Disability Wt.	DALY	Likelihood of permanent disability	Likelihood of treatment success	DALY averted
					Day 1					
1	9	77.27	F	Tendon adhesion	L wrist exploration w/tenolysis FDP	0.024	1.85448	0.7	0.7	0.9086952
2	16	70.3	M	Finger flexor tendon injury	R index finger Hunter rod placement	0.024	1.6872	0.7	0.7	0.826728
3	26	60.41	M	Finger flexor tendon injury and nerve laceration	R FPL repair w/tendon grafts; nerve repair with sural nerve graft	0.136	8.21576	0.7	0.7	4.0257224
4	60	27.81	M	Posttraumatic joint contracture	R long finger PIP joint arthrodesis	0.024	0.66744	0.7	0.7	0.3270456
5	68	20.68	F	Trigger finger	R LF trigger finger release	0.024	0.49632	0.7	0.7	0.2431968
6	3	83.23	F	Finger flexor tendon injury	L ring finger FDS/FDP-Hunter rod implant	0.024	1.99752	0.7	0.7	0.9787848
7	13	73.29	M	Cubitus varus	L lateral closing wedge osteotomy of supracondylar for cubitus varus	0.013	0.95277	0.7	0.7	0.4668573
8	14	72.29	M	Polydactyly	B/l thumb partial duplication repair; anlage excision	0.013	0.93977	0.7	0.7	0.4604873
9	47	39.9	M	Lipoma	Excision of L forearm mass	0.029	1.1571	0.7	0.7	0.566979
10	57	30.55	F	Trigger finger	R IF and LF trigger finger release	0.024	0.7332	0.7	0.7	0.359268
11	11	75.28	M	Burn scar contracture	L forearm excision of burn scar; STSG	0.018	1.35504	0.3	0.7	0.2845584
12	12	74.28	M	Burn scar contracture	R hand thumb webs space deepening with split thickness skin graft	0.024	1.78272	0.3	0.7	0.3743712
13	21	65.36	F	Partial traumatic amputation	L RF amputation completion	0.03	1.9608	0.7	0.7	0.960792
14	30	56.46	F	Nerve laceration	Nerve graft L ulnar nerve; anticlaw tendon transfer	0.136	7.67856	0.7	0.7	3.7624944
15	34	52.52	M	Skin contracture	L middle PIP contracture release and skin graft	0.024	1.26048	0.7	0.7	0.6176352
16	47	39.9	M	Radius and ulna fracture	ORIF L radius/ulna	0.065	2.5935	0.3	0.7	0.544635

TABLE 3: Continued.

Case #	Age	Remaining life expectancy	Sex	Diagnosis	Procedure	Disability Wt.	DALY	Likelihood of permanent disability	Likelihood of treatment success	DALY averted
					Day 2					
17	8	78.26	M	Metacarpal fracture	R LF pinning of metacarpal fracture	0.024	1.87824	0.7	0.7	0.9203376
18	11	75.28	M	Cubitus varus	R supracondylar osteotomy	0.013	0.97864	0.7	0.7	0.4795336
19	21	65.36	M	Burn scar contracture	R IF burn contracture release; FTSG	0.018	1.17648	0.7	0.7	0.5764752
20	45	41.8	M	Posttraumatic joint contracture	L index and long finger PIP fusion	0.024	1.0032	0.7	0.7	0.491568
21	48	38.95	M	Carpal tunnel syndrome	L carpal tunnel release	0.065	2.53175	0.7	0.7	1.2405575
22	51	36.12	F	Ganglion cyst	Excision of R wrist mass	0.029	1.04748	0.7	0.7	0.5132652
23	67	21.55	M	Dupuytren's contracture	L hand excision of Dupuytren's contracture	0.114	2.4567	0.7	0.7	1.203783
24	5	81.25	M	Burn scar contracture	R hand burn contracture release	0.018	1.4625	0.7	0.7	0.716625
25	7	79.26	M	Polydactyly	Reconstruction of R thumb polydactyly	0.013	1.03038	0.7	0.7	0.5048862
26	19	67.34	F	Tumor	Excision of L hand mass	0.029	1.95286	0.7	0.7	0.9569014
27	21	65.36	M	Tumor	Excision of bony tumor ×2 of L humerus	0.029	1.89544	0.7	0.7	0.9287656
28	31	55.48	M	Dorsal ganglion cyst	Excision of ganglion cyst	0.029	1.60892	0.7	0.7	0.7883708
29	42	44.71	F	Nonunion radius	Repair nonunion radius	0.05	2.2355	0.7	0.7	1.095395
30	56	31.47	F	De Quervain's syndrome	De Quervain's release	0.114	3.58758	0.7	0.7	1.7579142
31	11 mo	85.21	M	Thumb hypoplasia	R thumb amp, and pollicization	0.013	1.10773	0.7	0.7	0.5427877
32	23	63.38	M	Burn scar contracture	PIP arthrodesis; debulk flap	0.024	1.52112	0.7	0.7	0.7453488
33	33	53.5	M	Burn scar contracture	Contracture release of all fingers R hand; flexor tendon division	0.114	6.099	0.7	0.7	2.98851
34	37	49.58	F	Hook nail deformity	V-Y advancement L index fingertip	0.013	0.64454	0.7	0.7	0.3158246
35	48	38.95	M	Dupuytren's contracture	L little finger arthrodesis and k-wire for palmar scar revision w/FTSG	0.024	0.9348	0.7	0.7	0.458052

TABLE 3: Continued.

Case #	Age	Remaining life expectancy	Sex	Diagnosis	Procedure	Disability Wt.	DALY	Likelihood of permanent disability	Likelihood of treatment success	DALY averted
					Day 3					
36	8	78.26	M	Flexor tendon injury	2nd stage flexor tendon reconstruction; removal hunter rod and tendon graft from leg to finger	0.024	1.87824	0.7	0.7	0.9203376
37	10	76.27	F	Scar contracture	L hand scar revision; tenolysis; removal of k-wire	0.024	1.83048	0.7	0.7	0.8969352
38	20	66.35	M	Flexor tendon injury with nerve laceration	Repair flexor tendons wrist with tendon grafts, ulnar nerve repair with sural nerve graft	0.136	9.0236	0.7	0.7	4.421564
39	55	32.38	M	Carpal tunnel syndrome	R carpal tunnel release	0.065	2.1047	0.7	0.7	1.031303
40	5	81.25	M	Syndactyly	Syndactyly release L 4th web space	0.024	1.95	0.7	0.7	0.9555
41	17	69.32	M	Thumb hypoplasia	R thumb opponensplasty; R 1st web deepening; R thumb UCL reconstruction	0.114	7.90248	0.7	0.7	3.8722152
42	18	68.33	M	Foreign body with ulnar neuropathy	Excision of foreign body L hypothenar eminence; neurolysis ulnar nerve	0.065	4.44145	0.7	0.7	2.1763105
43	23	63.38	M	Foreign body	Bullet removal ×2 R hand	0.024	1.52112	0.7	0.7	0.7453488
44	34	52.52	M	Radial head fracture	L radial head excision	0.065	3.4138	0.7	0.7	1.672762
45	44	42.77	M	Posttraumatic joint contracture	L LF, RF, and SF PIP joint fusion	0.024	1.02648	0.7	0.7	0.5029752
46	49	38	M	Extensor tendon laceration	Tendon transfer for thumb extension PL → EPL	0.024	0.912	0.7	0.7	0.44688
47	20	66.35	M	Flexor tendon injury	Zone II IF, MF, and RF hunter rods	0.114	7.5639	0.7	0.7	3.706311
48	22	64.37	F	Posttraumatic joint contracture	L LF PIP joint arthrodesis	0.024	1.54488	0.7	0.7	0.7569912
49	22	64.37	M	Posttraumatic joint contracture	L thumb IP fusion	0.024	1.54488	0.7	0.7	0.7569912
50	47	39.9	M	Shoulder lipoma	Excision of R shoulder lipoma	0.029	1.1571	0.7	0.7	0.566979
51	61	26.91	F	Ganglion cyst and ulnocarpal abutment	R dorsal ganglion/L matched ulnar arthroplasty	0.114	3.06774	0.7	0.7	1.531926

TABLE 3: Continued.

Case #	Age	Remaining life expectancy	Sex	Diagnosis	Procedure	Disability Wt.	DALY	Likelihood of permanent disability	Likelihood of treatment success	DALY averted
					Day 4					
52	5	81.25	M	Burn scar contracture	R hand burn scar contracture release; FTSG	0.018	1.4625	0.7	0.7	0.716625
53	32	54.49	M	Flexor tendon injury	R FDS → FDP transfer 2–5	0.114	6.21186	0.7	0.7	3.043814
54	60	27.81	F	Ganglion cyst	L dorsal wrist excision of ganglion cyst	0.029	0.80649	0.7	0.7	0.395180l
55	61	26.91	M	Finger flexor tendon injury	L wrist ECRL to FDP; transfer of w/palmaris graft	0.114	3.06774	0.7	0.7	1.5031926
56	65	23.29	F	L ulna nonunion	ORIF with iliac crest bone graft	0.05	1.1645	0.7	0.7	0.570605
57	10	76.27	M	Syndactyly	Release syndactyly 2nd and 4th web spaces with flaps and grafts	0.024	1.83048	0.7	0.7	0.8969352
58	24	62.39	M	Malunion	R thumb MCP joint arthrodesis	0.114	7.11246	0.7	0.7	3.4851054
59	35	51.53	F	Nerve laceration	Tendon transfer for L wrist extension and thumb extension; FCU → ECRB, PL → EPL	0.136	7.00808	0.7	0.7	3.4339592
60	38	48.6	M	Nerve laceration	R forearm sural nerve graft	0.136	6.6096	0.7	0.3	1.388016
61	10 mo	85.21	M	L MF-RF syndactyly	L MF-RF syndactyly release	0.024	2.04504	0.7	0.7	1.0020696
62	17	69.32	M	Malunion	Thumb osteotomy and alignment-ORIF; removal of foreign body thumb	0.016	1.10912	0.7	0.7	0.5434688
63	18	68.33	M	Flexor tendon injury	L forearm FDS → FDP tendon transfer	0.114	7.78962	0.7	0.7	3.8169138
64	28	58.44	M	Radial nerve laceration	Tendon transfer radial nerve palsy; FCR → EDC; PT → ECRB; ring sublimis → EPL	0.136	7.94784	0.7	0.7	3.8944416
65	42	44.71	F	Carpal tunnel syndrome	L carpal tunnel release	0.065	2.90615	0.7	0.7	1.4240135

TABLE 3: Continued.

Case #	Age	Remaining life expectancy	Sex	Diagnosis	Procedure	Disability Wt.	DALY	Likelihood of permanent disability	Likelihood of treatment success	DALY averted
					Day 5					
66	14	72.29	M	Flexor tendon injury with nerve laceration	R FDS/FDP ring and small finger tenorrhaphy and digital nerve repair	0.114	8.24106	0.7	0.7	4.0381194
67	23	63.38	F	Burn scar contracture	L hand burn scar contracture release	0.018	1.14084	0.7	0.7	0.5590116
68	50	37.05	M	Radial nerve laceration	Tendon transfer of radial nerve palsy; FCR → EDC; PT → ECRB; ring sublimis → EPL	0.136	5.0388	0.7	0.7	2.469012
69	9	77.27	F	Burn scar contracture	Web space deepening and scar revision	0.018	1.39086	0.7	0.7	0.6815214
70	16	70.3	F	Malunion	R RF MCP arthrodesis	0.024	1.6872	0.7	0.7	0.826728
71	31	55.48	F	Ganglion cyst	Excision of R wrist dorsal ganglion	0.029	1.60892	0.7	0.7	0.7883708
72	47	39.9	F	Ulnocarpal abutment	L ulnar shortening	0.114	4.5486	0.7	0.7	2.228814
73	55	32.38	F	Carpal tunnel syndrome	R carpal tunnel release	0.065	2.1047	0.7	0.7	1.031303
74	14	72.29	F	Burn scar contracture	L LF PIP burn contracture release and fusion; FTSG; Z plasty L elbow burn scar	0.114	8.24106	0.7	0.7	4.0381194
75	39	47.62	F	Ganglion cyst	Excision of R volar wrist ganglion cyst	0.029	1.38098	0.7	0.7	0.6766802
76	42	44.71	M	Posttraumatic joint contracture	L thumb MCP arthrodesis	0.024	1.07304	0.7	0.7	0.5257896
77	46	40.85	M	Posttraumatic joint contracture	L long finger PIP joint arthrodesis	0.024	0.9804	0.7	0.7	0.480396
78	57	30.55	F	Carpal tunnel syndrome	L carpal tunnel release	0.065	1.98575	0.7	0.7	0.9730175
79	23	63.38	M	Finger mass	Excision of L ring finger mass	0.029	1.83802	0.7	0.7	0.9006298
80	62	26	M	Skin lesion	Excision of L hand skin lesion	0.029	0.754	0.7	0.7	0.36946
Mean:	30.759	55.938				Total:	220.009		Total:	104.349028

R = right; L = left; IF = index finger; LF = long finger; RF = ring finger; SF = small finger; PIP = proximal interphalangeal; MCP = metacarpal phalangeal; FPL = flexor pollicis longs; FDS = flexor digitorum superficialis; FDP = flexor digitorum profundus; FCR = flexor carpi radials; FCU = flexor carpi ulnaris; PL = palmaris longus; ECRL = extensor carpi radialis longus; ECRB = extensor; carpi radialis brevis; EDC = extensor digitorum communis; FCU = flexor carpi ulnaris; UCL = ulnar collateral ligament; STSG = split thickness skin graft; FTSG = full thickness skin graft; ORIF = open reduction internal fixation.

TABLE 4: Scoring system.

	Weight
Likelihood of permanent disability	
>95% go on to disability	1.0
<95 and >50%	0.7
<50 and >5%	0.3
<5%	0
Effectiveness of treatment	
>95% chance for cure	1.0
<95 and >50%	0.7
<50 and >5%	0.3
<5%	0

the literature that have ranged between $343 and $362 per DALY [14, 15]. Our cost per DALY is well within the two times per capita gross national income, an accepted metric for program cost-effectiveness as suggested by earlier studies [15]. We believe our slightly higher cost per DALY averted can be attributed to multiple factors. First, we have used conservative estimations for all DALY and disability weight. Second, previous studies did not use the 2010 version of the Global Burden of Disease (GBD) system to evaluate cost-effectiveness and consequently may have contributed to differences in the cost per DALY averted value. Third, bringing more staff, such as residents, anesthesiologists/anesthetist, pediatrician, nurses, and hand therapist, may have added to travel and lodging cost. As the availability of more locally trained medical professionals is available in Honduras, fewer anesthesiologists, or nurses, and therapists from the United States will be needed for each trip thus making each subsequent mission trip more cost-effective than the previous. With local capacity to care for simple cases like ganglion cyst removal, trigger finger release, and arthrodesis, subsequent trips can focus on more disabling complex conditions such as nerve injuries which require advance surgical training. Since a volunteer mission trip's costs are relatively fixed, focusing on these conditions can contribute to more DALYs averted lowering the trip's cost per DALY averted.

In addition to providing direct care, our team has been able to lecture at the medical school in San Pedro Sula and invite local surgeons to come and learn how to manage surgical hand cases. Our nurses and therapists have also worked with local staff to improve pre-, peri-, and postoperative care of patients. Such training and educational efforts are often difficult to quantify and are not reflected in the cost per DALY averted, but they are important in the long-term development of adequately trained local health care professionals and healthcare infrastructure. While the capacity to care for these surgical conditions is being developed in Honduras, surgical mission trips such as ours serve as an important bridge until that day arrives.

The limitations of this study include the inability to include certain costs, such as operating room, hospital stay, utilities, and building costs; however, given the large margin between the cost per DALY averted and the twice per capita gross national income (PCGNI) of Honduras ($3890 in 2012)

[4], we believe that the underreported costs have only a minor impact on the cost per DALY averted. Even if total costs (TC) were five times higher, the cost per DALY averted would still be the threshold value of $3890 ($2^*$ PCGNI), as illustrated in Table 1(e). As in previous cost-effectiveness studies, a rough trade-off is used to assign hand conditions with disability weights as the Global Burden of Disease 2010 study does not have many specific disability weights for various hand conditions. There are also instances where disability weights make little sense from a functional standpoint: amputation of finger(s) excluding thumb has a disability weight of 0.030 which compares poorly to disability weight of 0.013 for amputation of thumb, long term. One can argue that the loss of a thumb is more functionally debilitating than the loss of a finger as opposition-apposition function is lost in a thumb amputation and grip maybe minimally affected with a finger amputation [11]. The nature of short volunteer mission trip makes obtaining long-term outcomes data difficult. However, with greater capacity in host countries, prospective studies that assess patient outcomes will enable us to more objectively determine patient outcomes without relying on assumptions. Until then, we feel that using the correctional factor "probability of successful treatment" is needed to account for treatment success/failures as there is a lack of follow-up data. Imperfect as it maybe, the DALY method for assessing cost-effectiveness has been used in a number of previous studies in LMICs and offers a more objective and standardized way to assess the impact of surgical mission trips, cost-effectiveness and serves as a benchmark for future trips.

References

[1] P. Voche and P. Valenti, "Humanitarian surgery of the hand. Our experience in Vietnam," *Annales de Chirurgie Plastique et Esthétique*, vol. 44, no. 1, pp. 64–71, 1999.

[2] M. Beveridge and A. Howard, "The burden of orthopaedic disease in developing countries," *Journal of Bone and Joint Surgery A*, vol. 86, no. 8, pp. 1819–1822, 2004.

[3] C. N. Baran and Y. O. Tiftikcioglu, "Physicians for peace and interplast Turkiye: combined humanitarian surgical activities and conferences," *Plastic and Reconstructive Surgery*, vol. 119, no. 3, pp. 1077–1090, 2007.

[4] World Bank, http://www.worldbank.org/.

[5] World Health Organization, *Honduras*, 2013, http://www.who .int/countries/hnd/en/.

[6] D. S. Walsh, "A framework for short-term humanitarian health care projects," *International Nursing Review*, vol. 51, no. 1, pp. 23–26, 2004.

[7] S. Bunyavanich and R. B. Walkup, "US public health leaders shift toward a new paradigm of global health," *The American Journal of Public Health*, vol. 91, no. 10, pp. 1556–1558, 2001.

[8] K. C. Chung, "Volunteering in the developing world: the 2003-2004 sterling bunnell traveling fellowship to Honduras and Cambodia," *Journal of Hand Surgery*, vol. 29, no. 6, pp. 987–993, 2004.

[9] T. E. E. Goodacre, "Plastic surgery in a rural African hospital: spectrum and implications," *Annals of the Royal College of Surgeons of England*, vol. 68, no. 1, pp. 42–44, 1986.

[10] V. K. L. Yeow, S. T. Lee, T. J. Lambrecht et al., "International task force on volunteer cleft missions," *Journal of Craniofacial Surgery*, vol. 13, no. 1, pp. 18–25, 2002.

[11] C. J. Murray, T. Vos, R. Lozano et al., "Disability-adjusted life years (DALYs) for 291 diseases and injuries in 21 regions, 1990–2010: a systematic analysis for the Global Burden of Disease Study 2010," *The Lancet*, vol. 380, no. 9859, pp. 2197–2223, 2010.

[12] C. McCord and Q. Chowdhury, "A cost effective small hospital in Bangladesh: what it can mean for emergency obstetric care," *International Journal of Gynecology and Obstetrics*, vol. 81, no. 1, pp. 83–92, 2003.

[13] C. McCord, "Volunteer orthopedic surgical trips in Nicaragua: a cost-effectiveness evaluation," *World Journal of Surgery*, vol. 36, no. 12, pp. 2809–2810, 2012.

[14] R. A. Gosselin, G. Gialamas, and D. M. Atkin, "Comparing the cost-effectiveness of short orthopedic missions in elective and relief situations in developing countries," *World Journal of Surgery*, vol. 35, no. 5, pp. 951–955, 2011.

[15] A. T. Chen, A. Pedtke, J. K. Kobs, G. S. Edwards Jr., R. R. Coughlin, and R. A. Gosselin, "Volunteer orthopedic surgical trips in Nicaragua: a cost-effectiveness evaluation," *World Journal of Surgery*, vol. 36, no. 12, pp. 2802–2808, 2012.

[16] R. Gosselin, D. Ozgediz, and D. Poenaru, "A square peg in a round hole? Challenges with DALY-based "Burden of Disease" calculations in surgery and a call for alternative metrics," *World Journal of Surgery*, vol. 37, no. 11, pp. 2507–2511, 2013.

32

Basic Plastic Surgery Skills Training Program on Inanimate Bench Models during Medical Graduation

Rafael Denadai,[1,2] Andréia Padilha Toledo,[3] and Luis Ricardo Martinhão Souto[2]

[1] Institute of Plastic and Craniofacial Surgery, SOBRAPAR Hospital, Avenue Adolpho Lutz 100,
  Caixa Postal 6028, 13084-880 Campinas, SP, Brazil
[2] Division of Plastic and Reconstructive Surgery, Department of Surgery, School of Medical Sciences,
  University of Marília (UNIMAR), 17525-902 Marília, SP, Brazil
[3] School of Medical Sciences, University São Francisco (USF), 12916-900 Bragança Paulista, SP, Brazil

Correspondence should be addressed to Rafael Denadai, denadai.rafael@hotmail.com

Academic Editor: Georg M. Huemer

Due to ethical and medical-legal drawbacks, high costs, and difficulties of accessibility that are inherent to the practice of basic surgical skills on living patients, fresh human cadaver, and live animals, the search for alternative forms of training is needed. In this study, the teaching and learning process of basic surgical skills pertinent to plastic surgery during medical education on different inanimate bench models as a form of alternative and complementary training to the teaching programs already established is proposed.

1. Introduction

Recently there has been tremendous growth of ambulatory surgical procedures that general practitioners need to perform in order to treat cutaneous lesions [1–3]. In this context, as a large percentage of medical students do not acquire basic surgical skills during their training [4] and most of the general practitioners that perform ambulatory surgeries received no formal surgical training [5], it is necessary to establish a training program to teach and refine the basic surgical skills related to plastic surgery (e.g., to biopsy a cutaneous lesion and to reconstruct the defect by the rotation of a surgical flap) that are essential to perform these ambulatory surgical procedures during medical education [4–6].

Considering that surgical training on living patients (traditional learning) violates ethical and medical-legal aspects, that training on live animals and fresh human cadaver increases the risk of infections, involves high costs and limited access, requires specialized installations, and also contravenes ethical legal aspects, and that using virtual reality simulators involves high costs and restricted access [7, 8], the simulation-based basic surgical teaching on inanimate bench models is becoming widely used [9]. However, to date, it has not been established a teaching program that allows surgical

skills to be completely acquired [4, 5], and new opportunities in simulation-based surgical education need to be explored to positively impact quality and safety in surgical care [10].

Among all the surgical specialties, plastic surgery now occupies a negligible component of many undergraduate curricula, and there is much discussion in the worldwide literature regarding if there is a place for plastic surgery in the undergraduate curriculum [11–14]. Moreover, plastic surgery as a specialty is poorly understood by medical students and healthcare professionals [11, 15–18], and one of the important reasons for this is limited and inadequate plastic surgery exposure at undergraduate level [15–17]. Although undergraduate exposure is an important influential factor for subsequent career interest in plastic surgery [16, 19], many medical students are in favor of having plastic surgery teaching even though many may not necessarily want to pursue a career in the specialty [20]. So, as teaching undergraduate plastic surgery has potential benefits to all future physicians and ultimately patients, irrespective of career intentions [17], some authors [13, 14, 21, 22] have reported the need for plastic surgery education at undergraduate level.

Given the difficulties of changing the undergraduate curriculum [13, 23], simple solutions to increase plastic surgery exposure are required [13, 17]. Therefore, the aims of this study were to propose and to describe the teaching and learning process of basic surgical skills pertinent to plastic surgery during medical education using different inanimate bench models as a form of alternative and complementary training to the programs already established.

2. Simulation-Based Basic Plastic Surgical Skills Training

The proposal is based on self-directed training and feedback from instructors, distributed in several sessions (days, weeks, or months) of teaching and learning, interspersed with periods of rest [24, 25]. Each session consists of steps to be undertaken in subsequent ways: verbal teaching supervised by instructor and based on textbooks, online text, and online narrated expert demonstration videos; self-directed training on bench models with immediate feedback from the instructor in the classroom (or laboratory of simulation); self-directed training on bench models with posterior feedback from the instructor focused on extra-class procedures (the undergraduate must bring the bench model with the procedures carried out so that specific technical factors are assessed and constructive feedback is provided) [24–29].

3. Learning Goals

Once the basic skills training can lead to improved performance of more complex tasks [24], it is important to include teaching goals that are set before the beginning of the teaching and learning process in order of increasing difficulty, and these should be distributed in different training sessions [30]. Thus, as the student acquires simpler skills, more complex skills should be incorporated into the training. Initially, the goals may be similar for all group members. However, in subsequent sessions, proposals should vary according to individual needs. During the training steps, the instructor should explain the advantages and disadvantages of each technique, the proper choice of surgical materials, and proper use of surgical instruments.

In this training program, the basic plastic surgical skills are included (Figure 1) according to the analysis of the program for simulated training of surgical skills of the American College of Surgeons Program for Accreditation of Education Institutes performed by Rosen et al. [31].

4. Inanimate Bench Models

In recent years, different inanimate bench models have been proposed, discussed, and evaluated by our group [32–39] and by others [40–49]. In this training program, we adopted six inanimate bench models as teaching platforms (Table 1) because these enable the understanding of tridimensional procedures and also allow undergraduates to learn to respect the different layers of the skin (epidermis, dermis, subcutaneous cellular tissue, and muscles) during practice [32–49]. Such materials can be easily purchased from commercial outlets, such as craft shops and supermarkets. The parts of *postmortem* animals and organic materials must be gotten

fresh and stored in refrigeration to reduce the risks of infections and increase the feasibility time of models.

5. Surgical Knots

The surgical knots (interlace made between the ends of a tread in order to unite and fix them) should be part of the simulated surgical teaching because they are essential for hemostasis and synthesis (key surgical times). The knots can be performed with the aid of instruments or manually (one or two hands), such as the nodes of the index finger (second finger), the middle finger (third finger), of surgeon, and of shoemaker. The manual knots must follow these principles: (a) equal movements of opposed hands perform a perfect knot; (b) the tip of the tread that changes its side after the first semi-knot should return to the initial side to perform another semi-knot; (c) the knots should be firm but without tension on the tissue (*in vivo*, excessive strain can result, for example, in avulsion of a blood vessel) [50, 51]. The different types of surgical knots should be practiced repeatedly until they can be performed quickly, effectively and almost automatically [52].

6. Incision and Suture Techniques

The training of incisions (linear, circular, elliptical, vertical, and horizontal) and different sutures, such as simple interrupted sutures, vertical mattress suture according to Donati and McMillen, modified vertical mattress suture according to Allgöwer, horizontal mattress sutures, half-buried mattress sutures, subdermal interrupted sutures, running simple suture, running locked suture, and running subcuticular suture, can occur simultaneously (Figure 2). First, the undergraduate should mark the chosen material. The model is incised with the scalpel, which facilitates teaching the proper way to grip the instrument, its position with the "skin" (cutting angle between 30° and 60°), the way of the cut (firm and without "sawing" movements), and the depth of the incision [53, 54]. Following this, the created defects are repaired by placing points, also applying the technical aspects that are important to promote good healing, such as meticulous handling of tissues, proper positioning of the needle in the needle holder, angle of needle entry in the "skin," exit of the needle in an equidistant point in relation to its entry, and approximation and eversion of the "wound edges" with proper tension [5, 55].

7. Biopsy Techniques

The training of biopsy techniques (elliptical and circular; excisional and incisional; with and without safety margins) should be performed according to the previously set requirements. For example, for the practice of the classical elliptical incision (Figure 3), students should receive the following instructions [28, 53, 56–58].

Drawing of the Ellipse. The ellipse must be formed by two arcs that should be symmetrical in relation to the midline that separates them, and they should meet at the ends

TABLE 1: Advantages and disadvantages of inanimate bench models [8, 9, 31–49] adopted as learning tools in this basic plastic surgery training program.

Inanimate bench models	Fidelity	Infection risk	Financial costs*	Availability*	Easy handling	Reutilization**
Parts of *postmortem* animals						
Ox tongue	High	Present	+++	Variable	++	Possible
Cattle skin	High	Present	+++	Variable	++	Possible
Pig skin	High	Present	+++	Variable	++	Possible
Chicken skin	High	Present	+++	Variable	++	Possible
Organic material						
Fruits and vegetables	Low	Present	++	Variable	+++	Possible
Synthetic material						
Ethylene-vinyl acetate	Low	Absent	+	Variable	+++	Unlimited

*Varies according to seasonality and geographical region; **limited by risk of infections and natural deterioration of material.

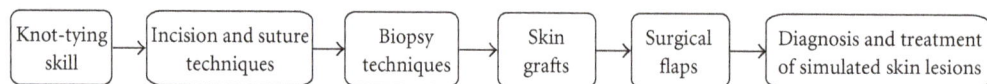

Knot-tying skill → Incision and suture techniques → Biopsy techniques → Skin grafts → Surgical flaps → Diagnosis and treatment of simulated skin lesions

FIGURE 1: Learning goals. Undergraduates should initially perform basic surgical knowledge and then be trained on the most complex surgical skills.

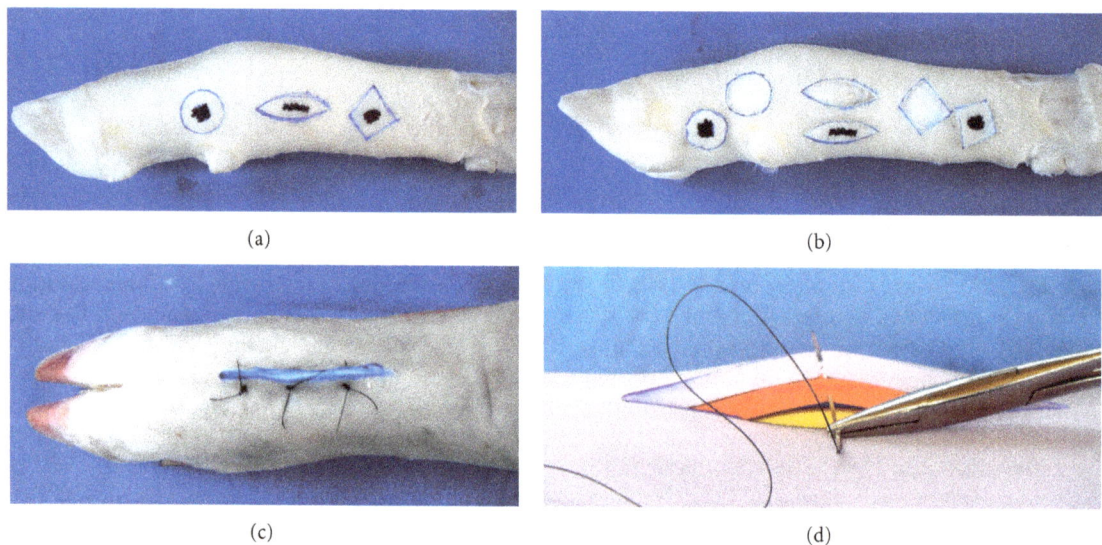

(a)

(b)

(c)

(d)

FIGURE 2: Inanimate bench models simulating incision and suture techniques. (a, b) Cattle-skin bench model simulating circular, linear and elliptic patterns of incision. (c) Pig-skin bench model simulating vertical mattress suture. (d) Synthetic ethylene-vinyl acetate bench model simulating subdermal interrupted suture; training should preferably be carried out near the edges of the material, and it is advisable to use multiple overlapping synthetic material plates aiming to mimic the different layers of the skin. Note that all the three bench models are simulating the procedures in a three-dimensional way.

forming a convexity; the used curvature should be based on a length-width ratio of 3 : 1 to 4 : 1; a 30° angle should be used at the ends of the ellipse (intersection of the arcs).

Safety Margins. A line should be marked around the periphery of the "skin lesion" to delimit the safety margins; according to current recommendations for surgical resection of most cases of nonmelanoma skin cancer, the safety margins should be of 2 to 10 mm.

Incision and Excision. Smooth movements with the scalpel (cut angle between 30° and 60°), cuts of "subcutaneous

tissue" with 1 or 2 movements, handling the tissue gently to avoid damaging the ellipse edges and the "epidermis," and resection of the same amount of "tissue" in all areas of the "wound" should be done.

8. Skin Grafts

Faced with a "skin" defect, students should plan a stamp graft in mesh or in strips with different diameters and thicknesses [59]. The graft should be removed intact from the donor area with a scalpel blade, Blair knife, or dermatome [46, 49, 59–63]; undergraduates should be trained on different

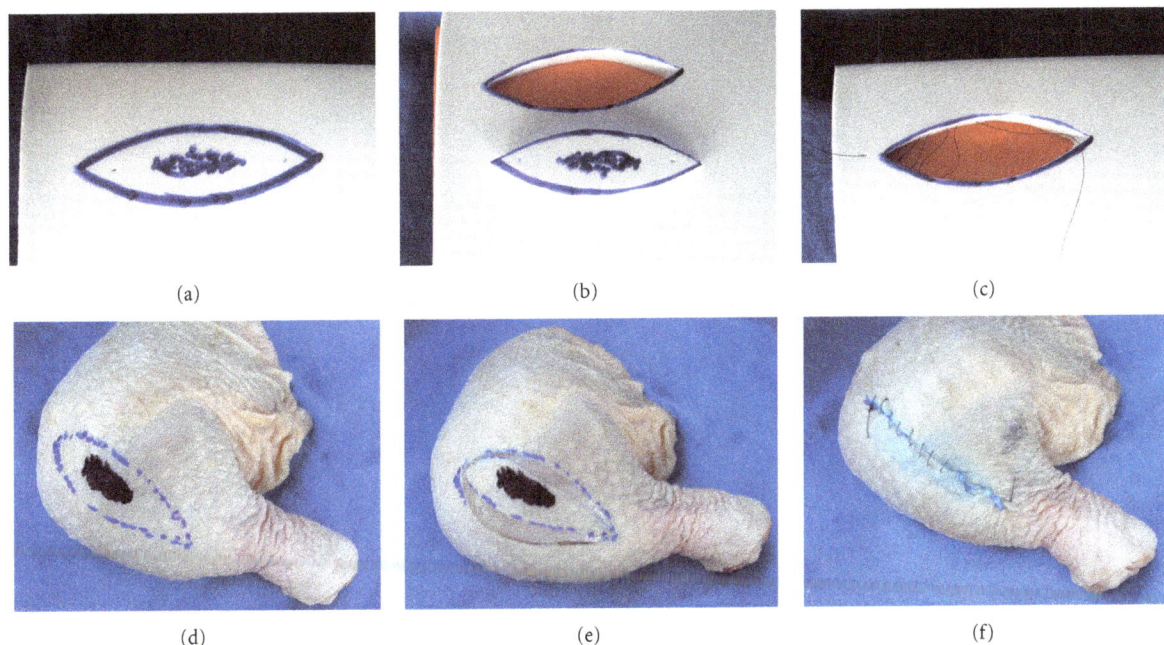

Figure 3: Inanimate bench models simulating elliptical biopsy technique. (a, b, and c) Synthetic ethylene-vinyl acetate bench model and (d, e, and f) chicken-skin bench model simulating (a, d) the safety margins forming an ellipse, (b, e) the intact removal of the "surgical piece", and repair of the surgical defects with the confection of (c) intradermal suture and (f) running simple suture. Note that both bench models allow three-dimensional understanding of the whole process of training.

pressures on the tissues and angulations between the blade and the "skin" in order to fabricate grafts of varying sizes and thicknesses [60–62]. After obtaining the graft, it should be placed and shaped in the receiving area so that the edges are well coadapted in all sides of the recipient area. Subsequently, the proper fixation of the graft should be carried out in order to reduce the dead space [59]. The simulation of the compressive dressing for skin grafts should also be part of the training [49].

9. Surgical Flaps

The bench models also allow the simulated practice of surgical flaps, such as transposition flaps (Z-plasty, W-plasty, rhomboid, and bilobed), of rotation, of advancement (V-Y and R-plasty), and in island (Figure 5). Faced with a "skin" defect, the carrying out of a flap based on schemas is planned [64]. From this, the markings are incised, the flap is moved to fill the defect, and simple stitches should fix the flap carefully, avoiding strain on its pedicle [65].

10. Diagnosis and Treatment of Simulated Cutaneous Lesions

Assuming the fact that the training of a complete procedure can be broken down into several components [66], following the acquisition of techniques of surgical knots, incisions, sutures, biopsies, grafts and flaps, the undergraduates can be trained on the diagnosis and treatment of simulated skin lesions by joining the learned skills. At this time, different "skin lesions" should be simulated on bench models, so that students make their respective diagnoses and/or treatments by using the previously learned principles and, then, the proper surgical repair. At this stage of the training, instructors should provide students with the cognitive aspects of decision making, such as which surgical procedure should be adopted in every kind of "skin lesion." Different skin lesions can be simulated on bench models.

Lipomas and Epidermoid Cysts. To simulate these lesions, styrofoam balls, mini-balloons filled with ink or projectiles of paintball. should be inserted through a subcutaneous tunnel on parts of *postmortem* animals bench models [67, 68]. Undergraduates must respect the simulated lesion completely, taking care not to leave parts of the lesion in the wound (Figure 4).

Necrotic Wounds. For training of tangential excision and surgical debridement (or escharotomy), the surface of the chosen bench model should be burned to simulate a necrotic area [69]. Undergraduates must respect the necrotic "tissue," taking care not to damage the healthy tissue (Figure 6).

Nonmelanoma Skin Cancer. The student should make an excisional biopsy with predetermined safety margins, since this is considered the standardized diagnostic therapeutic procedure for most cases of nonmelanoma skin cancer [58]. After the resection of different simulated skin lesions, undergraduates must make the appropriate repair of the created defect (primary approximation of the wound edges with stitch placing, graft or rotation, transposition or advancement of a flap) (Figure 7).

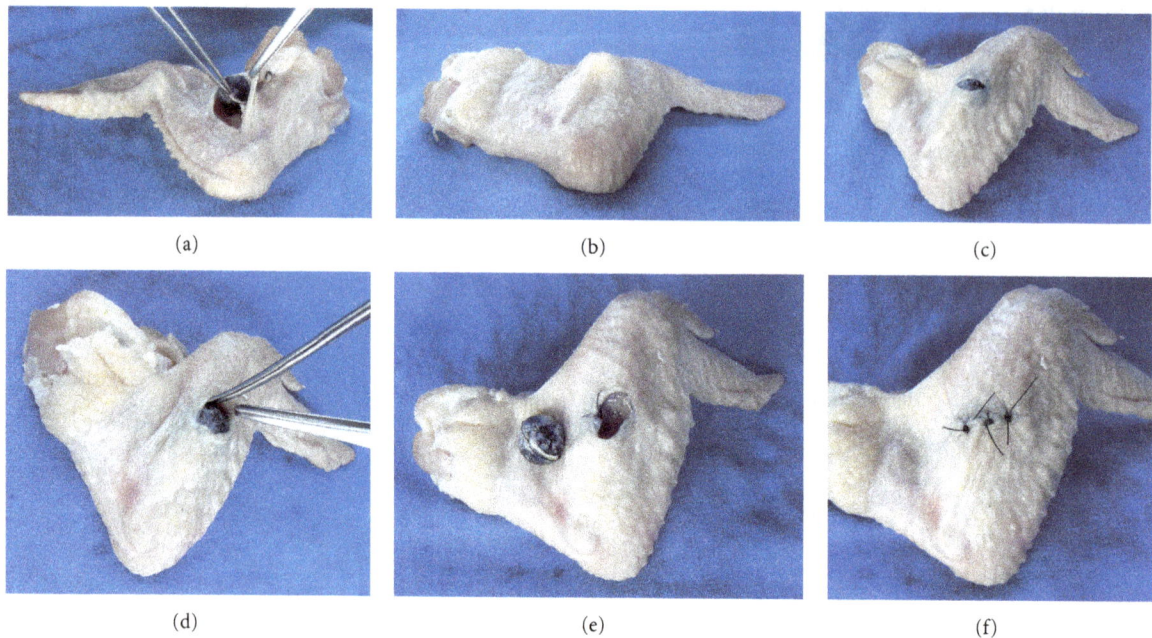

FIGURE 4: Chicken-skin bench model simulating a subcutaneous lipoma. (a) A small styrofoam ball should be placed in a subcutaneous tunnel made in the posterior portion of the model with the intention of (b) mimicking the cutaneous lesion. Following, students must (c) incise the skin, (d) carefully dissect the lesion, (e) resect it completely, and (f) repair the defect by means of single interrupted sutures.

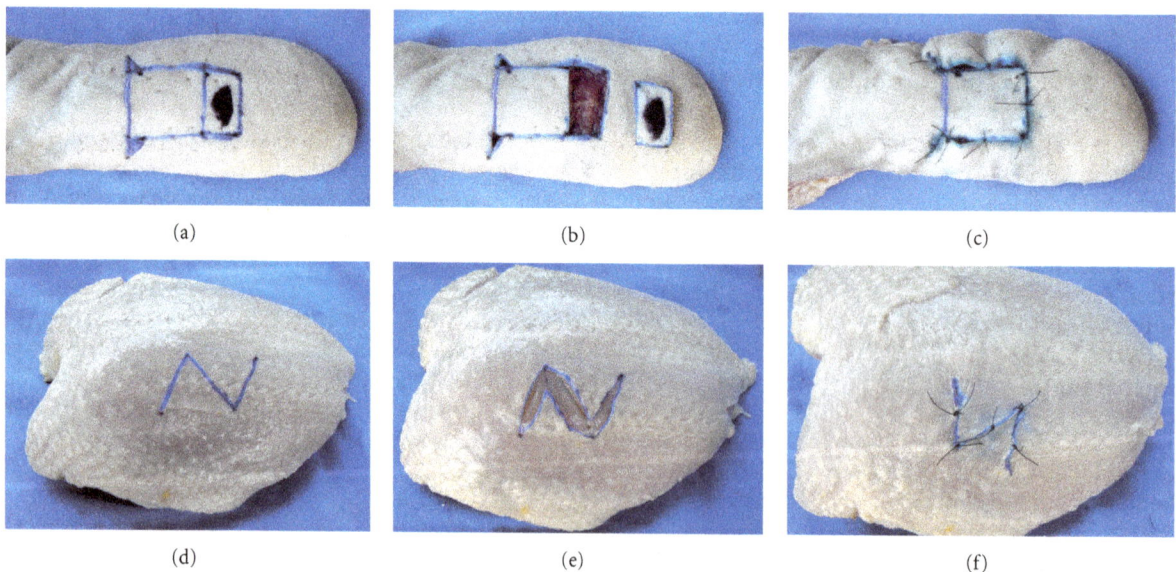

FIGURE 5: Inanimate bench models simulating flaps. (a, b, and c) Ox tongue bench model simulating a monopedicle advancement flap. (d, e, and f) Chicken-skin bench model simulating a Z-plasty. Note that students can easily see the advancement and transposition of surgical flaps, which often is hard to understand with the use of two-dimensional models. For example, it is simpler to explain that the center line of the Z-plasty should be placed along the scar, since it is this component that will be lengthened.

11. Training Time

There are no clear recommendations on the total number of hours that medical students must practice to acquire basic surgical skills. In this sense, in this basic plastic surgery training program, the number of training hours was distributed according to the complexities of skills (i.e., a longer training for those skills considered more complex) (Table 2). In general, the first week serves to introduce the subject (e.g., teaching issues such as clinical applicability of skills) and the other for the simulated training itself (hands-on training). It is important to take a break of one week between each of the six skills, totaling therefore six months of basic plastic surgery training (24 weeks, being 19 of teaching

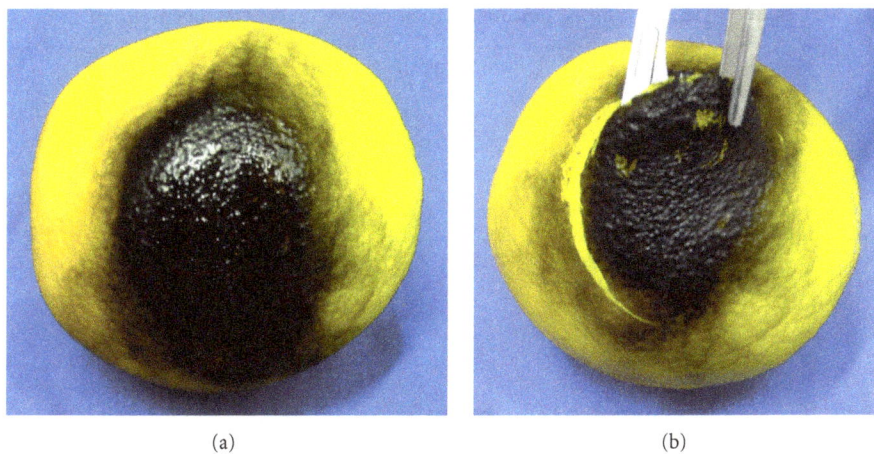

FIGURE 6: Organic bench model simulating (a) a necrotic wound and its (b) careful surgical debridement.

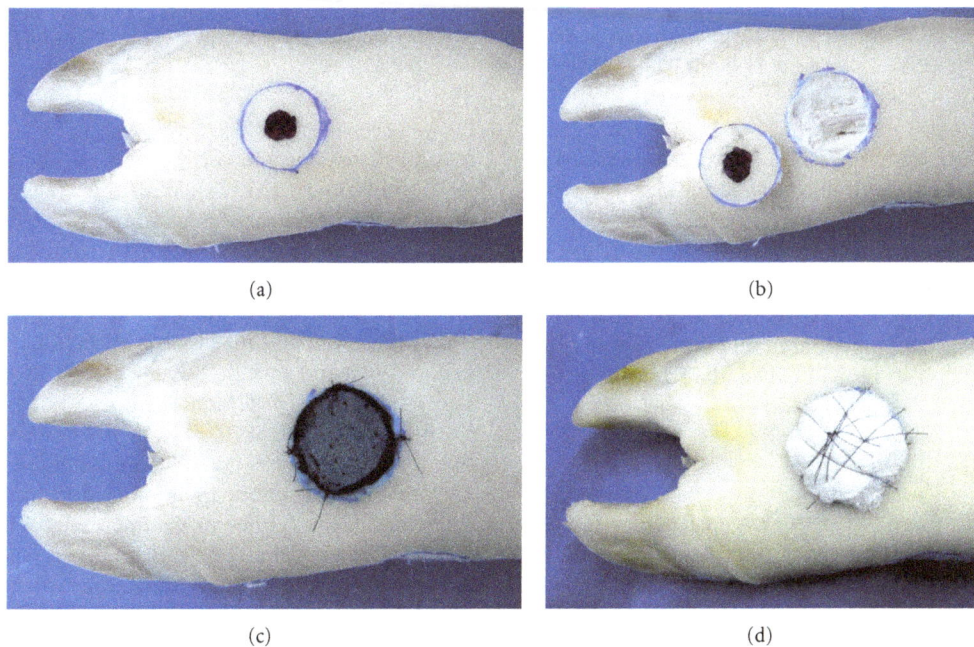

FIGURE 7: Cattle-skin bench model simulating (a) a nonmelanoma skin cancer with safety margins, (b) complete surgical excision of the "cutaneous tumor," (c) repair of the defect by placing an ox tongue graft, and (d) a pressure dressing fixed with braided suture over the gauze wad.

and learning and five of rest). A specific week or the total of weeks of a skill can be adjusted (i.e., increased or decreased) according to the individual or subgroups needs.

12. Self-Directed Training

During each training session, supervised by an instructor and at home, students should use the principles taught in an individualized, deliberate, repetitive, and participative way [30, 70]. Whenever there are doubts about a complete procedure or a particular step, they should seek for help from textbooks, online text, online narrated expert demonstration videos, and instructors [26–29].

13. Feedback

In the context of the acquisition of surgical skills based on simulation, feedback from instructors is associated with a better and faster learning and also with greater knowledge retention over time [30]. Thus, all undergraduates should receive feedback during and at the end of each training stage [30] in the classroom, or in specific times scheduled after the training at home [32–39]. Instructors must analyze specific movements, paying attention to inadequacies (e.g., mark lines and procedures already finished can serve as evaluation parameters), and following this, they should provide a constructive feedback (point and correct any technical errors) to

TABLE 2: Proposed training time in this basic plastic surgery training program.

| Learning goals | Training time (h) per week | | | | |
| | First day | | Second to sixth day | Seventh day | |
	Verbal teaching based on theoretical materials	Training on BM in the classroom (process feedback)	Training on BM outside the classroom*	Training on BM after practice outside the classroom (outcome feedback)	Total number of weeks**
Surgical knots	1	1	Variable	1	2
Incision and suture techniques	1	2	Variable	2	2
Biopsy techniques	1	3	Variable	3	3≈
Skin grafts	1	3	Variable	3	3¥
Surgical flaps	1	4	Variable	4	5°
Management of cutaneous lesions	2	4	Variable	4	4#

h: hour; BM: bench models; *each medical student must train repeatedly for as long as you feel necessary; instructor's role is to encourage this practice outside the classroom; **one week for introduction of the subject in each of the six skills; ≈ one week for incisional biopsies (without safety margins) and one for excisional biopsies (safety margins); ¥ one week for the handling of the surgical instruments for the preparation of graft (donor area) and one for graft placement on recipient area; °one week for each type of flap (transposition, rotation, advancement, and island flaps); #one week for each proposed cutaneous lesion (lipomas/epidermoid cysts, necrotic wounds, and non-melanoma skin cancer).

students [71]. Thus, undergraduates improve skills based on their mistakes and can be trained again and again, having, as a result, the gain of skills over time. Concurrent with the feedback, it is important to encourage students to resolve their doubts during practice and after extracurricular tasks.

To facilitate feedback, students should be distributed around rectangular tables, providing mobility to the instructor to clarify any doubts individually and also in subgroups [32, 42, 45].

14. Instructors

Feedback can be given by physician instructors (faculty expert or residents) and/or by nondoctors since they are qualified, such as laboratory technicians or medical students (monitoring format) [10, 24, 72, 73], without compromising the learning [72, 73]. The adoption of one instructor for each group of four undergraduates is recommended [74].

15. Assessment and Certification

Under simulated surgical teaching, we must emphasize the importance of an objective evaluation during and at the end of the whole teaching and learning process of each proposed surgical skill in order to measure the level of acquisition of the taught skills [75].

Among the various forms of the described assessments [31, 75], the Objective Structured Assessment of Technical Skills (OSATS) [76, 77] is currently considered as the gold standard for the objective evaluation of acquisition of surgical skills [75]. OSATS consists of two subscales: Task-Specific Checklist and Global Rating Scale (GRS) [76, 77].

Since GRS [76, 77] (Table 3) has the advantage of being used to assess generic aspects of technical performance and has a broad applicability, without the need to develop specific lists for each procedure [78], this scale has been adopted

as a measurement and certification tool by our group [32–39] and by others [53, 78]. With this scale, it is possible to evaluate the performances of students in eight main areas, through a 5-point scale, being 1 the minimum score and 5 the maximum one, so that the maximum score achieved is 40 [53, 76, 77]. Instructors can apply this scale at the end of each training session, and in subsequent sessions, they follow the gain of skills and specific points (among the eight evaluated ones) that deserve attention.

In addition, GRS [76, 77] can also be used as a certification tool; for an individual task, the candidate should achieve a score of 24 or more to be considered competent [78]. Therefore, if the trainee meets the predefined criteria based on objective assessment, he/she can progress to the next stage of training (considered as a more complex one). However, if the undergraduate is not able to proceed, the training should be repeated and focused on specific deficits, and, then, a new objective assessment should be carried out.

In the training evaluation, a characteristic of bench models that could be considered as a problem (they can tear) is actually an advantage because this occurs when students make a wrong movement (e.g., applying excessive force). This characteristic can serve as an evaluation mechanism with feedback for improving skills [32–34]. Moreover, the markings made on the surfaces of models also serve as an evaluation parameter [33].

16. Discussion

Over the last two decades, simulation-based education has emerged as an important innovation in medical learning and practice [31, 79]. In this context, surgical training is shifting from the traditional apprenticeship to a more objective standardized approach, using simulators to improve several medical aspects such as reducing errors and increasing patient safety [31]. Since currently the simulated acquisition

TABLE 3: Global rating scale adapted to evaluate the sutures and biopsies techniques [53, 76, 77].

Please rate the trainee's performance on the following scale.				
Respect for tissue	1	2 3	4 5	
	Frequently used unnecessary force on tissues or caused damage by inappropriate instrument use	Careful handling of tissue, but occasional inadvertent damage	Consistently handled tissues appropriately with minimal damage	
Time in motion	1	2 3	4 5	
	Many unnecessary moves	Efficient time and motion, but some unnecessary moves	Clear economy of movement and maximum efficiency	
Instrument handling	1	2 3	4 5	
	Repeatedly makes tentative or awkward moves with instruments	Competent use of instruments, but occasionally awkward	Fluid movements	
Elliptical excision skill*	1	2 3	4 5	
	Lacks knowledge of design parameters (<2 mm or >10 mm margins); angles *very* different than 30°; length-width ratio *very* different than 3-4 : 1	Adequate 2 to 10 mm margins; angles at ends of ellipse *slightly* different than 30°; length-width ratio *slightly* different than 3-4 : 1	Adequate 2 to 10 mm margins; 30° angles at both ends; length-width ratio 3-4 : 1	
Suture training**	1	2 3	4 5	
	Awkward and unsure with poor knot tying, and inability to maintain tension	Competent suturing with good knot placement and appropriate tension	Excellent suture control with correct suture placement and tension	
Flow of operation	1	2 3	4 5	
	Frequently stopped operating, seemed unsure of next move	Demonstrated some forward planning and reasonable progression of procedure	Obviously planned operation	
Knowledge of procedure	1	2 3	4 5	
	Inefficient knowledge of procedure. Looked unsure and hesitant	Knew all important steps of procedure	Demonstrated familiarity of all steps of procedure	
Final product	1	2 3	4 5	
	Final product of unacceptable quality	Final product of average quality	Final product of superior quality	
Overall performance	1	2 3	4 5	
	Very poor	Competent	Very good	
Maximum total score (40)				
Total score ( )				

*This parameter should be excluded for the evaluation of suture techniques; **this parameter should be excluded for the evaluation of biopsy techniques.

of basic surgical skills is recommended before any procedures on living patients [7], the main focus of this study was to propose a simulation-based basic plastic surgery training program during medical education, through the training on different inanimate bench models. In order to increase the arsenal of surgical skills of medical students during training, this teaching proposal and the way bench models are applied can be incorporated and adapted to complement the curriculum already established in different educational institutions [8, 30], and this,can be used in several disciplines such as surgical technique, plastic surgery, among others. Both novice medical students and students that master basic surgical skills partially, but that need to improve them, can benefit from this program. Similar to other studies [13], this training program also has the potential to introduce and improve students' plastic surgery skills, as well as develop personal career interests.

Based on the assumption recently described as the most effective method to teach surgical skills in simulation environments, a combination of self-directed training with instructors' feedback, intermittently distributed over a predetermined period (weeks or months) [24, 25], this was the teaching form adopted in the present study in order to retain and improve the learned surgical skills [24, 25]. However, some factors, such as high costs [25] (mainly in developing countries) [32, 33, 43], the lack of time, and shortage of faculty experts (traditional instructor) [10, 24] have been described as limiting factors for the implementation of this simulated training strategy.

One solution to partially reduce the financial cost is the use of low cost bench models, such as those described in the present study. The different inanimate bench models vary in relation to the fidelity level (realism) when compared to a live human being; there are high fidelity models, such as parts of *postmortem* animals (pig [37, 38, 40, 45, 46], chicken [38, 39, 44], and cattle [48] skins and ox tongue [40–42]) and others of low fidelity, such as plates of ethylene-vinyl acetate [32, 34–38, 47], organic material [33, 49], among others [40, 53].

Despite the intuitive belief that "the more realistic, the best," in the simulated training of surgical skills, the acquisition of skills should be measured by means of an objective method [75]. Therefore, since there are studies developed by our group [36–38] and by others [80–83] that demonstrate objectively that the surgical skills learned by novice undergraduate on bench models can result in improved performance in animals, corpses, and also in the operating room, regardless of the fidelity of bench model [9, 38, 39, 80–83], the choice of a specific bench model should not be based on its fidelity. Aspects such as availability, seasonal variability, and costs should be considered for this choice.

The authors believe that the bench models are complementary. In order to generate the interest of medical students in the practice of plastic surgery principles, the initial training in classrooms (or laboratories of surgical technique) should be preferably performed on bench models made from parts of *postmortem* animals, because it was shown that students feel more attracted by these bench models [40]. For the subsequent training sessions, low-fidelity bench models should be preferred because they are versatile, reusable, and easy to handle [32, 33, 35, 47, 49], unlike the *ex vivo* model that requires adequate space and conditions to be stored [7, 8], and it can make the training impracticable, for example, at home [35].

Although financial costs can be reduced by the previously described measures, time availability remains a problem for faculty experts [10, 24]. Feedback generated by computers could be an option to reduce the supervised learning time. However, besides the high cost for its acquisition, the retention of skills over time is significantly greater when learned from direct feedback from an instructor [84]. Similar to that described here, the incorporation of residents, trained medical students, or nonphysician skills laboratory [10, 72, 73] as instructors is an alternative that can reduce the number of faculty surgeons transferred from patient care to simulation environments. With this measure, faculty surgeon would focus on teaching complex tasks and cognitive aspects of clinical training (e.g., decision making) that are not duties of the nonmedical instructor [73]. Alternatives that can

also help reduce the time of supervised simulated teaching would be increased intervals between training sessions [85], to use concepts derived from blended learning [86], and to encourage the practice outside the classroom, for instance, at home, as it has been proposed by our group [32–39].

The present training program was structured especially to develop some basic plastic surgical skills. Therefore, it does not meet all the needs of medical students in training, which should include the acquisition of other basic surgical skills, as it is described by the American College of Surgeons/Association of Program Directors in Surgery National Skills Curriculum [31].

17. Conclusion

The proposal of simulation in basic plastic surgery training on inanimate bench models is a further complementary alternative to the arsenal of training programs already established in order to better prepare medical students before their contact with living patients which remains as the cornerstone of medical education.

Disclosure

The authors hereby certify that no financial support has been received from any commercial source by any coauthor, individual, or entity that is related directly or indirectly to the scientific work which is presented in this paper.

References

[1] D. A. Askew, D. Wilkinson, P. J. Schluter, and K. Eckert, "Skin cancer surgery in Australia 2001–2005: the changing role of the general practitioner," *Medical Journal of Australia*, vol. 187, no. 4, pp. 210–214, 2007.

[2] D. Wilkinson, P. Bourne, A. Dixon, and S. Kitchener, "Skin cancer medicine in primary care: towards an agenda for quality health outcomes," *Medical Journal of Australia*, vol. 184, no. 1, pp. 11–12, 2006.

[3] R. Gmajnić, S. Pribić, A. Lukić, B. Ebling, N. Čupić, and I. Marković, "Effect of surgical training course on performance of minor surgical procedures in family medicine physicians' offices: an observational study," *Croatian Medical Journal*, vol. 49, no. 3, pp. 358–363, 2008.

[4] S. S. Forbes, P. G. Fitzgerald, and D. W. Birch, "Undergraduate surgical training: variations in program objectives and curriculum implementation across Canada," *Canadian Journal of Surgery*, vol. 49, no. 1, pp. 46–50, 2006.

[5] A. M. Collins, P. F. Ridgway, M. S. U. Hassan, C. W. K. Chou, A. D. Hill, and B. Kneafsey, "Surgical instruction for general practitioners: how, who and how often?" *Journal of Plastic, Reconstructive and Aesthetic Surgery*, vol. 63, no. 7, pp. 1156–1162, 2010.

[6] M. Friedlich, T. Wood, G. Regehr, C. Hurst, and F. Shamji, "Structured assessment of minor surgical skills (SAMSS) for clinical clerks," *Academic Medicine*, vol. 77, no. 10, supplement, pp. S39–S41, 2002.

[7] I. Hammond and K. Karthigasu, "Training, assessment and competency in gynaecologic surgery," *Best Practice and Research*, vol. 20, no. 1, pp. 173–187, 2006.

[8] M. M. Hammoud, F. S. Nuthalapaty, A. R. Goepfert et al., "To the point: medical education review of the role of simulators in surgical training," *American Journal of Obstetrics and Gynecology*, vol. 199, no. 4, pp. 338–343, 2008.

[9] R. K. Reznick and H. MacRae, "Teaching surgical skills—changes in the wind," *The New England Journal of Medicine*, vol. 355, no. 25, pp. 2664–2669, 2006.

[10] D. J. Scott, C. M. Pugh, E. M. Ritter, L. M. Jacobs, C. A. Pellegrini, and A. K. Sachdeva, "New directions in simulation-based surgical education and training: validation and transfer of surgical skills, use of nonsurgeons as faculty, use of simulation to screen and select surgery residents, and long-term follow-up of learners," *Surgery*, vol. 149, no. 6, pp. 735–744, 2011.

[11] A. Burd, T. Chiu, and C. McNaught, "Plastic surgery in the undergraduate curriculum: the importance of considering students' perceptions," *British Journal of Plastic Surgery*, vol. 57, no. 8, pp. 773–779, 2004.

[12] A. R. Rowsell, "The place of plastic surgery in the undergraduate surgical curriculum," *British Journal of Plastic Surgery*, vol. 39, no. 2, pp. 241–243, 1986.

[13] C. R. Davis, J. M. O'Donoghue, J. McPhail, and A. R. Green, "How to improve plastic surgery knowledge, skills and career interest in undergraduates in one day," *Journal of Plastic, Reconstructive and Aesthetic Surgery*, vol. 63, no. 10, pp. 1677–1681, 2010.

[14] J. Mason, V. Androshchuk, and H. Morgan, "Re: Davis et al. How to improve plastic surgery knowledge, skills and career interest in undergraduates in one day, Journal of Plastic, Reconstructive and Aesthetic Surgery, vol. 63, pp. 1677–1681, 2010," *Journal of Plastic, Reconstructive and Aesthetic Surgery*, vol. 64, no. 3, article e87, 2011.

[15] C. S. J. Dunkin, J. M. Pleat, S. A. M. Jones, and T. E. E. Goodacre, "Perception and reality—a study of public and professional perceptions of plastic surgery," *British Journal of Plastic Surgery*, vol. 56, no. 5, pp. 437–443, 2003.

[16] Y. Al-Nuaimi, G. McGrouther, and A. Bayat, "Modernising medical careers in the UK and plastic surgery as a possible career choice: undergraduate opinions," *Journal of Plastic, Reconstructive and Aesthetic Surgery*, vol. 59, no. 12, pp. 1472–1474, 2006.

[17] N. Panse, S. Panse, P. Kulkarni, R. Dhongde, and P. Sahasrabudhe, "Awareness and perception of plastic surgery among healthcare professionals in Pune, India: do they really know what we do?" *Plastic Surgery International*, vol. 2012, Article ID 962169, 9 pages, 2012.

[18] B. Antoszewski, P. Kardas, A. Kasielska, and M. Fijalkowska, "Family physicians' perception of plastic surgery and its influence on referral. A survey from Poland," *European Journal of General Practice*, vol. 18, no. 1, pp. 22–25, 2012.

[19] A. K. Greene and J. W. May Jr., "Applying to plastic surgery residency: factors associated with medical student career choice," *Plastic and Reconstructive Surgery*, vol. 121, no. 3, pp. 1049–1053, 2008.

[20] R. G. Wade, M. A. Moses, and J. Henderson, "Teaching plastic surgery to undergraduates," *Journal of Plastic, Reconstructive and Aesthetic Surgery*, vol. 62, no. 2, p. 267, 2009.

[21] M. A. Prater and D. J. Smith Jr., "Determining undergraduate curriculum content in plastic surgery," *Plastic and Reconstructive Surgery*, vol. 84, no. 3, pp. 529–533, 1989.

[22] J. M. Porter, C. R. W. Rayner, and O. M. Fenton, "Teaching plastic surgery to medical students," *Medical Education*, vol. 26, no. 1, pp. 42–47, 1992.

[23] R. A. Agha, A. Papanikitas, M. Baum, and I. S. Benjamin, "The teaching of surgery in the undergraduate curriculum. Part II—importance and recommendations for change," *International Journal of Surgery*, vol. 3, no. 2, pp. 151–157, 2005.

[24] A. R. Jensen, A. S. Wright, A. E. Levy et al., "Acquiring basic surgical skills: Is a faculty mentor really needed?" *American Journal of Surgery*, vol. 197, no. 1, pp. 82–88, 2009.

[25] C. A. E. Moulton, A. Dubrowski, H. MacRae, B. Graham, E. Grober, and R. Reznick, "Teaching surgical skills: what kind of practice makes perfect? A randomized, controlled trial," *Annals of Surgery*, vol. 244, no. 3, pp. 400–409, 2006.

[26] C. Czarnowski, D. Ponka, R. Rughani, and P. Geoffrion, "Elliptical excision: minor surgery video series," *Canadian Family Physician*, vol. 54, no. 8, p. 1144, 2008.

[27] J. E. Janis, R. K. Kwon, and D. H. Lalonde, "A practical guide to wound healing," *Plastic and Reconstructive Surgery*, vol. 125, no. 6, pp. 230e–244e, 2010.

[28] L. H. Goldberg and M. Alam, "Elliptical excisions: variations and the eccentric parallelogram," *Archives of Dermatology*, vol. 140, no. 2, pp. 176–180, 2004.

[29] M. Tschoi, E. A. Hoy, and M. S. Granick, "Skin flaps," *Surgical Clinics of North America*, vol. 89, no. 3, pp. 643–658, 2009.

[30] J. A. Cannon-Bowers, C. Bowers, and K. Procci, "Optimizing learning in surgical simulations: guidelines from the science of learning and human performance," *Surgical Clinics of North America*, vol. 90, no. 3, pp. 583–603, 2010.

[31] J. M. Rosen, S. A. Long, D. M. McGrath, and S. E. Greer, "Simulation in plastic surgery training and education: the path forward," *Plastic and Reconstructive Surgery*, vol. 123, no. 2, pp. 729–740, 2009.

[32] É. M. Bastos and R. D. P. Silva, "Proposal of a synthetic ethylene-vinyl acetate bench model for surgical foundations learning. Suture training," *Acta Cirurgica Brasileira*, vol. 26, no. 2, pp. 149–152, 2011.

[33] R. Denadai and L. R. Souto, "Organic bench model to complement the teaching and learning on basic surgical skills," *Acta Cirurgica Brasileira*, vol. 27, no. 1, pp. 88–94, 2012.

[34] R. Denadai and E. M. Bastos, "Letter: the synthetic ethylene-vinyl acetate bench model," *Dermatologic Surgery*, vol. 38, no. 2, pp. 288–289, 2012.

[35] R. D. Silva and E. M. Bastos, "Cutaneous surgery workshop: some considerations," *Revista do Colégio Brasileiro de Cirurgiões*, vol. 38, no. 6, p. 452, 2011.

[36] R. Denadai, R. Saad-Hossne, M. Oshiiwa, and E. M. Bastos, "Training on synthetic ethylene-vinyl acetate bench model allows novice medical students to acquire suture skills," *Acta Cirurgica Brasileira*, vol. 27, no. 3, pp. 271–278, 2012.

[37] R. Denadai, M. Oshiiwa, and R. Saad-Hossne, "Does bench model fidelity interfere in the acquisition of suture skills by novice medical students?" *Revista Da Associacao Medica Brasileira*, vol. 58, no. 5, pp. 600–606, 2012.

[38] R. Denadai, M. Oshiiwa, and R. Saad-Hossne, "Teaching elliptical excision skills to novice medical students: a randomized controlled study comparing low- and high-fidelity bench models," *Indian Journal of Dermatology*. In press.

[39] R. Denadai, R. Saad-Hossne, and L. R. Souto, "Simulation-based cutaneous surgical-skill training on a chicken-skin bench model in a medicalundergraduate program," *Indian Journal of Dermatology*. In press.

[40] K. G. Tokuhara, D. W. Boldt, and L. G. Yamamoto, "Teaching suturing in a workshop setting: a comparison of several models," *Hawaii Medical Journal*, vol. 63, no. 9, pp. 258–259, 2004.

[41] J. M. Camelo-Nunes, J. Hiratsuka, M. M. Yoshida, C. A. Beltrani-Filho, L. S. Oliveira, and A. C. Nagae, "Ox tongue: an alternative model for surgical training," *Plastic and Reconstructive Surgery*, vol. 116, no. 1, pp. 352–354, 2005.

[42] D. Franco, J. Medeiros, A. Grossi, and T. Franco, "Suturing techniques teaching method using bovine tongue," *Revista do Colegio Brasileiro de Cirurgioes*, vol. 35, no. 6, pp. 442–444, 2008.

[43] S. Taché, N. Mbembati, N. Marshall, F. Tendick, C. Mkony, and P. O'Sullivan, "Addressing gaps in surgical skills training by means of low-cost simulation at Muhimbili University in Tanzania," *Human Resources for Health*, vol. 7, article 64, 2009.

[44] P. N. Khalil, M. Siebeck, W. Mutschler, and K. G. Kanz, "The use of chicken legs for teaching wound closure skills," *European Journal of Medical Research*, vol. 14, no. 10, pp. 459–460, 2009.

[45] K. S. Purim, "Cutaneous surgery workshop," *Revista do Colégio Brasileiro de Cirurgiões*, vol. 37, pp. 303–305, 2010.

[46] W. Y. Chan and M. Dalal, "Cost-effective plastic surgery skills training," *Journal of Plastic, Reconstructive and Aesthetic Surgery*, vol. 63, no. 2, pp. e136–e137, 2010.

[47] D. Gutiérrez-Mendoza, R. Narro-Llorente, M. E. Contreras-Barrera, V. Fonte-Ávalos, and J. Domíguez-Cherit, "Ethylene vinyl acetate (Foam): an inexpensive and useful tool for teaching suture techniques in dermatologic surgery," *Dermatologic Surgery*, vol. 37, pp. 1353–1357, 2011.

[48] P. N. Khalil, K. G. Kanz, M. Siebeck, and W. Mutschler, "Teaching advanced wound closure techniques using cattle digits," *Dermatologic Surgery*, vol. 37, no. 3, pp. 325–330, 2011.

[49] E. J. Whallett and J. C. McGregor, "An alternative model for teaching basic principles and surgical skills in plastic surgery," *Journal of Plastic, Reconstructive and Aesthetic Surgery*, vol. 64, no. 2, pp. 272–274, 2011.

[50] N. Dastur, "DIY surgical knot-tying tool," *Annals of the Royal College of Surgeons of England*, vol. 91, no. 3, p. 268, 2009.

[51] S. Sandwell, R. Hazani, and M. Kasdan, "An efficient hand-tying technique for vessel ligation," *American Surgeon*, vol. 75, no. 11, pp. 1098–1099, 2009.

[52] D. H. Oram, "Basic surgical skills," *Best Practice & Research Clinical Obstetrics & Gynaecology*, vol. 20, no. 1, pp. 61–71, 2006.

[53] C. Garcia, M. Neuburg, and K. Carlson-Sweet, "A model to teach elliptical excision and basic suturing techniques," *Archives of Dermatology*, vol. 142, no. 4, pp. 526–527, 2006.

[54] J. J. Vujevich, A. Kimyai-Asadi, and L. H. Goldberg, "The four angles of cutting," *Dermatologic Surgery*, vol. 34, no. 8, pp. 1082–1084, 2008.

[55] M. S. Khan, S. D. Bann, A. Darzi, and P. E. M. Butler, "Use of suturing as a measure of technical competence," *Annals of Plastic Surgery*, vol. 50, no. 3, pp. 304–308, 2003.

[56] P. C. Alguire and B. M. Mathes, "Skin biopsy techniques for the internist," *Journal of General Internal Medicine*, vol. 13, no. 1, pp. 46–54, 1998.

[57] W. Hussain, N. J. Mortimer, and P. J. M. Salmon, "Optimizing technique in elliptical excisional surgery: some pearls for practice," *British Journal of Dermatology*, vol. 161, no. 3, pp. 697–698, 2009.

[58] R. D. Silva and L. R. Souto, "Evaluation of the diagnosis and treatment of non-melanoma skin cancer and its impacts on the prevention habits in a specific population of southeastern Brazil," *European Journal of General Medicine*, vol. 8, pp. 291–301, 2011.

[59] R. Shimizu and K. Kishi, "Skin graft," *Plastic Surgery International*, vol. 2012, Article ID 563493, 5 pages, 2012.

[60] D. A. L. Watt, S. Majumder, and S. J. Southern, "Simulating split-skin graft harvest," *British Journal of Plastic Surgery*, vol. 52, no. 4, p. 329, 1999.

[61] P. A. Wilson, N. D. Rhodes, and S. J. Southern, "Surgical simulation in plastic surgery," *British Journal of Plastic Surgery*, vol. 54, no. 6, pp. 560–561, 2001.

[62] S. P. H. Bennett, P. Velander, P. A. McArthur, J. McPhail, R. Alvi, and K. E. Graham, "A novel model for skin graft harvesting," *Plastic and Reconstructive Surgery*, vol. 114, no. 6, pp. 1660–1661, 2004.

[63] T. C. S. Cubison and T. Clare, "Lesagne: a simple model to assess the practical skills of split-skin graft harvesting and meshing," *British Journal of Plastic Surgery*, vol. 55, no. 8, pp. 703–704, 2002.

[64] M. Tschoi, E. A. Hoy, and M. S. Granick, "Skin flaps," *Surgical Clinics of North America*, vol. 89, no. 3, pp. 643–658, 2009.

[65] O. Villafane, S. J. Southern, and I. T. H. Foo, "Simulated interactive local flaps: operating room models for surgeon and patient alike," *British Journal of Plastic Surgery*, vol. 52, no. 3, p. 241, 1999.

[66] J. D. Beard, B. C. Jolly, D. I. Newble, W. E. G. Thomas, J. Donnelly, and L. J. Southgate, "Assessing the technical skills of surgical trainees," *British Journal of Surgery*, vol. 92, no. 6, pp. 778–782, 2005.

[67] S. Sambandan, "The Norwich sebaceous cyst in surgical training," *Annals of the Royal College of Surgeons of England*, vol. 80, no. 4, pp. 274–275, 1998.

[68] J. Bowling and J. Botting, "Porcine sebaceous cyst model: an inexpensive, reproducible skin surgery simulator," *Dermatologic Surgery*, vol. 31, no. 8, part 1, pp. 953–956, 2005.

[69] A. A. Köse, Y. Karabağli, M. Arici, and C. Çetin, "Various materials may aid in teaching surgical procedures," *Plastic and Reconstructive Surgery*, vol. 114, no. 2, p. 611, 2004.

[70] K. A. Ericsson, "Deliberate practice and the acquisition and maintenance of expert performance in medicine and related domains," *Academic Medicine*, vol. 79, no. 10, supplement, pp. S70–S81, 2004.

[71] D. A. Rogers, G. Regehr, and J. MacDonald, "A role for error training in surgical technical skill instruction and evaluation," *American Journal of Surgery*, vol. 183, no. 3, pp. 242–245, 2002.

[72] S. C. Graziano, "Randomized surgical training for medical students: resident versus peer-led teaching," *American Journal of Obstetrics and Gynecology*, vol. 204, no. 6, pp. 542.e1–542.e4, 2011.

[73] M. J. Kim, M. L. Boehler, J. K. Ketchum, R. Bueno Jr., R. G. Williams, and G. L. Dunnington, "Skills coaches as part of the educational team: a randomized controlled trial of teaching of a basic surgical skill in the laboratory setting," *American Journal of Surgery*, vol. 199, no. 1, pp. 94–98, 2010.

[74] A. Dubrowski and H. MacRae, "Randomised, controlled study investigating the optimal instructor: student ratios for teaching suturing skills," *Medical Education*, vol. 40, no. 1, pp. 59–63, 2006.

[75] P. D. van Hove, G. J. M. Tuijthof, E. G. G. Verdaasdonk, L. P. S. Stassen, and J. Dankelman, "Objective assessment of technical surgical skills," *British Journal of Surgery*, vol. 97, no. 7, pp. 972–987, 2010.

[76] H. Faulkner, G. Regehr, J. Martin, and R. Reznick, "Validation of an objective structured assessment of technical skill for

surgical residents," *Academic Medicine*, vol. 71, no. 12, pp. 1363–1365, 1996.

[77] R. Reznick, G. Regehr, H. MacRae, J. Martin, and W. McCulloch, "Testing technical skill via an innovative "bench station" examination," *American Journal of Surgery*, vol. 173, no. 3, pp. 226–230, 1997.

[78] M. S. Khan, S. D. Bann, A. W. Darzi, and P. E. M. Butler, "Assessing surgical skill using bench station models," *Plastic and Reconstructive Surgery*, vol. 120, no. 3, pp. 793–800, 2007.

[79] T. Grunwald, T. Krummel, and R. Sherman, "Advanced technologies in plastic surgery: how new innovations can improve our training and practice," *Plastic and Reconstructive Surgery*, vol. 114, no. 6, pp. 1556–1567, 2004.

[80] E. D. Grober, S. J. Hamstra, K. R. Wanzel et al., "The educational impact of bench model fidelity on the acquisition of technical skill: the use of clinically relevant outcome measures," *Annals of Surgery*, vol. 240, no. 2, pp. 374–381, 2004.

[81] E. D. Grober, S. J. Hamstra, K. R. Wanzel et al., "Laboratory based training in urological microsurgery with bench model simulators: a randomized controlled trial evaluating the durability of technical skill," *The Journal of Urology*, vol. 172, no. 1, pp. 378–381, 2004.

[82] E. D. Matsumoto, S. J. Hamstra, S. B. Radomski, and M. D. Cusimano, "The effect of bench model fidelity on endourological skills: a randomized controlled study," *Journal of Urology*, vol. 167, no. 3, pp. 1243–1247, 2002.

[83] D. J. Anastakis, G. Regehr, R. K. Reznick et al., "Assessment of technical skills transfer from the bench training model to the human model," *American Journal of Surgery*, vol. 177, no. 2, pp. 167–170, 1999.

[84] M. C. Porte, G. Xeroulis, R. K. Reznick, and A. Dubrowski, "Verbal feedback from an expert is more effective than self-accessed feedback about motion efficiency in learning new surgical skills," *American Journal of Surgery*, vol. 193, no. 1, pp. 105–110, 2007.

[85] E. L. Mitchell, D. Y. Lee, N. Sevdalis et al., "Evaluation of distributed practice schedules on retention of a newly acquired surgical skill: a randomized trial," *American Journal of Surgery*, vol. 201, no. 1, pp. 31–39, 2011.

[86] U. M. Rieger, K. Pierer, J. Farhadi, T. Lehmann, B. Röers, and G. Pierer, "Effective acquisition of basic surgical techniques through Blended Learning," *Chirurg*, vol. 80, no. 6, pp. 537–543, 2009.

33

Nasal Septal Deviations: A Systematic Review of Classification Systems

Jeffrey Teixeira,[1] Victor Certal,[2,3] Edward T. Chang,[4] and Macario Camacho[5]

[1]Department of Otolaryngology Head and Neck Surgery, Walter Reed National Military Medical Center, Bethesda, MD, USA
[2]Department of Otorhinolaryngology/Sleep Medicine Centre, Hospital CUF, 4100-180 Porto, Portugal
[3]Centre for Research in Health Technologies and Information Systems (CINTESIS), University of Porto, 4200-450 Porto, Portugal
[4]Tripler Army Medical Center, Department of Surgery, Division of Otolaryngology, Tripler AMC, Honolulu, HI, USA
[5]Tripler Army Medical Center, Division of Otolaryngology, Sleep Surgery and Sleep Medicine, 1 Jarrett White Road,
 Tripler AMC, HI 96859, USA

Correspondence should be addressed to Macario Camacho; drcamachoent@yahoo.com

Academic Editor: Selahattin Özmen

Objective. To systematically review the international literature for internal nasal septal deviation classification systems and summarize them for clinical and research purposes. *Data Sources.* Four databases (including PubMed/MEDLINE) were systematically searched through December 16, 2015. *Methods.* Systematic review, adhering to PRISMA. *Results.* After removal of duplicates, this study screened 952 articles for relevance. A final comprehensive review of 50 articles identified that 15 of these articles met the eligibility criteria. The classification systems defined in these articles included C-shaped, S-shaped, reverse C-shaped, and reverse S-shaped descriptions of the septal deviation in both the cephalocaudal and anteroposterior dimensions. Additional studies reported use of computed tomography and categorized deviation based on predefined locations. Three studies graded the severity of septal deviations based on the amount of deflection. The systems defined in the literature also included an evaluation of nasal septal spurs and perforations. *Conclusion.* This systematic review ascertained that the majority of the currently published classification systems for internal nasal septal deviations can be summarized by C-shaped or reverse C-shaped, as well as S-shaped or reverse S-shaped deviations in the anteroposterior and cephalocaudal dimensions. For imaging studies, predefined points have been defined along the septum. Common terminology can facilitate future research.

1. Introduction

Nasal septal deviations play a critical role in nasal obstruction symptoms, aesthetic appearance of the nose, increased nasal resistance, and sometimes snoring [1]. Consequently, a comprehensive assessment of the nasal septum serves an essential role in preoperative planning, reestablishing function, and overall cosmetic appeal. Typically, a septoplasty suffices in addressing significant nasal septal deviations, but on occasion such deviations warrant a single-stage septorhinoplasty [2–4]. In 1954, Lindahl described nasal septal deviations as either developmental (usually smooth, "C-shaped" or "S-shaped" nasal septum with occurrence more often in the anterior septum) or traumatic (usually irregular, angulated, and sometimes dislocated) in origin [5].

Over the years, individual authors and groups studied the assessment and classification of internal nasal septal deviations but none to date conducted a systematic evaluation of these studies with a comprehensive summarization of the individual results. Because of the variation in classification systems, such as grading internal septal deflections in the anterior aspect versus along the entire nasal airway, utilizing physical examination versus computed tomography, a summary of the currently published international literature would help facilitate future research. The importance of a summary is notable when studies report the prevalence of nasal septal deviations, given that studies reporting findings by simply using a handheld otoscope will have a lower prevalence of nasal septal deviations than those that use endoscopy or computed tomography because the handheld otoscope fails to consider the internal nasal septum's entire length and subsequently undercategorized these deviations. This in turn led to underestimations of the true prevalence of nasal septal deviations [6]. In order to facilitate future research regarding the effect of internal nasal septal deviations with regard to both functional (nasal obstruction) and cosmetic outcomes, a summary of currently available methods for categorizing nasal septal deviations is a necessary first step. The objective of this study is to conduct a systematic review of internal nasal septal deviation classification systems that are currently published in the international literature and summarize them for both clinical and research purposes.

2. Methods

The authors (Macario Camacho and Jeffrey Teixeira) conducted a systematic review of the literature found within PubMed/MEDLINE, Scopus, Web of Science, and the Cochrane Library from inception of the respective databases through December 16, 2015. Various searches identified the pertinent articles in the current published literature. The authors used the following MeSH terms: "Nose Deformities, Acquired" or "Nose" in combination with search terms "classification," "classification system," "grading," and "grading system." A second search used the MeSH terms "Nose Deformities, Acquired" and "Classification." An additional search used the following phrases: "deviated nasal septum"; further searches used the following terms: "septal deviation" or "nasal deformity" in combination with search terms "classification," "classification system," "grading," and "grading system." The authors also reviewed "related citations" and "cited by" for relevant articles in order to identify additional possible studies to include. Further, the authors reviewed references cited within each article in order to identify additional studies.

The authors performed the literature search and independently reviewed the results to screen for relevant articles to include in the final review. The inclusion criteria included the following: studies which classify or grade internal nasal septal deviations, without regard to language. Exclusion criteria included the following: studies which do not classify or grade internal nasal septal deviations, or classification systems exclusively describing external nasal deformities. Statistical analysis was not applicable since there were no quantitative outcomes assessed, as this is a qualitative systematic review of classification systems. As part of the systematic review, the classification systems identified were each reviewed for commonalities, which could then be used to summarize the various classifications of nasal septal deviations.

3. Results

3.1. Study Selection. An example of a search in PubMed is (((("Nose Deformities, Acquired" [Mesh]) OR "Nose" [Mesh]) AND "Classification" [Mesh]) OR (((("Nose Deformities, Acquired" [Mesh]) OR "Nose" [Mesh]) AND "Classification system") OR (((("Nose Deformities, Acquired" [Mesh]) OR "Nose" [Mesh]) AND "Grading") OR (((("Nose Deformities, Acquired" [Mesh]) OR "Nose" [Mesh]) AND "Grading System") which yielded 541 results. Additional

searches applied to all the databases produced a grand total of 952 articles, and after reviewing the titles and the abstracts a total of 907 articles were excluded. Full texts were downloaded for 45 articles [2–46]. After retrieval and reviewing the references of those articles, an additional five articles were downloaded [19, 47–50]. Of the 50 articles reviewed in their entirety, the following are reasons for exclusion: two were letters to the editor [13, 49], one classified nasal defects based on subunits and corrective surgeries [24], one study correlated previously described systems in their patients [37], one used a previously published classification system [46], one described trauma and surgical techniques [2], two referenced their own previously described classification system [21, 28], one was a questions and answers article [17], two articles focused on the external nasal deformities [15, 39], fourteen articles focused on operative techniques [4, 18–20, 29–32, 35, 36, 38, 40, 47, 50], and ten articles failed to meet criteria as classification systems [5, 7, 9–12, 14, 22, 34, 42]. A total of fifteen articles met inclusion criteria for describing internal nasal septal deviation classification systems [3, 6, 8, 16, 23, 25–27, 33, 41, 43, 44, 48, 51]. Figure 1 demonstrates the flow diagram for study selection.

3.2. Individual Study Results. Salihoglu et al. included 9,835 patients in their study evaluating the effect of nasal examination, including nasal septal deviations (graded as 1, 2, and 3 based on 33% increments), on nasal obstruction using the visual analog scale (VAS) [45]. In their study, they noted that nearly half of the patients had nasal septal deviations and of those about 60% were bilateral and 40% were unilateral [45]. Vidigal et al. used a nasal septal deviation classification based on the relationship of the nasal septum to the inferior turbinate [41]. Degree I: the deviation did not reach the inferior turbinate, degree II: the deviation reached the inferior turbinate, and degree III: the deviation reached the lateral wall and compressed the inferior turbinate [41]. Several authors reported classification systems that focus on common deviation patterns, including septal tilt, S-shaped deviation, and C-shaped deviations. Lawson in 1978 proposed a classification of the twisted nose into two basic types: the C shaped and S-shaped twist [51]. That study placed a focus on identifying skeletal asymmetries secondary to nasal bone fractures [51]. Guyuron et al. divided septal deviations into six classes to include C- and S-shaped deviations in the anteroposterior and cephalocaudal direction as well as localized deviation with nasal spur and septal tilt [16]. Cerkes classified nasal deviations into five categories to include caudal nasal septal deviations (classic septal tilt), anteroposterior C-shaped deviation, cephalocaudal C-shaped deviation, anteroposterior S-shaped deviation, and cephalocaudal S-shaped deviation [33]. Similar to Guyuron's and Cerke's classification system, Lee and Baker described S- and C-shaped deviations in the vertical and horizontal plane [43]. In this instance, Lee and Baker equated vertical direction to cephalocaudal direction and horizontal plane to anteroposterior [43]. Rohrich et al. classified internal nasal septal deviations based on three broad categories to include caudal septal deviations, concave dorsal deviations, and concave/convex dorsal deviations (S-shaped) [3]. The authors further divided

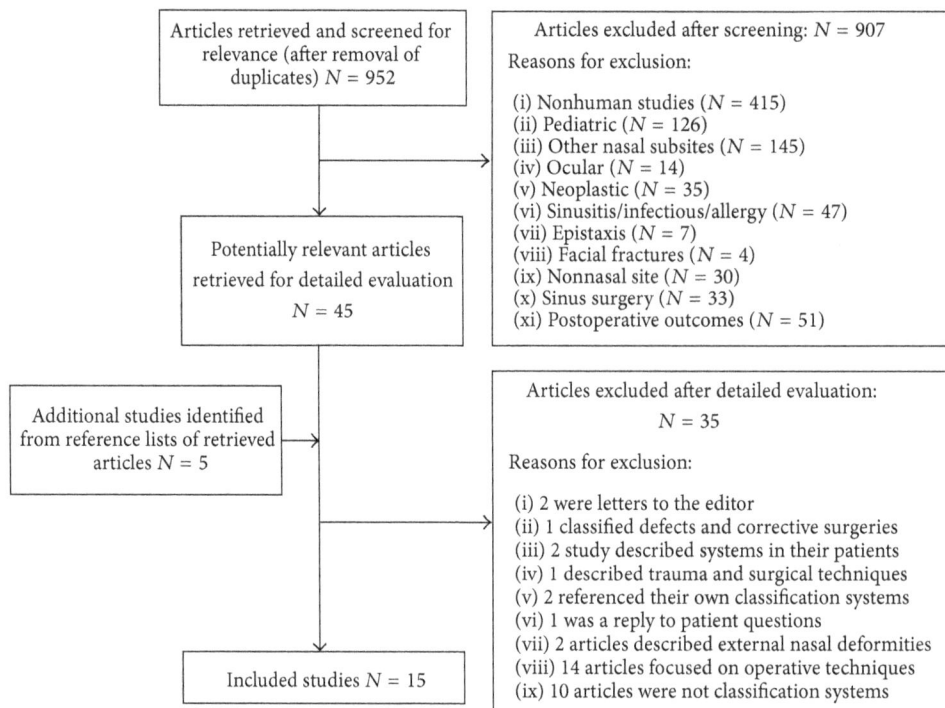

FIGURE 1: Flow diagram for the literature search and overall study selection.

caudal septal deviations and concave dorsal deformity into subtypes: straight septal tilt, concave deformity and S-shaped deformity for caudal septal deviation, and C-shaped dorsal deformity and reverse C-shaped dorsal deformity for concave dorsal deformity [3]. Parrilla et al. described corrective techniques for C- and S-shaped deformities and therefore by association recognized that these specific deformities exist, are reproducible, and require specific operative approach [4].

Rao et al. and Mladina used a similar classification system with a very precise description of the most common types of deviations seen in their practice [23, 27]. Mladina categorized the deviations into 7 types: Type 1: unilateral vertical septal ridge in the valve region that does not reach the valve itself, Type 2: unilateral vertical septal ridge in the valve region touching the nasal valve, Type 3: unilateral vertical ridge located more deeply in the nasal cavity, Type 4: S-shaped, Type 5: Almost horizontal septal spur, Type 6: massive unilateral bone spur, and Type 7: variation of these types [27]. Rao also classified septal deviations into 7 types: Type I: midline septum or mild deviations in vertical or horizontal plane, Type II: anterior vertical deviation, Type III: posterior vertical deviation, Type IV: S-septum, Type V: Horizontal spur on one side, Type VI: type V with a deep grove on the concave side, and Type VII: combination of II–VI [23].

I. Baumann and H. Baumann classified types of septal deviation into 6 types, where each type has several additional features: Type 1: septal crest, Type 2: cartilaginous deviated nose, Type 3: high septal crest deviation, Type 4: caudally inclined septum, Type 5: septal crest, and Type 6: caudally inclined septum [25]. Jin et al. followed a very similar format to Rao and Mladina by proposing four types of septal deviations: Type I: localized deviation including spur (spine), crest,

or caudal dislocation, Type II: curved/angulated deviation without localized deviation, Type III: curved/angulated deviation with localized deviation, and Type IV: curved/angulated deviation with associated external nasal deformity [26]. However, the authors further described septal deviation by including anatomic site as well as severity of septal deviation (mild, moderate, and severe) [26]. Sawhney and Sinha also emphasized the importance of classifying nasal septal deviation by the severity of deviation (marked, moderate, and mild) [8]. They integrated the following within the level of severity: cartilage and bony deflection, dislocation of septal cartilage, and level of deviation [8]. Buyukertan et al. divided the internal nasal septum into 10 segments: anterosuperior (AS), anteromedial (AM), anteroinferior (AI), mediosuperior (MS), mediomedia (MM), medioinferior (MI), posterosuperior (PS), posteromedial (PM), posteroinferior (PI), and caudal end (CE) of the septum nasi [48]. Lin et al. selected points on computed tomography imaging and analyzed them by computer software that compared contours of a deviated septum as compared to an ideal straight septum [44]. Points assessed included the perpendicular plate of the ethmoid bone and vomer bone junction, nasal spine, nasal bone, crista galli, and midpoint between the perpendicular plate-vomer junction and nasal spine [44]. Table 1 summarizes the various internal nasal septal deviation classification systems identified in this review, and Figures 2–7 demonstrate the combined internal classification systems.

4. Discussion

Septal deviations play a crucial role in functional nasal breathing. Unrecognized internal nasal septal deviations

TABLE 1: Studies meeting criteria for internal nasal septal deviation classification systems and a summary of the descriptions.

Author, year, location	Description of internal nasal septal deviation classification systems
Lin et al., 2014, USA [44]	Various points on computed tomography imaging which were analyzed by computer software that compared contours of a deviated septum as compared to an ideal straight septum. Points assessed included the perpendicular plate of the ethmoid bone and vomer bone junction, nasal spine, nasal bone, crista galli, and midpoint between the perpendicular plate-vomer junction and nasal spine.
Salihoglu et al., 2014, Turkey [45]	Grade 1: 0–33% deflection from midline toward lateral wall, Grade 2: 34–66% deflection from midline toward the lateral wall, and Grade 3: 67–100% deflection from the midline toward the lateral wall.
Vidigal et al., 2013, Italy [41]	Degree I: the deviation did not reach the lower nasal turbinate, Degree II: the deviation reached the lower nasal turbinate, and Degree III: the deviation reached the lateral wall and compressed the lower nasal turbinate.
Lee and Baker, 2013, USA [43]	Caudal septum is straight but deviated from the midline and is usually displaced from the maxillary crest, C-shaped septal deformity in the vertical plane, C-shaped septal deformity in the horizontal plane, S-shaped septal deformity in the horizontal plane, and S-shaped septal deformity in the vertical plane.
Reitzen et al., 2011, USA [6]	Tortuosity is measured at 4 defined points along the length of internal nasal septum. A ratio of the actual length of the septum (T) and the ideal length (I) is calculated as T/I.
Cerkes, 2011, Turkey [33]	Caudal septal deviation (septal tilt), anteroposterior C- and S-shaped deviation, and cephalocaudal C- and S-shaped deviations.
Jin et al., 2007, Korea [26]	Type I: localized deviation including spur (spine), crest, or caudal dislocation, Type II: curved/angulated deviation without localized deviation, Type III: curved/angulated deviation with localized deviation, and Type IV: curved/angulated deviation with associated external nasal deformity.
I. Baumann and H. Baumann, 2007, Germany [25]	Types based on primary deviation, each type has several additional features: Type 1: septal crest, Type 2: cartilaginous deviated nose, Type 3: high septal crest deviation, Type 4: caudally inclined septum, Type 5: septal crest, and Type 6: caudally inclined septum.
Rao et al., 2005, India [23]	Type I: midline septum or mild deviations in vertical or horizontal plane, Type II: anterior vertical deviation, Type III: posterior vertical deviation, Type IV: S-septum, Type V: horizontal spur on one side, Type VI: type V with a deep grove on the concave side, and Type VII: combination of II–VI.
Buyukertan et al., 2003, Turkey [48]	The septum is divided into 10 segments: anterosuperior (AS), anteromedial (AM), anteroinferior (AI), mediosuperior (MS), mediomedia (MM), medioinferior (MI), posterosuperior (PS), posteromedial (PM), posteroinferior (PI), and caudal end of the septum nasi (CE).
Rohrich et al., 2002, USA [3]	Caudal septal deviation (straight septal tilt, C-shaped, and S-shaped), concave dorsal deformity (C-shaped dorsal deformity and reverse C-shaped dorsal deformity), and concave/convex dorsal deformity (S-shaped).
Guyuron et al., 1999, USA [16]	C-shape anteroposterior deviation, C-shape cephalocaudal, S-shape anteroposterior, S-shape cephalocaudal, septal tilt deformity, and localized deviations or large spurs.
Mladina, 1987, Croatia [27]	Type 1: unilateral vertical septal ridge in the valve region that does not reach the valve itself, Type 2: unilateral vertical septal ridge in the valve region touching the nasal valve, Type 3: unilateral vertical ridge located more deeply in the nasal cavity, Type 4: S-shaped, Type 5: almost horizontal septal spur, Type 6: massive unilateral bone spur, and Type 7: variation.
Lawson, 1978, Canada [51]	C-shaped, S-shaped, and deviated nose, twisted nose, and skeletal asymmetry (depressed nasal fracture).
Sawhney and Sinha, 1964, India [8]	Grade deviations as mild, moderate, and marked (cannot see middle turbinate on side of the deviation). Cartilage and bony deflection, dislocation of septal cartilage, and level of deviation.

stand as the primary reason for failed rhinoplasty outcomes due to the pivotal role of the internal nasal septal deviation in migration and further deviation of nasal bones and lateral cartilage. Consequently, as many as 50% of cases of post-traumatic nasal deformity require subsequent revision rhinoplasty or septorhinoplasty [2, 4]. Parrilla et al. highlighted the importance in considering the anatomy behind the deviation and how preoperative nasal septal analysis guides the preoperative assessment and plan as well as operative technique,

reducing the risk of complication and repeat surgery which in themselves present with cumbersome challenges [4].

As stressed in the literature, identification of the C- and S-shaped deformities at the time of planning remains crucial to identifying potentially complex surgeries compared to less technically challenging operative interventions such as septal tilts [25, 43]. C- and S-shaped deformities are sometimes surgically scored on the convex side to silence the cartilaginous memory and frequently enhanced with grafting material

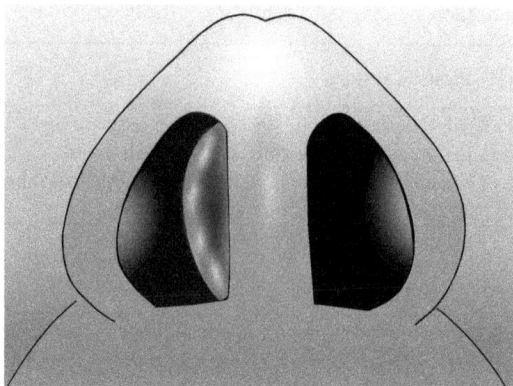

FIGURE 2: C-shaped nasal septal deviation in superoinferior dimension. Note: reverse C-shaped nasal septal deviation is the mirror image.

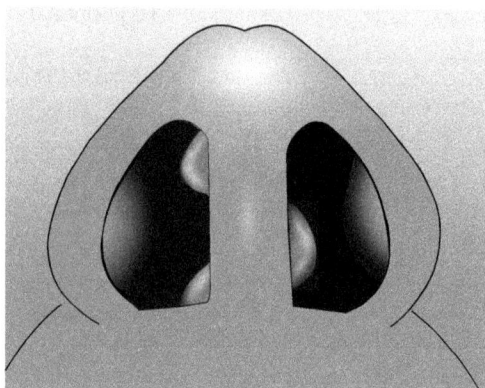

FIGURE 3: S-shaped nasal septal deviation in the superoinferior dimension. Note: reverse S-shaped nasal septal deviation is the mirror image.

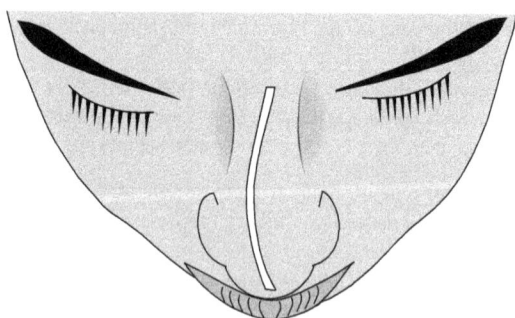

FIGURE 4: Internal and/or external nasal deviation in the anteroposterior dimension, C-shaped. Note: reverse C-shaped nasal septal deviation would be a mirror image.

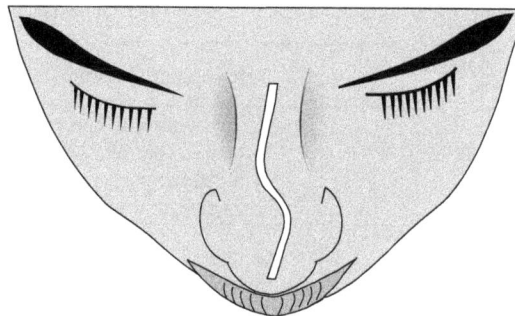

FIGURE 5: Internal and/or external nasal deviation in the anteroposterior dimension, S-shaped. Note: reverse S-shaped nasal septal deviation would be a mirror image.

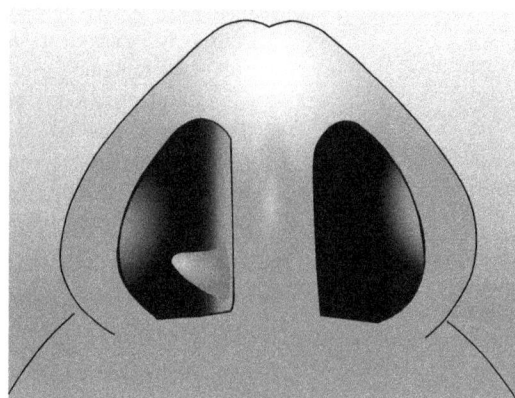

FIGURE 6: Outpouching (nasal septal spur).

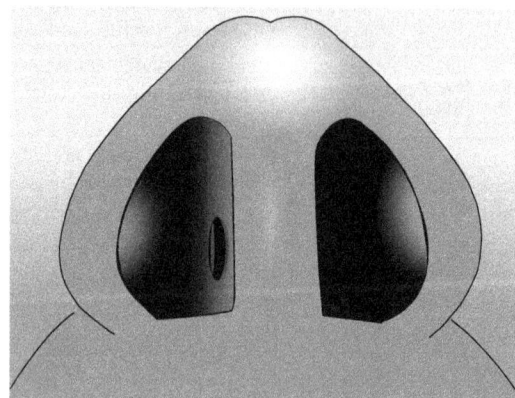

FIGURE 7: Open communication (nasal septal perforation).

to support and straighten the cartilaginous septum [3, 43]. Perforations also present with unique challenges, as the repair of a septal perforation usually necessitates bilateral elevation of the surrounding mucoperichondrium. While a unilateral perforation typically heals with no surgical intervention, bilateral opposing perforations can lead to permanent septal

perforation. Accurately identifying septal perforations further allows for appropriate preoperative planning including the need for grafting material versus flap.

Further, external nasal deformities and internal nasal septal deviations exist symbiotically. Accurately assessing these aspects and characteristics during the physical exam remains imperative to optimizing the assessment and preoperative planning process. Elicitation of a history of specific trauma and correlating the nuances of the injury with the specific findings on external exam and internal exam ensure accuracy of assessment. As pointed out by Cerkes, findings of antero-posterior C-shaped deviation correlate with an external deviation on the opposite side of the internal deviation while a cephalocaudal C-shaped deviation usually presents as a visible C-shaped external deformity [33]. Findings not consistent with such patterns should alert the clinician to other underlying forces that may be contributing to the noted deviation. Early identification of such forces and components allows for appropriate presurgical planning and therefore avoidance of surgical failure and further operative procedures. Evaluation of the external nose typically involves division of the nose into thirds with deviation of the upper third resulting from fractured nasal bones. Accurately identifying upper third deformities remains important, as correction of the septum alone typically fails to change the cosmetic appearance of the nose. Such deformities likely require osteotomies of the nasal bones for reapproximation and successful surgical management to improve the cosmetic appearance (i.e., rhinoplasty). However, the septum influences the middle and lower thirds of the nose to a greater degree with more emphasis on the latter. When imagining the biomechanics of the nose and septum, the quadrangular cartilage acts like a ridge board on a roof with the lateral cartilages functioning as the rafters. Consequently, an unstable quadrangular cartilage leads to unstable lateral cartilages contributing to external deformity or collapse. This analogy emphasizes the importance of assessing external deformity when evaluating the internal nasal septum.

Additionally, rhinomanometry and acoustic rhinometry evaluations reveal enhanced nasal resistance and diminished nasal volumes in patients with obstructive sleep apnea (OSA). Although a systematic review demonstrated that nasal findings have not been included in any of the 28 studies that used mathematical equations [52] to predict positive airway device treatment pressures (PAP pressures), it has been demonstrated in a meta-analysis that after nasal surgery (to include septoplasty) there is an associated decrease in PAP pressures and increased device use after septoplasty and/or additional nasal surgeries [53]. Vidigal et al. demonstrated that patients with OSA exhibit higher scores of nasal symptoms with higher frequency of complaints of nasal obstruction, nasal alterations, and inferior turbinate hypertrophy [41]. While acoustic rhinometric results appear statistically insignificant, the authors noted that rhinometric measurements fail to account for the dynamic changes of resistance, such as nasal cycling during wake and sleep [54]. Furthermore, acoustic rhinometry measurements demonstrated the greatest reproducible results in the first five centimeters (cm) of the nasal cavity, and as a result anterior deviations produce the greatest results while posterior deviations contribute little if anything to these measurements. To their credit, the authors of the study mentioned this discrepancy of failing to differentiate the deviations into posterior and anterior which likely affected their results [41]. As pointed out by Reitzen et al., turbinate hypertrophy as well as mucosal edema also appears to contribute to airflow resistance [6]. Preoperative identification of these contributing factors allows for categorization of additional areas of anatomical obstruction (inferior turbinate grades [55], nasal polyposis, etc.) and may demonstrate the

need for additional procedures such as bilateral inferior turbinoplasty, sinus surgery, or a rhinoplasty.

5. Conclusion

This systematic review ascertained that the majority of the currently published classification systems for internal nasal septal deviations can be summarized by C-shaped or reverse C-shaped, as well as S-shaped or reverse S-shaped, deviations in the anteroposterior and cephalocaudal dimensions. For imaging studies predefined points have been defined along the septum. Common terminology can facilitate future research.

Disclosure

The work was primarily performed at Tripler Army Medical Center, HI, USA.

References

[1] J. C. Hsia, M. Camacho, and R. Capasso, "Snoring exclusively during nasal breathing: a newly described respiratory pattern during sleep," *Sleep & Breathing*, vol. 18, no. 1, pp. 159–164, 2014.

[2] S. Higuera, E. I. Lee, P. Cole, L. H. Hollier Jr., and S. Stal, "Nasal trauma and the deviated nose," *Plastic and Reconstructive Surgery*, vol. 120, no. 7, pp. 64S–75S, 2007.

[3] R. J. Rohrich, J. P. Gunter, M. A. Deuber, and W. P. Adams Jr., "The deviated nose: optimizing results using a simplified classification and algorithmic approach," *Plastic and Reconstructive Surgery*, vol. 110, no. 6, pp. 1509–1523, 2002.

[4] C. Parrilla, A. Artuso, R. Gallus, J. Galli, and G. Paludetti, "The role of septal surgery in cosmetic rhinoplasty," *Acta Otorhinolaryngologica Italica*, vol. 33, no. 3, pp. 146–153, 2013.

[5] J. W. Lindahl, "The deviated nasal septum," *The Practitioner*, vol. 173, no. 1035, pp. 315–317, 1954.

[6] S. D. Reitzen, W. Chung, and A. R. Shah, "Nasal septal deviation in the pediatric and adult populations," *Ear, Nose and Throat Journal*, vol. 90, no. 3, pp. 112–115, 2011.

[7] A. G. Gibb, "Deviated nasal septum," *Nursing Times*, vol. 59, pp. 1569–1571, 1963.

[8] K. L. Sawhney and A. Sinha, "Diagnosis of deviated nasal septum," *Journal of the Oto-laryngological Society of Australia*, vol. 38, pp. 261–263, 1964.

[9] J. F. Birrell, "Nasal polypi and the deviated nasal septum," *The Practitioner*, vol. 205, no. 230, pp. 762–767, 1970.

[10] C. E. Iliades, "The deviated nasal septum indications for sub mucous resection," *Eye, Ear, Nose & Throat Monthly*, vol. 52, no. 4, pp. 136–140, 1973.

[11] K. Conrad, "Correction of crooked noses by external rhinoplasty," *The Journal of Otolaryngology*, vol. 7, no. 1, pp. 32–42, 1978.

[12] B. F. Jaffe, "Classification and management of anomalies of the nose," *Otolaryngologic Clinics of North America*, vol. 14, no. 4, pp. 989–1004, 1981.

[13] R. Bookman, "Deviated nasal septum as a diagnosis," *Annals of Allergy*, vol. 51, no. 4, pp. 465–466, 1983.

[14] R. G. Matschke and A. Fiebach, "Septum deviation and concomitant sinusitis," *HNO*, vol. 33, no. 12, pp. 541–544, 1985.

[15] D. A. F. Ellis and R. W. Gilbert, "Analysis and correction of the crooked nose," *The Journal of Otolaryngology*, vol. 20, no. 1, pp. 14–18, 1991.

[16] B. Guyuron, C. D. Uzzo, and H. Scull, "A practical classification of septonasal deviation and an effective guide to septal surgery," *Plastic and Reconstructive Surgery*, vol. 104, no. 7, pp. 2202–2209, 1999.

[17] "What's a deviated nasal septum? Does it need to be corrected?" *Mayo Clinic Health Letter*, vol. 18, no. 4, p. 8, 2000.

[18] D. G. Becker, "Septoplasty and turbinate surgery," *Aesthetic Surgery Journal*, vol. 23, no. 5, pp. 393–403, 2003.

[19] J. P. Gunter and R. J. Rohrich, "Management of the deviated nose. The importance of septal reconstruction," *Clinics in Plastic Surgery*, vol. 15, no. 1, pp. 43–55, 1988.

[20] H. S. Byrd, J. Salomon, and J. Flood, "Correction of the crooked nose," *Plastic and Reconstructive Surgery*, vol. 102, no. 6, pp. 2148–2157, 1998.

[21] B. Guyuron and R. A. Behmand, "Caudal nasal deviation," *Plastic and Reconstructive Surgery*, vol. 111, no. 7, pp. 2449–2457, 2003.

[22] E. Egeli, L. Demirci, B. Yazýcý, and U. Harputluoglu, "Evaluation of the inferior turbinate in patients with deviated nasal septum by using computed tomography," *Laryngoscope*, vol. 114, no. 1, pp. 113–117, 2004.

[23] J. J. Rao, E. C. V. Kumar, K. R. Babu, V. S. Chowdary, J. Singh, and S. V. Rangamani, "Classification of nasal septal deviations—relation to sinonasal pathology," *Indian Journal of Otolaryngology and Head and Neck Surgery*, vol. 57, no. 3, pp. 199–201, 2005.

[24] M. Bayramiçli, "A new classification system and an algorithm for the reconstruction of nasal defects," *Journal of Plastic, Reconstructive and Aesthetic Surgery*, vol. 59, no. 11, pp. 1222–1232, 2006.

[25] I. Baumann and H. Baumann, "A new classification of septal deviations," *Rhinology*, vol. 45, no. 3, pp. 220–223, 2007.

[26] H. R. Jin, J. Y. Lee, and W. J. Jung, "New description method and classification system for septal deviation," *Journal of Rhinology*, vol. 14, no. 1, pp. 27–31, 2007.

[27] R. Mladina, "The role of maxillar morphology in the development of pathological septal deformities," *Rhinology*, vol. 25, no. 3, pp. 199–205, 1987.

[28] R. Mladina, E. Čujić, M. Šubarić, and K. Vuković, "Nasal septal deformities in ear, nose, and throat patients: an international study," *American Journal of Otolaryngology: Head and Neck Medicine and Surgery*, vol. 29, no. 2, pp. 75–82, 2008.

[29] A. Seyhan, U. Ozaslan, E. Sir, and S. Ozden, "Three-dimensional modeling of nasal septal deviation," *Annals of Plastic Surgery*, vol. 60, no. 2, pp. 157–161, 2008.

[30] E. J. Dobratz and S. S. Park, "Septoplasty pearls," *Otolaryngologic Clinics of North America*, vol. 42, no. 3, pp. 527–537, 2009.

[31] J. Haack and I. D. Papel, "Caudal septal deviation," *Otolaryngologic Clinics of North America*, vol. 42, no. 3, pp. 427–436, 2009.

[32] H. M. T. Foda, "The crooked nose: correction of dorsal and caudal septal deviations," *HNO*, vol. 58, no. 9, pp. 899–906, 2010.

[33] N. Cerkes, "The crooked nose: principles of treatment," *Aesthetic Surgery Journal*, vol. 31, no. 2, pp. 241–257, 2011.

[34] A. Godoy, M. Ishii, P. J. Byrne, K. D. O. Boahene, C. O. Encarnacion, and L. E. Ishii, "The straight truth: measuring observer attention to the crooked nose," *Laryngoscope*, vol. 121, no. 5, pp. 937–941, 2011.

[35] T. Z. Shipchandler and I. D. Papel, "The crooked nose," *Facial Plastic Surgery*, vol. 27, no. 2, pp. 203–212, 2011.

[36] J. M. Sykes, J.-E. Kim, D. Shaye, and A. Boccieri, "The importance of the nasal septum in the deviated nose," *Facial Plastic Surgery*, vol. 27, no. 5, pp. 413–421, 2011.

[37] A. Sam, P. T. Deshmukh, C. Patil, S. Jain, and R. Patil, "Nasal septal deviation and external nasal deformity: a correlative study of 100 cases," *Indian Journal of Otolaryngology and Head and Neck Surgery*, vol. 64, no. 4, pp. 312–318, 2012.

[38] A. Boccieri, "The crooked nose," *Acta Otorhinolaryngologica Italica*, vol. 33, no. 3, pp. 163–168, 2013.

[39] Y. J. Jang, J. H. Wang, and B.-J. Lee, "Classification of the deviated nose and its treatment," *Archives of Otolaryngology—Head & Neck Surgery*, vol. 134, no. 3, pp. 311–315, 2008.

[40] G. S. Cho and Y. J. Jang, "Deviated nose correction: different outcomes according to the deviation type," *The Laryngoscope*, vol. 123, no. 5, pp. 1136–1142, 2013.

[41] T. D. A. Vidigal, F. L. M. Haddad, L. C. Gregório, D. Poyares, S. Tufik, and L. R. A. Bittencourt, "Subjective, anatomical, and functional nasal evaluation of patients with obstructive sleep apnea syndrome," *Sleep & Breathing*, vol. 17, no. 1, pp. 427–433, 2013.

[42] D. Karataş, F. Yüksel, M. Şentürk, and M. Dogan, "The contribution of computed tomography to nasal septoplasty," *The Journal of Craniofacial Surgery*, vol. 24, no. 5, pp. 1549–1551, 2013.

[43] J. W. Lee and S. R. Baker, "Correction of caudal septal deviation and deformity using nasal septal bone grafts," *JAMA Facial Plastic Surgery*, vol. 15, no. 2, pp. 96–100, 2013.

[44] J. K. Lin, F. C. Wheatley, J. Handwerker, N. J. Harris, and B. J. F. Wong, "Analyzing nasal septal deviations to develop a new classification system: a computed tomography study using MATLAB and OsiriX," *JAMA Facial Plastic Surgery*, vol. 16, no. 3, pp. 183–187, 2014.

[45] M. Salihoglu, E. Cekin, A. Altundag, and E. Cesmeci, "Examination versus subjective nasal obstruction in the evaluation of the nasal septal deviation," *Rhinology*, vol. 52, no. 2, pp. 122–126, 2014.

[46] S. Prasad, S. Varshney, S. S. Bist, S. Mishra, and N. Kabdwal, "Correlation study between nasal septal deviation and rhinosinusitis," *Indian Journal of Otolaryngology and Head and Neck Surgery*, vol. 65, no. 4, pp. 363–366, 2013.

[47] G. Francesconi and O. Fenili, "Treatment of deflection of the anterocaudal portion of the nasal septum," *Plastic and Reconstructive Surgery*, vol. 51, no. 3, pp. 342–345, 1973.

[48] M. Buyukertan, N. Keklikoglu, and G. Kokten, "A morphometric consideration of nasal septal deviations by people with paranasal complaints; a computed tomography study," *Rhinology*, vol. 41, no. 1, pp. 21–24, 2003.

[49] R. Mladina, "A morphometric consideration of nasal septal deviations by people with paranasal complaints; A computed tomography study," *Rhinology*, vol. 41, no. 4, pp. 255–255, 2003.

[50] M. H. Cottle, R. M. Loring, G. G. Fischer, and I. E. Gaynon, "The maxilla-premaxilla approach to extensive nasal septum surgery," *A.M.A. Archives of Otolaryngology*, vol. 68, no. 3, pp. 301–313, 1958.

[51] V. G. Lawson, "Management of the twisted nose," *The Journal of Otolaryngology*, vol. 7, no. 1, pp. 56–66, 1978.

[52] M. Camacho, M. Riaz, A. Tahoori, V. Certal, and C. A. Kushida, "Mathematical equations to predict positive airway pressures for obstructive sleep apnea: a systematic review," *Sleep Disorders*, vol. 2015, Article ID 293868, 11 pages, 2015.

[53] M. Camacho, M. Riaz, R. Capasso et al., "The effect of nasal surgery on continuous positive airway pressure device use and therapeutic treatment pressures: a systematic review and meta-analysis," *Sleep*, vol. 38, no. 2, pp. 279–286, 2015.

[54] A. Kimura, S. Chiba, R. Capasso et al., "Phase of nasal cycle during sleep tends to be associated with sleep stage," *The Laryngoscope*, vol. 123, no. 8, pp. 2050–2055, 2013.

[55] M. Camacho, S. Zaghi, V. Certal et al., "Inferior turbinate classification system, grades 1 to 4: development and validation study," *The Laryngoscope*, vol. 125, no. 2, pp. 296–302, 2015.

34

Plastic Surgery Inclusion in the Undergraduate Medical Curriculum: Perception, Challenges, and Career Choice—A Comparative Study

M. Farid,[1] R. Vaughan,[2] and S. Thomas[3]

[1]Department of Plastic and Reconstructive Surgery, The Royal London Hospital, Barts Health NHS, Whitechapel Road, London E1 1BB, UK
[2]Norwich Medical School, University of East Anglia, Chancellor Drive, Norwich NR4 7TJ, UK
[3]Department of Plastic and Reconstructive Surgery, University Hospital Birmingham NHS Foundation Trust, Queen Elizabeth Hospital Birmingham, Mindelsohn Way, Edgbaston, Birmingham, West Midlands B15 2GW, UK

Correspondence should be addressed to M. Farid; mohammed.farid@gmail.com

Academic Editor: Bishara Atiyeh

Objective. The undergraduate medical curriculum has been overcrowded with core learning outcomes with no formal exposure to plastic surgery. The aim of this study was to compare medical students from two educational settings for the basic understanding, preferred learning method, and factors influencing a career choice in plastic surgery. *Design and Setting.* A prospective cohort study based on a web-based anonymous questionnaire sent to final year medical students at Birmingham University (United Kingdom), McGill University (Canada), and a control group (non-medical staff). The questions were about plastic surgery: (1) source of information and basic understanding; (2) undergraduate curriculum inclusion and preferred learning methods; (3) factors influencing a career choice. A similar questionnaire was sent to non-medical staff (control group). The data was analysed based on categorical outcomes (Chi-square $\chi2$) and level of significance $p \leq 0.05$. *Results.* Questionnaire was analysed for 243 students (Birmingham, $n = 171/332$, 52%) (McGill $n = 72/132$, 54%). Birmingham students (14%) considered the word "plastic" synonymous with "cosmetic" more than McGill students (4%, $p < 0.025$). Teaching was the main source of knowledge for McGill students (39%, $p < 0.001$) while Birmingham students and control group chose the media (70%, $p < 0.001$). McGill students (67%) more than Birmingham (49%, $p < 0.010$) considered curriculum inclusion. The preferred learning method was lectures for McGill students (61%, $p < 0.01$) but an optional module for Birmingham (61%). A similar proportion (18%) from both student groups considered a career in plastic surgery. *Conclusions.* Medical students recognised the need for plastic surgery inclusion in the undergraduate curriculum. There was a difference for plastic surgery source of information, operations, and preferred method of learning for students. The study highlighted the urgent need to reform plastic surgery undergraduate teaching in collaboration with national educational bodies worldwide.

1. Introduction

There had been an overwhelming expansion in the core knowledge for medical subspecialities. This phenomenon led to the increased competition for plastic surgery inclusion in the undergraduate medical curriculum. The lack of educational opportunities for plastic surgery was noted with the clear decline in curriculum inclusion (13 out of 31 in 1986, 2 out of 34 in 2002) at undergraduate level in the United Kingdom (UK). Such exposure was imperative to help students make informed career decisions at an early stage about career choice [1–3]. Each medical student had unique reasons for pursuing a career in plastic surgery. The interaction with plastic surgeons was deemed the most influential factor while lifestyle and income were less important reasons for medical students [4].

Medical Students were not aware of the basic principles underpinning plastic surgery as a speciality. The complex dimension of "reconstructive" surgery had not been nurtured through medical education. This added to the misconception among public, medical students, and professionals due to the versatility of plastic surgery. Such image was worsened by the media negative role in labelling on plastic surgery as "cosmetic surgery" with rarely a reference to "reconstructive surgery." Nonetheless, future doctors should match patients' needs through awareness of the skills set offered by plastic surgeons [5]. The concern was public perception which equated plastic surgery with "cosmetic surgery" to be similar to students with no prior undergraduate teaching [6].

The tradition of teaching plastic surgery as an academic subject in the UK started during World War II by Sir Harold Gillies as "a fully fledged and desirable medical school subject for educating undergraduate students" [7]. This historical integration of plastic surgery continued to offer medical students a mixed skills set ranging from the key principles of wound healing to complex clinical scenarios in breast reconstruction, skin cancer, craniofacial anomalies, burns, lower limb trauma, and hand surgery. Nevertheless, neither the preferred learning methods for plastic surgery in the literature nor the reasons for a career choice had been investigated.

The construction of an educational model in plastic surgery was deemed crucial to be aligned with the undergraduate curriculum. The goals were to maximise exposure and help make informed career choices for those interested in pursuing a career in plastic surgery [8].

The main aim of this study was to investigate two different institutions (Birmingham, United Kingdom, and McGill, Canada) for knowledge, learning, and career factors for plastic surgery. It represented a landmark in comparing two unaffiliated universities for medical students underlying perception about plastic surgery.

2. Plastic Surgery Undergraduate Curriculum: Birmingham and McGill

Birmingham University had plastic surgery teaching predominantly incorporated within other surgical specialities. There was no formal teaching in the first two years. During the 4th year, there was an "optional" self-directed four-week clinical placement module. Throughout the 5th year (final year), plastic surgery teaching was in the form of a self-directed learning module without any clinical placement exposure for Birmingham medial students.

McGill University in Canada offered a more formal inclusion of plastic surgery in their curriculum with compulsory lectures and out-patients clinics in plastic surgery during the initial 2 years of medical studies. During 4th and 5th years, students were offered four clinical elective rotations lasting for 4 weeks each in plastic surgery. Overall, McGill students were more likely to be taught plastic surgery during their undergraduate studies compared to Birmingham students. The effect of the increased exposure to plastic surgery was explored in detail as part of this study.

3. Methods

3.1. Study Design. There was no academic affiliation between the two universities (McGill and Birmingham). The designed survey is based on the identification of integral aspects to plastic surgery teaching and career factors.

The permission to conduct the online survey (13 questions) was gained from both institutions. The questions were related to few parameters about plastic surgery (source of information and generic knowledge, operations, overlap with other specialities, preferred teaching method and clinical attachment period, and encouraging and discouraging factors for a career choice).

The survey was sent via a web-link (Survey Monkey) to final year medical students at Birmingham University (United Kingdom) and McGill University (Canada). There was a "control group" of non-medical administration staff at Queen Elizabeth University Hospital, Birmingham, United Kingdom. The selection was based on considering lay public views without prior medical knowledge or exposure. The exclusion criterion was based on failure to answer the entire survey questions by any student or control group staff.

The null hypothesis assumed no difference in the level of knowledge, method of learning, and career choice among students. All responses for the survey were analysed using SPSS* 15 software (Statistical Package for the Social Sciences). Statistical analysis was performed by a statistician using Chi-square ($\chi 2$) for categorical data and based on level of significance $p \leq 0.05$.

3.2. Study Aims. The study aimed to evaluate

(1) current understanding and source of plastic surgery knowledge;

(2) undergraduate curriculum inclusion and the preferred learning method;

(3) encouraging and discouraging factors for a career choice.

4. Results

A total of 243 students completed the questionnaire from both institutions (Birmingham = 171/332, McGill = 72/132), corresponding to 52% and 54%, respectively. The male : female ratio was (M : F 1 : 1.25) in Birmingham compared to (M : F 1.4 : 1) for McGill. The control group (non-medical staff) had 168 respondents (M : F 1 : 3) (Figure 1).

5. Birmingham versus McGill Students

5.1. Source of Information and Basic Knowledge in Plastic Surgery. Birmingham students mainly acquired their knowledge from the media (70%, $p < 0.001$) while McGill students had more formal teaching (39%, $p < 0.0001$) and exposure to clinical electives (13%, $p < 0.0001$). Friends were more a source of information for McGill (26%) than Birmingham students (16%, $p < 0.049$). The terms "plastic" and "cosmetic" surgery were viewed to be synonymous by

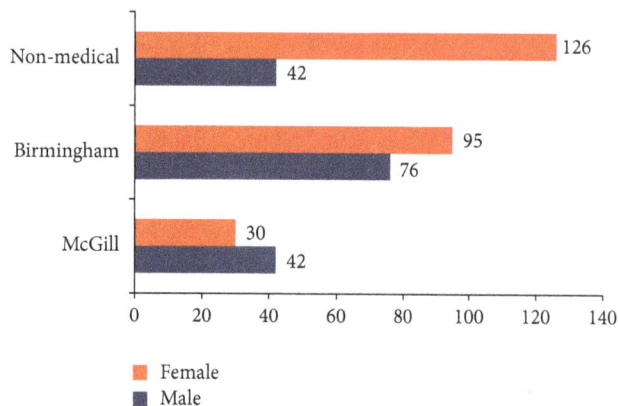

FIGURE 1: Gender distribution for medical students and non-medical staff.

only a small number of students at Birmingham (14%) and McGill (4%, $p < 0.025$). Plastic surgery did not have anatomical boundaries for a small number of students (McGill 1%, Birmingham 3%) and both groups were aware of the inclusion for emergency cases (McGill 99%, Birmingham 93%) (Tables 1(a) and 1(b)).

5.2. Operation Performed by Plastic Surgeons and Overlap with Surgical Specialties. Operations like facelift, abdominoplasty (tummy tuck), and breast augmentation (breast enlargement) were noticeably related to plastic surgery for both student groups. Skin lesions (McGill 7%, Birmingham 9%) and cleft palate (McGill 26%, Birmingham 21%) were the least linked to plastic surgery. More McGill students considered hand trauma (29%) exclusive to plastic surgeons compared to Birmingham students (12%, $p < 0.001$). A higher proportion of McGill (57%) compared to Birmingham (33%, $p < 0.001$) thought that breast reduction was solely performed by plastic surgeons (Table 1(c)). Although both groups (McGill and Birmingham) acknowledged an interspeciality overlap, it was the least for General surgery (69 & 59%) and most for maxillofacial surgery (93-94%) (Table 1(d)).

5.3. Curriculum Inclusion and Preferred Learning Method. McGill students (67%) expressed a stronger desire for plastic surgery inclusion in curriculum compared to Birmingham (49%, $p < 0.010$). The most popular learning methods were lectures (61%) and clinical placement (57%, $p < 0.001$) for McGill students, versus an optional module (61%) for Birmingham students. Both groups rated the optional module similarly (McGill 54%, Birmingham 61%) which ranked 3rd and 1st choice, respectively. Seminars and problem based learning had similar ratios (McGill 24%, Birmingham 26%). A research project was the least popular choice for both groups (McGill 11%, Birmingham 8%). The ideal module duration was 2 weeks (McGill 70%, Birmingham 77%) but the choice of 4 weeks had a lower response rate (McGill 31%, Birmingham 22%) (Tables 2(a) and 2(b)).

5.4. Factors Influencing a Career Choice in Plastic Surgery. A similar number of students considered plastic surgery for higher speciality training (McGill 18%, Birmingham 19%). The main encouraging factors for a career choice were specialised skills (McGill 85%, Birmingham 60%, $p < 0.0001$) and clinical diversity (McGill 61%, Birmingham 63%). Patient interaction rated 42% for Birmingham versus 28% for McGill ($p < 0.04$). Research was the least appealing factor for pursuing a plastic surgery career (McGill 15%, Birmingham 11%). Nearly two-thirds of both groups shared the lack of interest as a reason and over half the students were discouraged by the long training period and working hours. Working with other surgical specialists did not influence a career choice in plastic surgery (Tables 3(a) and 3(b)).

5.5. McGill and Birmingham Students Group versus Control Group

5.5.1. Source of Information and Basic Knowledge in Plastic Surgery. The main source of information was the media for the control group (85%, $p < 0.0001$) and Birmingham (70%) compared to McGill (31%). Friends were another common source of information for McGill (26%), Birmingham (16%), and control group (15%, $p < 0.0001$). Teaching and electives rated higher for McGill students compared to Birmingham ($p < 0.0001$) (Table 1(a)).

The control group perceived the term "cosmetic" to be synonymous with "plastic" (31%, $p < 0.001$) more than students (McGill 4%, Birmingham 14%). All 3 groups considered plastic surgery to have no anatomical boundaries (Control 7%, McGill 1%, and Birmingham 3%). Students (McGill 99%, Birmingham 93%) thought that plastic surgery involved emergency cases but a lower response for the control group (80%, $p < 0.0001$) (Table 1(b)).

The control group considered that 75% of medical students should apply for plastic surgery training while students had a significantly lower apply rate (McGill 18%, Birmingham 19%, $p < 0.001$) (Table 1(b)).

5.6. Operations Performed by Plastic Surgeons and Overlap with Surgical Specialities. Medical students (McGill 57%, Birmingham 61%) responses were higher than the control (46%, $p < 0.008$) for tummy tuck (abdominoplasty). A similar pattern was observed for facelift, cleft palate, hand trauma, skin lesions, and breast enlargement ($p < 0.01$). There was no significant difference ($p > 0.05$) for the 3 groups response to breast reduction and prominent ear procedures (Table 1(c)).

The students had a higher response for all subspeciality overlap compared to the control group ($p < 0.0001$). Trauma and orthopaedics, maxillofacial surgery, ENT, and dermatology were the top four overlapping surgical subspecialties choices for McGill and Birmingham students but had a consistently lower rating among control group ($p < 0.001$) (Table 1(d)).

All 3 groups preferred lectures, clinical placement, and an optional module as the top three learning methods. Lectures rated 61%, 38%, and 50% for McGill, Birmingham,

TABLE 1: Students' understanding of plastic surgery.

(a) Source of information for plastic surgery

Options	McGill % (n)	Birmingham % (n)	$\chi 2$, p value	Non-medical staff % (n)	$\chi 2$, p value
Elective	12.5 (9)	2.3 (4)	10.50, p < 0.001	7.74 (13)	NS
Media	30.55 (22)	69.59 (119)	30.41, p < 0.001	84.52 (142)	32.25, p < 0.0001
Teaching	38.89 (28)	17.54 (30)	13.06, p < 0.0001	3.57 (6)	31.12, p < 0.0001
Friends	26.39 (19)	15.79 (27)	3.87, p < 0.049	14.88 (25)	29.95, p < 0.0001

(b) Generic knowledge of plastic surgery

Question	McGill % (n)	Birmingham % (n)	$\chi 2$, p value	Non-medical staff % (n)	$\chi 2$, p value
Is the name "plastic" the same as "cosmetic"?	4.17 (3)	14.04 (24)	4.99, p < 0.025	30.95 (52)	25.18, p < 0.0001
Is plastic surgery limited to a specific part of the body?	1.4 (1)	2.92 (5)	NS	6.55 (11)	NS
Do plastic surgeons deal with emergency cases?	98.61 (71)	92.98 (159)	NS	79.76 (134)	21.739, p < 0.0001
Should plastic surgery be included in the undergraduate curriculum?	66.67 (48)	48.54 (83)	6.70, p < 0.010	70.83 (119)	11.94, p < 0.001
Is it appropriate to offer cosmetic surgery operations under the National Health Service?	40.27 (29)	56.14 (96)	5.10, p < 0.024	69.05 (118)	14.70, p < 0.001
Would you/students consider applying for plastic surgery training?	18.06 (13)	18.71 (32)	NS	75.00 (126)	130.43, p < 0.0001

(c) Operations performed by plastic surgeons only

Options	McGill % (n)	Birmingham % (n)	$\chi 2$, p value	Non-medical staff % (n)	$\chi 2$, p value
Prominent ear	37.5 (27)	43.86 (75)	NS	43.86 (73)	NS
Tummy tuck	56.94 (41)	60.82 (104)	NS	46.43 (78)	7.02, p < 0.008
Cleft palate	26.39 (19)	21.05 (36)	NS	38.69 (65)	12.39, p < 0.0001
Hand trauma	29.17 (21)	12.28 (21)	10.10, p < 0.001	28.57 (48)	7.4, p < 0.007
Facelift	72.22 (52)	76.02 (130)	NS	60.71 (102)	9.36, p < 0.002
Skin lesions	6.94 (5)	8.77(15)	NS	28.57 (48)	29.76, p < 0.0001
Breast Enlargement	70.83 (51)	60.23 (103)	NS	51.79 (87)	5.5, p < 0.019
Breast reduction	56.94 (41)	33.33 (57)	11.74, p < 0.001	41.66 (70)	NS

(d) Surgical specialties overlap with plastic surgery

Options	McGill % (n)	Birmingham % (n)	$\chi 2$, p value	Non-medical staff % (n)	$\chi 2$, p value
Trauma and orthopaedics	88.89 (64)	87.13 (149)	NS	69.64 (117)	20.36, p < 0.0001
Vascular	69.44 (50)	62.57 (107)	NS	23.21(39)	68.23, p < 0.0001
General surgery	69.44 (50)	59.65 (102)	NS	43.06 (72)	15.53, p < 0.0001
Dermatology	88.89 (64)	88.3 (151)	NS	55.36 (93)	58.02, p < 0.0001
Ear, nose, throat (ENT)	93.06 (67)	80.7 (138)	5.86, p < 0.015	56.55 (95)	38.98, p < 0.0001
Maxillofacial	91.67 (66)	94.74 (162)	NS	79.17 (133)	19.97, p < 0.0001

and control group, respectively. Clinical placement (64%) was the 1st choice for control group ($p < 0.001$), 2nd for McGill (57%), and 3rd for Birmingham (37%, $p < 0.0001$). A research project was the least favourable choice in all three groups, with a higher response for control group (27%, $p < 0.0001$) versus students (McGill 11%, Birmingham 8%) (Table 2(a)).

The control group (71%, $p < 0.001$) and students (McGill 67%, Birmingham 49%) shared the view that plastic surgery should be taught in the undergraduate curriculum. A clinical rotation for 5-6 weeks was the appropriate learning duration for control group (62%, $p < 0.0001$) but students opted for 2-week placement (McGill 69%, Birmingham 77%) (Table 2(b)).

5.7. Factors Influencing a Career Choice in Plastic Surgery. The most encouraging factor for a career in plastic surgery was specialised skills for the control group (78%, $p < 0.01$)

TABLE 2: Undergraduate plastic surgery teaching.

(a) Method for plastic surgery teaching

Options	McGill % (*n*)	Birmingham % (*n*)	χ^2, *p* value	Non-medical staff % (*n*)	χ^2, *p* value
Seminars	23.61 (17)	25.73 (44)	NS	40.48 (68)	*10.91, p < 0.001*
Clinical attachment	56.94 (41)	36.84 (63)	*8.363, p < 0.004*	64.29 (108)	*18.36, p < 0.0001*
Lectures	61.11 (44)	38.01 (65)	*10.93, p < 0.001*	50 (84)	NS
Problem based learning	15.72 (11)	13.45 (23)	NS	36.9 (62)	*29.13, p < 0.0001*
Research project	11.11 (8)	8.12 (14)	NS	27.38 (46)	*42.41, p < 0.0001*
Optional module	54.17 (39)	61.4 (105)	NS	42.86 (72)	NS

(b) Duration for an optional module in plastic surgery

Weeks	McGill % (*n*)	Birmingham % (*n*)	χ^2, *p* value	Non-medical staff % (*n*)	χ^2, *p* value
0–2	69.44 (50)	76.74 (132)	NS	7.14 (12)	*182.96, p < 0.0001*
3-4	30.56 (22)	21.64 (37)	NS	30.36 (51)	NS
5-6	0%	1.17 (2)	NS	61.9 (104)	*193.63, p < 0.0001*

TABLE 3: Career choice in plastic surgery.

(a) Encouraging factors for a career in plastic surgery

Options	McGill % (*n*)	Birmingham % (*n*)	χ^2, *p* value	Non-medical staff % (*n*)	χ^2, *p* value
Patient interaction	27.78 (20)	42.11 (72)	*4.42, p < 0.036*	42.26 (71)	NS
Clinical diversity	61.11 (44)	63.16 (108)	NS	34.52 (58)	*31.23, p < 0.0001*
Research	15.28 (11)	11.69 (20)	NS	22.62 (38)	NS
Specialised skills	84.72 (61)	59.64 (102)	*14.42, p < 0.0001*	77.98 (131)	*5.79, p < 0.016*

(b) Discouraging factors for a career in plastic surgery

Options	McGill % (*n*)	Birmingham % (*n*)	χ^2, *p* value	Non-medical staff % (*n*)	χ^2, *p* value
Long working hours	45.83 (33)	52.05 (89)	NS	32.14 (54)	*13.27, p < 0.0001*
Lack of interest	68.06 (49)	64.32 (110)	NS	67.26 (113)	NS
Long training	54.17 (39)	59.65 (102)	NS	38.1 (64)	*15.78, p < 0.0001*
Working with other specialists	1.40 (1)	2.34 (4)	NS	4.17 (7)	NS

Note. NS = not significant, *p* > 0.05.

and McGill students (85%). Clinical diversity was more popular for students (McGill 61%, Birmingham 63%) than the control group (35%, *p* < 0.001). Patient interaction was similar at 42% for both the control group and Birmingham compared to 28% for McGill (*p* < 0.0001). Research was the least encouraging factor among students (McGill 15%, Birmingham 12%) and control (23%) as a career incentive (Table 3(a)).

The discouraging factors were long working hours (32%) and long training (16%) for the control group (*p* < 0.001) with a higher response in Birmingham (52%, 60%) and McGill (46%, 54%), respectively. Working with other specialists was the least discouraging factor for the control group, McGill and Birmingham (4%, 1%, and 2%, resp.). Two-thirds of all 3 groups considered the lack of interest in plastic surgery as the most discouraging factor (Table 3(b)).

6. Discussion

The main aim of this study was to determine the perception of medical students of plastic surgery, undergraduate curriculum inclusion, and influencing career choice. Students' prior clinical exposure, knowledge, and educational needs formed the basis for responses.

6.1. Source of Information and Basic Knowledge in Plastic Surgery. The name plastic originated from the Greek *"plastikos"* or Latin *"plasticus,"* meaning to mould. Nevertheless, the meaning of the word had been misunderstood by medical students. More Birmingham students than McGill considered the term "plastic" and "cosmetic" to have a similar meaning. The concerning fact that the knowledge about plastic surgery for students was predominantly from the media shared similar views to non-medical staff. This was echoed by Hamilton III et al. (2004) who revealed that medical students gained plastic surgery knowledge in equal proportion from the media and formal medical school teaching. On the other hand, McGill students had formal teaching and clinical electives throughout undergraduate years and a third of their intake did a plastic surgery rotation in their final year. This explained the significantly lower response for media as a source of information for this group [9–11].

Cosmetic surgery was perceived to be technically less challenging, associated with less operative risk, a shorter recovery, and less postoperative pain compared to "plastic or reconstructive" surgery. Reid and Malone (2008) reiterated that the media had a tendency to misrepresent cosmetic surgery as plastic or reconstructive surgery because the term "cosmetic" was considered synonymous to "plastic" or "reconstructive" surgery [12].

The funding of cosmetic surgery by the national health system was considered acceptable by non-medical staff more than Birmingham or McGill students. This fact reflected on the different understanding for the meaning of cosmetic surgery. The issue of funding remains a matter of political contention due to the financial challenges to meet patients' clinical needs [13, 14].

6.2. Operations Performed by Plastic Surgeons and Overlap with Surgical Specialties.

The scope of surgical operations performed solely by plastic surgeons had not been determined in-depth in terms of students' perception. A relevant study by Agarwal et al. (2014) reported the poor understanding of medical students about the role of plastic surgeons for hand surgery. As part of the study, a list of operations was included to whether performed solely by plastic surgeons. Face lifts, tummy tucks, and breast enhancement were recorded as the top three operations for all three groups while skin lesions, hand trauma, and cleft surgery were the bottom three operations. There had been no limit to the range of plastic surgery operations and the extent of pathological breadth from the crown of the head to the sole of the foot. Hence, the expected overlap with different surgical subspecialties was highlighted in the 3 groups response. Maxillofacial surgery ranked the highest for Birmingham and control group versus ENT for McGill. Vascular surgery ranked the least for the control. Medical students were more aware of emergency cases in plastic surgery than the control group. This trend supported Agarwal et al. (2013) who concluded the need to improve medical students' education about the scope of plastic surgery [9, 15–17]. It seemed apparent that students showed better awareness of the overlap with other specialties than control group. Another pattern was noted for the type of operations performed by plastic surgeons. Breast enhancement was one of the top choices for all groups while breast reduction ranked lower for Birmingham students and control group compared to McGill. This difference highlighted the in-depth differing perception between students groups due to the underlying level of teaching and exposure to plastic surgery.

The scope of undergraduate teaching, curriculum inclusion, and preferred method of plastic surgery teaching was supported by students and control group. Nevertheless, there was a variable difference for these parameters among students and control group. Seminars were more valued among the control than students. A research project was the least popular teaching method for students and ranked last for control group. Lectures and clinical placement were more popular among McGill and noncontrol group compared to Birmingham. All these modalities in terms of didactic lectures, electives, and clinical rotations can be supported

with career workshops, open days, and e-learning modules [10]. Nonetheless, this should be tailored and explored with students during early undergraduate years prior to deciding the range of teaching methods. The teaching could be targeted through subspeciality areas like burns, head and neck, skin and breast cancer, trauma, congenital anomalies, and their reconstruction. These are often linked to many "charities" that medical students can join earlier in their medical journey for long term mutual benefit.

An optional module was one of the top choices for all 3 groups but the interesting aspect was that the preferred duration was 2 weeks for students compared to 6 weeks for the control. It reflected on students understanding of the challenges in curriculum to accommodate a longer rotation and the lack of sufficient hospital allocations for continually increased student intake [18, 19]. Regardless of the clinical rotation period, the exposure to a plastic surgery ward would give medical students the opportunity to observe a range of pathologies including lumps, ulcers, pressure sores, lymphadenopathy, head and neck masses, burns, and soft tissue injuries. This knowledge is deemed essential for today's doctors to appreciate the scope of plastic surgery.

6.3. Factors Influencing a Career Choice.

The students showed a similar response for a career in plastic surgery. One of the potential factors would be a varied possible personal preference to other specialities. This was an unusual finding considering that McGill students have more exposure and teaching for the speciality. Mahalingam et al. (2014) reported that increased plastic surgery exposure during undergraduate studies correlated with a career choice [20]. We further investigated the influencing factors to choose plastic surgery as a career. Specialised skills seemed a commonly favourable encouraging factor for all 3 groups. Research was the least popular reason for a career choice. This theme should be considered by educators to meet students' needs as it also meets public opinion. Similarly, a lack of interest was most discouraging factor for a career choice in all 3 groups. Long training and lengthy working hours were less appealing for students than the control group. Previous work by Ek et al. (2005) reiterated that the increasing desire of medical students to maintain a healthy work-life balance had reduced the choice of surgery as a career. May et al., 2005, also reported that this was associated with a better sense of career satisfaction. The perception of a better lifestyle associated with cosmetic private practice was a motivating factor among student in previous research. Working with other specialties did not discourage students or the public reflecting the awareness for team work in present day medicine [21–23]. All groups were unified in research being the most discouraging reason for a career in plastic surgery. The latter fact was striking as research had been deemed key to a surgical career choice and progression. Students preferred to pursue a career without undertaking research who put more value on clinical diversity and skills.

The phenomenon regarding why students made such choices can be underlined by exploring their medical curriculum. McGill University encouraged student participation in plastic surgery in all academic years which was endorsed by the Canadian postgraduate training scheme. Students at McGill were better informed through enhanced teaching and clinical placements to make a career choice earlier. On the other hand, the structure of medical training in the UK might influence Birmingham students' choice. Wade et al. (2009) reported that most plastic surgeons (67%) in the United Kingdom chose their career during postgraduate training. It strengthens the rationale that exposure to plastic surgery further helps such choice which is likely to be in postgraduate period in the UK. Other researchers like Sutton et al. (2014) reported a recent shift in the United Kingdom that a similar percentage of medical students (65%) were choosing their specialty earlier at undergraduate medical studies. Hence, the lack of exposure to plastic surgery at the undergraduate level was deemed a disadvantage for those interested in such choice [24–26].

In terms of gender variation, surgical specialities may not be popular among female students possibly due to lack of interest and work-life balance. Few strategies can be implemented to encourage higher enrolment among this group. Role models, mentoring, a positive clinical posting, and early exposure to career fairs and taster days positively influenced female trainees to choose a surgical career. There is a current trend over recent years that more female trainees are encouraged to choose surgery as a career in the future. This has been endorsed by the Royal Colleges and national higher surgical training scheme [27–30].

The strengths of this project were multifaceted and aimed to raise global awareness about plastic surgery teaching and career choice. There has been no previous research comparing two educational settings for their underlying knowledge in relation to curriculum exposure. Previous literature highlighted the issue for the lack of teaching in plastic surgery but failed to determine a causal link to curriculum or career factors. The two institutions were not affiliated in any academic setting so there is no bias in this research. The study was validated by comparing the student group to non-medical staff to strengthen the finding for curriculum comparison and career choice. It highlighted the need for a more formal introduction of plastic surgery teaching at an early stage for medical students. Nevertheless, few weaknesses were inherent to the nature of any survey based cohort study. The response rate was over 50% for students at both institutions and deemed acceptable. The authors did not think that a higher response would achieve considerably a variable outcome but may strengthen the study findings. This statement is supported by the clear statistical difference for obtained results. Another weakness was the study represented a snapshot for final year students at two institutions. Further research should be considered worldwide for a greater in-depth understanding for the variable patterns in teaching and career choice. This would be truly important for countries with a considerable practice in plastic surgery and more public awareness (e.g., Brazil, Korea, and USA) [31, 32]. Furthermore, our study determined the public opinion for the United Kingdom only. It would be more valuable to collect data from Canadian public even though the aim was not to compare public views.

The study also determined the need for medical schools, surgeons, and students to work in close partnership to deliver the best plastic surgery education. A good example of such partnership was "The Medical Student Learning Centre," a web-based project aimed at teaching plastic surgery delivered by the Dalhousie Faculty of Medicine, Division of Plastic and Reconstructive Surgery, Halifax, Canada [33]. This method ensured a diverse learning experience within the limited time in the undergraduate curriculum and set an example for future learning. The emphasis for this platform was on providing both formal and self-directed undergraduate teaching in plastic surgery. Another suggestion from this study would be to integrate plastic surgery with other curriculum components. This crucial step was initiated by the Canadian Carnegie Foundation (2004) with recommendations for the advancement of teaching in undergraduate medical education. It emphasised the need to standardise learning outcomes, integrate formal knowledge with clinical experience, and focus on progression of professional identity [34–39].

7. Conclusions

This study was a snapshot of medical students' perception and teaching of plastic surgery in the United Kingdom and Canada. Students at both medical schools had a different level of understanding about plastic surgery and factors for career choice which was reflected by their undergraduate medical curriculum.

Educational and regulatory organisations exemplified by the Royal College of Surgeons in both countries, the British Association of Plastic & Reconstructive Surgeons (BAPRAS), and the Canadian Society of Plastic Surgeons need to introduce and monitor formal plastic surgery teaching at the undergraduate level within the curriculum. These organisations should liaise with key educators including the Deans of medical schools and government institutions to facilitate this process.

Acknowledgments

The exceptional role model and a real inspiration is Professor Bruce Williams, Chief of Plastic Surgery Division, McGill University. No words would describe the author's sincere appreciation for his encouragement with this project and pursuing a career path in plastic surgery. The statistical analysis was assisted by Mr. Gavin Rudge, a research fellow in the Department of Public Health, Epidemiology and Biostatics, University of Birmingham.

References

[1] A. R. Rowsell, "The place of plastic surgery in the undergraduate surgical curriculum," *British Journal of Plastic Surgery*, vol. 39, no. 2, pp. 241–243, 1986.

[2] R. Denadai and C. Raposo-Amaral, "Undergraduate plastic surgery education: problems, challenges, and proposals," *Ann Med Health Sci Res.*, vol. 4, supplement 3, pp. 169-170, 2014.

[3] C. R. Davis, J. M. O'Donoghue, J. McPhail, and A. R. Green, "How to improve plastic surgery knowledge, skills and career interest in undergraduates in one day," *Journal of Plastic, Reconstructive and Aesthetic Surgery*, vol. 63, no. 10, pp. 1677–1681, 2010.

[4] R. G. Wade, M. A. Moses, and J. Henderson, "Teaching plastic surgery to undergraduates," *Journal of Plastic, Reconstructive and Aesthetic Surgery*, vol. 62, article 267, no. 2, 2009.

[5] C. S. J. Dunkin, J. M. Pleat, S. A. M. Jones, and T. E. E. Goodacre, "Perception and reality—a study of public and professional perceptions of plastic surgery," *British Journal of Plastic Surgery*, vol. 56, no. 5, pp. 437–443, 2003.

[6] C. De Blacam, D. Kilmartin, C. Mc Dermott, and J. Kelly, "Public perception of plastic surgery," *Journal of Plastic, Reconstructive and Aesthetic Surgery*, vol. 68, no. 2, pp. 197–204, 2015.

[7] A. Bamji, "Sir Harold Gillies: surgical pioneer," *Trauma*, vol. 8, no. 3, pp. 143–156, 2006.

[8] A. K. Greene and J. W. May Jr., "Applying to plastic surgery residency: factors associated with medical student career choice," *Plastic and Reconstructive Surgery*, vol. 121, no. 3, pp. 1049–1054, 2008.

[9] J. P. Agarwal, S. D. Mendenhall, and P. N. Hopkins, "Medical student perceptions of plastic surgeons as hand surgery specialists," *Ann Plast Surg.*, vol. 72, no. 1, pp. 89–93, 2014.

[10] Y. Al-Nuaimi, G. McGrouther, and A. Bayat, "Modernising medical careers in the UK and plastic surgery as a possible career choice: undergraduate opinions," *Journal of Plastic, Reconstructive and Aesthetic Surgery*, vol. 59, no. 12, pp. 1472–1474, 2006.

[11] G. S. Hamilton III, J. S. Carrithers, and L. H. Karnell, "Public perception of the terms 'cosmetic,' 'plastic,' and 'reconstructive' surgery," *Archives of Facial Plastic Surgery*, vol. 6, no. 5, pp. 315–320, 2004.

[12] A. J. Reid and P. S. Malone, "Plastic surgery in the press," *J Plast Reconstr Aesthet Surg*, vol. 61, no. 8, pp. 866–869, 2008.

[13] "Professional Standards for Cosmetic Practice," Royal College of Surgeons, England, UK, 2013, https://www.rcseng.ac.uk/standards-and-research/standards-and-guidance/service-standards/cosmetic-surgery/professional-standards-for-cosmetic-surgery/.

[14] "Review of the Regulation of Cosmetic Interventions," Department of Health, England, UK, 2016, https://www.gov.uk/government/publications/review-of-the-regulation-of-cosmetic-interventions.

[15] A. Burd, T. Chiu, and C. McNaught, "Plastic surgery in the undergraduate curriculum: the importance of considering students' perceptions," *British Journal of Plastic Surgery*, vol. 57, no. 8, pp. 773–779, 2004.

[16] J. P. Agarwal, S. D. Mendenhall, L. A. Moran, and P. N. Hopkins, "Medical student perceptions of the scope of plastic and reconstructive surgery," *Ann Plast Surg.*, vol. 70, no. 3, pp. 343–349, 2013.

[17] R. B. Berggren, "Role of the plastic surgeon in undergraduate medical education," *Plastic and Reconstructive Surgery*, vol. 50, no. 1, pp. 75-76, 1972.

[18] A. Jain and J. Nanchahal, "Research options for plastic surgical trainees," *British Journal of Plastic Surgery*, vol. 55, no. 5, pp. 427–429, 2002.

[19] R. Geoffrion, J. W. Choi, and G. M. Lentz, "Training surgical residents: The current Canadian perspective," *Journal of Surgical Education*, vol. 68, no. 6, pp. 547–559, 2011.

[20] S. Mahalingam, P. Kalia, A. Nagendran, and P. Oakeshott, "Undergraduate exposure to plastic surgery: the medical student perspective," *Journal of Plastic, Reconstructive and Aesthetic Surgery*, vol. 67, no. 5, pp. e125-e126, 2014.

[21] E. R. Dorsey, D. Jarjoura, and G. W. Rutecki, "The influence of controllable lifestyle and sex on the specialty choices of graduating U.S. medical students, 1996–2003," *Academic Medicine*, vol. 80, no. 9, pp. 791–796, 2005.

[22] T. Maiorova, F. Stevens, A. Scherpbier, and J. Van Der Zee, "The impact of clerkships on students' specialty preferences: what do undergraduates learn for their profession?" *Medical Education*, vol. 42, no. 6, pp. 554–562, 2008.

[23] E. W. Ek, E. T. Ek, and S. D. Mackay, "Undergraduate experience of surgical teaching and its influence on career choice," *ANZ Journal of Surgery*, vol. 75, no. 8, pp. 713–718, 2005.

[24] N. T. Mabvuure, J. Rodrigues, S. Klimach, and C. Nduka, "A cross-sectional study of the presence of United Kingdom (UK) plastic surgeons on social media," *Journal of Plastic, Reconstructive and Aesthetic Surgery*, vol. 67, no. 3, pp. 362–367, 2014.

[25] P. A. Sutton, J. Mason, D. Vimalachandran, and S. McNally, "Attitudes, motivators, and barriers to a career in surgery: a national study of uk undergraduate medical students," *Journal of Surgical Education*, vol. 71, no. 5, pp. 662–667, 2014.

[26] R. G. Wade, E. L. Clarke, S. Leinster, and A. Figus, "Plastic surgery in the undergraduate curriculum: a nationwide survey of students, senior lecturers and consultant plastic surgeons in the UK," *Journal of Plastic, Reconstructive and Aesthetic Surgery*, vol. 66, no. 6, pp. 878–880, 2013.

[27] D. C. Marshall, J. D. Salciccioli, S.-J. Walton, J. Pitkin, J. Shalhoub, and G. Malietzis, "Medical student experience in surgery influences their career choices: a systematic review of the literature," *Journal of Surgical Education*, vol. 72, no. 3, pp. 438–445, 2015.

[28] "Women in Surgery," Royal College of Surgeons, England, UK, 2016, https://www.rcseng.ac.uk/careers-in-surgery/women-in-surgery/.

[29] H. A. Sanfey, A. R. Saalwachter-Schulman, J. M. Nyhof-Young, B. Eidelson, and B. D. Mann, "Influences on medical student career choice: gender or generation?" *Archives of Surgery*, vol. 141, no. 11, pp. 1086–1094, 2006.

[30] M. S. Patel, D. S. Mowlds, B. Khalsa, J. E. Foe-Parker, A. Rama, and F. Jafari, "Early intervention to promote medical student interest in surgery and the surgical subspecialties," *J Surg Educ.*, vol. 70, no. 1, pp. 81–86, 2013.

[31] "The British Association of Aesthetic Plastic Surgeons—Annual Audit," 2014, http://baaps.org.uk/about-us/audit/2040-auto-generate-from-title.

[32] The International Society of Aesthetic Plastic Surgery (ISAPS), "International Survey on Aesthetic/Cosmetic Procedures," 2014, http://www.isaps.org/Media/Default/global-statistics/2015%20ISAPS%20Results.pdf.

[33] Dalhousie Faculty of Medicine, Division of Plastic and Reconstructive Surgery, Halifax, Canada, 2016, https://medicine.dal.ca/departments/department-sites/surgery/divisions/plastic-reconstructive-surgery/education/undergraduate.html.

[34] A. Au and J. B. Kim, "Integration of plastic surgery into the undergraduate medical curriculum: the Norwich model and experience," *Int J Med Educ.*, vol. 3, pp. 14–16, 2012.

[35] N. Bremner, M. Davies, and S. Waterston, "Experience of plastic surgery as an undergraduate—vital for the future of the specialty!," *Journal of Plastic, Reconstructive and Aesthetic Surgery*, vol. 61, no. 2, pp. 235-236, 2008.

[36] M. J. Goldacre, L. Laxton, E. M. Harrison, J. M. J. Richards, T. W. Lambert, and R. W. Parks, "Early career choices and successful career progression in surgery in the UK: prospective cohort studies," *BMC Surgery*, vol. 2, article 32, no. 10, 2010.

[37] M. Khatib, B. Soukup, O. Boughton, K. Amin, C. R. Davis, and D. M. Evans, "Plastic surgery undergraduate training: how a single local event can inspire and educate medical students," *Annals of Plastic Surgery*, vol. 75, no. 2, pp. 208–212, 2015.

[38] K. Walsh, "Plastic surgery in the curriculum," *J Plast Reconstr Aesthet Surg.*, vol. 67, no. 7, pp. 1015-1016, 2014.

[39] D. Irby, "Educating physicians for the future: carnegie's calls for reform," *Medical Teacher*, vol. 33, no. 7, pp. 547–550, 2011.

35

A Comparison of Barbed Sutures and Standard Sutures with regard to Wound Cosmesis in Panniculectomy and Reduction Mammoplasty Patients

Kristen Aliano,[1] **Michael Trostler,**[2] **Indira Michelle Fromm,**[2] **Alexander Dagum,**[2] **Sami Khan,**[2] **and Duc Bui**[2]

[1]*Department of Plastic Surgery, University of Texas Medical Branch, Galveston, TX, USA*
[2]*Department of Plastic Surgery, Stony Brook University Hospital, Stony Brook, NY, USA*

Correspondence should be addressed to Michael Trostler; michael.trostler@stonybrookmedicine.edu

Academic Editor: Nicolo Scuderi

Cosmesis is a vital concern for patients undergoing plastic and reconstructive surgery. Many variations in wound closure are employed when attempting to minimize a surgical scar's appearance. Barbed sutures are one potential method of achieving improved wound cosmesis and are more common in recent years. To determine if barbed sutures differ from nonbarbed in wound cosmesis, we conducted a single-blinded, randomized, controlled trial of 18 patients undergoing bilateral reduction mammoplasty or panniculectomy. Patients were their own controls, receiving barbed sutures on one side and standard sutures on the contralateral side. Surgical scars were evaluated postoperatively by patient preference self-assessment and an observer. Ten patients were evaluated at 3 months postoperatively, yielding a mean Stony Brook Scar Evaluation Scale (SBSES) rating of 4.4 for barbed suture and 3.5 for regular suture ($p = 0.15$). At 6 months, 8 patients performed self-assessment to determine their preference; 4 preferred the barbed sutures, 1 preferred the regular sutures, and 3 had no preference. Further research with larger sample sizes is needed to determine if barbed sutures convey any advantage over standard sutures in wound healing. However, our results suggest that barbed sutures are a reasonable alternative to standard sutures particularly with regard to wound cosmesis.

1. Introduction

For patients who undergo plastic and reconstructive surgery, the appearance of surgical scars is an important consideration. Particularly, in the realm of aesthetic surgery, patients want scars that are easily camouflaged, have minimal hypertrophy and hyper- or hypopigmentation, and are not irregular in contour. Selecting an appropriate method of wound closure is consequently of paramount importance to surgeons, who seek to optimize postoperative scar appearance while minimizing surgical complications. To achieve these goals, surgeons employ a wide variety of options for wound closure, including topical adhesives, absorbable staples, and at least 5,269 types of sutures [1]. Barbed sutures present one such option, differing from most types of standard (smooth, nonbarbed) sutures in their ability to anchor tissues without the use of knots. Whereas the use of standard sutures is thought to increase risk of tissue ischemia due to increased tension at individual suture loops, the use of barbed sutures distributes tension across the length of a wound [2, 3]. By reducing mechanical stress on the skin, particularly at the wound edges, barbed sutures may potentially result in improved scar cosmesis. Prospective studies comparing the use of standard sutures and barbed sutures suggest that complication rates between the two are not significantly different or that the complications are lower in procedures involving barbed sutures [4–6]. Additionally, the use of barbed sutures may decrease operative times, in turn decreasing operative costs and increasing surgical efficiency.

Both unidirectional and bidirectional barbed sutures are available, including the unidirectional V-Loc™ (Covidien) and the bidirectional Quill™ (Angiotech). Bidirectional barbed sutures differ from unidirectional in that they have needles on both ends; the direction of the barbs changes

TABLE 1: Patient demographics.

Demographics	
	N (%)
Age (years)	38 (range 20–59)
Gender	
Female	18 (100)
Procedures	
Panniculectomy	5 (27.8)
Reduction mammoplasty	10 (55.6)
Unknown/incomplete chart	3 (16.7)
Race	
White	11 (61.1)
Black/African American	2 (11.1)
Hispanic	1 (5.6)
Unknown/not recorded	4 (22.2)

TABLE 2: SBSES, Stony Brook Scar Evaluation Scale [10].

	Scar category	Points
Width	>2 mm	0
	≤2 mm	1
Height	Elevated/depressed in relation to surrounding skin	0
	Flat	1
Color	Darker than surrounding skin	0
	Same color or lighter than surrounding skin	1
Hatch marks/suture marks	Present	0
	Absent	1
Overall appearance	Poor	0
	Good	1

at the midpoint of the suture [7]. Bidirectional barbed sutures have not been studied previously in panniculectomy patients, although there have been studies using them in abdominoplasty patients [8, 9]. The use of unidirectional barbed sutures in reduction mammoplasty patients has been previously reported in a study involving multiple types of procedures [5]. We performed a prospective matched-pairs study comparing postoperative scar cosmesis, complication profiles, and operative time for incisions closed with barbed sutures and incisions closed with standard sutures.

2. Methods

Over a period of 18 months, patients undergoing bilateral reduction mammoplasty or panniculectomy were recruited from the practice of two plastic surgeons. A total of 27 patients were initially enrolled in the study, all of whom were female, with 18 patients completing at least one follow-up visit with survey and scar evaluation. Panniculectomy was performed in 5 patients, with bilateral mammoplasty performed in the remaining 13 patients. Demographic data was collected and is shown in Table 1. Inclusion criteria were age >18 years old and patients undergoing panniculectomy or bilateral reduction mammoplasty. Exclusion criteria were age <18 years old, unilateral procedure, or no follow-up visits. To allow patients to act as their own controls, each reduction mammoplasty patient was randomized to have barbed sutures used on either the right or the left breast; standard sutures were used on the contralateral breast. Panniculectomy patients were randomized to have barbed sutures used on either the right or left half of the surgical incision; standard sutures were used on the contralateral side. Bidirectional Quill™ sutures were used for incisions closed with barbed sutures; monocryl or vicryl sutures were used for incisions closed with standard sutures. All patients were blinded as to which type of suture was used on which breast or incision half. Intraoperative details by type of suture, including incision length and time to achieve closure, were recorded. At one week postoperatively, patients were

evaluated for complications. At 3-, 6-, and 12-month follow-up visits, patients rated their scars' overall appearances using a visual analog scale. At the time of these follow-ups, an observer also evaluated the patients' scars using the Stony Brook Scar Evaluation Scale (SBSES) which can be seen in Table 2 [10]. This observer was meant to be blinded to the side as well but had access to the patient charts and could potentially check which side had barbed and nonbarbed sutures. Statistical comparison of standard and barbed sutures was performed using dependent t-tests for paired samples, and ANOVA testing was used to compare across time points. This study was reviewed and approved by the IRB and informed consent was obtained from all subjects.

3. Results

The length of the incision closed by each type of suture was recorded for 11 patients with mean incision length not statistically different between groups: 26.6 cm for standard and 26 cm barbed sutures ($p = 0.24$). The amount of time to close each incision was recorded for 14 patients. Mean time to achieve closure significantly differed by type of suture used: 36.3 minutes for standard sutures and 24.4 minutes for barbed sutures ($p = 0.003$). Complications from the procedures and results of the follow-up evaluations are shown in Table 3.

At 1 week postoperatively, 11 patients' incision sites were evaluated for complications. One adverse event was recorded for incisions closed with each type of suture. One bilateral mammoplasty patient reported nipple numbness and bruising on the breast closed with barbed sutures, while another bilateral mammoplasty patient was found to have 3 cm vertical dehiscence of the breast closed with standard sutures.

At 3 months postoperatively, a nonblinded observer used SBSES to rate the appearance of 10 patients' scars on a scale of 0 to 5. Observer evaluation yielded a mean rating of 4.4 for barbed sutures and 3.5 for standard sutures, but this was not statistically significant ($p = 0.15$). Additionally, the patients performed a self-assessment of their scars, with 6 patients preferring side closed with barbed sutures, 1 patient slightly preferring the standard sutures, and 3 patients expressing no

TABLE 3: Complications and patient evaluation (SBSES, Stony Brook Scar Evaluation Score).

	Barbed	Nonbarbed	p value
1 week	Nipple numbness and ecchymosis	3 cm vertical dehiscence	
Time to suture (minutes)	24.4	36.3	0.003
SES			
3 months	4.4	3.5	0.15
6 months	3.75	3.125	0.44
12 months	4.75	4.25	0.39
Total across time	4.23	3.5	*0.08*
Patient preference			0.19
3 months	6 (60)	1 (10)	
6 months	4 (50)	1 (12.5)	
12 months	1 (25)	2 (50)	
ANOVA testing between different time points	$p = 0.34$	$p = 0.5$	

preference. The patient who slightly preferred the standard suture was also the patient who experienced nipple numbness in the side with barbed suture.

At 6 months postoperatively, a nonblinded observer again rated the appearance of 8 patients' scars, which was not statistically significant, with a mean rating of 3.75 for barbed sutures and 3.13 for standard sutures ($p = 0.44$). The patients self-assessed their scars, with 4 patients preferring the incision closed with barbed sutures, 1 patient with slight preference for the incision closed with standard sutures, and 3 patients expressing no preference. Two of the 3 patients with no current preference had no preference previously, and the 1 patient with slight preference for standard previously reported no preference.

At 12 months postoperatively, a nonblinded observer recorded a final rating for the appearance of 4 patients' scars, yielding a mean rating of 4.75 for barbed sutures and 4.25 for nonbarbed sutures ($p = 0.39$). On self-assessment 1 patient preferred the barbed sutures, 2 patients preferred standard sutures, and 1 patient expressed no preference. Only one of the patients in the 12-month group had follow-up at all time points and preferred the Quill suture at each point. One of the two patients who preferred standard suture was also the patient who had nipple numbness on the barbed suture side at the initial follow-up visit. The one patient who expressed no preference had previously expressed no preference.

When attempting to compare the SBSES across the time points for the barbed suture group, it was found on ANOVA test that there was no statistically significant difference between the 3-, 6-, and 12-month time points: 4.4, 3.75, and 4.75, respectively ($p = 0.34$). When comparing the nonbarbed suture groups with ANOVA testing at 3-, 6-, and 12-month time points, 3.5, 3.13, and 4.25, respectively, there was similarly no statistically significant difference ($p = 0.5$).

4. Discussion

A previous study of barbed suture closure of the Pfannenstiel incision in 188 patients suggests that scar cosmesis in wounds closed with Quill™ sutures is comparable to that of wounds closed with standard sutures [6]. Scar cosmesis in wounds closed with unidirectional barbed sutures is also comparable or superior to that of standard sutures in studies involving blinded evaluators [4, 11]. The results of our study similarly suggest that, at 3, 6, and 12 months postoperatively, there is no significant difference in mean cosmesis scores between wounds closed with barbed sutures and wounds closed with standard sutures. However, the possibility of scoring bias in our study cannot be discounted as the observer who assigned scar cosmesis scores was not blinded as to which type of suture was used on each side. Of additional note, at least 5 scar evaluation scales, including the scale used in this study, are available to clinicians/researchers, and it has been suggested that these scales are more suited to assess change in an individual than between individuals [12]. The existence of multiple scar scales also may complicate comparison of results between studies that use different scales.

To our knowledge, this is the first study of scar cosmesis in wounds closed with barbed sutures in which patients were asked to evaluate their own scars. At 3 months postoperatively, 10 patients evaluated their scars, of which 9 preferred the barbed suture closure or had no preference. Likewise, at 6 months postoperatively, 8 patients evaluated their scars, of which 7 preferred the barbed suture closure or had no preference. Patients did appear to show a slight preference for the standard suture closure at 12 months postoperatively; however, the small size with only 4 patients with follow-up records at this time lacks the power to make a definitive statement. Two of the four patients at the 12-month time point had not been previously evaluated. While our sample sizes at each stage are too small to be statistically significant or to adequately power the study, these results anecdotally suggest that patient satisfaction is no worse for barbed suture closure than for standard suture closure as scar maturation proceeds. It is also important to note that in contrast to the outside evaluator who assigned scar cosmesis scores, patients were blinded as to which sutures were used on which side, thereby minimizing bias.

Despite the shortcomings of a small sample size, complication profiles for both types of sutures used in this study appeared comparable. Two patients in this study experienced postoperative complications, including one instance of wound dehiscence in an incision closed with standard sutures and one instance of nipple numbness and ecchymosis in an incision closed with barbed sutures. Tissue ischemia may result in wounds closed with standard sutures, as the knots necessary for closure cause unequal distribution of tension. This is important to note as pressure-induced ischemia and necrosis are major contributors to wound dehiscence [6]; however, due to the small sample size of this study and the low overall complication rate, it is not possible to determine whether wound dehiscence was prevented by the use of barbed sutures. Conversely, several retrospective reviews have reported complication rates that were significantly higher among wounds closed with barbed sutures [13, 14]. This conflict in clinical opinion indicates that additional research with a larger patient base is necessary to discern whether complications from incisions closed with barbed sutures differ significantly from standard sutures.

An important consideration for any surgical procedure is the duration, as shorter procedure times may be more cost-effective due to decreased operating room fees, anesthesia charges, and time the patient spends under general anesthesia. In our study, the use of barbed sutures decreased the time to closure over that of standard sutures by 32.8% (24.4 minutes versus 36.3 minutes, $p = 0.003$). In a 2011 study, Jandali and colleagues reported that use of barbed sutures decreased the duration of unilateral breast reconstruction by 50 minutes, although there was no significant difference in the duration of bilateral breast reconstruction [13]. According to their cost analysis, despite the increased cost of barbed sutures over standard sutures, a 50-minute decrease in operative time would save a total of $7600 in operating room and anesthesia charges. Studies of abdominal closure in deep inferior epigastric perforator (DIEP) flap breast reconstruction and donor site quilting in latissimus dorsi flap breast reconstruction found no significant differences in operating times [15, 16]. Moreover, it is important to note that although our results show a significant difference in incision closure times, this difference may not correspond to shorter operative times overall. Additional research is necessary to determine whether the use of barbed sutures actually significantly decreases operative time and, consequently, operating costs.

Major limitations of this study are the small population size, the lack of blinding by the scar evaluator, and the incomplete follow-up by the patients for all time points and completion of the surveys. Future directions would include expanding the procedures done with barbed sutures and including a large population size to increase the power of the study.

5. Conclusion

It is advantageous for surgeons to have multiple options for wound closure, to allow for complex closure situations, to reduce the risk of postoperative complications, and to maximize patient satisfaction with the appearance of their surgical scars. The results of this study suggest that barbed sutures provide a reasonable alternative to standard sutures, with similar complication rates, shorter operative times, and comparable cosmetic outcomes. However, further investigation is needed to assess the validity of these results.

Competing Interests

The authors declare that there is no conflict of interests regarding the publication of this paper.

References

[1] J. Hochberg, K. M. Meyer, and M. D. Marion, "Suture choice and other methods of skin closure," *The Surgical Clinics of North America*, vol. 89, no. 3, pp. 627–641, 2009.

[2] M. D. Paul, "Bidirectional barbed sutures for wound closure: evolution and applications," *The Journal of the American College of Certified Wound Specialists*, vol. 1, no. 2, pp. 51–57, 2009.

[3] J. A. Greenberg, "The use of barbed sutures in obstetrics and gynecology," *Reviews in Obstetrics & Gynecology*, vol. 3, pp. 82–91, 2010.

[4] V. Grigoryants and A. Baroni, "Effectiveness of wound closure with V-Loc 90 sutures in lipoabdominoplasty patients," *Aesthetic Surgery Journal*, vol. 33, no. 1, pp. 97–101, 2013.

[5] J. P. Rubin, J. P. Hunstad, A. Polynice et al., "A multicenter randomized controlled trial comparing absorbable barbed sutures versus conventional absorbable sutures for dermal closure in open surgical procedures," *Aesthetic Surgery Journal*, vol. 34, no. 2, pp. 272–283, 2014.

[6] A. P. Murtha, A. L. Kaplan, M. J. Paglia, B. B. Mills, M. L. Feldstein, and G. L. Ruff, "Evaluation of a novel technique for wound closure using a barbed suture," *Plastic and Reconstructive Surgery*, vol. 117, no. 6, pp. 1769–1780, 2006.

[7] G. Ruff, "Technique and uses for absorbable barbed sutures," *Aesthetic Surgery Journal*, vol. 26, no. 5, pp. 620–628, 2006.

[8] J. P. Warner and K. A. Gutowski, "Abdominoplasty with progressive tension closure using a barbed suture technique," *Aesthetic Surgery Journal*, vol. 29, no. 3, pp. 221–225, 2009.

[9] A. D. Rosen, "Use of absorbable running barbed suture and progressive tension technique in abdominoplasty: a novel approach," *Plastic and Reconstructive Surgery*, vol. 125, no. 3, pp. 1024–1027, 2010.

[10] A. J. Singer, B. Arora, A. Dagum, S. Valentine, and J. E. Hollander, "Development and validation of a novel scar evaluation scale," *Plastic and Reconstructive Surgery*, vol. 120, no. 7, pp. 1892–1897, 2007.

[11] S. Koide, N. R. Smoll, J. Liew et al., "A randomized 'N-of-1' single blinded clinical trial of barbed dermal sutures vs. smooth sutures in elective plastic surgery shows differences in scar appearance two-years post-operatively," *Journal of Plastic, Reconstructive & Aesthetic Surgery*, vol. 68, no. 7, pp. 1003–1009, 2015.

[12] R. Fearmonti, J. Bond, D. Erdmann, and H. Levinson, "A review of scar scales and scar measuring devices," *Eplasty*, vol. 10, article e43, 2010.

[13] S. Jandali, J. A. Nelson, M. R. Bergey, S. S. Sonnad, and J. M. Serletti, "Evaluating the use of a barbed suture for skin closure during autologous breast reconstruction," *Journal of Reconstructive Microsurgery*, vol. 27, no. 5, pp. 277–286, 2011.

[14] R. Cortez, E. Lazcano, T. Miller et al., "Barbed sutures and wound complications in plastic surgery: an analysis of outcomes," *Aesthetic Surgery Journal*, vol. 35, no. 2, pp. 178–188, 2015.

[15] C. de Blacam, S. Colakoglu, A. O. Momoh, S. J. Lin, A. M. Tobias, and B. T. Lee, "Early experience with barbed sutures for abdominal closure in deep inferior epigastric perforator flap breast reconstruction," *Eplasty*, vol. 12, article e24, 2012.

[16] D. K. Thekkinkattil, T. Hussain, T. K. Mahapatra, P. L. McManus, and P. J. Kneeshaw, "Feasibility of use of a barbed suture (V-Loc 180) for quilting the donor site in latissimus dorsi myocutaneous flap breast reconstruction," *Archives of Plastic Surgery*, vol. 40, no. 2, pp. 117–122, 2013.

36

Single Stage Nipple-Sparing Mastectomy and Reduction Mastopexy in the Ptotic Breast

M. E. Pontell (iD),[1] **N. Saad,**[2] **A. Brown,**[3] **M. Rose,**[4] **R. Ashinoff,**[4] **and A. Saad**[4]

[1]*Department of Surgery, Drexel University College of Medicine, Philadelphia, PA, USA*
[2]*Department of Surgery, University of Maryland, Baltimore, MD, USA*
[3]*Department of Breast Surgery, Cancer Care Institute, Egg Harbor Township, NJ, USA*
[4]*The Plastic Surgery Center, The Institute for Advanced Reconstruction, Egg Harbor Township, NJ, USA*

Correspondence should be addressed to M. E. Pontell; matthewpontellmd@gmail.com

Academic Editor: Nicolò Scuderi

Purpose. Given the proposed increased risk of nipple-areolar complex (NAC) necrosis, nipple-sparing mastectomy (NSM) is generally not recommended for patients with large or significantly ptotic breasts. NAC preserving strategies in this subgroup include staged or simultaneous NSM and reduction mastopexy. We present a novel approach towards simultaneous NSM and reduction mastopexy in patients with large, ptotic breasts. *Methods.* Literature pertaining to NSM for women with large, ptotic breasts was reviewed and a surgical approach was designed to allow for simultaneous NSM and reduction mastopexy in such patients. *Results.* Eight patients underwent bilateral NSM with simultaneous reduction mammaplasty and immediate reconstruction. The majority of breasts demonstrated advanced ptosis (69% grade III, 31% grade II) and the average breast volume excised was 760 grams. In those patients without a history of smoking, NAC necrosis rates were 0%. In those patients with a history of smoking, 83% of breasts experienced NAC necrosis (60% total, 40% partial). One hundred percent of patients who smoked experienced some degree of NAC necrosis. Among breasts with grade II versus grade III ptosis, NAC necrosis rates were roughly equal. *Conclusions.* Historically, patients with large, ptotic breasts were excluded from NSM due to the proposed increased risk of NAC necrosis. This study demonstrates a safe approach towards NSM and reduction mastopexy using an inferior, wide-based, epithelialized pedicle. While all patients eventually achieved satisfactory results, there was an association between smoking and NAC necrosis. Smoking cessation is paramount to the operation's success.

1. Introduction

Nipple-sparing mastectomy (NSM) is a contemporary derivative of subcutaneous mastectomy (SCM), which was originally performed for fibrocystic disease of the breast [1, 2]. NSM is an increasingly popular alternative to skin-sparing mastectomy (SSM), as it allows for preservation of the nipple-areolar complex (NAC) [1, 3, 4]. With proper patient selection, NSM can be used in both the prophylactic and the therapeutic settings [1, 4–6]. Regardless of the indication, the central tenets of NSM are to remove the glandular breast tissue while maximizing structural preservation of the breast and adhering to oncologic standards [1, 3]. The trend towards the development of more advanced NSM modifications is driven by patient demand and an increasing amount of literature documenting its therapeutic success [7].

From an oncologic perspective, NSM is reserved for patients with tumors that do not involve the skin, are less than three centimeters in diameter, and are at least two centimeters away from the NAC [4, 8]. This procedure is a safe option for the treatment of breast carcinoma, and tumor recurrence rates are low [4, 5, 8–10]. Patients with excessively large and/or ptotic breasts or clinically palpable locoregional lymphadenopathy are generally excluded from therapeutic NSM [4, 8]. From a prophylactic standpoint, bilateral mastectomy remains a point of controversy and some surgeons do advocate for its use in high-risk patients who have a strong genetic predisposition towards developing

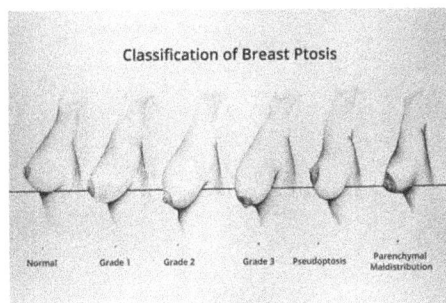

FIGURE 1: Artist's depiction of the breast ptosis grading system proposed by Regnault et al. *Normal*: areola above the inframammary fold (IMF) and above the gland contour; *Grade I*: areola at the IMF and above the gland contour; *Grade II*: areola below the IMF and above the gland contour; *Grade III*: areola below the IMF and below the gland contour; *Pseudoptosis*: areola at the IMF with glandular ptosis; *Parenchymal Maldistribution*: areola at the IMF with loose, hypoplastic glandular skin.

breast cancer [10, 11]. On the other hand, contralateral prophylactic mastectomy (CPM) for risk reduction in patients with primary breast cancer is well supported [10, 11]. For appropriately selected patients, prophylactic mastectomy can reduce the risk of developing breast cancer by 80–95%, even in the presence of a retained NAC [4, 5, 10, 12]. As such, NSM is an important option in the prevention and treatment of breast cancer [12]. Additionally, NAC preservation has a positive impact on patient satisfaction [13, 14].

Nevertheless, the ability to perform a NSM can be restricted by patient anatomic factors. The procedure is generally not recommended for patients with breast volume exceeding 500 grams or grade II or III ptosis given the proposed increased risk of NAC necrosis (Figure 1) [4, 8]. Potential strategies for this patient subgroup include staged NSM and reduction mastopexy or NSM with simultaneous reduction mastopexy [1, 10, 13, 15–21]. Here, we present an alternate way to perform a simultaneous NSM and reduction mastopexy with breast reconstruction for females with large, ptotic breasts. This technique may provide a suitable option for such women who seek NAC preservation and wish to avoid multiple operations. Additionally, implant-based reconstruction may obviate a longer procedure for those who cannot tolerate a free-flap transposition.

2. Methods

A review of the literature was conducted on all cases of NSM and reduction mastopexy for women with large-volume, ptotic breasts. Based on the results, a modified surgical approach was created, designed to allow for simultaneous NSM and reduction mastopexy for women with high-grade ptosis and large-volume breasts. This study was conducted under the approval of the institutional review board of AtlantiCare Medical Center. All of the NSMs were performed by a single breast surgeon (AB) and the reconstructive procedures were performed by one, or occasionally two, of the plastic surgeons (AS, RA, and MR).

All mastectomies were nipple-sparing and were performed simultaneously with a reduction mammaplasty. Eight patients were included in this study, for a total of sixteen mastectomies (n = 16). Inclusion criteria consisted of patients with grade II or III breast ptosis who were candidates for prophylactic (five patients, ten breasts) or therapeutic (three patients, six breasts) NSM. After NSM and simultaneous reduction mammaplasty, patients underwent immediate placement of tissue expanders or reconstruction by deep inferior epigastric perforator (DIEP) flaps. In the tissue expander group, implants were inserted during the second-stage procedure. Additional minor revisions were made as necessary.

Data collection included patient demographics, preoperative indications, and active comorbid conditions at the time of surgery. All technical data, perioperative complications, and revision procedures were recorded and patients were followed up until all wounds had healed.

2.1. Surgical Technique. Nipple-sparing mastectomy with this technique involved a supra-areolar incision with lateral and medial extensions (Figure 2). Retroareolar breast tissue was sent for frozen section to rule out carcinoma involvement of the NAC and thin mastectomy flaps were raised superiorly and inferiorly with the NAC being thus carried on a broad, inferior-based epithelialized dermal pedicle. A variable amount of skin above the supra-areolar incision was excised in a pattern akin to a boomerang, with the width of the boomerang adjusted based upon how much lift was needed to bring the NAC into a more normal anatomic position. After raising the skin flaps up to the level of the clavicle superiorly, the inframammary fold inferiorly, the sternal border medially, and the anterior edge of the latissimus muscle laterally, the breast tissue was sharply dissected off of the pectoralis major muscle.

At this point, if expanders were used, the pectoralis major muscle was lifted off of the chest wall sharply to allow for a submuscular pocket to cover the superior and superior-medial portions of the expander. Various acellular-dermal matrix (ADM) products were utilized to create the inferior and inferolateral coverage over the expander. Expander size was chosen based upon base width of the native breast and other chest-wall measurements. The ADM was sutured into place along the inframammary fold, the lower border of the pectoralis muscle, and the lateral chest wall with 2-0 Vicryl sutures. The expander was placed and a drain was placed below the skin but above the expander pocket. All expanders were partially inflated with sterile saline and the SPY Intraoperative Perfusion Assessment System (distributed in North America by LifeCell Corp., Branchburg, NJ; manufactured by Novadaq Technologies Inc., Richmond, British Columbia, Canada) was used at this point to confirm NAC and mastectomy flap viability. Closure consisted of two layers of 3-0 and 4-0 monocryl followed by Dermabond.

If a DIEP flap was used, then a two-team approach was used with one team member dissecting out the recipient vessels in the chest while a second team member was raising and dissecting out the DIEP flap on the abdominal wall.

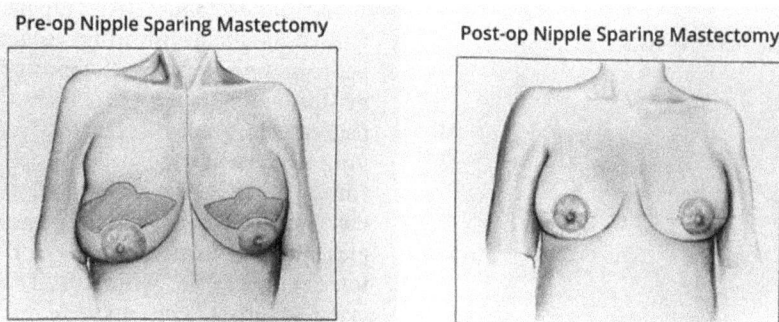

FIGURE 2: Artist's depiction of pre- and postoperative markings for simultaneous nipple-sparing mastectomy and reduction mastopexy. A "boomerang" shaped supra-areolar incision is made, through which breast tissue and a variable amount of skin are excised. The edges are reapproximated after insertion of a tissue expander.

Coupled venous anastomoses were used in all cases and hand-sewn arterial anastomoses were used in all cases with 8-0 nylon sutures. Flaps were stabilized onto the chest wall with 3-0 Vicryl sutures after restoration of blood flow. Abdominal fascia was repaired with 1-0 PDS sutures and the abdominal flap was closed with 0-0 PDS for the fascial layer, 3-0 monocryl for the dermal layer, and 4-0 monocryl for the skin. Ten-millimeter flat channel drains were used in the abdomen and behind the DIEP flaps in all cases. Flaps were monitored with Doppler ultrasound and clinical exam every fifteen minutes for 3 hours and then hourly thereafter.

3. Results

Eight patients underwent bilateral NSM with simultaneous reduction mammaplasty and breast reconstruction. A total of sixteen mastectomies were performed. Average age was 49 years, 75% of patients had comorbid conditions, and 63% of patients were actively smoking at the time of surgery. Five patients met criteria for prophylactic resection and three patients met criteria for therapeutic resection. Sixty-nine percent of breasts demonstrated grade III ptosis and the remainder were grade II. Seventy-five percent of patients had bilateral nipple-sparing mastectomies with immediate reconstruction with a tissue expander and implant insertion on a later date. The remaining 25% of patients underwent immediate reconstruction with DIEP flap. Average volume of breast tissue excised was 760 grams. In the tissue expander group, the average expander size was 560 cc with average initial expander volumes of 240 cc (Table 1). SPY intraoperative perfusion confirmed viable mastectomy flaps and nipple-areolar complexes.

There were a total of 11 mastectomies that were not complicated by NAC necrosis. One patient developed unilateral hematoma. The average age in this group was 49 years, one patient was actively smoking at the time of surgery, and 91% of patients had active comorbid diseases. Twenty-seven percent of procedures were therapeutic, and 73% were prophylactic. Breast ptosis grades were 81% grade III and 19% grade II. Eighty-one percent of mastectomies were reconstructed initially with tissue expanders and 19%

underwent immediate DIEP flap reconstruction. In those patients who were nonsmokers, NAC necrosis rates were 0% (Table 2).

There were a total of five mastectomies that were complicated by NAC necrosis (60% total, 40% partial). Of these, two breasts also developed seromas and one developed mastectomy flap necrosis. Average age in the NAC necrosis group was 59 years. All patients who developed NAC necrosis were smokers and only one patient had active comorbidities. Forty percent of procedures were prophylactic and 60% were therapeutic. Ptosis grades were 40% grade III and 60% grade II. Sixty percent of patients in this group underwent reconstruction by a tissue expander and the remaining 40% underwent immediate DIEP flap-based reconstruction (Table 3).

Rates of partial and total NAC necrosis rates were 12.5% and 18.7%, respectively. Comparison of the breasts that experienced NAC necrosis with those that did not revealed average ages of 59 and 49 years, respectively. One hundred percent of patients who experienced NAC necrosis were smokers versus 9% in the NAC intact group. Twenty percent of cases of NAC necrosis had associated comorbidities versus 91% in the NAC intact group. On average, the percentage of therapeutic mastectomies was slightly higher in the NAC necrosis group; however, the percentage of grade III ptosis was lower. Reconstruction methods were similar in both groups (Table 4). All patients were eventually able to heal their incisions and postoperative wounds (Figure 3).

4. Discussion

Female patients with large-volume, severely ptotic breasts who are candidates for NSM pose a specific challenge to reconstructive surgeons. Most surgeons are reluctant to perform a simultaneous NSM and reduction mastopexy given the supposed increased risk of NAC and skin flap necrosis [1, 4, 7, 12, 13, 22]. Some authors argue that advanced breast ptosis may further contribute to the development of this complication and may also impair NAC repositioning and management of the skin envelope when necessary [1, 4, 7, 12, 22]. Studies propose that high-grade ptosis and/or

TABLE 1: Patient characteristics and procedural specifics.

Pt	Age	Sex	Smoker	PMH	Indication	Ptosis grade	Technique	Expander size	Breast volume excised (R/L)
1	55	F	No	Hypertension	Biopsy with atypical cells in the setting of bilateral silicone injections	III (B/L)	Bilateral NSM with reduction mammaplasty and expander insertion	350 cc	665 gr/740 gr
2	30	F	No	Asthma, depression	BRCA mutation	III (B/L)	Bilateral NSM with reduction mammaplasty and expander insertion	800 cc	1240 gr/1316 gr
3	54	F	No	Gastric cancer, thyroid disease, peripheral neuropathy	BRCA mutation	III (B/L)	Bilateral NSM with reduction mammaplasty and expander insertion	400 cc	429 gr/449 gr
4	58	F	No	Thyroid disease	BRCA mutation	III (B/L)	Bilateral NSM with reduction mammaplasty and expander insertion	800 cc	1006 gr/776 gr
5	52	F	Yes	None	Unilateral, multifocal DCIS	III (B/L)	Bilateral NSM with reduction mammaplasty and DIEP flap reconstruction	N/A	NR
6	58	F	No	Hypertension, diabetes mellitus	Unilateral invasive breast cancer, BRCA	III/II (R/L)	Bilateral NSM with reduction mammaplasty and DIEP flap reconstruction	N/A	546 gr/436 gr
7	32	F	Yes	None	Unilateral invasive breast cancer	II (B/L)	Bilateral NSM with reduction mammaplasty and expander insertion	500 cc	NR
8	55	F	Yes	Ovarian cancer, thyroid disease	BRCA	II (B/L)	Bilateral NSM with reduction mammaplasty and expander insertion	500 cc	NR

PMH: past medical history; R: right; L: left; B/L: bilateral; NSM: nipple-sparing mastectomy; BRCA: breast cancer susceptibility gene; DCIS: ductal carcinoma in situ; N/A: not applicable; DIEP: deep inferior epigastric perforator; NR: not reported.

TABLE 2: Breasts that did not experience NAC necrosis stratified by individual mastectomy.

Pt.	NAC necrosis	Wound complications	Age	Smoker	PMH	Indication	Ptosis grade	Reconstruction
1 (R)	No	Hematoma	55	N	Y	Prophylactic	III	Expander
1 (L)	No	None	55	N	Y	Prophylactic	III	Expander
2 (R)	No	None	30	N	Y	Prophylactic	III	Expander
2 (L)	No	None	30	N	Y	Prophylactic	III	Expander
3 (R)	No	None	54	N	Y	Prophylactic	III	Expander
3 (L)	No	None	54	N	Y	Prophylactic	III	Expander
4 (R)	No	None	58	N	Y	Prophylactic	III	Expander
4 (L)	No	None	58	N	Y	Prophylactic	III	Expander
6 (L)	No	None	58	N	Y	Therapeutic	II	DIEP
6 (R)	No	None	58	N	Y	Therapeutic	III	DIEP
7 (L)	No	None	32	Y	N	Therapeutic	II	Expander

Pt.: patient number; NAC: nipple-areolar complex; PMH: past medical history; N: no; Y: yes; R: right breast; L: left breast; DIEP: deep inferior epigastric perforator.

excessive breast volume may increase the length of the skin flap required to supply the NAC, thereby compromising vascular supply [22]. Additionally, some argue that substantial amounts of breast tissue need to be left behind to ensure NAC and flap perfusion resulting in an inadequate mastectomy [13]. Nevertheless, several studies have reported options for women with large breasts and/or advanced ptosis who meet criteria for NSM [1, 13]. These techniques can be broadly

TABLE 3: Breasts that experienced NAC necrosis stratified by individual mastectomy.

Pt.	NAC necrosis	Wound complications	Age	Smoker	PMH	Indication	Ptosis grade	Reconstruction
5 (R)	Partial	None	52	Y	N	Therapeutic	III	DIEP
5 (L)	Total	Flap necrosis	52	Y	N	Therapeutic	III	DIEP
7 (R)	Partial	None	32	Y	N	Therapeutic	II	Expander
8 (R)	Total	Seroma	55	Y	Y	Prophylactic	II	Expander
8 (L)	Total	Seroma	55	Y	Y	Prophylactic	II	Expander

Pt.: patient number; NAC: nipple-areolar complex; R: right breast; L: left breast; Y: yes; N: no; DIEP: deep inferior epigastric perforator.

TABLE 4: Breasts that experienced NAC necrosis compared to those that did not.

Group	Number of breasts	Avg. age	Smokers	Comorbidities present	Therapeutic versus prophylactic	Ptosis grade (II versus III)	Expander versus DIEP
NAC necrosis	5	59 years	100%	20%	60% versus 40%	60% versus 40%	60% versus 40%
NAC intact	11	49 years	9%	91%	27% versus 73%	19% versus 81%	81% versus 19%

NAC: nipple-areolar complex; Avg.: average; DIEP: deep inferior epigastric perforator.

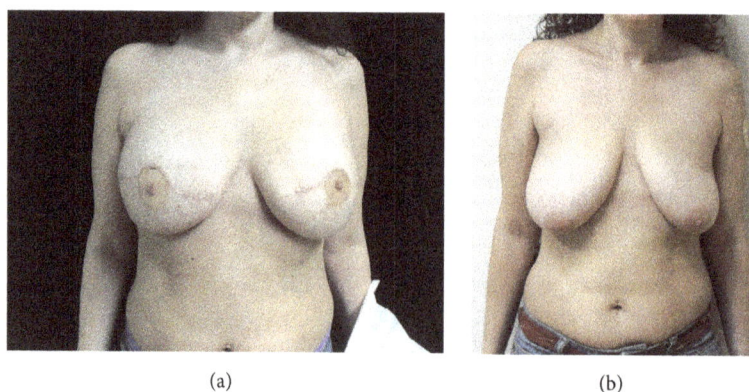

(a)   (b)

FIGURE 3: Pre- (a) and postoperative (b) photographs after simultaneous nipple-sparing mastectomy and reduction mastopexy with implant-based reconstruction.

subdivided into staged NSM and reduction mastopexy [1, 13, 23] or simultaneous reduction mastopexy with NSM [10, 16–21].

Review of the literature revealed three studies that focused on staged reduction mastopexy and NSM for women with large, ptotic breasts [1, 13, 23]. Spear et al. published a series of cases in which such patients were offered staged NSM and reduction mastopexy [13]. Partial NAC necrosis rates were roughly 12.5% and there were no cases of total NAC necrosis [13]. While results were promising, the authors felt this procedure would be best suited for patients with medium-volume breasts with moderate ptosis [13]. Two other studies employed the use of immediate flap-based reconstruction after NSM with a delayed reduction mastopexy [1, 23]. These studies used various free flaps to support NAC perfusion after NSM, and reduction mastopexy for moderately to severely ptotic breasts was performed on a later date [1, 23]. The main disadvantage in the staged approach is that the patient requires two major surgeries. Additionally,

patients with active comorbid conditions may not be able to tolerate a lengthy free-flap procedure. The mean percentages of partial and total NAC necrosis in the staged group were 4.16% and 1%, respectively (Table 5).

In the 1970s, several studies examined the utility of SCM with NAC preservation with simultaneous reduction mastopexy for patients with large breasts and/or severe ptosis [16–19, 21]. While these studies showed promising results regarding NAC preservation, several failed to specify the breast size or degree of ptosis [16, 19]. Additionally, early studies focused on SCM with NAC preservation, which likely resulted in a less comprehensive mastectomy as indications at that time were strictly prophylactic. The literature suggests that breast tissue quantities now considered unacceptable for conventional NSM were left behind during SCM to support NAC and flap perfusion [1]. Nevertheless, there has been a resurgence of interest in simultaneous NSM and reduction mastopexy, likely reflecting the increase in patient demand [7]. Two studies in 2010 and 2011 demonstrated good results

Table 5: Table reviewing all of the studies published on nipple-sparing mastectomy in large-volume, ptotic breasts from 1970 to 2016.

	Technique	Reconstruction	Sample size (number of breasts)	Indication	Ptosis/breast volume	Partial NAC necrosis	Total NAC necrosis	Other complications
Simultaneous mastopexy and NSM								
Goulian & McDivitt, 1972	SCM with reduction mastopexy	Implant None	24	Risk reduction	Medium-large Not specified	None	None	Hematoma (NR)
Biggs et al., 1977	SCM with reduction mastopexy	Implant	33	NR	Not specified Min-Mod ptosis	None	None	Partial flap necrosis (1) Capsular contractures (8) Atrophy requiring excision (1) Explant (1)
Jarrett et al., 1978	SCM, reduction mastopexy, and free nipple graft	Implant	44	Risk reduction	Large volume Severe ptosis	None	None	NR
Gibson, 1979	SCM with reduction mastopexy	NR	NR	Risk reduction	Not specified	None	None	NR
Rusby & Gui, 2010	NSM with reduction mastopexy	Expander	16	Risk reduction	NR NR	NR	6.3%	None
Nava et al., 2011	NSM with reduction mastopexy	Implant	13	Therapeutic	NR NR	NR[#]	NR[#]	NR[#]
Rivolin et al., 2012	NSM with periareolar pexy	Implant	22	Therapeutic	Medium-large volume Moderate ptosis	13.6%	4.6%[*]	None
Al-Mufarrej et al., 2013	NSM with reduction mastopexy	Expander Implant	48	Risk reduction	Large volume Moderate	8.3%	4.2%	Infected implant (2.1%) Implant rupture (14.6%) Hematoma (2.1%) Capsular contracture (4.2%)
Pontell et al., 2016 (this report)	NSM with reduction mastopexy	Expander DIEP Flap	16	Risk reduction Therapeutic	Large volume Grade II/III ptosis	0%[**]	0%[**]	Hematoma Seroma Mastectomy flap necrosis
Staged mastopexy and NSM								
Schneider et al., 2012	NSM with immediate flap placement and staged reduction mastopexy	TUG Flap DIEP Flap	34	NR	Large volume Grade II/III ptosis	None	3%	Hematoma (3%)
DellaCroce et al., 2015	NSM with immediate flap placement and staged reduction mastopexy	DIEP Flap SGAP Flap	110	Risk reduction Therapeutic	Medium-large volume Grade II/III ptosis	None	None	Partial mastectomy flap necrosis (3.6%) Incisional dehiscence (8%) Hematoma (2.7%) Partial flap necrosis (1.8%)

TABLE 5: Continued.

Technique	Reconstruction	Sample size (number of breasts)	Indication	Ptosis/breast volume	Partial NAC necrosis	Total NAC necrosis	Other complications
Spear et al., 2012	Reduction mastopexy followed by NSM	Implant Tissue expander	24	Risk reduction Therapeutic	Medium volume Grade II/III ptosis	12.5%	None	Breast infection (8%) Skin flap necrosis (17%) Explant (4%)

NAC: nipple-areolar complex; NSM: nipple-sparing mastectomy; SCM: subcutaneous mastectomy; NR: not reported; DIEP: deep inferior epigastric perforator; TUG: transverse upper gracilis; SGAP: superior gluteal artery perforator. #Complications were not stratified by NSM (SRM) versus SSM status. *This study mentions the exclusion of one patient who had total NAC necrosis. **These rates exclude the patients who were smokers, including patients with partial and total NAC necrosis rates of 12.5% and 18.7%, respectively.

regarding NAC preservation; however, the data reported did not allow any conclusions to be drawn regarding the breast size or degree of ptosis [7, 24]. Al-Mufarrej et al. and Rivolin et al. reported on two series of patients with medium- to large-volume breasts and moderate ptosis who underwent NSM with simultaneous reduction mastopexy [10, 15]. Results of these studies demonstrated excellent NAC preservation in prophylactic and therapeutic scenarios; however, the issue of severe breast ptosis did not appear to be addressed [10, 15]. Average partial and total NAC necrosis rates in the simultaneous group were 3.65% and 2.16%, respectively (Table 5).

The pedicled flap used in this study is a wide-based, epithelialized version of the traditional inferiorly based flaps used during reduction mammaplasty. The base of the flap was widened in attempt to preserve the natural arterial and venous supply to the NAC. The NAC receives arterial perfusion from a periareolar network that is supplied by perforating branches of the internal thoracic artery, the anterior intercostal arteries, and the lateral thoracic artery [25]. The most important contribution arises from the third internal thoracic artery perforator [25]. All of these arterial networks course towards the NAC in a medio- or lateroinferior direction (Figure 4). After formation of the periareolar plexus, the cutaneous perforators travel within the subcutaneous tissue before reaching the NAC and after mastectomy the NAC relies solely on these cutaneous branches as the underlying breast tissue has been removed [1, 26]. With respect to vascular outflow, the NAC is drained through a superior and inferior horizontal venous sling (Figure 4) [27]. After mastectomy, the NAC drainage relies heavily on the superficial, inferiorly coursing venous network [27]. The cutaneous venous system is even more superficial than the arterial network and as such is more likely to be damaged during deepithelialization [27]. Necrosis of the NAC results from either arterial or venous insufficiency and the latter appears to be even more prevalent with larger breast resection volumes [13, 27–29]. Given the vascular anatomy of the NAC, expanding the base of the pedicle in a lateral fashion should theoretically preserve more of the arterial supply and venous drainage. In addition, by maintaining an epithelialized pedicle, the cutaneous vascular perforators that nourish the NAC should also be better preserved. The importance of

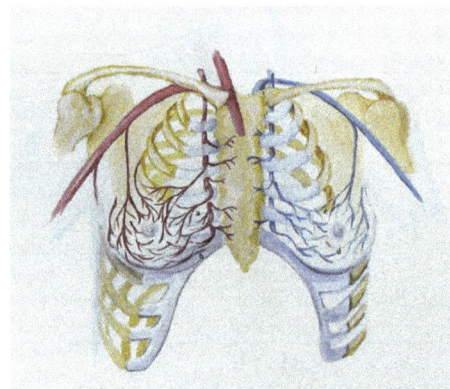

FIGURE 4: Artist's depiction of the arterial supply *(right breast)* and venous drainage *(left breast)* to the nipple-areolar complex (NAC). The most important contributor to NAC perfusion arises from the third internal thoracic artery perforator (a). This branch travels medially from its origin and courses just under the NAC where it gives off tributaries to the periareolar network. The anterior intercostal arteries originate more inferiorly and course along the inframammary fold before giving their contributions to the arterial supply of the NAC (b). The NAC is drained through superior (c) and inferior (d) horizontal venous slings that ultimately drain into the thoracic and subclavian veins [17, 19].

vascular preservation is amplified with larger breast volumes [27, 28]. In theory, such dissection should offer anatomical advantages when compared to other techniques that use narrow, deepithelialized pedicles to support NAC perfusion after NSM and reduction mammaplasty.

Limitations of this study include the small sample size and thus an inability to draw statistically significant conclusions. In addition, while the average breast volume excised was 760 grams, several of the patients did not have excised breast volumes recorded and therefore NAC necrosis could not be analyzed alongside breast volumes. Overall rates of partial and total NAC necrosis were 12.5% and 18.7%, respectively. The discordance between SPY perfusion results and NAC survival may represent either a lack of diagnostic accuracy on behalf of the SPY system or, more likely, the complex microvascular disease that develops in active smokers. While these complication rates do appear high, subset analysis reveals that all patients who had NAC necrosis were smokers and all patients who smoked developed NAC necrosis. Excluding the subset of patients who smoked, partial and total NAC necrosis rates were 0%. Such complications did not appear to be related to patient age, the presence or absence of comorbidities, indication for procedure, grade II versus III ptosis, or the type of reconstruction performed.

In summary, this study presents an alternate technique for simultaneous NSM and reduction mastopexy for women with large, ptotic breasts. Using this method, comparable amounts of NAC preservation were able to be achieved in what has historically been considered a high-risk patient group for this procedure. While NSM has traditionally been avoided in this patient subgroup, this study supports its inclusion when considering a patient for either prophylactic or therapeutic NSM. Using a wide, inferior, epithelialized pedicle based on the vascular anatomy of the NAC, comparable rates of NAC preservation are possible, even in patients with large-volume, severely ptotic breasts. Options for immediate reconstruction exist, and a staged approach may not be necessary. Emphasis on smoking cessation is paramount to the success of the operation.

References

[1] F. J. DellaCroce, C. A. Blum, S. K. Sullivan et al., "Nipple-Sparing Mastectomy and Ptosis: Perforator Flap Breast Reconstruction Allows Full Secondary Mastopexy with Complete Nipple Areolar Repositioning," *Plastic and Reconstructive Surgery*, vol. 136, no. 1, pp. 1–9, 2015.

[2] S. Spear, "Nipple sparing mastectomy and reconstruction: Indications, techniques, and outcomes," in *Surgery of the Breast: Principles and Art*, S. Spear, Ed., vol. 1, pp. 287–297, Wolters Kluwer/Lippincott WIlliams & Wilkins, 3rd edition, 2011.

[3] H. R. Moyer, B. Ghazi, J. R. Daniel, R. Gasgarth, and G. W. Carlson, "Nipple-sparing mastectomy: Technical aspects and aesthetic outcomes," *Annals of Plastic Surgery*, vol. 68, no. 5, pp. 446–450, 2012.

[4] S. L. Spear, S. C. Willey, E. D. Feldman et al., "Nipple-sparing mastectomy for prophylactic and therapeutic indications," *Plastic and Reconstructive Surgery*, vol. 128, no. 5, pp. 1005–1014, 2011.

[5] L. C. Hartmann, D. J. Schaid, J. E. Woods et al., "Efficacy of bilateral prophylactic mastectomy in women with a family history of breast cancer," *The New England Journal of Medicine*, vol. 340, no. 2, pp. 77–84, 1999.

[6] P. Maxwell, P. Whitworth, and A. Gabriel, "Nipple sparing mastectomy," in *Surgery of the Breast: Principles and Art*, S. Spear, Ed., vol. 1, pp. 298–307, Wolters Kluwer/Lippincott WIlliams & Wilkins, 3rd edition, 2011.

[7] JE. Rusby and GP. Gui, "Nipple-sparing mastectomy in women with large or ptotic breasts," *Journal of Plastic, Reconstructive and Aesthetic Surgery*, vol. 125, pp. 818–829, 2010.

[8] S. L. Spear, C. M. Hannan, S. C. Willey, and C. Cocilovo, "Nipple-sparing mastectomy," *Plastic and Reconstructive Surgery*, vol. 123, no. 6, pp. 1665–1673, 2009.

[9] C. M. Chen, J. J. Disa, V. Sacchini et al., "Nipple-sparing mastectomy and immediate tissue expander/implant breast reconstruction," *Plastic and Reconstructive Surgery*, vol. 124, no. 6, pp. 1772–1780, 2009.

[10] F. M. Al-Mufarrej, J. E. Woods, and S. R. Jacobson, "Simultaneous mastopexy in patients undergoing prophylactic nipple-sparing mastectomies and immediate reconstruction," *Journal of Plastic, Reconstructive & Aesthetic Surgery*, vol. 66, no. 6, pp. 747–755, 2013.

[11] L. Lostumbo, N. E. Carbine, and J. Wallace, "Prophylactic mastectomy for the prevention of breast cancer," *Cochrane Database of Systematic Reviews*, vol. 11, Article ID CD002748, 2010.

[12] S. L. Spear, M. E. Carter, and K. Schwarz, "Prophylactic mastectomy: Indications, options, and reconstructive alternatives," *Plastic and Reconstructive Surgery*, vol. 115, no. 3, pp. 891–909, 2005.

[13] S. L. Spear, S. J. Rottman, L. A. Seiboth, and C. M. Hannan, "Breast reconstruction using a staged nipple-sparing mastectomy following mastopexy or reduction," *Plastic and Reconstructive Surgery*, vol. 129, no. 3, pp. 572–581, 2012.

[14] D. K. Wellisch, W. S. Schain, R. Barrett Noone, and J. W. Little, "The psychological contribution of nipple addition in breast reconstruction," *Plastic and Reconstructive Surgery*, vol. 80, no. 5, pp. 699–704, 1987.

[15] A. Rivolin, F. Kubatzki, F. Marocco et al., "Nipple-areola complex sparing mastectomy with periareolar pexy for breast cancer patients with moderately ptotic breasts," *Journal of Plastic, Reconstructive & Aesthetic Surgery*, vol. 65, no. 3, pp. 296–303, 2012.

[16] E. W. GIBSON, "Subcutaneous mastectomy using an inferior nipple pedicle," *ANZ Journal of Surgery*, vol. 49, no. 5, pp. 559-560, 1979.

[17] J. E. Woods, "Detailed technique of subcutaneous mastectomy with and without mastopexy," *Annals of Plastic Surgery*, vol. 18, no. 1, pp. 51–61, 1987.

[18] J. R. Jarrett, R. G. Cutler, and D. F. Teal, "Subcutaneous mastectomy in small, large, or ptotic breasts with immediate submuscular placement of implants," *Plastic and Reconstructive Surgery*, vol. 62, no. 5, pp. 702–705, 1978.

[19] D. Goulian and R. W. McDivitt, "Subcutaneous mastectomy with immediate reconstruction of the breasts, using the dermal mastopexy technique," *Plastic and Reconstructive Surgery*, vol. 50, no. 3, pp. 211–215, 1972.

[20] N. G. Georgiade and W. Hyland, "Technique for subcutaneous mastectomy and immediate reconstruction in the ptotic breast," *Plastic and Reconstructive Surgery*, vol. 56, no. 2, pp. 121–128, 1975.

[21] T. M. Biggs, R. O. Brauer, and L. E. Wolf, "Mastopexy in conjunction with subcutaneous mastectomy," *Plastic and Reconstructive Surgery*, vol. 60, no. 1, pp. 1–5, 1977.

[22] P. Chirappapha, J.-Y. Petit, M. Rietjens et al., "Nipple sparing mastectomy: Does breast morphological factor related to necrotic complications?" *Plastic and Reconstructive Surgery*, vol. 2, no. e99, pp. 1–7, 2014.

[23] L. F. Schneider, C. M. Chen, A. J. Stolier, R. L. Shapiro, C. Y. Ahn, and R. J. Allen, "Nipple-sparing mastectomy and immediate free-flap reconstruction in the large ptotic breast," *Annals of Plastic Surgery*, vol. 69, no. 4, pp. 425–428, 2012.

[24] M. B. Nava, J. Ottolenghi, A. Pennati et al., "Skin/nipple sparing mastectomies and implant-based breast reconstruction in

patients with large and ptotic breast: oncological and reconstructive results," *The Breast*, vol. 21, no. 3, pp. 267–271, 2012.

[25] P. V. van Deventer, "The blood supply to the nipple-areola complex of the human mammary gland," *Aesthetic Plastic Surgery*, vol. 28, no. 6, pp. 393–398, 2004.

[26] H. Nakajima, N. Imanishi, and S. Aiso, "Arterial anatomy of the nipple-areola complex," *Plastic and Reconstructive Surgery*, vol. 96, no. 4, pp. 843–845, 1995.

[27] C. M. Le Roux, W.-R. Pan, S. A. Matousek, and M. W. Ashton, "Preventing venous congestion of the nipple-areola complex: An anatomical guide to preserving essential venous drainage networks," *Plastic and Reconstructive Surgery*, vol. 127, no. 3, pp. 1073–1079, 2011.

[28] G. Gravante, A. Araco, R. Sorge et al., "Postoperative wound infections after breast reductions: The role of smoking and the amount of tissue removed," *Aesthetic Plastic Surgery*, vol. 32, no. 1, pp. 25–31, 2008.

[29] P. V. van Deventer, B. J. Page, and F. R. Graewe, "The safety of pedicles in breast reduction and mastopexy procedures," *Aesthetic Plastic Surgery*, vol. 32, no. 2, pp. 307–312, 2008.

Permissions

List of Contributors

P. Agbenorku
Reconstructive Plastic Surgery and Burns Unit, Komfo Anokye Teaching Hospital, School of Medical Sciences, Kwame Nkrumah University of Science and Technology, Kumasi, Ghana

E. Otupiri
Department of Community Health, School of Medical Sciences, Kwame Nkrumah University of Science and Technology, Kumasi, Ghana

S. Fugar
Department of Surgery, Komfo Anokye Teaching Hospital, Kumasi, Ghana

Raffaele Serra, Gianluca Buffone and Stefano de Franciscis
Department of Medical and Surgical Science, University Magna Graecia of Catanzaro, Viale Europa, 88100 Catanzaro, Italy

Anna Maria Miglietta and Sergio Abonante
Breast Unit, Annunziata Hospital, 87100 Cosenza, Italy

Vincent Giordano
Plastic Surgery Unit, Annunziata Hospital, 87100 Cosenza, Italy

Yoshiko Iwahira and Yoshio Tanaka
Tokyo Breast Surgery Clinic, Japan

Tomohisa Nagasao
Department of Plastic and Reconstructive Surgery, Faculty of Medicine/Graduate School of Medicine, Kagawa University, Kida County, Miki-Cho, Ikenobe 1750-1, Takamatsu, Kagawa 761-0793, Japan

Yusuke Shimizu
Department of Plastic and Reconstructive Surgery, Ryukyu University Hospital, Japan

Kumiko Kuwata
Department of Plastic Surgery, Aichi Children's Health and Medical Center, Japan

Arash Momeni, Derrick C. Wan and Gordon K. Lee
Division of Plastic and Reconstructive Surgery, Stanford University Medical Center, 770 Welch Road, Suite 700, Palo Alto, CA 94305-5715, USA

Rebecca Y. Kim
Division of General Surgery, Stanford University Medical Center, Stanford, CA 94305, USA

Ali Izadpanah
Division of Plastic and Reconstructive Surgery, McGill University Health Centre, Montreal, Canada

Ibrahim Abdulrasheed and Asuku Malachy Eneye
Division of Plastic Surgery, Department of Surgery, Ahmadu BelloUniversity Teaching Hospital, Shika, Kaduna State, Zaria 810001, Nigeria

W. M. Rdeini
Seventh Day Adventist Hospital, Kumasi, Ghana

P. Agbenorku
Kwame Nkrumah University of Science and Technology, Kumasi, Ghana

V. A. Mitish
Russian Peoples' Friendship University of Russia, Moscow, Russia

Trinh Cao Minh and Do Xuan Hai
Practical and Experimental Surgery Department, Vietnam Military Medical University (HVQY), K58, Hadong, Hanoi, Vietnam

Pham Thi Ngoc
Veterinary Hygiene Department, National Institute of Veterinary Research (NIVR), Truong Chinh, Dong Da, Hanoi, Vietnam

Wani Sajad
Department of Plastic Surgery, SKIMS, Srinagar, Jammu and Kashmir 190011, India

Raashid Hamid
Department of Plastic Surgery, SKIMS, Srinagar, Jammu and Kashmir 190011, India
Married Doctors Hostel, Block A, Room No. S2, SKIMS, Soura, Jammu and Kashmir 190011, India

Mansoor Khan, Abdul Majeed, Waqas Hayat, Hidayat Ullah, Shazia Naz, Syed Asif Shah, Tahmeedullah Tahmeed, Kanwal Yousaf and Muhammad Tahir
Plastic and Reconstructive Surgery, Hayatabad Medical Complex, IV Hayatabad, Peshawar, Pakistan

Mitsuru Nemoto, Shinsuke Ishikawa, Natsuko Kounoike, Takayuki Sugimoto and Akira Takeda
Department of Plastic and Reconstructive Surgery, Kitasato University Hospital, 1-15-1 Kitasato, Minami-ku, Sagamihara, Kanagawa 252-0374, Japan

Samrat Mukherjee, Sachin Kamat and Samuel Adegbola
Bariatric Surgery Unit, Homerton University Hospital, Homerton Row, Homerton, London E9 6SR, UK

Sanjay Agrawal
Bariatric Surgery Unit, Homerton University Hospital, Homerton Row, Homerton, London E9 6SR, UK
Centre for Digestive Diseases, Blizard Institute, Queen Mary University of London, London E1 2AT, UK

Jamal Omran Al Madani
Plastic Surgery Unit, Plastic Surgery Resident, Security Forces Hospital, Riyadh, Saudi Arabia

Akihiro Ogino and Kiyoshi Onishi
Department of Plastic and Reconstructive Surgery, 6-11-1, Omori-nishi, Ota-ku, Tokyo 143-8541, Japan

Brian P. Tierney
Tierney Plastic Surgery, 2011 Church Street, Suite 805, Nashville, TN 37203, USA

Jason P. Hodde and Daniela I. Changkuon
Cook Biotech Incorporated, 1425 Innovation Place, West Lafayette, IN 47906, USA

Michael S. Hu
Hagey Laboratory for Pediatric Regenerative Medicine, Department of Surgery, Division of Plastic and Reconstructive Surgery, Stanford University School of Medicine, Stanford, CA 94305, USA
Institute for Stem Cell Biology and Regenerative Medicine, Stanford University School of Medicine, Stanford, CA 94305, USA
Department of Surgery, John A. Burns School of Medicine, University of Hawaii, Honolulu, HI 96813, USA

Tripp Leavitt, Samir Malhotra, Zeshaan N. Maan, Alexander T. M. Cheung and H. Peter Lorenz
Hagey Laboratory for Pediatric Regenerative Medicine, Department of Surgery, Division of Plastic and Reconstructive Surgery, Stanford University School of Medicine, Stanford, CA 94305, USA

Dominik Duscher
Hagey Laboratory for Pediatric Regenerative Medicine, Department of Surgery, Division of Plastic and Reconstructive Surgery, Stanford University School of Medicine, Stanford, CA 94305, USA
Section of Plastic, Aesthetic and Reconstructive Surgery, Johannes Kepler University, Linz, Austria

Michael S. Pollhammer, Manfred Schmidt and Georg M. Huemer
Section of Plastic, Aesthetic and Reconstructive Surgery, Johannes Kepler University, Linz, Austria

Graham G. Walmsley and Michael T. Longaker
Hagey Laboratory for Pediatric Regenerative Medicine, Department of Surgery, Division of Plastic and Reconstructive Surgery, Stanford University School of Medicine, Stanford, CA 94305, USA
Institute for Stem Cell Biology and Regenerative Medicine, Stanford University School of Medicine, Stanford, CA 94305, USA

William H. C. Tiong, Mohd Ali Mat Zain and Normala Hj Basiron
Department of Plastic and Reconstructive Surgery, Hospital Kuala Lumpur, Jalan Pahang, 50586 Kuala Lumpur, Malaysia

Luigi Valdatta and Mario Cherubino
Department of Biotechnology and Life Science (DBSV), University of Insubria, 21100 Varese, Italy
Plastic and Reconstructive Surgery Division, Ospedale di Circolo di Varese, Viale Borri 57, 21100 Varese, Italy

Anna Giulia Cattaneo and Anna Minuti
Department of Biotechnology and Life Science (DBSV), University of Insubria, 21100 Varese, Italy

Igor Pellegatta and Stefano Scamoni
Plastic and Reconstructive Surgery Division, Ospedale di Circolo di Varese, Viale Borri 57, 21100 Varese, Italy

Reem Dina Jarjis, Lone Bak Hansen and Steen Henrik Matzen
Department of Plastic Surgery and Breast Surgery, Zealand University Hospital, Sygehusvej 10, 4000 Roskilde, Denmark

Luis Bermudez, Kristen Trost and Ruben Ayala
Research and Outcomes Department, Operation Smile, Inc., Norfolk, VA 23509, USA

Mark Gorman
Castle Hill Plastic Surgery Unit, Hull HU16 5JQ, UK

James Coelho and Sameer Gujral
Department of Plastic Surgery, Royal Devon and Exeter Hospital, UK

Alastair McKay
Canniesburn Plastic Surgery Unit, Glasgow, UK

Pratik B. Patel, Marguerite Hoyler and John G. Meara
Program in Global Surgery and Social Change, Department of Global Health and Social Medicine, Harvard Medical School, Boston, MA 02115, USA
Department of Plastic and Oral Surgery, Boston Children's Hospital, 300 Longwood Avenue, Enders 1, Boston, MA 02115, USA

Rebecca Maine
Program in Global Surgery and Social Change, Department of Global Health and Social Medicine, Harvard Medical School, Boston, MA 02115, USA
Department of Plastic and Oral Surgery, Boston Children's Hospital, 300 Longwood Avenue, Enders 1, Boston, MA 02115, USA
Department of Surgery, University of California San Francisco Medical Center, San Francisco, CA 94131, USA

Christopher D. Hughes
Program in Global Surgery and Social Change, Department of Global Health and Social Medicine, Harvard Medical School, Boston, MA 02115, USA
Department of Plastic and Oral Surgery, Boston Children's Hospital, 300 Longwood Avenue, Enders 1, Boston, MA 02115, USA
Department of Surgery, University of Connecticut Health Center, Farmington, CT 06030, USA

Lars Hagander
Program in Global Surgery and Social Change, Department of Global Health and Social Medicine, Harvard Medical School, Boston, MA 02115, USA
Department of Plastic and Oral Surgery, Boston Children's Hospital, 300 Longwood Avenue, Enders 1, Boston, MA 02115, USA
Department of Pediatric Surgery and International Pediatrics, Faculty of Medicine, Lund University, Lund SE-221 00, Sweden

K. Carroll and P. A. Mossey
Dental Hospital and School, University of Dundee, 1 Park Place, Dundee DD1 4HR, UK

K. S. Houschyar
Division of Plastic and Reconstructive Surgery, Department of Surgery, Stanford School of Medicine, Stanford, CA 94305, USA
Clinic for Plastic and Reconstructive Surgery, Bergmannstrost Halle, 06112 Halle, Germany
Clinic for Hand Surgery, Rhon-Klinikum AG, 97616 Bad Neustadt an der Saale, Germany

A. Momeni, M. N. Pyles, Z. N. Maan and O. S. Jew
Division of Plastic and Reconstructive Surgery, Department of Surgery, Stanford School of Medicine, Stanford, CA 94305, USA

J. Y. Cha
Division of Plastic and Reconstructive Surgery, Department of Surgery, Stanford School of Medicine, Stanford, CA 94305, USA
Orthodontic Department, College of Dentistry, Yonsei University, Seoul, Republic of Korea

D. Duscher
Section of Plastic and Reconstructive Surgery, Department of Surgery, Johannes Kepler University Linz, 4040 Linz, Austria

F. Siemers
Clinic for Plastic and Reconstructive Surgery, Bergmannstrost Halle, 06112 Halle, Germany
Clinic for Hand Surgery, Rh"on-Klinikum AG, 97616 Bad Neustadt an der Saale, Germany

J. van Schoonhoven
Clinic for Hand Surgery, Rh"on-Klinikum AG, 97616 Bad Neustadt an der Saale, Germany

Giovanni Francesco Marangi, Tiziano Pallara, Barbara Cagli and Paolo Persichetti
Department of Plastic and Reconstructive Surgery, "Campus Bio-Medico di Roma" University, Via A. del Portillo 200, 00128 Rome, Italy

Emiliano Schena
Laboratory of Research in Biomedical Instrumentation and Measurements, "Campus Bio-Medico di Roma" University, Via A. del Portillo 200, 00128 Rome, Italy

Francesco Giurazza, Elio Faiella and Bruno Beomonte Zobel
Division of Radiology, "Campus Bio-Medico di Roma" University, Via A. del Portillo 200, 00128 Rome, Italy

YsselMendoza Marí, Maday Fernández Mayola, Ariana García Ojalvo and Jorge Berlanga Acosta
Wound Healing and Cytoprotection Group, Biomedical Research Direction, Center for Genetic Engineering and Biotechnology, Avenue 31/158 and 190, Playa, 10600 Havana, Cuba

Ana Aguilera Barreto and Yilian Bermúdez Alvarez
Formulation Department, Technological Development Direction, Center for Genetic Engineering and Biotechnology, Avenue 31/158 and 190, Playa, 10600 Havana, Cuba

Ana Janet Mir Benítez
Esthetic Surgery Department, "Joaqu´ın Albarr´an" Hospital, Avenue 26 and Boyeros, Plaza de la Revoluci´on, 10600 Havana, Cuba

Niels Hammer-Hansen, Javed Akram and Tine Engberg Damsgaard
Plastic Surgical Research Unit, Department of Plastic Surgery, Aarhus University Hospital, 8000 Aarhus, Denmark

Kashif Abbas
Islam Medical College, Sialkot, Pakistan
H No. 88 K-1, Wapda Town, Lahore, Pakistan

Masood Umer and Haroon ur Rashid
Aga Khan University Hospital, Karachi, Pakistan

Macario Camacho
Otolaryngology-Head and Neck Surgery, Tripler Army Medical Center, Honolulu, HI 96859, USA
Department of Psychiatry and Behavioral Sciences, Sleep Medicine Division, Stanford Hospital and Clinics, Stanford, CA 94063, USA

Soroush Zaghi
Otolaryngology-Head and Neck Surgery, Division of Sleep Surgery and Medicine, Stanford Hospitals and Clinics, Stanford, CA 94304, USA
Department of Head and Neck Surgery, David Geffen School of Medicine at UCLA, Los Angeles, CA 90095, USA

Victor Certal
Department of Otorhinolaryngology, Sleep Medicine Centre, Hospital CUF, 4100-180 Porto, Portugal
Centre for Research in Health Technologies and Information Systems (CINTESIS), University of Porto, 4200-450 Porto, Portugal

Jose Abdullatif
Department of Otorhinolaryngology, Hospital Bernardino Rivadavia, C1425ASQ Buenos Aires, Argentina

Rahul Modi
Department of Otolaryngology-Head and Neck Surgery, Dr. L. H. Hiranandani Hospital Mumbai, Maharashtra 400076, India
Otolaryngology-Head and Neck Surgery, Division of Sleep Surgery and Medicine, Stanford Hospitals and Clinics, Stanford, CA 94304, USA

Shankar Sridhara
Otolaryngology-Head and Neck Surgery, Dwight D. Eisenhower Army Medical Center, Fort Gordon, GA 30905, USA

Anthony M. Tolisano, Edward T. Chang and Benjamin B. Cable
Otolaryngology-Head and Neck Surgery, Tripler Army Medical Center, Honolulu, HI 96859, USA

Robson Capasso
Otolaryngology-Head and Neck Surgery, Division of Sleep Surgery and Medicine, Stanford Hospitals and Clinics, Stanford, CA 94304, USA

Christopher Vashi
The Plastic Surgery Group, Chapel Place II, 340Thomas More Parkway, Crestview Hills, KY 41017, USA

The Plastic Surgery Group of Greater Cincinnati, 4850 Red Bank Expressway, Cincinnati, OH45227, USA

Libby R. Copeland-Halperin
Department of Surgery, Inova Fairfax Hospital, 3300 Gallows Road, Falls Church, VA 22042, USA

Vincenza Pimpinella
Division of Nursing, Mount Sinai Beth Israel Medical Center, 245 5th Avenue, New York, NY 10016, USA

Michelle Copeland
Division of Plastic and Reconstructive Surgery, Icahn School ofMedicine atMount Sinai, 1001 5th Avenue, New York, NY 10028, USA

Kashyap K. Tadisina
College of Medicine, University of Illinois at Chicago, Chicago, IL 60612, USA

Karan Chopra
Department of Plastic and Reconstructive Surgery, Johns Hopkins University, Baltimore, MD 21287, USA

John Tangredi and J. Grant Thomson
Section of Plastic and Reconstructive Surgery, Yale University School of Medicine, New Haven, CT 06511, USA

Devinder P. Singh
Division of Plastic Surgery, University of Maryland Medical Center, Wing S8D, 22 South Greene Street, Baltimore, MD 21201, USA

Rafael Denadai
Institute of Plastic and Craniofacial Surgery, SOBRAPAR Hospital, Avenue Adolpho Lutz 100, Caixa Postal 6028, 13084-880 Campinas, SP, Brazil
Division of Plastic and Reconstructive Surgery, Department of Surgery, School of Medical Sciences, University of Mar´ılia (UNIMAR), 17525-902 Mar´ılia, SP, Brazil

Andŕeia Padilha Toledo
School of Medical Sciences, University São Francisco (USF), 12916-900 Bragança Paulista, SP, Brazil

Luis Ricardo Martinhão Souto
Division of Plastic and Reconstructive Surgery, Department of Surgery, School of Medical Sciences, University of Mar´ılia (UNIMAR), 17525-902 Mar´ılia, SP, Brazil

Jeffrey Teixeira
Department of Otolaryngology Head and Neck Surgery, Walter Reed National Military Medical Center, Bethesda, MD, USA

Victor Certal
Department of Otorhinolaryngology/Sleep Medicine Centre, Hospital CUF, 4100-180 Porto, Portugal
Centre for Research in Health Technologies and Information Systems (CINTESIS), University of Porto, 4200-450 Porto, Portugal

Edward T. Chang
Tripler Army Medical Center, Department of Surgery, Division of Otolaryngology, Tripler AMC, Honolulu, HI, USA

Macario Camacho
Tripler Army Medical Center, Division of Otolaryngology, Sleep Surgery and Sleep Medicine, 1 Jarrett White Road, Tripler AMC, HI 96859, USA

M. Farid
Department of Plastic and Reconstructive Surgery, The Royal London Hospital, Barts Health NHS, Whitechapel Road, London E1 1BB, UK

R. Vaughan
Norwich Medical School, University of East Anglia, Chancellor Drive, Norwich NR4 7TJ, UK

S. Thomas
Department of Plastic and Reconstructive Surgery, University Hospital Birmingham NHS Foundation Trust, Queen Elizabeth Hospital Birmingham, Mindelsohn Way, Edgbaston, Birmingham, West Midlands B15 2GW, UK

Kristen Aliano
Department of Plastic Surgery, University of Texas Medical Branch, Galveston, TX, USA

Michael Trostler, Indira Michelle Fromm, Alexander Dagum, Sami Khan and Duc Bui
Department of Plastic Surgery, Stony Brook University Hospital, Stony Brook, NY, USA

M. E. Pontell, N. Saad, A. Brown, M. Rose, R. Ashinoff and A. Saad
Department of Surgery, Drexel University College of Medicine, Philadelphia, PA, USA
Department of Surgery, University of Maryland, Baltimore, MD, USA
Department of Breast Surgery, Cancer Care Institute, Egg Harbor Township, NJ, USA
The Plastic Surgery Center, The Institute for Advanced Reconstruction, Egg Harbor Township, NJ, USA

Index